Stress and Mental Disorders

Stress and Mental Disorders

Insights from Animal Models

RICHARD McCARTY

Department of Psychology
Vanderbilt University

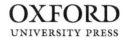

OXFORD

UNIVERSITY PRESS

OXFORD
UNIVERSITY PRESS

Oxford University Press is a department of the University of Oxford. It furthers the University's objective of excellence in research, scholarship, and education by publishing worldwide. Oxford is a registered trade mark of Oxford University Press in the UK and certain other countries.

Published in the United States of America by Oxford University Press
198 Madison Avenue, New York, NY 10016, United States of America.

Library of Congress Cataloging-in-Publication Data
Names: McCarty, Richard, 1947– author.
Title: Stress and mental disorders : insights from animal models /
Richard McCarty.
Description: New York, NY : Oxford University Press, 2020. |
Includes bibliographical references and index.
Identifiers: LCCN 2019048689 (print) | LCCN 2019048690 (ebook) |
ISBN 9780190697266 (hardback) | ISBN 9780190697280 (epub) |
ISBN 9780190697297
Subjects: LCSH: Stress (Physiology) | Stress (Psychology) |
Neuroendocrinology.
Classification: LCC QP82.2.S8 M33 2020 (print) | LCC QP82.2.S8 (ebook) |
DDC 616.9/8—dc23
LC record available at https://lccn.loc.gov/2019048689
LC ebook record available at https://lccn.loc.gov/2019048690

1 3 5 7 9 8 6 4 2

Printed by Integrated Books International, United States of America

Dedicated to my two wonderful mentors:

Charles H. Southwick, Ph.D. (1928–2015)
and
Irwin J. Kopin, M.D. (1929–2017)

Contents

Acknowledgments

The idea for this book developed during the spring semester of 2016 when I returned as a faculty member to the Department of Psychology after 13 years as a full-time administrator, first as Dean of the College of Arts and Science for seven years and then as Provost for six years. At that point, I was faced with developing new course offerings within my home department. For the spring semester, I decided to offer a new seminar for advanced undergraduates, *Stress and Mental Disorders*. After searching unsuccessfully for a text that could supplement assigned readings for my seminar, I thought it might be an ideal challenge for me to write a monograph that could be used for a course like the one I was developing. Toward the end of the spring semester of 2016, I called my friend and colleague, Professor David Barlow, to ask for his advice given his remarkable record of achievement as a writer of textbooks and monographs. With his encouragement, I started to pull together my ideas for this book. I was fortunate to be guided in this effort by Sarah Harrington, Senior Editor for Psychology at Oxford University Press. The advice and suggestions of three reviewers that Sarah engaged were critical in shaping the final plan for this book. These reviewers provided incredibly valuable feedback and advice on my original prospectus, and I am deeply grateful to them.

As the contract for the book was finalized, I had knee-replacement surgery in January 2017 in the middle of a year-long sabbatical leave. Because of the time required for rehabilitation and a bit of time for feeling sorry for myself, I was not able to start on the book until March 2017. Twenty-five months later, the manuscript was done and the review process started. Along the way, I benefited from advice and suggestions from several colleagues on drafts of chapters. They included Vanderbilt colleagues John Gore, Steve Hollon, Kathryn Humphreys, Bunmi Olatungi, Sohee Park, Bill Petrie, Sandy Rosenthal, and Elisabeth Sandberg, as well as Dave Barlow (Boston University), Kim Johnson (University of Iowa), Terry Keane (VA Boston Healthcare System and Boston University School of Medicine), and Bob Stewart (Washington and Lee University). Their comments and suggestions were extremely helpful, but of course, any shortcomings in the book or errors of omission or commission are my responsibility. I also received outstanding support from the staff of the Jean and Alexander Heard Library system at Vanderbilt in securing materials that were not available electronically.

When I was working on illustrations for two review papers in 2015–2016, I had the good fortune to meet an incredibly talented medical illustrator here in Nashville, Megan Rojas. As I started on the book, I discovered that she and her family were being transferred to Bucharest, Romania. Fortunately, Megan continued to do her magic from her new home and she provided all of the original illustrations for this book. Thank you so much, Megan!

When I was a graduate student at The Johns Hopkins University School of Hygiene and Public Health (now the Bloomberg School of Public Health), I had the good fortune to meet a new faculty member, Joseph T. Coyle, M.D. In the course of asking for Joe's advice on experiments I was planning on the role of brain catecholamines in aggressive behavior, he suggested I consider applying for a postdoctoral fellowship at the National Institute of Mental Health to work with Irwin J. Kopin, M.D. After finishing at Hopkins in 1976, I was lucky enough to be accepted into Irv's laboratory and I remain grateful to this day to Joe for his advice and counsel. Forty-five years after those initial meetings, I reached out to Joe to ask if he would write an introduction for this book. Joe is not only a distinguished leader in academic psychiatry, but he has also published ground-breaking research using animal models of various mental and neurodegenerative disorders. He quickly accepted my invitation and for me, it was a way to connect back and thank him for all of the many good things that have flowed from his excellent advice.

Two friends at Vanderbilt have enriched my professional life considerably. John Gore, Director of the Vanderbilt University Institute for Imaging Sciences, has been a close friend for 17 years and has hosted me at his summer home in Woods Hole, Massachusetts, over spring break on several occasions. The weather was not always favorable on the Cape in March, but the food, drink, and fellowship were always beyond comparison, and several chapters in this book took shape there. Sandy Rosenthal, Professor of Chemistry, has encouraged me every step of the way as I wrote this book and has been a source of inspiration and insights along the way. I always look forward to our regular lunches at Sportsman's Grill.

My wife, Sheila, has made it possible for me to work on this book by her endless supplies of encouragement, patience, and love. I have been an absentee partner too often to tally, and a major challenge going forward is for me to focus more on our time together.

Working on this book has been a most stimulating and enriching adventure for me personally. I have also come to appreciate at a deeper level how vital basic research with animal models is to improving the lives of the millions of people who suffer from mental disorders. I am confident that some of the experimental approaches described in this book will lead to breakthroughs in the treatment and prevention of mental disorders in the not-too-distant future. In the end, that is why so many talented researchers have devoted so much energy to this global effort in research and discovery. This book is a celebration of their continuing efforts.

Richard McCarty
Nashville, Tennessee
January 2020

Introduction

A challenge that has confronted clinicians since the time of Hippocrates is understanding of the causes of mental disorders. The late Leon Eisenberg, M.D., the founding chairman of the Department of Social Medicine at Harvard Medical School, had a keen eye for the pendulum swings in the dominant theories. He saw the 1960s as a period of "brainless" psychiatry as psychoanalysis reigned over the academic departments of Psychiatry with the belief that unconscious conflicts explained all psychopathology (Eisenberg & Guttmacher, 2010). By the 1990s, he bemoaned the rise of "mindless" psychiatry. Psychiatrists were seen primarily as diagnosticians, who prescribed medications to correct inferred neuronal dysfunction linked to mental disorders categorized by the American Psychiatric Association's *Diagnostic and Statistical Manual of Mental Disorders* (*DSM*). The provision of psychotherapy was largely restricted to less costly psychologists and social workers, if offered at all.

The most recent pendulum swing has gone off in the direction of molecular genetics as the most effective strategy to understand the pathophysiology of mental disorders (McCarroll et al., 2014). Rigorous, sufficiently powered genome-wide association studies (GWAS) with the bar for statistical significance set high at 5×10^{-8} (because of the large number of comparisons) indicate that most single nucleotide polymorphisms (SNPs) associated with risk for a mental disorder are located in non-coding regions of the genome (Harrison, 2015). Furthermore, each site appears to confer a small amount of risk, typically less than 5%. In addition, as the number of mental disorders subject to GWAS expands, it has become clear that many of these SNPs are associated with risk for more than one disorder (Lee et al., 2013). Even in the case of rare but highly penetrant copy number variants, in which mega-base portions of the genome containing several genes are deleted or duplicated, pleiotropic psychopathology is the rule (Marshall et al., 2017).

This lack of disorder specificity indicates that the methods that we use to "diagnose" or categorize psychiatric disorders have little relationship to their etiology. This poor correlation between genetic risk and mental disorder undermines some of our most revered theories about the etiology of mental disorders that were "reverse engineered" from the mechanism of actions of drugs serendipitously found to treat them nearly 60 years ago. For example, the dopamine hypothesis has dominated thinking about the pathophysiology of schizophrenia for more than 40 years (Snyder, 1976). Nevertheless, few risk genes for schizophrenia are associated with dopaminergic neurotransmission, whereas multiple genes, which encode proteins within two degrees of separation from the N-methyl-D-aspartate (NMDA) receptor, are represented in the schizophrenia GWAS (Balu & Coyle, 2015). The fallibility of the diagnostic categories likely accounts for the lack of success in developing mechanistically novel treatments, the failure of clinical trials of new psychotropic drugs, and the desertion of psychiatry by major pharmaceutical companies.

The most recent research indicates psychopathology results from an interaction between genetic vulnerabilities and environmental insults (Geschwind & Flint, 2015). Environment is defined quite broadly, ranging from prenatal vitamin deficiencies to childhood abuse and neglect. Notably, childhood abuse and neglect have been associated with increased risk for anxiety disorders, posttraumatic stress disorder, major depressive disorder, and schizophrenia (Chen et al., 2010). Thus, it appears that the environmental insults are also not "disorder" specific, but rather are manifest in the context of intrinsic vulnerabilities. Furthermore, emerging evidence from epigenetic studies indicate that environmental insults can modify the structure of the genome through DNA methylation and histone acetylation, resulting in persistent alterations in the expression of affected genes (Sharma et al., 2016). These epigenetic alterations of the genome can persist through many cell divisions, enter the germ line, and propagate to subsequent generations, as suggested by studies on the children of Holocaust survivors (Yehuda et al., 2016).

In *Stress and Mental Disorders: Insights from Animal Models*, Richard McCarty, Ph.D., a Professor of Psychology at Vanderbilt University, takes a fresh look at the basic assumptions about how to categorize mental disorders. Professor McCarty draws upon his 40-year experience as an experimental psychologist and neuroscientist with a deep interest in the pathophysiology of psychiatric disorders to address how we might approach a radical realignment of psychiatric diagnosis with documented etiology. He acknowledges the Research Domain Criteria (RDoC), which was put forth by the National Institute of Mental Health as a matrix for organizing research around five symptomatic domains observed in several "disorders" and linking them to risk genes, environmental risk factors, and brain circuits (Cuthbert & Insel, 2013). However, instead of moving from risk gene to phenotype, McCarty focuses on environmental risk factors that are much more salient than risk genes in common mental disorders such as major depressive disorder, anxiety disorders, and phobias (Geschwind & Flint, 2015). In particular, his approach is to focus on one of the most robust environmental risk factors: *stress.* Stress is a fundamental risk factor or exacerbating factor for virtually every mental disorder.

He reviews the evolution of the theories of stress from the time of the pre-Socratic philosophers in Greece to the present. He presents evidence that the stress effector system impacts the hypothalamic pituitary axis, the sympathetic and parasympathetic neural systems, critical brain circuits including the amygdala, prefrontal cortex, and the hippocampus, and the immune/inflammation processes. He then reviews the interplay of stress in the pathophysiology of common mental disorders (i.e., schizophrenia, autism, bipolar disorder, etc.) linking human research to models in experimental animals. Finally, he explores the nature of resilience as a protective factor that mitigates both intrinsic and environmental risk factors.

Joseph T. Coyle, M.D.
Eben S. Draper Chair of Psychiatry and Neuroscience
Harvard Medical School and McLean Hospital

References

Balu, D. T., & Coyle, J. T. (2015). The NMDA receptor 'glycine modulatory site' in schizophrenia: D-serine, glycine and beyond. *Current Opinion in Pharmacology, 20,* 109–115.

Chen, L. P., Murad, M. H., Paras, M. L., Colbenson, K. M., Sattler, A. L., Goranson, E. N., . . . Zirakzadeh, A. (2010). Sexual abuse and lifetime diagnosis of psychiatric disorders: systemic review and meta-analysis. *Mayo Clinic Proceedings, 85,* 618–629.

Cuthbert, B. N., & Insel, T. R. (2013). Toward the future of psychiatric diagnosis: The seven pillars of RDoC. *BMC Medicine, 11,* 126.

Eisenberg, L., & Guttmacher, L. B. (2010). Were we all asleep at the switch? A personal reminiscence of psychiatry from 1940 to 2010. *Acta Psychiatrica Scandanavica, 122,* 89–102.

Geschwind, D. H., & Flint, J. (2015). Genetics and genomics of psychiatric disease. *Science, 349,* 1489–1494.

Harrison, P. J. (2015). Recent genetic findings in schizophrenia and their therapeutic relevance. *Journal of Psychopharmacology, 29,* 85–96.

Lee, S. H., Ripke, S., Neale, B. M., Faraone, S. V., Purchell, S. M., Perlis, R. H., & Wray, N. R. (2013). Genetic relationship between five psychiatric disorders estimated from genome-wide SNPs. *Nature Genetics, 45,* 984–994.

Marshall, C. R., Howrigan, D. P., Merico, D., Thiruvahindrapuram, B., Wu, W., Greer, D. S., & CNV and Schizophrenia Working Groups of the Psychiatric Genomics Consortium. (2017). Contribution of copy number variants to schizophrenia from a genome wide study of 41,321 subjects. *Nature Genetics, 49,* 27–35.

McCarroll, S. A., Feng, G., & Hyman, S. E. (2014). Genome-scale neurogenetics: methodology and meaning. *Nature Neuroscience, 17,* 756–763.

Sharma, S., Powers, A., Bradley, B., & Ressler, K. J. (2016). Gene X environment determinants of stress and anxiety-related disorders. *Annual Review of Psychology, 67*, 239–261.

Snyder, S. H. (1976). The dopamine hypothesis of schizophrenia: focus on the dopamine receptor. *American Journal of Psychiatry, 133*, 187–202.

Yehuda, R., Daskalakis, N. P., Bierer, L. M., Bader, H. N., Klengel, T., Holsboer, F., & Binder, E. B. (2016). Holocaust exposure induced intergenerational effects of *FKBP5* methylation. *Biological Psychiatry, 80*, 372–380.

1

Psychiatric Illnesses

An Overview

This book seeks to highlight the critical role that stressful life events play in the onset and recurrence of mental disorders in humans. However, the approach I will take is an indirect one. The majority of research that I will feature is from animal models of mental disorders, especially models that have employed laboratory strains of mice and rats. Animal models afford investigators an opportunity to study underlying mechanisms related to a given behavioral phenotype that models aspects of a human psychiatric disorder, including how stressful experiences impact the expression of that disease-related phenotype.

As you will see, this broad field of research has been an intensely explored area over the past 40 years, and has benefited from major conceptual and methodological advances in neuroscience, endocrinology, genetics, and developmental psychobiology. Unfortunately, these basic research advances have not been matched by advances in the realm of clinical psychiatry. The need for breakthroughs in understanding the etiology, pathophysiology, treatment, and prevention of mental disorders has never been greater given the enormous toll these disorders take at the level of individuals, family units, communities, and nations. The case has been made convincingly that mental disorders are diseases of the brain, but psychiatry still stands alone among medical specialties in being more art than science. Psychiatrists still cannot call upon reliable biomarkers as part of their diagnostic processes. Drugs currently approved for the treatment of the most prevalent psychiatric disorders, including depression, bipolar disorder, and schizophrenia, have advanced little over the past 50 years in spite of significant investments of money and talent relating to research funding. Of great concern is the fact that many of the major pharmaceutical companies have pulled back on their research investments devoted to developing new drugs for the treatment of psychiatric disorders, even though these classes of drugs remain among the most heavily prescribed across all illnesses (Hyman, 2012; Insel, 2012; Karayiorgou et al., 2012). Simply put, patients the world over are desperately in need of breakthroughs in the treatment of mental disorders!

As we will see throughout this book, all is not lost. There is reason for optimism, as basic and clinical research advances combine to identify new targets for drug discovery and unmask some of the neural, genetic, and epigenetic complexities of these devastating illnesses. In addition, new discoveries are being made in the area of resilience to psychiatric disorders, and these findings will inform approaches for their prevention.

The remainder of this introductory chapter will serve as an overview of several key issues relating to psychiatric disorders. They include: (i) the nature of psychiatric disorders, (ii) a brief history of psychiatric diagnosis, and (iii) the global burden of psychiatric illnesses.

The Challenge of Diagnosis in Psychiatry

What Is a Psychiatric Disorder?

The answer to this question is not as simple as one might expect, as it comes down to a problem of defining where "normal" ends and "abnormal" begins. Most nosological systems take a categorical (qualitative) approach to mental illnesses. That is, an individual is classified as "well" or is diagnosed with a mental disorder based upon a checklist of symptoms. As will be discussed in the following, a different approach is represented by dimensional systems of diagnosis, where a given mental illness is defined as being above a stated threshold on one or more scales that are continuous with the state of being "well" (Krystal & State, 2014).

Also contributing to the challenge of a widely accepted definition is the issue of culturally defined norms for behavior, as well as societal problems relating to the stigma of mental illness. Fully aware of these and other complications, Stein et al. (2010) suggested changes in the definition of a mental/psychiatric disorder in advance of the completion of the fifth edition of the *Diagnostic and Statistical Manual* (*DSM-5*; American Psychiatric Association, 2013). Their key defining criteria of a mental/psychiatric disorder are summarized in Table 1.1.

A simpler definition of a mental disorder is found in Chapter V of the 10th edition of the *International Classification of Diseases and Related Health Problems* (*ICD-10*). It states that a mental disorder is "a clinically recognizable set of symptoms or behaviours associated in most cases with distress and with interference with personal functions."

German Contributions to Nosology

Kahlbaum and Hecker. The advent of modern diagnostic systems in psychiatry dates to the mid-19th century in Germany, as represented by the work of two leading psychiatrists of that period, Karl Ludwig Kahlbaum (1828–1899) and

Table 1.1 *DSM-5* Definition of a Mental/Psychiatric Disorder*

Features

A. A behavioral or psychological syndrome or pattern that occurs in an individual.

B. The consequences include clinically significant distress (e.g., a painful symptom) or disability (i.e., impairment in one or more important areas of functioning).

C. It must not be merely an expected response to common stressors and losses (e.g., the loss of a loved one) or a culturally sanctioned response to a particular event (e.g., trance states in religious rituals).

D. It reflects an underlying psychobiological dysfunction.

E. It is not primarily a result of social deviance or conflicts with society.

Other considerations

F. It has diagnostic validity on the basis of various diagnostic validators (e.g., prognostic significance, psychobiological disruption, response to treatment).

G. It has clinical utility (e.g., contributes to better conceptualization of diagnoses or to better assessment and treatment).

H. No definition perfectly specifies precise boundaries for the concept of either "medical disorder" or "mental/psychiatric disorder."

I. Diagnostic validators and clinical utility should help to differentiate a disorder from diagnostic "nearest neighbors."

J. When considering whether to add a mental/psychiatric condition to the nomenclature or delete a mental/psychiatric condition from the nomenclature, potential benefits (e.g., provides better patient care or stimulates new research) should outweigh potential harms (e.g., hurts particular individuals, is subject to misuse).

---

*Modified from Stein et al. (2010).

his protégé, Ewald Hecker (1843–1909). Both Kahlbaum and Hecker reported that the plethora of psychiatric diagnostic systems in use in the mid-1800s in Germany were based upon symptom clusters that were so heterogeneous as to prevent advances in understanding the etiology and prognosis of a given condition, and then developing a plan for its treatment (Bräunig & Krüger, 1999; Kendler & Engstrom, 2017).

Another issue that Kahlbaum and Hecker confronted was the role of neuropathological studies of brains at autopsy for gaining insights into the etiology of mental disorders. Both argued that neuroanatomical findings were of little use without an accurate system of classification of psychiatric disorders. Hecker in particular suggested that only by carefully following the entire course of illness in a broad array of patients could a psychiatrist gain sufficient insight to subdivide broad symptom complexes into specific disease entities.

Kahlbaum and Hecker were not well known during their careers as they did not hold prestigious university professorships and, in fact, spent the majority of their careers working in private insane asylums. However, their writings on psychiatric diseases and classification systems had a major impact on Emil Kraepelin (1856–1926), whose influence on psychiatric nosology continues to the present (Kendler & Engstrom, 2017).

The impact of Kraepelin. An important aspect of Kraepelin's academic training was the 18 months he spent in the experimental psychology laboratory of Professor Wilhelm Maximilian Wundt (1832–1920) at the University of Leipzig. His exposure to Wundt and the new methods and approaches for measuring aspects of human perception, motivation, and cognition were to remain a key part of Kraepelin's approach to psychiatry for the remainder of his career. In 1886, during the lecture to celebrate his appointment to a professorship at the University of Tartu in Russian Estonia, Kraepelin presented his vision for the future of psychiatry. He believed strongly that psychiatry should remain a branch of the medical sciences. He expressed serious reservations about the overemphasis at the time on studies of post-mortem brain anatomy as a means of understanding psychiatric illnesses. Indeed, he argued that few if any advances had been made by using neuropathological findings to understand the etiology of psychiatric disorders. As an alternative, he argued forcefully for the value of the emerging tools of experimental psychology for characterizing psychiatric illnesses and unmasking aspects of their etiology (Engstrom & Kendler, 2015; Kendler, 2016).

Kraepelin's continuing influence on the development of psychiatry in Europe and the United States was enhanced by his widely read textbook (*Psychiatry: A Textbook for Students and Physicians*) that was published in nine editions, with the first edition published in 1883 and the ninth edition, comprising four volumes, published in 1927, the year after his death (see Kraepelin, 2002). His textbook included his nosology of psychiatric disorders, which was based largely on his own clinical observations that expanded continuously over the course of his long and distinguished career. One of his fundamental beliefs was that patients who shared the same symptom profile and course might be affected by the same disease. He was constantly attempting to highlight differences between diagnostic categories and to improve the prediction of the course of a given disorder (Mack et al., 1994).

Kraepelin also believed that his diagnostic system was imperfect, and that any diagnostic system should evolve over time as new information became available (Engstrom & Kendler, 2015). He included three validators of psychiatric diagnoses, clinical features, brain pathology, and etiology, all of which intersected with psychiatric diseases that were ultimately defined by Nature. Unfortunately, more than 100 years after Kraepelin's initial proposals, Nature has failed to reveal the essential elements of psychiatric illnesses to us (Heckers, 2015).

The Emergence of American Psychiatry

The Swiss connection. Adolf Meyer (1866–1950), who emigrated from his native Switzerland to the United States in 1892, served as a valuable interface between European and American psychiatry in the late 1800s and early 1900s and was a strong initial proponent of Kraepelin's classification system of psychiatric illnesses. Fluent in German, Meyer provided American psychiatrists with an early introduction to Kraepelin's popular textbook prior to the availability of the first translation into English (Meyer, 1896). After working as a psychiatrist in Chicago, Worchester, Massachusetts, and New York, he was appointed the first psychiatrist-in-chief of The Johns Hopkins Hospital in 1910. Over time, Meyer became disenchanted with Kraepelin's system of classification, and developed his own theories that posited that psychiatric disorders were psychobiologic reactions to the environment. He later developed his own classification system of psychiatric disorders that emphasized these reactions to the environment (Mack et al., 1994).

There were many concerns in the United States in the late 19th century regarding the challenges of creating a psychiatric nosology. In many respects, psychiatrists of that time were focused more on the individual patient than on creating diagnostic categories that would subsume particular patients under each category. Psychiatric disorders were thought to arise when the balance between the individual, the environment, and the larger society was disrupted. These imbalances were thought to occur in individuals who were in some way predisposed or susceptible to the effects of external forces. Rarely was a behavioral disturbance linked to overt pathology, such as a brain tumor (Grob, 1991).

A nudge from the social sciences. A major impetus for the development of a consistent nomenclature for psychiatric disorders arose in the United States, not from psychiatry, but rather, from the emerging fields of the social sciences. In particular, the census of 1880 sought to quantify the number of dependent persons, including those with mental disorders, to inform public policy and to quantify the requirements for appropriately scaled public welfare programs. Given the inconsistencies in psychiatric classification systems at the time, a simple system of seven forms of "insanity" were employed in the census: mania, melancholia, monomania, paresis, dementia, dipsomania, and epilepsy. A similar classification system was employed in the census of 1890 (Wilson, 1993).

Early in the 20th century, census officials urged the American Medico-Psychological Association (the forerunner of today's American Psychiatric Association) to develop a uniform classification system for collecting information on mental diseases and patients in asylums. The Committee on Statistics of the American Medico-Psychological Association stated early in its report that the ". . . present condition with respect to the classification of mental diseases is chaotic." Referring to the lack of uniformity in the methods for reporting statistics across asylums and states, the report went on to say, "This condition of affairs discredits the science of psychiatry and reflects unfavorably upon our Association, which should serve as a correlating and standardizing agency for the whole country." The work of the Committee on Statistics was focused on the following major projects: (i) consider the benefits of uniform statistics for mental diseases and the operation of insane asylums, (ii) develop a system for the classification of mental diseases, (iii) produce forms for reporting such data, and (iv) take appropriate measures to ensure uniform statistical reports (Salmon et al., 1917, p. 256).

The advent of diagnostic categories. Based in large measure on the work of the Committee on Statistics, the American Medico-Psychological Association and the National Committee for Mental Hygiene jointly issued the first standardized system of classification of mental diseases in the United States, *Statistical Manual for the Use of Institutions for the Insane* (1918). This publication included 22 major diagnostic categories, many of which included multiple subcategories, and emphasis was placed on the biological basis of most mental diseases. One measure of success of this publication was that it went through ten editions between 1918 and 1942 (Wilson, 1993).

During the years between the two world wars, the *Statistical Manual* had little impact on the practice of psychiatry. For the most part, therapeutic approaches were eclectic and nonspecific, with clinical judgment and intuition serving as the guiding stars in the treatment of psychiatric patients (Grob, 1991).

The impact of World War II. During the involvement of the United States in World War II (1941–1945), a major shift occurred in the provision of medical services for the armed forces. At the beginning of the war, psychiatrists were few in number in all branches of the armed forces. By the end of the war, the number of positions for psychiatrists had greatly expanded, and some physicians from other specialties were pulled into psychiatry services to meet the critical need for treatment, especially from combat-related traumas. Psychiatrists learned many valuable lessons from their service in World War II, and they brought these hard-won lessons back with them when they left the armed services and returned to civilian life and the practice of psychiatry in their local communities. First and foremost, they learned that the stress of combat could contribute greatly to problems of maladjustment. They found that immediate treatment of service members in settings near the front lines and in close proximity to the social support networks of their combat units often yielded positive outcomes. Many of the psychiatrists with wartime experiences adopted psychodynamic and psychoanalytic approaches to therapy, and they were not supportive of their patients having extended stays in institutional settings. This major deviation in the provision of services marked a dramatic point of departure away from a focus on mentally ill patients in institutional settings and toward a much broader and more inclusive vision of psychiatry's relevance to many problems of adjustment within society (Grob, 1991; Wilson, 1993).

The Birth of the *Diagnostic and Statistical Manual of Mental Disorders*

Soon after the end of World War II, two new systems of classification for psychiatric disorders were developed. One emerged from the now renamed American Psychiatric Association (APA), and eventually led to the publication of the first edition of the *DSM-I*. The second came from the World Health Organization (WHO), a branch of the newly created United Nations, which assumed responsibility for the production of the sixth edition of the *ICD-6* (Mack et al., 1994).

The early years. In 1948, the APA Committee on Nomenclature and Statistics released a call for suggestions to aid in the revision of its statistical manual. This request for input from the membership was made in recognition of the changing demographics of the APA, the proliferation of diagnostic classifications, and the recent dominant position of psychoanalytic and psychodynamic approaches to therapy. Within two years, mimeographed copies of a revised psychiatric classification system were distributed to individuals and interested organizations, and the final version was presented for approval to the APA Council. In 1952, the APA published the first edition of *DSM* with a clear aim of improving the treatment of patients by enhancing the accuracy of diagnoses of psychiatric disorders (Raines, 1953).

DSM-I divided mental disorders into two broad categories. In the first category, the group of mental disorders was thought to have resulted from a primary disruption of brain function, which was precipitated by infection, poison, alcohol intoxication, or genetic disorders such as Huntington's chorea. The second category represented disorders associated with an individual's inability to adjust to his or her environment, including psychotic disorders (e.g., manic-depressive and paranoid reactions and schizophrenia) and psychoneurotic disorders (e.g., anxiety, depression, obsessive-compulsive disorder, antisocial behavior, stress reactions, alcohol and drug abuse disorders, and compulsiveness) (Grob, 1991).

DSM-II was published in 1968, and reflected a vigorous effort to sustain the success of *DSM-I* and to collaborate with those responsible for the creation of *ICD-8*, which was approved in 1966 and became effective in 1968 (Gruenberg, 1968). In addition, there was a concerted effort encouraged by the US Surgeon General to develop a standard international classification system for psychiatric diagnoses that would facilitate an exchange of information among psychiatrists from many nations (Spitzer & Wilson, 1968).

The crisis in psychiatry. The publication of *DSM-III* in 1980 followed broad-based challenges from many corners of society in the 1970s to the legitimacy of psychiatry (Nesse & Stein, 2012). At the heart of these criticisms was the dependence of psychiatry on clinical impressions and the unreliability and possible social construction of diagnostic categories. Two events in 1973 serve to illustrate these overt challenges to legitimacy. In the first, the Board of Trustees of the APA voted to eliminate homosexuality as a disease category in *DSM*. While history has shown this was, in fact, the correct action to take, it appeared at the time to be a response to political pressure from an increasingly vocal gay rights lobby, rather than a decision that was based upon scientific merit. And for those who supported the action to remove homosexuality as a *DSM* disease category, the question arose as to why homosexuality was ever viewed as a mental disorder in the first place (Wilson, 1993).

The second event was the publication of an article by David Rosenhan, a professor of psychology at Stanford University. Rosenhan (1973, p. 251) addressed a critical issue relating to psychiatric diagnosis in his study: "the question of whether the sane can be distinguished from the insane (and whether degrees of insanity can be distinguished from each other)." Briefly, Rosenhan designed an experiment in which eight sane individuals (pseudopatients, including Rosenhan) gained admission to 12 psychiatric hospitals in different parts of the United States. Upon arrival at the admissions office, each pseudopatient complained of recently hearing voices that were unfamiliar and, though unclear, the words that each remembered were "empty," "hollow," and "thud." Once admitted, the pseudopatients ceased reporting any overt symptoms and behaved as they normally would have. Each kept notes about the experiences on the ward, often in view of staff members. With one exception, the pseudopatients were admitted with a diagnosis of schizophrenia (one was diagnosed as having manic-depressive psychosis) and all were discharged with the same diagnosis, but with the notation "in remission." Strangely enough, a number of inpatients suspected that the pseudopatients were journalists or undercover investigators, but the staff members never suspected them of faking their symptoms.

In a second part of the Rosenhan experiment, the staff members at a teaching hospital were told that one or more pseudopatients would seek admission to their facility in the coming 3 months. The staff members were aware of the results of the previous study and expressed doubt that pseudopatients would escape detection within their facility. Unfortunately, they were wrong. Although no pseudopatients were sent to the hospital, many staff members, including psychiatrists, suspected that some of those seeking admission were pseudopatients (Rosenhan, 1973).

Although the Rosenhan experiments were criticized on methodological grounds (see, for example, Spitzer, 1975), the damage was done, given the broad impact of the journal *Science*, where the article was published. One psychiatrist (Szasz, 1961) had already staked out the extreme view that mental illness was a "myth." Seymour Kety, professor of psychiatry at Harvard Medical School, was one of several leaders in the field of psychiatry who countered these arguments with the strongly expressed view that psychiatry was a branch of medicine and that the medical model was the optimal approach for the diagnosis and treatment of mental illnesses, especially given the importance of genetics in their etiology (Kety, 1974).

The rise of the medical model in psychiatry. From this crisis of confidence in psychiatry was born the impetus for the next revision of *DSM*. Critical input for the task force responsible for drafting *DSM-III* was the Research Diagnostic Criteria (RDC) developed at Washington University by a group of research-oriented psychiatrists. The RDC was based upon the Feighner criteria (Feighner et al., 1972; Kendler et al., 2010), named after Dr. John Feighner, who, as a resident in psychiatry at Washington University, encouraged the formation of a study group to work on issues relating to psychiatric nosology. The efforts of the study group resulted in clearly stated diagnostic criteria for 14 psychiatric syndromes that yielded high levels of agreement between clinicians, but without a role for clinical inference. No hypotheses concerning the etiology of these 14 syndromes were offered.

The publication of *DSM-III* was a critical moment in the history of American psychiatry. It marked the rise of the medical model and established the central role of research activities in departments of psychiatry. It also signaled a dramatic reduction in influence of the psychodynamic and psychoanalytic forces that had controlled the profession for most of the 20th century. For the first time, post-traumatic stress disorder (PTSD) was recognized as a new diagnostic category, due in part to intense lobbying efforts by Viet Nam veterans groups and their supporters. The addition of PTSD to *DSM-III* also opened up the field of psychiatry to the importance of trauma studies, and stimulated the development of diagnostic instruments for assessing PTSD in service members as well as civilians (Keane et al., 1987). None of these changes came easily, and there were many tense moments and disagreements leading up to the ultimate approval of *DSM-III* by the APA (Wilson, 1993).

As experience with *DSM-III* increased, some of its weaknesses were revealed. For example, comorbidity between disorders was found to be prevalent, and this continues to be an issue of concern in the present. That is, individuals diagnosed with one mental disorder also qualified for one or more additional diagnoses. Within diagnostic groups, there was significant heterogeneity of patients, such that two patients could be in the same diagnostic grouping but have few or no symptoms in common. This difficulty pointed to the problem of using symptom checklists to define diagnostic categories. In addition, the boundaries separating individuals without mental illness from those with a disorder were not distinct, and at times appeared arbitrary (Nesse & Stein, 2012). Finally, diagnostic categories had evolved based upon studies of individuals with middle- to late-stage illnesses. This presented difficulties for identifying high-risk individuals early in the course of their illnesses and delivering appropriate levels of care to them (McGorry, 2013). It was argued by some leaders in the field that adopting a clinical staging model for psychiatric diagnosis would afford an opportunity to intervene with early-stage treatments that tended to be more benign and more effective compared to later-stage treatments (Scott et al., 2013).

The publication of *DSM-IV*. Following a major revision to *DSM-III* in 1987, *DSM-IV* was published in 1994, followed by a text revision (*DSM-IVTR*) in 2000. In the preparation of *DSM-IV*, a high threshold was maintained for any changes that were made from *DSM-III*. In addition, a concerted effort was made to have *DSM-IV* as consistent as possible with *ICD-10*, which was released in 1995. How successful were these efforts to ensure diagnostic consistency across the two systems?

To address this important issue, Andrews et al. (1999), using the Composite International Diagnostic Interview (CIDI, Version 2.1), compared the concordance rates for psychiatric diagnoses in a clinical sample with twice the prevalence of a given disorder compared to the general population. The CIDI from the WHO is a structured diagnostic interview that addresses each criterion from *ICD-10* and *DSM-IV*. The results of this comparative study revealed high rates of diagnostic concordance for dysthymia, depression, substance dependence, and generalized anxiety disorder (77%–87%); moderate rates of concordance for social phobia, agoraphobia with panic disorder, obsessive-compulsive disorder, and panic disorder (56%–66%); and low rates of concordance for agoraphobia without panic disorder, PTSD, and substance use or abuse (33%–45%). Minor differences in wording between the two systems accounted for these differing rates of concordance, and it remains a continuing challenge to bring the description of diagnostic criteria in the two systems into alignment to the greatest extent possible.

The development of *DSM-5*. The relative calm surrounding the publication of *DSM-IV* in 1994 was a distant memory when *DSM-5* was published in 2013. Six years before the publication of *DSM-5*, Dr. Steven E. Hyman (2007) offered his personal views on how basic and clinical research in neuroscience might be usefully incorporated into the new edition. His views did not originate from a dispassionate observer with little interest in the next editions of *DSM* and *ICD*. Rather, his opinions carried the added weight of his dual involvement as a member of the *DSM-5* Task Force and his position as chair of the International Advisory Group to the WHO for the revision of *ICD-10*, Chapter V, "Mental and Behavioural Disorders." In addition, he served as director of the National

Institute of Mental Health in the United States during 1996–2001, and was intimately involved in mental health policies and oversaw a large research portfolio designed to reduce the burden of mental disorders on patients, their families, and American society.

Hyman emphasized that any new diagnostic criteria, including those related to neuroscience, neuroimaging, and psychiatric genetics, must be validated to a very high standard. His suggestions for improvements in *DSM-5* were as follows:

- Create experimental diagnostic criteria for some mental disorders that could be included in research studies and evaluated for their reliability and effectiveness. When a given experimental criterion held considerable promise, the relevant data could be posted for public comment and then evaluated by a standing committee, with authority to edit the *DSM-5* or *ICD-11* standards. In this manner, new information would not have to sit on the shelf until the next editions of the two diagnostic manuals appeared.
- Experimental diagnostic approaches for some mental disorders could involve the following dimensional strategies:
  - Identify clinically significant symptom clusters for which there were relevant data from animal models and clinical studies regarding underlying neural circuitry.
  - Create larger groupings of patients based upon clustering of symptoms, patterns of familial transmission, and pathophysiological changes. Such an approach recognized the high rates of comorbidity for some psychiatric disorders and the sharing of risk genes across disorders.

Unfortunately, these and other changes in *DSM-5*, including the introduction of biomarkers for some disorders, did not materialize. Valid criticisms of *DSM-5* have arisen from many leading psychiatrists (refer to Casey et al., 2013; Nemeroff et al., 2013), but the time for radical change in the diagnosis of mental disorders had not yet arrived. One hopes that *DSM-6* will bring the changes that are long overdue, but only time will tell. Refer to the section on Research Domain Criteria (RDoC), later in this chapter, as a follow-up to one of Dr. Hyman's suggestions for change. Apparently, someone was paying attention.

History of the *International Statistical Classification of Diseases and Related Health Problems*

The critical early role of statisticians. This section is based in large part on the excellent historical overview of Moriyama et al. (2011) on the initial development and continued updating of the statistical classification of diseases and causes of death. At the meeting of the International Statistical Institute (ISI) in Vienna in 1891, Jacques Bertillon, chief of statistics for the City of Paris, was asked to chair a committee that would prepare a listing of causes of death for presentation at the next ISI meeting in Chicago in 1893. Bertillon had been working on the classification of causes of death since 1885, and his committee presented three versions of the listing of causes of death for consideration by the delegates to the meeting. All three versions were approved, and formed the basis for the *International List of Causes of Death*. In a brief period of time, Bertillon's classification was translated into several languages and was adopted for use in many countries, including all of North America, some countries in South America, and some cities in Europe.

At the urging of the American Public Health Association, ISI approved a plan to revise the *International List of Causes of Death* on a 10-year cycle. Revisions were approved in 1900, 1909, 1920, 1929, and 1938, with the League of Nations serving as a contributing partner for the three revisions that occurred following World War I.

Enter the WHO. At the end of World War II, the Interim Commission of the WHO was involved in drafting the sixth revision, which represented a major expansion over previous editions due to the addition of listings for causes of morbidity. In 1948, the two-volume publication, *Statistical Classification of Diseases, Injuries, and Causes of Death*, was approved and went into effect in participating countries in 1950. It contained a limited section on morbidity associated with mental disorders.

Given the extensive changes that were approved for the sixth edition, it was agreed by the involved partners that the seventh edition, which was approved in 1955, would be more limited in scope to allow member countries an opportunity to become more familiar with the classification systems for morbidity and mortality. Major revisions were made in several areas of the eighth edition, including mental illnesses, which was approved in 1965. The ninth edition, approved in 1975, started out to include minor revisions, but demands of medical specialists for greater ease of retrieval of data made the changes more extensive than originally planned.

The tenth revision of the *International Statistical Classification of Diseases and Related Health Problems* (*ICD-10*) was approved in 1989, but implementation was delayed until 1995. Extensive revisions were made in several sections, including Chapter V, "Mental and Behavioural Disorders." *ICD-10* will have remained in force for more than 25 years, and this is the longest period the publication has gone without a major revision. Many health-care professionals throughout the world are looking forward to the next revision (Moriyama et al., 2011); *ICD-11* was approved in 2019, but its full implementation will not occur until the beginning of 2022.

The international scope of *ICD*. Recent editions of the *ICD* have played a critical role in identifying people who are in need of mental health services. Such individuals often seek treatment in primary care settings, especially in low- and middle-income countries. As *ICD-11* moved through the review process, there was a focus on supporting health-care providers in primary care clinics in these low- and middle-income countries, where there are few psychiatrists available, but the disease burden of mental illnesses is substantial. In addition, a high priority was placed on developing a diagnostic system that could be used with relative ease in a wide array of clinical settings (International Advisory Group for the Revision of *ICD-10* Mental and Behavioural Disorders, 2011; Stein et al., 2013).

Research Domain Criteria

Consistent with the recommendations offered by Dr. Hyman regarding *DSM-5* (Hyman, 2007), in early 2009 the National Institute of Mental Health (NIMH) proposed a new dimensional classification system that would be deployed to support research on mental disorders that was well in advance of the publication of *DSM-5* (Insel et al., 2010). This new research-based classification system was a direct outgrowth of the 2008 NIMH Strategic Plan that included the following Strategy 1.4: "Develop, for research purposes, new ways of classifying mental disorders based on dimensions of observable behavior and neurobiological measures." Termed the Research Domain Criteria (RDoC) project, it represents one of the few times that a new project has been launched at NIMH without a catchy acronym (National Institute of Mental Health, 2008, p. 9).

Brain circuits. Three underlying assumptions guided the development of the RDoC project. First and foremost, mental illnesses were viewed as disorders of brain circuits. Next, the disorders in brain circuits should be discoverable using the tools of clinical neuroscience, including functional brain imaging, electrophysiology, and in vivo methods for studying brain connections. Finally, at some point in the future, findings from psychiatric genetics and clinical neuroscience will augment traditional diagnostic symptoms and inform the management of individual patients. Implicit in the RDoC conceptualization was the importance of a dynamic interplay between the developing individual and the environment, both prenatally and postnatally (Cuthbert, 2014; Morris & Cuthbert, 2012).

The matrix. A summary of the five domains and associated constructs that make up the headings for the rows of the RDoC matrix are included in Table 1.2. The column headings for the RDoC matrix include genes, molecules, cell circuits, physiology, behaviors, self-report measures, and laboratory experimental paradigms (e.g., Trier Social Stress Test, cold pressor test, fear conditioning). Cross-cutting themes include prenatal and postnatal environmental

Table 1.2 The Five Primary Domains of the Research Domain Criteria (RDoC) and Their Associated Constructs and Subconstructs

---

Domain: Negative Valence Systems

Construct: Acute threat (fear)

Construct: Potential threat (anxiety)

Construct: Sustained threat

Construct: Loss

Construct: Frustrative non-reward

Domain: Positive Valence Systems

Construct: Approach motivation

Subconstruct: Reward valuation

Subconstruct: Effort valuation/Willingness to work

Subconstruct: Expectancy/Reward prediction error

Subconstruct: Action selection/Preference-based decision making

Construct: Initial responsiveness to reward attainment

Construct: Sustained/Longer term responsiveness to reward attainment

Construct: Reward learning

Construct: Habit

Domain: Cognitive Systems

Construct: Attention

Construct: Perception

Subconstruct: Visual perception

Subconstruct: Auditory perception

Subconstruct: Olfactory/Somatosensory/Multimodal perception

Construct: Declarative memory

Construct: Language

Construct: Cognitive control

Subconstruct: Goal selection; updating, representation, and maintenance

Subconstruct: Response selection; inhibition/suppression

Subconstruct: Performance monitoring

Construct: Working memory

Subconstruct: Active maintenance

Subconstruct: Flexible updating

Table 1.2 Continued

    Subconstruct: Limited capacity

    Subconstruct: Interference control

Domain: Social Processes

  Construct: Affiliation and attachment

  Construct: Social communication

    Subconstruct: Reception of facial communication

    Subconstruct: Production of facial communication

    Subconstruct: Reception of non-facial communication

    Subconstruct: Production of non-facial communication

  Construct: Perception and understanding of self

  Subconstruct: Agency

  Subconstruct: Self-knowledge

  Construct: Perception and understanding of others

  Subconstruct: Animacy perception

  Subconstruct: Action perception

  Subconstruct: Understanding mental states

Domain: Arousal and Regulatory Systems

  Construct: Arousal

  Construct: Circadian rhythms
  Construct: Sleep-wakefulness

---

influences on the individual (refer to the NIMH website relating to RDoC for a complete description).

In the near term, RDoC is likely to be most relevant for clinical research projects and for preclinical studies with animal models. However, the great hope is that this new approach to developing a diagnostic system for mental illnesses will make possible a set of biosignatures that correspond to the various mental disorders and their subtypes, and that will ultimately lead to improvements in diagnosis, clinical care, and patient outcomes (Insel et al., 2010; Stein et al., 2013). One early positive development was the launch of a new journal in 2017, *Chronic Stress*, that encourages active discussion from all points of view about the place of research on chronic stress within the RDoC framework, to serve as a forum for educating interested individuals and organizations about RDoC, and to address gaps in the current RDoC framework (Abdullah et al., 2017).

The pillars of RDoC. The RDoC project represents a revolutionary approach to psychiatric diagnosis that will either inform future revisions of *DSM* and *ICD*, or perhaps replace them altogether (Yee et al., 2015). The following seven pillars of RDoC (Cuthbert & Insel, 2013; Morris & Cuthbert, 2012) capture some of the dramatic changes that continue to unfold for researchers interested in mental disorders. They include:

1. The RDoC project adopts a translational research perspective by starting with basic research findings in genetics, neuroscience, and behavioral science and progressing to questions concerning how disruptions in these systems lead to mental illnesses. Symptom-based definitions of mental disorders are not a part of this approach.
2. The RDoC project is unapologetically dimensional in its approach to mental disorders, and seeks to study the full range of variation in a given variable, from normal to abnormal. Such an approach is especially helpful for instances when a given variable changes in a nonlinear fashion.
3. A significant commitment of the RDoC project is to develop measures that are equally valid along the full range of the distribution of symptoms. Such a commitment ensures that data will be available to determine appropriate cut-points where clinical intervention is desirable.
4. *DSM-5* diagnostic criteria do not dictate or otherwise limit the generation of patient samples for RDoC studies. Rather, investigators might recruit from a group that includes all individuals who go to a particular clinic, and supplement that group with other individuals (i.e., healthy controls) who capture the full range of distribution of a given phenotype.
5. The RDoC project promotes a tight coupling between behavioral processes and their underlying neural circuits. To be included in the matrix, a behavioral process must map onto a brain circuit or some other biological system. Similarly, a brain circuit is included in the matrix only if it has a clearly defined relationship to behavioral endpoints.
6. At the outset, there was recognition that RDoC could not tackle all of the *DSM-5* diagnostic categories. Instead, there was a focus on those areas of psychopathology for which there were already sufficient data sets to support further research.
7. Going forward, a key aspect of RDoC must be its flexibility in making changes to the matrix as research advances are made. In addition, there must be an openness to fund research projects that seek to establish new constructs or modify existing ones.

Concerns arise. No revolution has ever been started without a healthy measure of criticism. This was certainly true for RDoC (Berenbaum, 2013; Bilder et al., 2013; Cuthbert & Kozak, 2013; Frances, 2014; Patrick et al., 2013). One overriding concern for some has been that the US governmental agency that initiated the RDoC project is also one of the largest funders of research in mental disorders in the world, with a total budget in FY2019 of more than $1.6 billion. It is understandable that many investigators would worry about where their current research programs fit, if at all, within the RDoC matrix. Another funding-related concern is to what extent NIMH would earmark a significant portion of its funding for projects with an explicit focus on RDoC (Weinberger et al., 2015). Related to the previous issue is whether RDoC would limit the scope of clinical research to those behavioral parameters that are most readily studied in animal models (Berenbaum, 2013).

More focused concerns have centered on areas that are absent from the RDoC. For example, Weinberger et al. (2015, p. 1161) argued that RDoC failed to capture the "remarkable difference between well and sick", or "the critical importance of time in defining course or prognosis and in clinical decision making." They also worried about superficial similarities across *DSM-5* diagnostic categories, and the fact that much of the input into and control of RDoC was in the hands of non-clinicians. Another concern they expressed was that mixing *DSM-5* diagnostic groups presents difficulties for reconciling findings from psychiatric genetics. They conclude by suggesting that a better use of scarce research funds would be to support a pilot program to determine if research using the RDoC matrix actually results in an improvement in the well-being of patients. It is evident that many were having a difficult time letting go of the current diagnostic categories, however flawed they may be.

Kraemer (2015) viewed RDoC and *DSM-5* through a methodological lens. She began by noting the interchangeability of dimensional and categorical diagnoses and argued that clinical researchers and clinicians should be free to select a categorical or a dimensional form for the same diagnosis, based upon what is optimal for a given purpose. She was unwavering in her opposition to having a dimensional approach to diagnosis (e.g., RDoC) for research studies and a categorical approach to diagnosis (e.g., *DSM*) in clinical settings. This, she said (Kraemer, 2015, p. 1163), "would be a recipe for disaster for patients with mental health problems." She also expressed concern about the promises of RDoC not being fulfilled, the construction of clinical samples for RDoC studies, and the inability of RDoC-inspired studies to detect a pattern of genetic susceptibility to a particular environmental influence during the course of development. For Kraemer (2015), the ultimate measure of a diagnostic approach, whether categorical or dimensional, is whether it reduces the burden of mental disorders on the individual and on society.

A signature beginning. One exciting development that has emerged from discussions of *DSM-5* and RDoC was the establishment in November 2012 of the Signature Bank by the Institut Universitaire en Santé Mentale de Montréal (IUSMM) that takes a dimensional and trans-nosological approach to mental illnesses (Lupien et al., 2017). The Signature Bank is involved in an ongoing effort to collect data on biological, psychological, and social behavioral signatures of patients who are seen at IUSMM and agree to participate in the project. In addition, blood, saliva, and hair samples are collected for measurement of various hormonal, metabolic, immune, and genetic markers. In a second phase, researchers at the Signature Bank recruited a control group that was matched on several dimensions to the original patient group. This exciting effort and others like it will provide fertile ground for discoveries that will improve the diagnosis, treatment, and prevention of mental disorders in the future.

A great deal hinges on the success of RDoC. The inherent flexibility of the project suggests that mid-course corrections should be made relatively quickly and easily. In time, more voices will be brought into the conversation and some of the criticisms that have been leveled will be addressed. In the end, if RDoC brings about needed changes in the diagnostic systems for mental disorders, then the initial visionary work of Dr. Insel and his colleagues will be validated.

Unfortunately, Dr. Insel will not oversee the continued expansion of RDoC, as he resigned as director of NIMH in 2015. His replacement, Dr. Joshua Gordon, came to NIMH as the new director in 2016, and he commented on RDoC at the end of his first year as director (Gordon, 2017). Dr. Gordon views RDoC as an excellent initiative for all of the reasons that have been discussed earlier. However, he also views RDoC as a grand hypothesis with plenty of promises but, at this point, few deliverables that have shed light on the etiology of mental disorders. Stay tuned for further developments.

A Dimensional Alternative to RDoC

Conway et al. (2019) described a dimensional system to understand psychopathology that is based upon quantitative analyses of the co-occurrence of psychological symptoms to establish a set of dimensions that have been proposed to reflect the natural architecture of mental disorders. This system, the Hierarchical Taxonomy of Psychopathology (HiTOP), includes broad, heterogeneous constructs, progressing to more specific and homogeneous dimensions. In this system, comorbidity of mental disorders is represented by dimensions (e.g., internalizing) that span multiple *DSM* diagnostic categories. It also captures diagnostic heterogeneity by incorporating processes such as worry and panic that make up the building blocks of mental disorders.

Proponents of the HiTOP framework argue that it has the potential to unify genetic and neurobiological findings relevant to mental disorders; it provides an enhanced framework for understanding how stressful stimuli affect various levels of the hierarchy from super-spectra to spectra and down to subfactors; and it provides a convenient framework for evaluating the impact of symptom components, syndromes, spectra, and super-spectra for the onset and treatment of mental disorders. Like RDoC, HiTOP is constantly undated as new data appear, but it is much closer to direct clinical implementation than RDoC (Conway et al., 2019).

The Power of One

Could it really be that simple? Could a single dimension accurately reflect an individual's risk for psychopathology, comorbidity across mental diagnoses, persistence of disorders over the life span, and symptom severity? Caspi and Moffitt (2018) have presented a compelling case in support of a single dimension of psychopathology, referred to as p, which represents increasing severity of symptoms of psychopathology. The use of p directly confronts some of the many challenges facing psychiatry today, including the weaknesses of a symptom-based categorical diagnostic system, high rates of comorbidity, significant overlap between diagnostic categories and their environmental and genetic risk factors, and the fact that the same drugs may be used to treat multiple psychiatric disorders. Finally, as we will see in the later chapters of this volume, there is also considerable overlap in behavioral, neuroendocrine, physiological, and molecular measurements across animal models of specific psychiatric disorders.

As appealing as the concept of p may be to those who are frustrated with the *DSM*-based approach to psychiatric diagnosis, there is a great deal of work that must be done to validate this approach. For one, a system to measure p must be developed that that is sensitive and specific and that captures an individual's liability to develop psychopathology across the life span. In time, measures of p could be employed to document the effectiveness of behavioral and pharmacological treatments of mental disorders as well as to track patients in clinical interventions aimed at primary prevention of mental disorders (Caspi & Moffitt, 2018). This is a development that bears watching over the coming years.

An alternative to a single dimension of psychopathology is the view that psychiatric illnesses are best understood in terms of a transdiagnostic factor reflecting general levels of psychopathology combined with a set of symptoms that are disorder-specific. To investigate this possibility, Gong et al. (2019) obtained magnetic resonance imaging (MRI) scans from 404 patients with a diagnosis of schizophrenia, major depressive disorder, PTSD, or obsessive-compulsive disorder; 201 healthy controls; and 20 unaffected first-degree relatives. Compared to healthy controls, the four diagnostic groups had significantly greater gray matter volume in the putamen, and the volume of this region was positively correlated with symptom severity across diagnostic groups. Increased size of putamen was also evident in first-degree relatives compared to controls. These investigators concluded that greater volume of the putamen may represent a transdiagnostic marker of a general familial risk for psychopathology.

Precision Medicine and Psychiatry

On January 30, 2015, President Barack Obama announced major federal support for an Initiative in Precision Medicine (Collins & Varmus, 2015). This initiative marked the beginning of a new strategy for the practice of medicine that could benefit individual patients as well as the health-care system more broadly. The wheels were set in motion for precision medicine by an influential US National Academy of Sciences committee report (National Research Council, 2011). The ultimate success of this ambitious effort will hinge on a host of interrelated challenges, including the creation and maintenance of health-care databases that include relevant and accurate health-related and environmental information on individuals, with attention to ethical concerns about assiduous protection of the privacy of patient medical information. In addition, decision support for physicians must be available at the moment when patients are seen in physician offices, clinics, or hospitals. Finally, the benefits of precision medicine should be cost-sensitive and inclusive of all segments of the multiethnic society of the United States. These challenges are substantial and will require considerable buy-in from patients, health-care providers, scientists, insurers, and policymakers in the coming years (Ashley, 2015; Buckley & Miller, 2017; Kohane, 2015).

A key advantage of precision medicine is that drug selection and dosage may be optimized based upon a patient's genetic profile. Significant progress has already been made in bringing precision medicine approaches to oncology and cardiovascular medicine (Wang et al., 2011; Weeke & Roden, 2014; Zeggini et al., 2019). The determination of appropriate doses of the anticoagulant warfarin serves as an excellent case in point.

Warfarin and Precision Medicine

Warfarin is an oral anticoagulant that is frequently prescribed to prevent the formation of blood clots. However, if doses of warfarin are too high, there is the risk of hemorrhage and emergency visits to the hospital. Warfarin comes as a racemic mixture of S-warfarin and R-warfarin. The former is 3–5 times more potent as an anticoagulant, has a shorter half-life in the circulation, and is metabolized to a large extent by a cytochrome P-450 enzyme, CYP2C9. Compared to the wild-type allozyme, CYP2C9*1, two allozyme variants have significantly less enzyme activity (12% for CYP2C*2 and 5% for CYP2C*3). Those individuals with the allozyme variants must receive lower doses of warfarin to avoid medical complications (Weeke & Roden, 2014).

Another factor that influences the dose of warfarin is its molecular target, vitamin K epoxide reductase complex subunit 1 (VKORC1). Single-nucleotide polymorphisms (SNPs) in *VKORC1* influence the attainment of an effective dose of warfarin. Finally, another cytochrome P450 gene, *CYP4F2*, has been shown to catalyze vitamin K oxidation. The variant *CYP4F2* allozyme shows decreased ability to catalyze the reaction, and as a result, individuals with the relevant genetic variant in *CYP4F2* require an increase in the warfarin dose. If genetic information is included in prediction algorithms for warfarin dosing, patients tend to have greatly improved outcomes (Wang et al., 2011; Weeke & Roden, 2014).

Increasing Precision in Psychiatry

The American effort. The big questions is: can psychiatry be an integral part of the Precision Medicine Initiative? This vital question was addressed in part by Insel and Cuthbert (2015) soon after the Precision Medicine Initiative was announced by President Obama. For psychiatry to catch up to other medical specialties, they argued, psychiatry must move beyond a symptom-based classification of mental disorders and embrace an approach that includes advances in genomics, neuroscience, and behavioral sciences (Akil et al., 2010). In this way, subgroups of patients can be identified that map onto biological and behavioral measures and that inform appropriate selections of therapies. Needless to say, the RDoC project was viewed as integral to this overall effort. In fact, in the year prior to President Obama's announcement, Insel (2014, p. 396) revealed that "RDoC's ultimate goal is precision medicine for psychiatry—a diagnostic system based on a deeper understanding of the biological and psychosocial bases of a group of disorders that is unambiguously among the most disabling disorders in medicine."

The European effort. The European Commission has also supported a new program, "Stratified Medicine for Mental Disorders" (Schumann et al., 2014). Stratified medicine may be viewed as a link in the path to precision medicine in that it seeks to identify subgroups of patients with distinct mechanisms of disease or distinct responses to various drugs (Trusheim et al., 2007). The program in stratified medicine for mental disorders is complementary to RDoC in that it focuses on basic and clinical research strategies to advance understanding of the basic pathophysiology of mental disorders without tying the research efforts to the current *DSM* and *ICD* systems of classification. This stratified approach may also facilitate the identification of biological tests that will contribute to greater precision in psychiatric diagnosis (Kapur et al., 2012).

Decision Support Tools for Psychiatry

Even at this early stage in the march toward precision medicine for psychiatry, there are developments worthy of scrutiny. One is the marketing of pharmacogenetic decision-support tools to aid clinicians in their selection of antidepressants. When these products first came to market in 2004, they were of limited use and generally provided information for a limited number of serotonin-related genes and gene variants. Second-generation decision-support tools include tests for multiple genes and provide information on gene-gene interactions as well as drug-drug interactions. This information is designed to reduce toxicity and increase efficacy of antidepressants (Bousman et al., 2017). Unfortunately, the various commercially available tools have not been carefully evaluated for their medical or cost effectiveness in supporting a prescribing physician's decisions (Bousman & Hopwood, 2016; Hicks et al., 2013).

Zeier et al. (2018) provided a detailed evaluation of evidence gathered on several commercially available kits that provide combinatorial pharmacogenetics decision-support tools to guide psychiatrists in choosing which among several antidepressants to prescribe for individual patients. These kits generate data on known risk gene variants and, in some cases, genetic variation in hepatic cytochrome P450 genes involved in peripheral drug metabolism. These authors concluded that these kits, which number more than 30, are not quite at a stage where they provide highly effective information to physicians, except in cases where knowledge of possible drug side effects is critical for patient management.

The decision-support tools described in the preceding are obviously a long way from being a part of a full implementation of precision medicine in psychiatry. However, these first small steps do foreshadow a time when the full extent of a patient's genomic information, brain imaging studies, and other medical test results will be combined with his or her demographic, psychosocial, and environmental profiles and will be available at the point of care, wherever that might be, to optimize decisions about drug selection and dosing as well as cognitive behavioral therapies and related lifestyle changes that would contribute to a personalized treatment protocol following a given diagnosis (Miller & O'Callaghan, 2013; Silbersweig & Loscalzo, 2017; Trivedi, 2016).

Davis et al. (2015) have presented a broader conceptualization of biomarkers of psychiatric disorders, even in the absence of a definitive understanding of brain circuit disruptions. Biomarkers could be useful in several ways: (i) quantifying risk of developing a disorder, (ii) confirming the diagnosis of a disorder,

(iii) rating the severity of a disorder, (iv) determining the stage of a disorder, (v) assessing the response to a given therapy, and (vi) providing a prognosis for a given patient. In some instances, a single biomarker may apply to more than one category, and even more than one disorder.

Mental Disorders and the Global Burden of Disease

The Burden of Mental Disorders

In the last decade of the twentieth century, the Harvard School of Public Health, the World Health Organization, and the World Bank joined forces to quantify causes of disability worldwide, using the measure disability-adjusted life years (DALYs). A DALY is a measure of the number of healthy years lost due to an illness or injury (Murray, 1994). The goal of this substantial undertaking was to provide accurate data on who dies and from what causes across the globe (Murray & Lopez, 1996). The data from this effort are critical to establishing priorities for global public health initiatives as well as the allocation and deployment of health-care resources within countries around the globe.

Given its timing, the broad-based study captured the "epidemiological transition," whereby non-communicable diseases caused a greater number of deaths than communicable diseases, even in the developing world. In the developed world, more than 85% of all deaths were attributed to non-communicable diseases. In addition, quantification of causes of disability unmasked the dramatic global impact of mental and substance use disorders in 1990, with 5 of the 10 leading causes of disability falling into this category (Table 1.3).

Using data from the Global Burden of Diseases, Injuries, and Risk Factors Study 2010, Whiteford et al. (2013) estimated the burden of diseases linked specifically to mental and substance use disorders. They reported that mental and substance use disorders combined were the fifth leading cause of DALYs worldwide in 2010 (7.4% of total disease burden), with depressive disorders having the greatest impact. The prevalence of mental disorders remained relatively constant from 1990 to 2010, with increases explained primarily by population growth and aging.

Because death records do not typically list mental disorders as the primary cause of death or even a contributing factor, Walker, McGee, and Druss (2015) conducted a meta-analysis of cohort studies that compared all-cause mortality estimates for groups with mental disorders compared to control groups that were free of mental disorders. They reported that the relative risk of death in the groups with mental disorders was 2.22. For those with mental disorders, 67% of deaths resulted from natural causes, 18% from unnatural causes, and 15% from other or unknown causes. They estimated that a median of 10 years of potential

Table 1.3 The Leading Causes of Disability Worldwide in 1990 as Measured by Years of Life Lived with a Disability (YLD)

	Total YLDs (millions)	Percent of Total
All causes of disability	472.7	
1. Unipolar major depression	50.8	10.7
2. Iron-deficiency anemia	22.0	4.7
3. Falls	22.0	4.6
4. Alcohol use	15.8	3.3
5. Chronic obstructive pulmonary disease	14.7	3.1
6. Bipolar disorder	14.1	3.0
7. Congenital anomalies	13.5	2.9
8. Osteoarthritis	13.3	2.8
9. Schizophrenia	12.1	2.6
10. Obsessive-compulsive disorders	10.2	2.2

life were lost due to mental disorders, and that 14% of deaths worldwide (8 million deaths) were due to mental disorders.

Grand Challenges in Global Mental Health

The Grand Challenges in Global Mental Health initiative was launched in 2010 to address the significant global burden of disease from mental, neurological, and substance use (MNS) disorders. MNS disorders contribute 13% of the global burden of disease as measured by DALYs, exceeding the impact of cancer or cardiovascular disease. The initiative, which is to run through 2020, is a collaborative effort led by the NIMH in the United States and the Global Alliance for Chronic Disease, based at University College London, in partnership with the Welcome Trust, the McLaughlin-Rotman Centre for Global Health of the University of Toronto, and the London School of Hygiene and Tropical Medicine.

A Delphi panel of more than 400 advocates, clinicians, researchers, and program implementation experts from more than 60 countries was surveyed to establish priorities for the Grand Challenges initiative. The Delphi method involves an iterative process, with structured questioning of and controlled feedback to panelists such that a consensus develops (Jones & Hunter, 1995). A Grand Challenge was defined as a specific barrier that, when removed, would help to address an important health problem. If successfully implemented, the intervention would have a high likelihood of success for being scaled up and impactful. The first pass resulted in 1,565 suggestions, which were distilled down to 154 unique challenges. From this compressed list, the panelists then rank-ordered their top 40 Grand Challenges. In the final step, panelists were asked to rate each of the challenges on a four-point scale for its potential to reduce disease burden, its impact on equity, the anticipated immediacy of impact, and its feasibility. The five highest rated challenges are presented in Table 1.4.

Table 1.4 The Five Highest-Ranked Grand Challenges from the Grand Challenges in Global Mental Health Initiative

Grand Challenge	Stage 2 Ranking	Final Ranking
Integrate core packages of mental health services into routine primary health care (2.375)	3	1
Reduce the cost and improve the supply of effective psychotropic drugs for mental, neurological, and substance use disorders (2.343)	11	2
Train health professionals in low- and middle-income countries to provide evidence-based care for children with mental, neurologic, and substance use disorders (2.294)	5	3
Provide adequate community-based care and rehabilitation for people with chronic mental illness (2.247)	14	4
Strengthen the mental health component in the training of all health-care personnel to create an equitable distribution of mental health providers (2.134)	16	5

Notes: These challenges were initially identified through a Delphi panel exercise that yielded a final list of 40 Grand Challenges from an initial list of 1,565 suggestions. The 40 highest-ranked Grand Challenges were then rated (1–4 scale) based upon their ability to reduce disease burden, impact equity, have an immediate impact, and be feasible to implement. Numbers in parentheses are the mean ratings for the top five Grand Challenges. Refer to the supplementary information in Collins et al. (2011) for additional details.

Several themes emerged from the top-ranked Grand Challenges, including the following:

- There was a strong life-span developmental focus, including the prenatal period, and recognition that efforts to identify MNS disorders as early as possible would reduce their adverse impact on individuals and their families.
- MNS disorders require a health systems-wide approach to deal with the impact of MNS disorders on family units, communities, and nations. Integration of services could improve patient outcomes and reduce health-care costs.
- A strong base of research effectiveness should undergird all methods for providing care to patients (e.g., pharmacological, psychological, or psychosocial) with MNS disorders.
- The panel members clearly recognized the impact of adverse and highly stressful environments (e.g., forced migration, war, torture, natural disasters, and extreme poverty, among others) on MNS disorders. However, additional research is needed to determine how these stressors stimulate the onset of MNS disorders or increase their severity (Collins et al., 2011).

Given the successes of previous Grand Challenges for infectious diseases (begun in 2003) and for chronic non-communicable diseases (begun in 2007), there is reason for optimism regarding this most recent global effort in the area of MNS disorders (Daar et al., 2007; Varmus et al., 2003). The global burden of disease for MNS disorders and the gap in treatment options between developed and developing countries have, for the most part, been well-kept secrets. Involving policymakers and global health funding agencies is a critical first step in reducing the punishing burden of MNS diseases on people across the globe (Collins et al., 2011).

Summary

It is clear from the material covered in this chapter that psychiatry has lagged behind other medical disciplines in taking full advantage of advances in genetics and neuroscience to improve the diagnosis, treatment, and prevention of mental disorders. In addition, the current approach to psychiatric diagnosis is still rooted in the late 19th century, and has not fully embraced findings in psychiatric genomics that suggest significant shared heritability among *DSM-5* diagnostic categories (The Brainstorm Consortium, 2018).

The two primary diagnostic systems that are employed by clinical psychiatrists, *DSM-5* and *ICD-10* (soon to be *ICD-11*), present significant challenges to basic researchers interested in developing animal models of specific psychiatric disorders. How does one begin to model a given psychiatric disorder that does not represent a natural kind? The advent of the NIMH RDoC system has already had a positive impact on basic researchers, and there is hope that this research-based diagnostic system will deliver a much-needed infusion of new ideas into basic as well as clinical research in psychiatry.

Psychiatric patients are clearly in need of the same level of precision relating to their care as patients in oncology or cardiology. A major premise of this book is that research with animal models will greatly accelerate the development and validation of biomarkers for psychiatric disorders that will ultimately improve the accuracy of diagnosis. In addition, animal models have the potential to reveal novel molecular targets for drug discovery, leading to improvements in treatment. Today, many patients are treated with first-line therapies that were developed more than 40 years ago. Breakthroughs in drug development are urgently needed!

There is clearly a greater sense of urgency than ever before associated with the need for drastic improvements in the care of psychiatric patients. Psychiatric disorders exert a devastating impact that is felt within families, communities, and nations around the world. The high rates of disability associated with psychiatric disorders also exact a severe economic toll on patients as well as the larger economies of nations.

I hope to convey a sense of cautious optimism as we move through the following chapters. Precision medicine in psychiatry in one clear and compelling goal for the future, such that each patient receives an accurate diagnosis and is prescribed the right medication(s) at the right dose at the right time and delivered to the right target in the brain to achieve the best possible clinical outcome. An additional goal is to develop a coordinated effort to prevent the occurrence of psychiatric disorders through early identification of and intervention with individuals who are at high risk of developing a given disorder.

2

Making the Case

Stress and Mental Disorders

In this chapter, I will focus on three mental disorders—schizophrenia, bipolar disorder, and major depressive disorder. For each, I will review studies on the heritability of these disorders, and then highlight the impact of stressful life experiences in their onset and maintenance. Stressful life experiences will be broadly defined to include the stress associated with maternal infections during fetal development. My goal is a simple one; I wish to craft airtight cases that stress has a major role in the etiology of each of these disorders. Armed with this background information, we will then be well positioned to tackle the exciting body of research on these and other mental disorders using experimental results obtained from animal models.

Why pick these three mental disorders and not others? One reason was a practical one; due to limitations of space, I could only summarize the involvement of stress in three mental disorders. I also considered mental disorders that varied across several critical dimensions and where the literature was rich enough to draw firm conclusions regarding the etiologic role of stress in disease onset, maintenance, and recurrence (Table 2.1). As you can see, these three mental disorders differ across several dimensions relating to prevalence in the population, heritability, sex differences, level of disability in a typical patient, and impact of the disorder on morbidity at the population level.

Genetics of Mental Disorders

The Garden as a Laboratory

Oh, for the simple life of an Augustinian monk tending his garden and conducting experiments on pea plants that would later revolutionize the study of genetics. Gregor Mendel was a low achiever for most of his adult life, having failed on two occasions to pass the certification test to be a teacher of science. But did he ever have a green thumb, and good fortune smiled on him when he decided upon the seven true-breeding characteristics of the pea plants that became the focus of his revolutionary experiments. Among the seven characteristics (seed texture, seed color, flower color, flower position, color of pea pod, shape of pea pod, and plant height), he selected only two variants for each (one dominant

Table 2.1   Distinguishing Features of Three Mental Disorders: Schizophrenia, Bipolar Disorder, and Major Depressive Disorder (MDD)

Distinguishing Feature	Schizophrenia	Bipolar Disorder	MDD
Prevalence	1%	2%–3%	17%
Heritability	High	High	Moderate
Sex differences	♂ >> ♀	♀ > ♂	♀ >> ♂
Individual disability	Very high	Very high	Moderate
Global burden of disease	Low	Low	Very high

trait and one recessive trait), and then cross-bred them to produce hybrids. These experiments were conducted from 1857 until 1868, when Mendel was appointed abbot of the monastery in Brno, in what is now the Czech Republic. He was quickly overwhelmed with administrative duties, and his plant experiments were soon abandoned (Mukherjee, 2016; Weiling, 1991).

The rest, as they say, is history. By the beginning of the twentieth century, Mendel's paper that was published in 1866 in the obscure journal *Verhandlungen des Naturforschenden Vereines in Briinn* (*Proceedings of the Brno Natural Science Society*) was rediscovered multiple times and widely praised for introducing the concept of "units of heredity," a critical feature of the new science of genetics (Hartl & Orel, 1992).

Now, let's contrast the elegant simplicity of Mendel's experiments with the astounding complexity characteristic of contemporary studies of psychiatric genomics. If Mendel had to contend with this level of complexity, he would surely have lost his religion and made extra visits to the confessional! And this level of complexity is not amenable to a lone and highly motivated scientist locked away in a laboratory (or a monastery garden, for that matter). These are big challenges that often require a "big science" approach.

Psychiatric Genetics

At the beginning of the new millennium, the publicly funded and privately funded components of the Human Genome Project were brought to completion and a first draft of the 2.91 billion base-pair sequence of human DNA was published (Venter et al., 2001). This remarkable multinational effort has opened up new opportunities for the diagnosis, treatment, and prevention of many diseases, including psychiatric disorders (Cowan et al., 2002). Smoller et al. (2015) has provided a superb overview of methods to explore the genetics of major psychiatric disorders (refer to Figure 2.1). The initial question to be considered is the

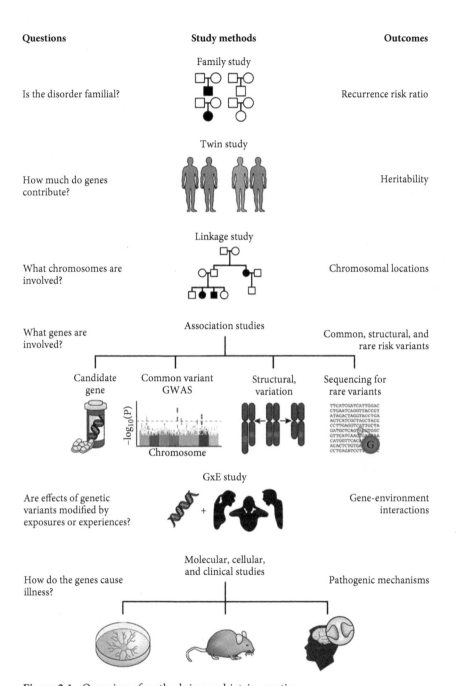

Questions	Study methods	Outcomes

Family study

Is the disorder familial?

Recurrence risk ratio

Twin study

How much do genes
contribute?

Heritability

Linkage study

What chromosomes are
involved?

Chromosomal locations

Association studies

What genes are
involved?

Common, structural, and
rare risk variants

Candidate
gene

Common variant
GWAS

Structural,
variation

Sequencing for
rare variants

$-\log_{10}(P)$

Chromosome

GxE study

Are effects of genetic
variants modified by
exposures or experiences?

Gene-environment
interactions

**Molecular, cellular,
and clinical studies**

How do the genes cause
illness?

Pathogenic mechanisms

Figure 2.1. Overview of methods in psychiatric genetics.
Reproduced from Smoller et al. (2015) and used with permission of Dr. Smoller.

extent to which a given disorder is heritable (refer to Table 2.2). Family and twin studies have been especially useful in addressing the contributions of genotype and environment to complex traits of interest (Polderman et al., 2015; Sullivan et al., 2003).

Big science comes to psychiatry. Given that a disorder is heritable, then molecular genetic studies can pinpoint the chromosomal locations of a small number of defects. However, it is now clear that psychiatric disorders are influenced by many susceptibility loci, each with a small effect size, and the optimal experimental approach to identify a large number of loci is through genome-wide association studies (GWAS). By examining genetic variation at millions of single-nucleotide polymorphisms (SNPs) in an individual genome using microarrays, one can quickly scale up and conduct GWAS in tens of thousands of individuals with a specific diagnosis and compare the results with disorder-free controls (Corvin et al., 2010).

There are a number of subtleties associated with GWAS that are important to keep in mind. Sample sizes are extremely large, often greater than 25,000, and may reach as high as 100,000 or more given the need for statistical power to detect many risk variants, each with a low effect size. Levels of significance in GWAS are very different from typical laboratory-based empirical studies, where the threshold for statistical significance is often set at $P <0.05$. A genome-wide significance level is typically set at 5×10^{-8}, reflecting a Bonferroni correction

Table 2.2 Prevalence and Heritability Estimates of Eight Major Mental Disorders

Psychiatric Disorder	Population Prevalence	Heritability
Schizophrenia	1%	0.70–0.85
Bipolar disorder	2%–3%	0.60–0.85
Major depressive disorder	~17%	0.40
ASDs	0.04%–0.8%	0.90
Anorexia nervosa	0.6%	0.55
Anxiety disorders	29%	0.40–0.50 (panic disorder)
Obsessive compulsive disorder	1.6%	0.60–0.70
ADHD	8%	0.60–0.90

Note: For calculations of heritability, a score of 1.0 indicates that 100% of the variance for a given disorder is explained by genotype alone, whereas a score of 0.0 indicates that none of the variance for a given disorder is explained by genotype.

Abbreviations: ASDs: autism spectrum disorders; ADHD: attention deficit hyperactivity disorder.

Based upon information originally reported by Burmeister et al. (2008).

given that the number of independent statistical tests conducted in a typical GWAS exceeds 1 million. In most cases, loci that have significant associations with a given disorder are located in regulatory regions of the genome, and do not always clearly implicate a specific gene (Maurano et al., 2012). Most investigators report the nearest gene to an identified locus, but this may not always be accurate (Smemo et al., 2014). Attempts are underway to catalogue how changes in the genome affect changes in gene expression (Koester & Insel, 2016).

Studies employing microarrays have also been used to detect rare structural chromosomal variants, including copy number variants (CNVs), insertions/deletions, and balanced translocations. Finally, extremely rare pathogenic variants can occur de novo in a gamete, a fertilized ovum, or a developing fetus. These pathogenic variants are typically more highly penetrant than common variants. Taken together, the combination of all genetic risk factors, including their number, allelic frequencies, and effect sizes, constitutes the genetic architecture of a given psychiatric disorder (Geschwind & Flint, 2015; Smoller, 2016).

Combining forces. The organization that is coordinating this global effort to explore genetic contributions to psychiatric disorders is the Psychiatric Genomics Consortium (PGC), an international collaboration that was launched in 2007. It now includes over 800 investigators from 40 countries, with nearly 1,000,000 samples undergoing analyses. There are currently 15 workgroups devoted to specific disorders/diseases and methodologies. From the outset, the consortium insisted on aggregating data from across laboratories and maintaining an open database of results that can be shared with appropriate individuals and groups. As the field progressed, it became obvious that much larger sample sizes were required to detect the small effect sizes of many genetic loci of interest (O'Donovan, 2015; Sullivan et al., 2012).

Breakthough in schizophrenia. In many ways, schizophrenia is the Gordian knot for psychiatry. Many of the symptoms of schizophrenia are uniquely human (e.g., hallucinations, delusions, disordered thoughts), and disability associated with a diagnosis of schizophrenia is the highest for any mental disorder. Heritability estimates for schizophrenia are high—81% based on a meta-analysis of 12 twin studies (Sullivan et al., 2003). Current antipsychotic drugs were first developed more than 60 years ago, and many patients do not respond favorably.

In 2014, a major GWAS reported by the PGC identified 108 genetic regions that played a significant role in susceptibility to schizophrenia (Schizophrenia Working Group of the Psychiatric Genomics Consortium, 2014). These associations were often linked to genes expressed in the brain. This study was successful in part because of the statistical power afforded by a sample of nearly 37,000 individuals with schizophrenia and more than 113,000 controls. The 108 loci that attained genome-wide significance only explained 3.4% of the variance in liability to schizophrenia.

The major findings confirmed some suspected defects in schizophrenia and revealed several new ones. There was a significant association with the gene that codes for the D_2 dopamine receptor (*DRD2*), the major target for most antipsychotic drugs (Urs et al., 2017). Additional associations were detected for genes involved in glutamatergic transmission, synaptic plasticity, and functioning of calcium channels. Finally, significant associations were detected for genes expressed in tissues that have a role in immune function. The immune system has long been hypothesized to play a role in the etiology of schizophrenia, and these genomic findings indicated that the connection is worthy of further exploration (Horváth & Kirnics, 2014).

Follow-up studies determined that there was no obvious connection between immune loci and schizophrenia, save for the major histocompatibility (MHC) region. This finding was in stark contrast to GWAS results for five autoimmune diseases (Crohn's disease, multiple sclerosis, psoriasis, rheumatoid arthritis, and ulcerative colitis), in which there were significant associations with several non-MHC immune genes that were not expressed in brain tissue. Of the six immune genes previously associated with schizophrenia (*DPP4, HSPD1, EGR1, CLU, ESAM,* and *NFATC3*), each gene encodes proteins that have non-immune-related functions in brain tissue. In this case, the relationship of these six "immune" genes to schizophrenia may be explained by their pleiotropic effects on neural development and plasticity, and not through their effects on the immune system per se. These findings, while consistent with a pleiotropic effect, are not definitive, and additional studies to probe the role of the immune system in schizophrenia were still needed (Pouget et al., 2016). And the wait wasn't very long.

A major breakthrough occurred when Sekar et al. (2016) probed the MHC region on chromosome 6, where the strongest risks associated with schizophrenia were previously reported. Within the MHC region, the strongest risks were associated with the gene *C4*, which codes for a complement factor involved in acquired immunity. There are two versions of *C4, C4A* and *C4B*, which are influenced by insertion of a human endogenous retroviral in a non-coding region of the gene. These investigators developed methods to quantify the number of copies of the two genes and their expression. Their findings indicated that the higher the expression of *C4A,* the greater the risk of schizophrenia. The complement system plays an important role in synaptic pruning, a process whereby synaptic connections in brain are pared back during central nervous system development (Stephan et al., 2012). Up-regulation of *C4A* may lead to excessive synaptic pruning, and explain some of the structural deficits in brain associated with schizophrenia.

In a related study, MacDonald et al. (2017) reported a selective reduction ($\downarrow$19%) of dendritic spine density on pyramidal neurons in layer 3 of primary auditory cortex in schizophrenic patients compared to matched healthy controls.

The selective loss of immature spines may be related to *CACNB4*, which was one of the 108 risk genes identified in the GWAS. Related experiments with *C4* through gene x environment paradigms in animal models may reveal new pathways for therapeutic interventions (Nimgaonkar et al., 2017).

An interesting approach taken by Sellgren et al. (2019) involved cellular reprogramming of monocytes from schizophrenic patients and healthy controls. The reprogrammed monocytes resembled microglia morphologically and were capable of engulfing dendritic spines of co-cultured neurons. The greater engulfment of dendritic spines by those cells obtained from schizophrenia patients was indeed associated with the risk variant *C4A*. In addition, these investigators demonstrated that pretreatment of microglia-like cell cultures with minocycline resulted in a dose-dependent decrease in dendritic spine engulfment. In a review of electronic health records of Partners Healthcare system in Boston, Massachusetts, the authors determined that individuals 10–18 years of age who were prescribed minocycline or a similar brain-penetrant antibiotic with anti-inflammatory properties for cases of acne for at least 3 months had significant reductions in risk of developing schizophrenia later in life. These investigators concluded that excessive synaptic pruning may be a viable target for delaying or preventing the onset of schizophrenia in high-risk individuals (Sellgren et al., 2019).

Combining data from GWAS and expression of quantitative trait loci, Zhao et al. (2018) identified 49 genes significantly associated with schizophrenia as revealed by Summary Data-Based Mendelian Randomization (SMR) software analysis. In addition, 80 gene sets associated with schizophrenia were identified by gene expression association analysis. Of particular note was a gene associated with endoplasmic reticulum functioning (*CRELD2*) and a gene that may be involved in DNA methylation (*DIP2B*), as well as a gene set critical for normal brain development.

Focusing on the role of CNVs in the etiology of schizophrenia, the PGC pooled microarray data from most of the available genomic studies of schizophrenia at the time of the study. The results, based on data from 21,094 cases of schizophrenia and 20,227 controls, identified eight risk loci that exceeded the genome-wide level of significance after correcting for multiple comparisons. Collectively, these loci were carried by a small percentage (1.4%) of the cases, and only 0.85% of the variance in schizophrenia risk was explained by carrying one of these eight identified loci. CNV burden was higher for genes involved in synaptic function and neurobehavioral disruptions in mouse models. Ever greater sample sizes are required to provide statistical power sufficient to detect variants of modest effect sizes or extremely rare variants (CNV and Schizophrenia Working Groups of the Psychiatric Genomics Consortium, 2017).

GWAS informs nosology. Genome-wide techniques have been or are being applied to other psychiatric disorders, including bipolar disorder (Psychiatric

GWAS Consortium Bipolar Disorder Working Group, 2011), major depressive disorder (Major Depressive Disorder Working Group of the Psychiatric GWAS Consortium, 2013; Network and Pathway Analysis Subgroup of Psychiatric Genomics Consortium, 2015; Wong et al., 2017), post-traumatic stress disorder (Logue et al., 2015), anxiety disorders (Otowa et al., 2016), autism spectrum disorder (Robinson et al., 2016; The Autism Spectrum Disorders Working Group of the Psychiatric Genomics Consortium, 2017), and attention deficit hyperactivity disorder (Demontis et al., 2019). Many roadblocks have been encountered, especially related to the need for significant increases in sample sizes for some disorders. Sample sizes in the range of 100,000 or more may be needed to detect the small effect sizes of variants for some of these disorders (Smoller, 2016). With major depressive disorder, there are also challenges with low heritability, heterogeneity of the disorder, interactions of genotype with environmental stressors, and the high likelihood of misdiagnoses in the individuals making up the population under study (Levinson et al., 2014).

Cross-disorder comparisons. Genome-wide studies have also called into question the validity of current diagnostic categories in psychiatry. Focusing on five psychiatric disorders (autism spectrum disorder, attention deficit hyperactivity disorder, bipolar disorder, major depressive disorder, and schizophrenia), the Cross-Disorder Group of the PGC (2013) examined possible shared genetic variants among some or all of these disorders. The results clearly pointed to shared genetic risk factors among the two childhood-onset and three adult-onset psychiatric disorders. These included four SNPs that exceeded the corrected level of statistical significance ($P < 5 \times 10^{-8}$), two of which were within two subunits of L-type voltage-gated calcium channels. Variants of calcium channel genes appear to exert pleiotropic effects on a range of disorders, and may be valuable new targets in drug discovery. These cross-disorder genetic effects may explain in part the comorbidity of disorders observed in many psychiatric patients (Cross-Disorder Group of the Psychiatric Genomics Consortium, 2013). These important genomic findings further blur the boundaries between diagnostic categories, even those that were thought to have little in common (O'Donovan & Owen, 2016; Smoller et al., 2019).

Another approach to unpacking shared genetic risk across multiple psychiatric disorders is through an investigation of risk genes that affect central nervous system development during the fetal period using the iPSYCH Danish birth cohort (Schork et al., 2019). Using this database, four GWAS-significant loci were identified that influence the function of radial glia cells and interneurons during the development of the neocortex in the second trimester of pregnancy through effects on calcium channels, other neurotransmitter receptors, and multiple aspects of synaptic plasticity. These findings suggest that a critical period may exist during fetal development when susceptibility to development of mental disorders in later life is established. Once established, the timing of these gene x environment interactions during fetal development may stimulate interventions to reduce risk prior to birth (Schork et al., 2019).

Probing etiology. Using a validated technique for estimating genetic correlations that only requires GWAS summary statistics, Bulik-Sullivan and coworkers (2015) examined several human diseases and complex traits in a database of 1.5 million unique phenotypic measurements for possible etiologic connections. Focusing only on the results with direct relevance to psychiatric disorders, this report noted significant positive genetic correlations between schizophrenia and bipolar disorder, schizophrenia and depression, schizophrenia and anorexia nervosa, schizophrenia and Crohn's disease, bipolar disorder and depression, and bipolar disorder and years of education. These results underscore further the blurred boundaries among psychiatric diagnoses, and point to new etiologic connections that are worthy of further investigation (Figure 2.2).

Focusing on schizophrenia and bipolar disorder, the Bipolar Disorder and Schizophrenia Working Group of the Psychiatric Genomics Consortium (2018) examined genetic data from more than 53,000 cases of the two disorders combined and a comparable number of controls. As expected, these results revealed considerable genetic overlap, with 114 loci shared between schizophrenia and bipolar disorder. For the first time, this group identified specific loci that distinguish between the two disorders, as well as polygenic components that contribute to shared symptom dimensions within the two disorders. The findings pointed to the possibility of employing genomic data to characterize patients at a finer-grained level and lead to more personalized treatments for a given constellation of risk factors.

Sharing risk. These conclusions are further supported by a major GWAS from the Brainstorm Consortium (2018). Drawing on the combined statistical power of GWAS representing more than 265,000 patients and more than 780,000 controls, this consortium reported that psychiatric disorders share a significant portion of their common variant genetic risk. This shared risk was especially evident for five psychiatric disorders: schizophrenia, major depressive disorder, bipolar disorder, anxiety disorders, and attention deficit hyperactivity disorder. That the genetic architecture of these psychiatric disorders does not reflect accurately on the current system for diagnosing psychiatric disorders is an understatement. This team of researchers argued strongly for an effort to recast psychiatric nosology to reflect the genetic reality as revealed by the continuing avalanche of GWAS findings.

Blurred boundaries. There are several ways to explain these positive genetic correlations between what many consider distinct psychiatric disorders. For example, there may be some level of genetic risk that is shared across many psychiatric disorders, with the final symptom clusters of a given disorder being shaped

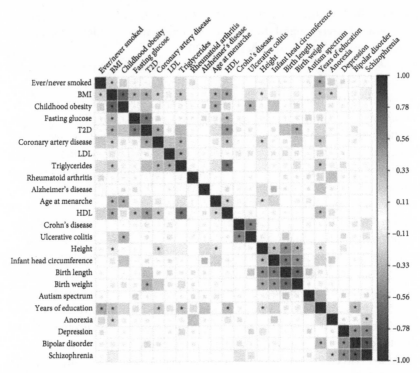

Figure 2.2. Genetic correlations among 24 traits analyzed by genome-wide association. Blue, positive genetic correlation; red, negative genetic correlation. Larger squares correspond to more significant *P* values. Genetic correlations that are different from zero at a false discovery rate (FDR) of 1% are shown as full-sized squares. Genetic correlations that are significantly different from zero after Bonferroni correction for the 300 tests in this analysis are marked with an asterisk. Results that did not pass multiple-testing correction are shown as smaller squares, to avoid obscuring positive controls, where the estimates point in the expected direction but do not achieve statistical significance owing to small sample sizes. The correction for multiple testing is conservative as the tests are not independent. To keep this figure to a reasonable size, representatives of several clusters of highly correlated traits were presented. Additional details and supplemental materials are available in the original publication (see also Plate 1).
Reproduced from Bulik-Sullivan et al. (2015) and used with permission of the publisher.

by other genetic, epigenetic, and environmental variables. A second possibility is that the phenotypic overlap between any two disorders may involve shared risk variants that have direct influence on those specific phenotypic traits. Finally, a shared cognitive dysfunction (e.g., delusional thought patterns) driven by common risk variants may lead to multiple disorder-specific outcomes due to pleiotropic effects. If these findings and others like them from GWAS data sets are employed to drive improvements in psychiatric diagnostic systems, then the care and clinical outcomes for patients will be greatly enhanced (The Brainstorm Consortium, 2018).

It is clear from the summary on the genetics of mental disorders that risk alleles are an important component in the etiology of the various disorders. However, risk alleles present only a part of the critical interaction between a susceptible genotype and a stressful environment. In the section that follows, I present an overview of the contributions of stressful life events to the development of three mental disorders: schizophrenia, bipolar disorder, and depression. As we will see, the dynamic interplay between a susceptible genotype and a stressful environment is a critical feature of many conceptions of the etiology of various mental disorders.

Stress and Psychiatric Disorders

In this section, I will draw on selected studies from the human literature that point clearly to a substantial contribution of environmental stressors in the etiology of psychiatric disorders. To keep the scope of this section to a manageable level, I will limit this presentation to three disorders—schizophrenia, bipolar disorder, and major depressive disorder—as discussed at the beginning of this chapter. I did not include post-traumatic stress disorder as, by definition, a diagnosis requires prior exposure to a traumatic or highly stressful event. This information builds a strong case for the chapters that follow; namely, that much can be learned about the mechanisms by which stress influences the expression of genetic risk for psychiatric disorders by studying appropriate animal models. Further, this information may be translated in various ways that are of direct benefit to patients and their families.

Stress and Schizophrenia

For the first half of the twentieth century, most psychiatrists adopted the view that schizophrenia was caused by a single etiologic agent. Others incorrectly asserted that the environment was responsible, given that the lower social classes had a much higher rate of schizophrenia than the upper classes (Hollingshead & Redlich, 1958). However, this difference evaporated when the social classes of the parents were considered. Bleuler (1963, p. 949) suggested "that hereditary disposition and life history act together in the genesis of schizophrenia," an idea that remains attractive today.

In their landmark paper, Gottesman and Shields (1967, p. 204) posited that most cases of schizophrenia were polygenically determined, and that the appearance of the schizophrenic phenotype "would depend on both the number of genes present and the amount of stress." Stress appears to impact vulnerable individuals at two distinct periods of development—during the prenatal/neonatal periods (e.g., obstetric complications, including perinatal hypoxia) and in later life around the time when symptoms of psychosis are first detected (Boksa, 2004; Mittal et al., 2008; Moghaddam, 2002).

Focus on the placenta. The intrauterine environment may play a critical role in the expression of risk genes for schizophrenia. The risk of developing schizophrenia explained by polygenic risk scores derived from GWAS is increased 5-fold in individuals who were exposed to early life complications. In this study (Ursini et al., 2018), early life complications were defined as somatic complications and conditions occurring during pregnancy, labor-delivery, and the neonatal period that were potentially harmful to the offspring, with special focus on the disruptions in development of the central nervous system. In addition, schizophrenic patients who experienced early life complications had significantly higher polygenic risk scores than patients without early life complications. Additional studies have revealed that schizophrenia risk loci that interact with early life complications are highly expressed in the placenta. In addition, these risk loci are more highly expressed in complicated pregnancies and are up-regulated in placentae from male versus female offspring. From this study, the placenta emerged as a critical interface between a stressful intrauterine or early postnatal environment and a fetus or neonate at high risk of developing schizophrenia. These findings also underscore the importance of high quality prenatal care as one means of reducing the risk of developing schizophrenia in early adulthood (Ursini et al., 2018).

Prenatal stress. Let's next consider how genes and environmental perturbations interact to shape the developmental trajectory of the schizophrenic phenotype.

Prenatal infections. One approach has been to explore the impact of outbreaks of infectious diseases on risk of schizophrenia in the offspring. For example, Suvisaari et al. (1999), using data from the Finnish Health Ministry, reported an association between the incidence of poliomyelitis and the occurrence of live births 5 months later of individuals who later developed schizophrenia. The effect of poliomyelitis on later development of schizophrenia was limited to the second trimester of pregnancy. Similarly, O'Callaghan et al. (1994) examined in two data sets the number of deaths per month during 1937–1965 for 16 infectious diseases in England and Wales. Next, they determined the number of children born during this period who later developed schizophrenia. Their results indicated that increased deaths from bronchopneumonia but not from 15 other infectious diseases preceded by 3 or 5 months (for the two data sets) an increase in births of children who later developed schizophrenia.

A more precise approach for exploring prenatal determinants of schizophrenia was adopted by the Prenatal Determinants of Schizophrenia (PDS) Study, which included a cohort of pregnant women who gave birth during 1959–1967, and were part of the pre-paid Kaiser Foundation Health Plan in its various clinics in Alameda County, California (Susser et al., 2000). Initially, more than 12,000 live births were included in this large-scale prospective study. This study was unusual in that regular sampling of blood from patients allowed investigators to confirm exposure of mothers to various pathogens.

Brown and Derkits (2010) have reviewed evidence that prenatal maternal infections may place the fetus at enhanced risk for later development of schizophrenia. Using data from the PDS Study, an early report demonstrated that maternal respiratory infections during the second trimester, but not the first or third trimesters, resulted in an increased risk for schizophrenia spectrum disorders in the offspring (Brown et al., 2000). Later studies documented that maternal influenza exposure during the first trimester of pregnancy was attended by a 7-fold increase in risk for schizophrenia in the offspring. No elevations in risk occurred if exposure to influenza was limited to the second half of gestation (Brown et al., 2004). Similar results have been reported for toxoplasmosis infections, which carried a 2-fold greater risk for schizophrenia in offspring (Brown et al., 2005), and herpes simplex type 2 infections, which carried a 1.8-fold increase in risk for schizophrenia in offspring (Buka et al., 2008). Brown and Derkits (2010) proposed a biological pathway from infectious agent → immune response → susceptibility genes → altered synaptic plasticity in fetal brain that could be involved in the increased risk for schizophrenia in offspring of infected mothers. These possible pathways connecting maternal exposure to offspring psychosis will be discussed further in Chapter 8.

War is hell. Van Os and Selten (1998) took an unusual approach to examine the role of prenatal stress in the later development of schizophrenia. They made use of the National Psychiatric Case Register to follow over their life spans individuals who were exposed during the first, second, or third trimester of pregnancy to the May 1940 invasion of The Netherlands by the German army. The 5-day invasion resulted in significant destruction of property and the deaths of several thousand civilians and several thousand Dutch soldiers. Their findings indicated that the incidence of schizophrenia was higher in the invasion-exposed birth cohort, especially in the first trimester of pregnancy, compared to controls. It appeared that the sensitivity of male but not female fetuses to prenatal stress extended into the second trimester.

A more severe tragedy occurred in The Netherlands at the end of World War II, when German forces imposed a tight blockade on western cities, leading to acute famine and what was termed the "Hunger Winter" (October 1944 to May 1945). For those babies conceived from October 15 to December 31, 1944, there was a 2-fold greater risk of developing schizophrenia later in life compared to birth cohorts before ($N = 10$ cohorts) and after ($N = 6$ cohorts) this 2.5-month period. The cumulative incidence of schizophrenia was approximately 1.9 cases/1,000 subjects in the 16 birth cohorts, compared to 3.8 cases/1,000 subjects in the highest risk group with occurrence of intense famine during the first trimester (Susser et al., 1996).

A more recent study examined the risk of schizophrenia in a cohort of almost 90,000 babies born in Jerusalem during 1964–1976. A particular focus of this study was on babies born to women who were pregnant during the Arab-Israeli war in 1967. There was an elevated relative risk of schizophrenia for those who were in the second month of fetal life in June 1967, and the risk was greater in females than in males. These findings are consistent with maternal stress during pregnancy serving as a risk factor for later onset of schizophrenia (Malaspina et al., 2008).

Stress during infancy through adolescence. Stressful experiences during childhood can also have a lasting impact on brain development and mental health outcomes (Ruby et al., 2014). In a comprehensive meta-analysis of childhood adversities/trauma and later development of psychosis, Varese et al. (2012) conducted a detailed review of the literature during 1980–2011 and identified 36 studies that qualified for further analysis. Psychosis included the following diagnoses: psychotic disorder, schizophrenia, or schizoaffective disorder. Across all 36 published studies, there was a significant association between childhood adversity and later psychosis (odds ratio = 2.78). In the 18 case-control studies, patients with psychosis were 2.7 times more likely to have been a victim of childhood adversity than controls. Odds ratios for the following types of adversity and abuse were as follows: emotional abuse (3.40), physical abuse (2.95), neglect (2.90), bullying (2.39), sexual abuse (2.38), and parental death (1.70). All odds ratios were significant at $P < 0.001$ with the exception of parental death ($P > 0.15$). Strikingly, if the various types of adversity and trauma were magically removed from the population, with all other factors remaining constant, the number of people suffering from psychosis would have been reduced by 33%!

Stress and disease onset. Adverse events in adulthood may also impact the onset of schizophrenia in at-risk individuals. Two early studies (Brown & Birley, 1968; Birley & Brown, 1970) concluded that stressful life events, especially those in the 3 weeks prior to the onset of symptoms, may play a role in the onset and recurrence of schizophrenic symptoms in up to 50% of patients. Several investigators have concluded that vulnerability to stressors and not frequency of exposure to stressors is a key aspect of the developmental course of schizophrenia. Vulnerable individuals would progress into a schizophrenic episode when their capacity to cope with especially intense life stressors was suboptimal (Horan et al., 2005; Norman & Malla, 1993; Nuechterlein & Dawson,

1984; Nuechterlein et al., 1994; Rabkin, 1980; Zubin & Spring, 1977). Stressful life events might serve as an environmental trigger that would move these otherwise vulnerable individuals into a phase of disease onset or relapse (Ventura et al., 1989).

A major study sponsored by the World Health Organization (Day et al., 1987) was stimulated by the studies of Brown and Birley described earlier. A sample of 386 patients who experienced a recent episode of schizophrenia was studied using semi-structured interviews. The patients were drawn from five developed countries and four developing countries spanning five continents. Results from eight of the nine centers were consistent with the hypothesis of an increase in significant life events in the 2–3-week period preceding the onset of psychotic symptoms for 40%–60% of the patients. Many of these individuals were also experiencing ongoing difficulties with family members or loved ones, and the significant life events could have been the triggering events to move patients into a florid psychotic state (Day et al., 1987).

Beards et al. (2013) conducted a meta-analysis of the role of life events occurring in adulthood on psychosis. The analysis included 16 published studies carefully selected from the literature over the period 1968–2012. Fourteen of these studies reported positive associations between exposure to stressful life events in adulthood and onset of psychosis, with an overall odds ratio of 3.19. The authors had reservations about the overall quality of the studies, and expressed the hope that more rigorous studies on this topic would be conducted in the future.

How do individuals at high risk for psychosis experience stressful life events and the daily hassles of conducting one's affairs compared to healthy controls? This important issue was addressed by Trotman et al. (2014) as part of the North American Prodrome Longitudinal Study, Phase 2 (NAPLS-2). Their results indicated that high-risk individuals reported significantly more stress associated with stressful life events and daily hassles compared to healthy controls. In addition, high-risk adolescents and young adults reported being exposed to higher levels of stressful life events compared to healthy controls. Further, high-risk individuals rated stressful events as more subjectively intense compared to controls. The findings of this study were also consistent with stress sensitization in high-risk individuals, such that more frequent exposure to stressors resulted in higher stress ratings related to daily hassles experienced later in life (Trotman et al., 2014).

The diathesis-stress model. Based upon the extensive body of research conducted since the 1960s on schizophrenia and stress, several theories have emerged to account for the findings. Early on, the diathesis-stress model (Bleuler, 1963; Rosenthal, 1963) presented schizophrenia as resulting from a complex interaction between multiple genes and an accumulation of adverse experiences that exceeded some threshold level. Walker and her colleagues (Corcoran et al., 2003; Pruessner et al., 2017; Walker & Diforio, 1997; Walker et al., 2008) and others (van Winkel et al., 2008) have supplemented the diathesis-stress model by linking the enhancing effects of hypothalamic-pituitary-adrenocortical (HPA) responses to stressful life events on up-regulation of brain dopamine systems and alterations in inflammatory processes. Howes and McCutcheon (2017) further modified the diathesis-stress model to include a critical role for stress-induced activation of brain microglia in the onset of schizophrenia. The diathesis-stress model has also been expanded somewhat to a three-hit theory of schizophrenia, in which genetic risk factors (Hit 1) interact with early-life stressors (Hit 2), resulting in a high-risk phenotype that is susceptible to adverse stressors in adolescence or adulthood (Hit 3) (Daskalakis & Binder, 2015; Daskalakis et al., 2013).

In summary, there is convincing evidence that stress plays an important role at multiple time points in the developmental course of schizophrenia (Mondelli, 2014). Stressors acting on a susceptible genotype may be critically involved during the prenatal period, during the postnatal period from just after birth through adolescence, and into adulthood.

Stress and Bipolar Disorder

As summarized by Angst and Sellaro (2000), Kraepelin (1899) included bipolar disorder, mania, single episode depression, and recurrent depression in a single diagnostic category, manic-depressive insanity. Others, including the French physician Ballet (1903), maintained that these were distinct illnesses. Kraepelin (2002) was among the first psychiatrists to suggest a link between stressful life events (e.g., illness or death of a loved one) and the onset and clinical course of bipolar disorder. In addition, he suggested that a point was reached where the onset of the disorder did not require a precipitating event. These important observations have been replicated many times over the past 100+ years, and theories relating to the etiology of bipolar disorder have been constructed around them.

Prenatal stress. A host of studies has investigated the impact of adverse events during the prenatal period on the later development of bipolar disorder. I will omit from further discussion any adverse events that have yielded inconsistent results (e.g., maternal smoking, difficult childbirth, etc.).

Using the Child Health and Development Study birth cohort, Canetta et al. (2014) compared 85 individuals with bipolar disorder with 170 matched controls. Their results indicated that serologically confirmed maternal influenza infections were associated with a 5-fold greater risk of bipolar disorder with psychotic features compared to controls that were not exposed to the virus.

The increased risk of bipolar disorder in children exposed prenatally to influenza could not be explained by higher maternal levels of circulating cytokines (Cheslack-Postava et al., 2017).

Drawing from the Third National Health and Nutrition Survey, Pearce et al. (2012) reported a significant association between antibodies for *Toxoplasma gondii* and bipolar disorder type I in which both depressive and manic features occurred. However, it should be noted that the number of cases of toxoplasmosis with bipolar disorder type I was very small in this study, so the results should be interpreted with some caution.

Stress during infancy through adolescence. Moving to factors occurring after birth, stressful life events prior to age 15, including parental illness, unemployment, imprisonment, psychopathology, death from natural or unnatural causes, family disruption, or living away from the family may impact the development of bipolar disorder later in life. Bergink et al. (2016) explored these issues using a database of all individuals born in Denmark during 1980–1998 ($N = 980,554$). With the exception of parental natural death and parental illness, a single exposure to an early life stressor resulted in increased risk for bipolar disorder. Of all variables investigated, a mental disorder in a parent was the greatest risk factor for later development of bipolar disorder (hazard ratio = 3.53). Life stressors added marginally to the effect of having a parent with a mental disorder. An earlier study using data from the Danish Psychiatric Central Research Register found that suicide of the mother or a sibling and other major life events were associated with an increased risk of first hospitalization with manic symptoms (Kessing et al., 2004).

Childhood maltreatment, including exposure to multiple traumatic events, was also highly prevalent in patients with bipolar disorder (Etain et al., 2010). Agnew-Blais and Danese (2016) conducted a systematic review and meta-analysis to explore further the relationship between childhood maltreatment and the clinical course of bipolar disorder. Maltreatment included instances of physical, sexual, or emotional abuse; neglect; or family conflict. After a detailed review of articles published up to January 1, 2015, these investigators selected 30 published articles from an initial pool of 527 articles for use in the meta-analysis. Compared to patients with bipolar disorder but without experiences of childhood maltreatment, bipolar patients with a history of maltreatment were more susceptible to and had greater severity of symptoms of bipolar disorder. Specifically, bipolar patients who experienced childhood maltreatment were characterized by the following: greater severity of mania, depression, and psychosis scores; higher risk of comorbidity with post-traumatic stress disorder, anxiety disorders, and substance and alcohol misuse disorders; earlier age of onset of bipolar disorder; greater risk of rapid cycling; greater number of manic and depressive episodes; and greater risk of suicide attempts. These findings have important implications for improving the diagnosis and treatment of bipolar patients (Aas et al., 2016; Agnew-Blais & Danese, 2016; Leverich & Post, 2006; Post et al., 2001).

Stress in adulthood. Many studies have examined the impact of stressful life events in precipitating or triggering bipolar illness. One early study subdivided 53 bipolar patients into two groups: early onset and late onset of the disorder, with 20 years of age being the cut-point. In the late onset but not in the early onset group, there were more self-reported stressful events in the year prior to the first episode of illness and the most recent illness (Glassner & Haldipur, 1983).

In a carefully controlled prospective study, Ellicott et al. (1990) followed 61 outpatients with a diagnosis of bipolar disorder for a 2-year period. There were frequent assessments of stressful life events, symptoms relating to the disorder, and compliance with treatment. The results revealed a significant association between the highest levels of stressful life events and relapse or recurrence of the disorder. In addition, Hammen and Gitlin (1997) reported that bipolar patients experienced more intense stressors and greater levels of total stress in the 6 months prior to an acute episode of illness.

Similarly, Johnson and Miller (1997) reported that bipolar patients who experienced significant negative life events took more than 3 times as long to recover from an episode as those without significant negative life events. In these and related studies, Johnson (2005) argued that studies of life events and bipolar disorder must achieve greater levels of specificity with respect to the impact of goal attainment activities, schedule-disrupting events, and stressful negative events on depressive and manic episodes.

Several reviews have considered the findings on psychosocial factors, including life stressors, which influence the onset or recurrence of bipolar disorder. The relevant literature is a mixed bag of cross-sectional and retrospective studies, some studies have lacked appropriate control groups, and many studies have suffered from small sample sizes (Alloy et al., 2005). Johnson and Roberts (1995) were among the first to situate life events stressors within the larger context of etiological theories of bipolar disorders. Based upon their review of the literature, they concluded that life events stressors have an important impact on the course of bipolar disorder. In particular, they suggested that stressors that disrupt normal activity rhythms, alter behavioral engagement, or might be susceptible to sensitization through recurring exposures have the greatest impact on bipolar disorder. More recent reviews have drawn attention to spring/summer seasonal disruptions, drug use, parental loss, and the stress of attaining life goals as factors that influence the course of bipolar disorder (Marangoni et al., 2016; Proudfoot et al., 2011).

To address these complex issues more directly, Lex et al. (2017) conducted a meta-analysis to address the central question of whether stress plays a role in bipolar disorder. Their meta-analysis, which included a detailed review of the literature published up to September 2014, included 53 articles that reported findings from 42 samples. They found that bipolar patients reported significantly more stressful life events prior to an acute episode compared to symptom-free intervals. In addition, bipolar patients also reported more stressful life events in the 12 months prior to an acute episode compared to levels in healthy controls. Childbirth may be an especially stressful event in bipolar patients because it tends to disrupt normal biological and behavioral circadian rhythms. The frequency of stressful life events did not differ between bipolar patients and those with schizophrenia, unipolar depression, or chronic illnesses.

Biological bases of bipolar disorder. Several investigations have probed the underlying neural, endocrine, and molecular alterations associated with bipolar disorder.

Adrenal steroids. Ostiguy et al. (2011) examined cortisol levels in saliva of 62 offspring of parents with bipolar disorder (mean age = 20.3 years) and compared them to 60 offspring without a family history of bipolar disorder (mean age = 18.7 years). The findings revealed that salivary cortisol levels were significantly higher in young adults with a bipolar parent at the following sampling times: mean daytime levels (average of 7 sample points); mean awakening levels; and levels at 13:00, 15:00 and 20:00 hours. In addition, offspring with a bipolar parent were more sensitive to naturally occurring interpersonal stressors compared to controls. These findings suggest that at-risk individuals may be especially vulnerable to the effects of daily stressors, and that their adrenal cortical responses to stress may contribute to the onset of bipolar disorder (Ostiguy et al., 2011).

Dopamine. The dopamine hypothesis of affective disorders dates from more than 50 years ago, and yet it remains a prominent feature of theories of bipolar disorder today (Schildkraut, 1965). In a detailed review of the field, Ashok et al. (2017) suggested that a state of increased dopaminergic transmission, with elevations in D2 and D3 receptors in the striatum, and a hyperactive reward-processing network underlie the manic phase of bipolar disorder. In contrast, a consistent finding in relation to the depressive phase of bipolar disorder has been an elevation of striatal dopamine transporter levels. The authors recognized the limitations of the dopamine hypothesis of bipolar disorder, as much of the evidence to date is based upon pharmacological responses.

BDNF. Brain-derived neurotrophic factor (BDNF) is a newer molecular element of theories of bipolar disorder (Post, 2007). Duman and Monteggia (2006) summarized research that connects exposure to stress with reduced expression of the *BDNF* gene in limbic brain regions that are involved in regulation of mood and cognition. In addition, they suggested that up-regulation of BDNF synthesis may be involved in the actions of antidepressants. Consistent with this hypothesis was the report that prior exposure to traumatic events in bipolar patients was associated with a significant decrease in serum BDNF levels (Kauer-Sant'Anna et al., 2007). In addition, Hosang et al. (2010) examined the interaction between stressful life events and the val66met polymorphism in the *BDNF* gene in bipolar patients and healthy controls. The val66met polymorphism is located in the non-coding 5'pro-BDNF sequence, and appears to affect intracellular processing and secretion of the mature protein, but not its intrinsic activity (Egan et al., 2003). The results from the study revealed a significant interaction between stressful life events and the val66met polymorphism for the worst depressive episode, but not for the worst manic episode experienced by bipolar patients (Hosang et al., 2010). Similar results have been reported for an interaction between stressful life events and the val158met polymorphism in the catechol-O-methyl-transferase (*COMT*) gene in bipolar patients and their worst depressive episodes (Hosang et al., 2016).

GWAS. The hypothesized complex polygenic architecture of bipolar disorder has been confirmed in a GWAS of Japanese bipolar patients and controls and a meta-analysis of a larger data set that included European patients and controls (Ikeda et al., 2018). Two risk loci were identified, and three others were confirmed. Newly identified risk loci included one in a region that corresponds to genes coding for fatty acid desaturase (*FADS*), and the other located near *NFIX*, a gene in the nuclear factor 1 family that is involved in transcription and replication. Three other confirmed gene variants included *MAD1L1*, which is involved in regulation of mitosis; *TRANK1*, which encodes tetratricopeptide repeat and ankyrin repeat; and *ODZ4*, which encodes teneurin transmembrane protein. All five of these gene variants attained genome-wide statistical significance. Finally, rare deleterious genomic variants have also been suggested to play a role in multigenerational families with bipolar disorder (Rao et al., 2017). A final aspect of genetic susceptibility in bipolar disorder concerns changes in methylation of DNA, which modifies gene expression patterns (Fries et al., 2016, 2017; Kebir et al., 2017). Additional details of these epigenetic aspects of disease suscepti-bility will be discussed in Chapter 7.

Stress and the kindling hypothesis of bipolar disorder. Dr. Robert M. Post, who spent most of his career at the National Institute of Mental Health in Bethesda, Maryland, combined clinical and basic research findings into a com-prehensive framework to explain how psychosocial stress could contribute to recurring episodes of unipolar or bipolar affective disorders (Post, 1992). Central to his efforts were results from animal experiments on behavioral sen-sitization to stimulant drugs and electrophysiological kindling. Behavioral sensitization refers to the augmented locomotor responses of laboratory ani-mals following repeated injections of stimulant drugs such as amphetamine or cocaine. Importantly, there was also evidence of cross-sensitization between psychostimulant drugs and stressors (Kalivas & Stewart, 1991). Kindling was first reported by Goddard et al. (1969), and consisted of repeated low-level electrical stimulation of the amygdala. These sub-threshold stimulations led to progressive increases in amplitude, duration, and complexity of after-discharges, eventually culminating in spontaneous limbic seizures.

Drawing from these two separate lines of basic research with animal models, Post (1992) suggested that exposure of humans to stressful experiences could result in unipolar or bipolar illness, and lead to long-lasting changes in gene expression that persist over time and lead to vulnerabilities to further episodes of affective illness. Eventually, Post argued, the episodes of illness would occur with minimal or no stressful life experiences. In recent updates of his original theory, Post and colleagues (Kapczinski et al., 2008; Post, 2016) incorporated newer findings from allostasis and epigenetics research that provide a broader view of the impact of chronic exposure to stressful stimuli, and a compelling molecular mechanism to explain long-term pathophysiological changes in gene regulation that are thought to influence the clinical course of bipolar disorder.

The "kindling model" has been tested by several groups of investigators, and the results are somewhat inconsistent. Hlastala et al. (2000) focused their attention on a critical aspect of the kindling model, that major stressful life events should play a diminishing role over time in bipolar patients. Employing a carefully selected study population of 64 patients with bipolar I disorder, they found that the number of episodes of illness did not predict the level of stress experienced by patients before the onset of illness. In addition, there was no evidence that minor stressors played a greater role prior to the onset of later episodes of illness. Thus, their results failed to support a kindling model or a sensitization model. However, their results did favor an involvement of age at the time of episode onset, such that high levels of life stressors prior to an illness episode decreased as age increased, and low levels of stressors before an illness episode increased as age increased (Hlastala et al., 2000).

In a test of the stress sensitization hypothesis, Dienes et al. (2006) evaluated 59 participants with a diagnosis of bipolar I disorder every 3 months for one year. Stressful life events and early life adversity were assessed using a structured interview protocol. They reported a lack of interaction between stressful life events and number of prior illness episodes on recurrence of illness. However, participants with early life adversity had a significantly younger age of onset of bipolar disorder, and reported lower levels of stress prior to illness episode recurrence compared to participants who did not experience early life adversity. The latter findings were generally consistent with a sensitization-like process.

In a related study, Shapero et al. (2017) examined the effects of early life adversity in a group of bipolar individuals that included 112 bipolar II participants and 33 cyclothymic disorder participants. Their results indicated that early life stressors sensitized bipolar individuals to the effects of minor negative life stressors for depressive illness episodes but not for hypomanic illness episodes.

Weiss et al. (2015) followed a group of 102 participants with bipolar II disorder in an attempt to compare the kindling model of Post (1992) with the autonomy model of Monroe and Harkness (2005). The kindling model suggests that sensitization to life stressors occurs over time, such that even minor stressors will precipitate recurrence of an illness episode. In contrast, the autonomy model posits that major and minor forms of life stressors decrease in frequency over the course of bipolar disorder, and have little or no impact upon the recurrence of illness episodes. Their findings partially supported the kindling model but did not support the autonomy model. Specifically, they found that with increasing lifetime episodes of depression, a prospective bout of depression was associated with an increase in minor but not major negative life event stressors. With increasing lifetime episodes of hypomania, prospective bouts of hypomania were associated with an increase in minor but not major positive life event stressors. A major inconsistency in their findings was the fact that major positive or negative valence life events stressors did not decrease in frequency with increasing lifetime episodes of hypomania or depression, respectively (Weiss et al., 2015).

Summary. The role of life stressors in the etiology of bipolar disorder remains an active area of investigation. The methodological challenges in this field of research are significant, and the perfect study has not yet been conducted. What is clear is that the seminal kindling theory of Post (1992) still influences this field of investigation, although the results to date are not uniformly consistent in support of the theory (Bender & Alloy, 2011).

Stress and Depression

Studies of stressful life events and depression have a long history. One of the first well-controlled studies was conducted by Paykel et al. (1969), using a sample of 185 depressed patients and a group of matched controls. Their findings indicated that depressed patients experienced approximately three times as many stressful life events (e.g., increase in marital discord, marital separation, serious illness of the patient or a family member, death of a family member, etc.) in the six months prior to onset of a depressive episode compared to controls over a comparable time period.

Twin studies. A critical study that established a causal relationship between stressful life events and the onset of major depressive disorder was conducted by Kendler et al. (1999), based upon a 1-year study of female twins from the Virginia Twin Registry. This research addressed the thorny issue of the degree to which genetic and familial factors influenced exposure to stressful life experiences. That is, some individuals tend to favor environments or situations that lead them to experience stressful events (Kendler et al., 1993). The sample included more than 24,000 person-months of exposure and 316 confirmed episodes of depression. The results provided conclusive evidence that stressful life events were significantly associated with the onset of depression. However, approximately one-third of the association between stressful life events and the onset of major depression was dependent (i.e., related to the individual's own behaviors or choices). The remaining two-thirds of the association were clearly connected to independent stressful life experiences (Kendler et al., 1999).

A remarkably consistent finding over the years has been the higher incidence of major depression in women than men. Based on data from the National Comorbidity Survey, women were approximately 1.7 times more likely than men to experience an episode of depression over the life span (Kessler et al., 1993). Might this sex difference in prevalence of depression result from greater sensitivity to stressful life events and/or more frequent exposure to stressful life events in females?

Using a population-based sample of female-female, male-male, and female-male twin pairs, Kendler, Thornton, and Prescott (2001) found no evidence that females and males differed in their frequency of exposure or in their sensitivity to stressful life events. However, women did report higher rates of exposure to some stressful life events (e.g., difficulties with housing, loss of a confidant, challenges with individuals in their proximal network, illness of individuals in their distal network) and men reported higher rates of exposure to other life stressors (e.g., job loss, legal problems, robbery, difficulties at work).

Silberg et al. (1999) followed a sample of male and female twin pairs from childhood into adolescence to examine genetic and stressful environmental contributions to the onset of depression. There was a significant increase in depression among adolescent girls compared to boys. Stressful life events were evident for boys and girls, with a greater impact evident in girls. Genetic factors were dominant in girls, such that some girls in the study experienced an episode of depression in the absence of a significant stressful life event.

Kendler and his colleagues also explored developmental pathways to the onset of depression in women and in men using structural equation modeling. Using a sample of female twins, Kendler et al. (2002) reported that three major pathways led to depression, one of which was psychosocial adversity. This pathway included childhood sexual abuse, parental loss, family disruptions, traumatic experiences, marital difficulties, and stressful life events. In their study of male twins, Kendler et al. (2006) also noted three major pathways to depression, one of which included adversity and interpersonal difficulties (e.g., childhood sexual abuse, loss of a parent, traumatic experiences, and stressful life events). In both men and women, genetic risk contributed to each of the three sex-specific pathways.

Stress from infancy to adolescence. Data from the National Survey of Health and Development (encompassing the March 3–9, 1946, British birth cohort) were also studied to explore the relationship between stress and later development of depression (Colman et al., 2014). The findings from this study pointed to direct and indirect effects of early life adversity and later life stressors on depression. In addition, there was evidence of a cumulative impact of stressful experiences throughout development on the onset of major depressive disorder in adulthood.

The impact of childhood adversity prior to age 17 on later development of mental disorders was studied using the National Epidemiological Survey of Alcohol and Related Conditions (McLaughlin et al., 2010). Childhood adversity included instances of emotional and physical abuse, violence within the family, neglect, endangerment, sexual abuse, mental illness in the family, and incarceration of a parent. Stressful life events over the preceding year were associated with a significant increase in risk for depression and other disorders. However, the risk for depression in women and men was approximately 2 times greater in those individuals with 3 or more experiences of adversity during childhood compared to those without experiences of childhood adversity. Further, those individuals who experienced childhood adversity tended to perceive stressors in adulthood as more overwhelming and unmanageable.

These results were presented as evidence that childhood adversities sensitize individuals to the deleterious impact of exposure to stressful life events in adulthood. In addition, the authors suggested that childhood adversities may serve as a broad-based diathesis for several categories of psychopathology over the life span (McLaughlin et al., 2010). Finally, Heim and Bender (2012) have pointed to the existence of sensitive periods during postnatal development when early life stressors exert their greatest effects in humans.

The stress-diathesis theory. Several theories relating to the etiology of major depressive disorder have been advanced over the years. I will limit this discussion to a subset of these theories. The diathesis-stress theory of depression has evolved from conceptualizations of the etiology of schizophrenia (see earlier discussion), and emphasizes a process whereby stressful stimulation activates or interacts with a specific diathesis (e.g., vulnerability), resulting in the transformation of a predisposition into the onset of a depressive episode (Monroe & Simons, 1991). The diathesis could be cognitive (Lewinsohn et al., 2001) or genetic (Caspi et al., 2003).

Consistent with the diathesis-stress model, a seminal report by Caspi et al. (2003) was the first to demonstrate that a polymorphism in the promoter region of the serotonin transporter (5-HTT) gene could moderate the effects of major life stressors on depressive symptoms, major depressive disorder, and suicide attempts. Using a large representative birth cohort in New Zealand (Dunedin Multidisciplinary Health and Development Study), these investigators reported that individuals with one or two short (*s*) alleles in the promoter region of the *5-HTTLPR* gene were affected to a greater extent by exposure to major life stressors than individuals with two long (*l*) alleles. The *s* allele is less efficient transcriptionally compared to the *l* allele. Major life stressors included child maltreatment and financial, health, relationship, and housing issues.

These basic findings of a gene x environment effect on depression have been replicated by several groups (e.g., Kendler et al., 2005; Vrshek-Schallhorn et al., 2014) and confirmed by a major meta-analysis of 54 studies published through November 2009 (Karg et al., 2011). In addition, Gotlib et al. (2008) provided evidence that girls 9–14 years old with two copies of the *s* allele had significantly greater levels of cortisol in saliva immediately and up to 45 minutes after exposure to laboratory stressors (serial subtraction followed by a stressful interview for a total of 15 minutes) compared to girls with at least one *l* allele, providing a potential mechanism to explain the increased susceptibility to depression in individuals homozygous for the *s* allele. A subsequent meta-analysis covering the literature published through October 2011 confirmed a significant association between *5-HTTLPR* genotype and cortisol reactivity to acute psychosocial stress, with levels of reactivity significantly greater in individuals homozygous for the *s* allele compared to those homozygous for the *l* allele or heterozygotes (Miller et al., 2013).

To address the inconsistencies in the literature, Culverhouse et al. (2018) conducted a collaborative meta-analysis of 31 data sets that contained more than 38,000 subjects of European ancestry that were genotyped for the *5-HTTLPR* and evaluated for depression and childhood maltreatment as well as other stressful life events. This study did not confirm a gene x environment interaction or a main effect of the *s* allele on occurrence of depression. However, there were significant main effects for sex and for the impact of stressors on depression. Given the findings noted earlier by Caspi et al. (2003), Culverhouse et al. (2018) concluded that if an interaction effect does occur, it is not generalizable from the Dunedin data set, is of modest effect size, and only occurs in limited situations.

Kindling and depression. Another prominent theory of major depressive disorder (and bipolar disorder; see earlier discussion) is the kindling hypothesis originally presented by Post (1992). In his landmark paper, Post developed a framework to explain recurring episodes of depression that linked sensitization to repeated exposure to stressful stimulation, with persistent molecular changes in stress-sensitive brain circuits. He has expanded his theory to include epigenetic changes that would have profound influences on regulation of gene activity (Post, 2016).

Monroe and Harkness (2005) evaluated the kindling hypothesis from the perspective of life stress research, focusing particular attention on whether recurring episodes of depression become autonomous of input from life stressors, or sensitized to them. In a test of the kindling hypothesis, Kendler, Thornton, and Gardner (2000, 2001) examined the relationship between stressful life events and occurrences of depression in a population-based study of female twins. In the first study, the results indicated that with each new episode of depression, the association between stressful life events and the onset of depression declined. This effect was especially strong for up to 9 episodes of depression, and confirmed the kindling hypothesis of Post (1992). Beyond 9 episodes of depression, there was no evidence of further sensitization to stressful life events.

In their second study, these investigators considered whether enhanced genetic risk increased the rate of kindling, or rendered individuals "pre-kindled." Their results clearly favored the pre-kindled model, such that those individuals with highest genetic risk demonstrated a weak association between stressful life events and the first episode of major depression compared to individuals with low genetic risk. With subsequent episodes of depression, the relationship between stressful life events and onset of depression changed little in those at high genetic risk, but decreased markedly in those at low genetic risk (Kendler, Thornton, & Gardner, 2001).

The cognitive model. The most comprehensive theory of depression by far is the cognitive model advanced by Beck and Bredemeier (2016). This model (refer to Figure 2.3), which has been updated and expanded several times over the past 40 years, argues that depression results from a tendency to perceive events in a negative fashion and to evince exaggerated biological responses to stressful experiences. These disruptions in cognitive processing and regulation of stress responsiveness are regulated by specific brain circuits that render an individual susceptible to experiences of loss, such as those related to intimate relationships, membership in a group, or valued resources. The classic symptoms of depression, including lack of pleasure derived from such activities as eating, drinking, and social interactions, as well as loss of energy to engage in daily activities, are manifestations of these disruptions in cognitive processing and regulation of stress-responsive biological systems (autonomic, endocrine, and immune).

An attractive feature of the expanded cognitive theory is its incorporation of an evolutionary framework for interpreting the potential survival value of the symptoms of depression. Beck and Bredemeier (2016) posit that "the perceived loss of an investment in a vital resource" leads to activation of the depression program, resulting in behavioral and physiological adaptations designed to reduce energy expenditures as a means of compensating in part for the loss. They

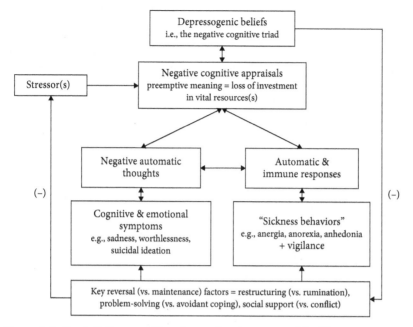

Figure 2.3. Precipitation, manifestation, and maintenance of the "depression program." According to the model, precipitating stressors and depressogenic beliefs interact to generate negative cognitive appraisals. If the individual perceives that he or she has lost a vital investment, various processes are initiated in service of energy conservation to compensate for this loss. Specifically, these processes consist of (a) negative automatic thoughts that generate cognitive and emotional symptoms (e.g., sadness, feelings of worthlessness) and (b) autonomic and immune responses resulting in "sickness behaviors" (e.g., anorexia, anhedonia) coupled with vigilance. Furthermore, depressogenic beliefs are reinforced/strengthened. Once this program is activated, a number of factors can determine if/when it is terminated, including the individual's available support as well as engagement in cognitive restructuring or problem-solving. However, these processes are undermined by depressogenic beliefs. The converse processes that serve to maintain the depression program (e.g., ruminative thinking, social conflict) can generate additional stress for the individual.

Note: (–) indicates proposed negative relationships/effects.

Reproduced from Beck & Bredemeier (2016) and used with permission of the publisher.

argue that efforts to reduce energy expenditures in the face of a loss of a vital resource may well have been adaptive in the evolutionary history of our species, but clearly are not in the present times. An evolutionary interpretation of depression in included in Chapter 12.

Summary

In this chapter, I have used three psychiatric disorders—schizophrenia, bipolar disorder, and major depressive disorder—to marshal evidence that clearly points to interactions between a susceptible genotype and stressful life events in the etiology of these devastating diseases. For each disorder, there is a significant contribution from genotype, ranging from 0.40 for major depressive disorder to >0.70 for schizophrenia. For each of the three psychiatric disorders, there is also a rich literature on the role played by stressful life experiences in the onset and recurrence of illness episodes.

Given the obvious limitations of research with human cohorts, further advances in understanding the mechanisms by which stressful life experiences interact with a susceptible genotype to result in a psychiatric disorder will be hastened by experiments with animal models. Later in this volume, I will include individual chapters to showcase what has been learned about several of the most prevalent psychiatric disorders by reviewing research on a variety of animal models. These experiments provide a fertile ground for designing intervention strategies to prevent psychiatric disorders from occurring, and if they do occur, for revealing new molecular targets for drug discovery and other advances in treatment options.

3

Evolution of the Stress Concept

Early Conceptions of Health and Disease

Since humans have lived in fixed and stable communities with the capacity to maintain domesticated animals and cultivate crops for reliable sources of food, sufficient leisure time has been available for the elites of the community to consider the qualities of a life well lived and the ways in which one could enhance one's quality of life. Common themes run through the formulations of human health and disease from the original philosophical and medical traditions of Egypt, China, India, and Greece. A brief description of each follows.

Ancient Egyptian Medicine

Ancient Egyptian medicine (1630–1350 BCE) was infused with a strong element of the supernatural. The belief system held that there were 36 gods of the atmosphere and an equal number of demons, and the human body was divided into as many parts. If a specific part of the body was not in optimal health, the corresponding demon had to be appeased for a cure to occur. Although plant-based medicines and other natural products were employed by the ancient Egyptians, they were used only in conjunction with an effort to appease the demons through the use of magic rites, amulets, and other approaches (Subbarayappa, 2001; Ritner, 2000).

Traditional Chinese Medicine

Traditional Chinese medicine has been practiced for more than 3,000 years and is based upon two foundational principles—yin-yang and the five elements (*wu xing*). These two theories were thought to explain all changes and all of the natural phenomena in the universe, including those associated with humans. The human body, like the universe, was thought to be composed of two opposites, yin and yang, that are confronting as well as interdependent and that can transform into each other. If the two forces were balanced and in harmony, then the body was healthy. However, if there was disharmony, then illness occurred. Five element theory, which may be traced back to an ancient Chinese philosophical system, suggested that the universe consisted of five basic elements: wood, fire, earth, metal, and water. This theory also described the relationship between the human body and the external environment and the pathophysiological interactions among the internal organs of the body (Lao et al., 2012).

Ancient Indian Medicine

Within ancient Indian medicine, Ayurveda emphasized the interrelatedness of mind and body, of food and medicine, and within the body, of the various physiological processes, all conceived and explained in terms of the five elements. Central to all of these beliefs was a holistic approach, with an emphasis on balance or equilibrium. The equilibrium or the harmony of both the mind and the physical body was required for a healthy and purposeful life, and for the realization of personal goals. Recognizing the dynamic interaction between humans (microcosm) and the universe (macrocosm), the Ayurvedic theory of equivalence of macrocosm and microcosm posited that an individual's health would be sound and vibrant if the interaction was natural and wholesome, while a disharmonious interaction would result in disease (Subbarayappa, 2001).

The Early Greeks

For the ancient Greeks, humans as a biological entity and as an integral part of the biology of nature demanded a new understanding of, and a new insight into, healthy living. Heracleitus was among the first to suggest that the natural state of all things was one of constant flux. As an early cosmologist, he supported this view by stating that the primary element, or *physis*, of the universe was fire, an agent of change. The flux constantly occurred between two poles (e.g., happiness and sadness, illness and health, etc.) as people lived their lives. Soon thereafter, Empedocles proposed the corollary idea that the four elements (water, earth, fire, and air) were assembled into all matter, including living things, by love and were disassembled by strife. Thus, balance or harmony (assembly) was a necessary condition for the survival of all living organisms. Similarly, the philosopher and physician Alcmaeon of Croton defined health as a balance of forces within the body, which constituted a state of "political isonomy." In contrast, poor health resulted from an asymmetry of these forces within the body. He was also one of the first early physicians to ascribe mental functions to the brain.

The Hippocratic legacy. One hundred years later, the works of Hippocrates (probably from multiple authors between 450 and 350 BCE) spelled out in the magnum opus, *Corpus Hippocraticum*, a scientific approach to diseases and their cures, generally referred to as the Hippocratic method. There was an insistence on prognosis and the notion that disease was a natural process of abnormality. To the Hippocratic writers, life processes involved a constant interaction between the individual and his or her environment. They also built on the classical theory of Greek medicine from the late 5th century BCE involving the four humors: blood, phlegm, yellow bile, and black bile. Thus, health in the body meant the interplay of proper proportions of the four humors; when one humor was in a state of excess, disease would result. An individual's propensity for disease was also thought by Hippocrates to be inherited.

The Hippocratic writers also thought that in a majority of cases the body would be able to resolve the harmful effects of a disease by itself; a physician should step in only when the condition deteriorated. Three groups of causative factors were recognized in Hippocratic medicine: (i) the vitiation of natural dispositions or temperaments; (ii) improper environmental conditions, food, and drink; and (iii) an individual's own habits, actions, or functions. Hippocrates and his followers were careful observers, and they believed in recording observations during the systematic examination of each patient. They did not conceive of a sharp divide between normal and pathological states; rather, they viewed the disease state as one which would be less capable of overcoming the effects of a harmful environment. They stressed the importance of climate vis-à-vis physiological and pathological states. The teachings of Hippocrates and the works of his followers became the canon of medicine in the centuries that followed, and were distinguished by a dependence on reason and a lack of association with supernatural beliefs regarding human health.

Enter Galen. In the second century CE, Galen of Pergamum, located in Asia Minor, rose to prominence as a physician. A Greek by birth, he spent much of his professional life in Rome, although he was forced to leave Rome later in life because of professional conflicts. He held Hippocrates in high esteem and enriched Greek and Roman medicine with his own clinical, anatomical, and physiological studies. It was Galen who suggested that a spirit, *pneuma*, was drawn inside by the act of breathing and was responsible for the various faculties of the *physis*, the internal creative essence of an organism. Galen's physiology encompassed what he called the *natural spirit* (in the liver), the *vital spirit* (in the heart), and the *animal spirit* (in the brain), as well as the *pneuma* that circulated throughout the body. He also thought the liver was the center of the venous blood system. He suggested that in some individuals there was a natural tendency toward having one of the four humors in excess, and that these natural imbalances would lead to inherent differences in temperament (e.g., sanguinous, phlegmatic, bilious, or melancholic). His assertion that anatomical structures and bodily functions were designed by the Creator later received the approval of the Catholic Church (by about the eighth century CE). It was, therefore, Galen, more than Hippocrates, who greatly influenced European medicine until the birth of the Renaissance (Chrousos & Gold, 1992; Jackson, 2014a; Temkin, 1953).

Summary

Putting aside the Egyptians and their focus on magic, the traditions of ancient Chinese, Indian, and Greek medicine emphasized the importance of harmony and balance in relation to health, and set the stage many centuries later for studies that examined the health consequences of disturbing harmony and balance via stressful stimuli. There was also an appreciation for the challenges presented by an ever-changing environment and the need to adjust physiologically and behaviorally to these challenges (i.e., stressors) to maintain good health.

Modern Foundations of Stress Research

The French Connection

During the latter half of the 19th century, Claude Bernard (Figure 3.1) established himself as the preeminent scientist in France. The impact of his experiments and publications was felt across Europe, Russia, and the United States during his lifetime and continued following his death. While completing his medical training, Bernard was fortunate to come under the influence of the noted physician and physiologist François Magendie, professor of medicine at the Collège de France and an attending physician at the Hôtel-Dieu de Paris. In spite of being an unremarkable medical student, Bernard displayed an early aptitude for working with laboratory animals, and fully embraced Magendie's enthusiasm for rigorous experimentation as the only means to advance knowledge in physiology (Boullerne, 2011; Coleman, 1985; Gross, 1998).

Career trajectory. With his career path as a physiologist set, Bernard progressed from a laboratory assistant to a deputy professor to professor and director of the laboratory upon the death of Professor Magendie in 1855. This career path was a bumpy one, however, as Bernard had no official position for the three years following his service as a laboratory assistant (1842–1844). During this challenging period, he was forced to conduct experiments at his home or in the private laboratories of his colleagues. In 1847, he returned to Magendie's laboratory, but the facilities remained inadequate, and financial support for research was all but lacking. Finally, in 1852, he began to receive a small stipend for his work as a scientist. In 1854, he was appointed to the Chair of General

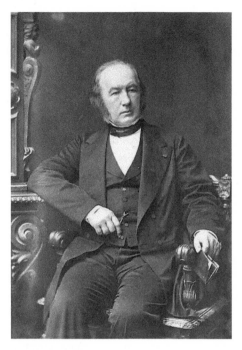

Figure 3.1. Claude Bernard, M.D.

Physiology at the Faculty of Science, but this position provided no laboratory facilities and was largely a teaching position (Coleman, 1985; Gross, 1998).

Upon Magendie's death in 1855, Bernard returned to the Collège de France as the holder of the Chair of Medicine. It was not until 1868, however, that Bernard received new, though still modest, laboratory facilities at the National Museum of Natural History. The laboratory did not become functional until 1873, and Bernard never took an active role in the administration and direction of the facility. Bernard carried memories of these difficult times with him to the end of his life, and he became a powerful and passionate advocate for the establishment of an independent discipline of physiology that was provided with adequate funding and laboratory facilities from the state. Such support would permit French scientists to compete on an equal footing with scientists from other countries (Gross, 1998).

A rich legacy. Bernard's major research findings resulted from experiments that were conducted in less than ideal laboratory facilities from 1843 until 1858. Four major discoveries during this especially productive period included: (i) the role of the pancreas in digestion; (ii) the role of vasomotor nerves in body temperature regulation through effects on vasodilation and vasoconstriction; (iii) the importance of the liver in glycogen synthesis/storage and glucose regulation; and (iv) vagal control of the heart. Although he remained an active presence in the laboratory for the remainder of his career, Bernard transitioned to produce several important monographs on physiology, including *Introduction to the Study of Experimental Medicine*, published in 1865, and *Lectures on the Phenomena Common to Animals and Plants*, published in 1878 (Boullerne, 2011; Cooper, 2008; Gross, 1998).

A national hero. At the time of his death in 1878, Claude Bernard was the most celebrated scientist in all of France. He had received several national honors for his research, he was a *commandeur* of the Ordre National de la Légion d'honneur, he was an elected member of the Academy of Science and the Academy of Medicine, he was a member of the Senate, and he was elected one of the 40 "immortals" and later served as president of the Académie française. This group, founded in 1635, is responsible for all matters pertaining to the French language. Upon his death in 1878, Bernard was honored with a public funeral, the first time such an honor was bestowed upon a French scientist, and he was buried in Père Lachaise cemetery (Gross, 1998).

A big idea. We now come to Bernard's most enduring scientific contribution—the constancy of *le milieu intérieur*, or the internal environment. His views on this concept probably evolved from the mid-1850s until his death in 1878, and encompassed his studies of regulation of glucose levels in blood and maintenance of a stable body temperature. He argued that an ability to maintain a constancy of the internal environment allowed for the development of the most complex forms of life, as reflected in the following quote from Bernard (1927, p. 84):

> The constancy of the internal environment is the condition for free and independent life . . . The constancy of the environment presupposes a perfection of the organism such that external variations are at every instant compensated and brought into balance. In consequence, far from being indifferent to the external world, the higher animal is on the contrary in a close and wise relation with it, so that its equilibrium results from a continuous and delicate compensation established as if by the most sensitive of balances.

Bernard also pointed out the critical role played by the nervous system in ensuring the harmonious functions of the body's vital systems. These ideas were emphasized in Bernard's public lectures and in his widely disseminated writings, but they had little impact on the field of physiology until 50 years later (Gross, 1998; Wasserstein, 1996). Indeed, there was no mention of the *le milieu intérieur* in the extensive obituary published in the United States in the year of Bernard's death (Flint, 1878). Why such a significant delay?

Bernard's most detailed description of his thoughts on *le milieu intérieur* appeared in the monograph published just after his death (Bernard, 1974). Here, he advanced the notion that higher animals are in close and constant contact with the external environment, and they must constantly compensate for and adjust to the changes in the external environment to sustain life. And for Bernard, only the nervous system was positioned to maintain the harmony that existed among all of the monitored variables in *le milieu intérieur*. Finally, as Cooper (2008) has pointed out, it was not a great leap to envision that a loss of this harmonious balance could lead to disease. With regard to this latter point, Bernard became the bridge (le Pont Neuf, perhaps) that connected early beliefs on balance and harmony in the body in Greece with the development of stress and diseases of adaptation by Selye in the 20th century.

Although Bernard never fully embraced Darwin's views on evolution by natural selection (Darwin, 1859), it was an evolutionary interpretation of experimental data from marine organisms that brought Bernard's concept of *le milieu intérieur* into a position of scientific prominence. As Gross (1998) summarized so nicely, experiments on electrolyte composition of body fluid in various marine species revealed that more highly evolved species (e.g., bony fish) had sodium levels that differed significantly from seawater, whereas less highly evolved species (e.g., crabs and lobsters) had sodium levels that were similar to seawater. These qualitative findings were followed by more sophisticated studies that supported the evolution of ever more sensitive mechanisms to protect the internal environment from the external world.

English-speaking supporters. Early in the 20th century, there were well-placed champions of Bernard's concept of *le milieu intérieur* in both the United Kingdom and the United States. British scientists who situated their studies in the context of Bernard's regulation of the internal environment included William Bayliss and Ernest Starling, co-discoverers of the first hormone, secretin; J. S. Haldane and Joseph Barcroft, who studied respiratory physiology; and C. S. Sherrington, the eminent British neurophysiologist. In the United States, Lawrence J. Henderson and Walter Bradford Cannon, both professors at Harvard Medical School, supported the critical nature of Bernard's research for the life sciences. Henderson (1927) wrote the introduction to the American translation of Bernard's *Introduction to the Study of Experimental Medicine*. His own research on the maintenance of blood pH also drew extensively on the work of Bernard. As will be discussed in the following, Cannon's research on the sympathetic nervous system and his introduction of the term *homeostasis* were strongly influenced by Bernard's studies, and Cannon introduced Bernard's work to a much wider audience (Cooper, 2008; Gross, 1998; Schiller, 1967).

Stress: The Early Years

The distinguished physician and historian of medicine, Dr. Mark Jackson (2013), has provided an illuminating summary of efforts during the late 19th and early 20th centuries to link stressful experiences and health status in Great Britain and the United States. The stresses and strains of modern life, including overcrowded living conditions, competition for limited resources, and the exhausting pace of life, were thought to be associated with increases in mortality from heart disease in Great Britain as early as the 1870s. Others suggested connections between mental stress and cancer, and excessive workplace demands on the development of angina pectoris (Jackson, 2013).

The importance of Crile. Based in part on his experiences as a battlefield surgeon during the Spanish-American War of 1898 and later service during World War I in France, George Crile (1915, 1922) crafted a theory of disease that emphasized the demands placed upon the body to adapt to environmental conditions, especially emotionally provoking stimuli. He suggested that physiological responses to emotional stimuli were contributing factors in cardiovascular disease; digestive diseases; Graves' disease; and other disorders of the thyroid gland, diabetes, and mental disorders. According to Jackson (2013, pp. 57–58), "Stress constituted a key concept within Crile's physiological framework of disease. Like many of his contemporaries, Crile believed that the physiological system was being driven at 'an overwhelming rate of speed' by the 'stress of our present-day life.'"

Preparing the way. In many ways, Crile's theories of stress and disease foreshadowed the emergence of Walter Bradford Cannon and Hans Selye as the leading architects of modern stress theory. Besides being a highly skilled surgeon and an innovator in developing surgical instruments and procedures and the use of anesthetics, Crile was a cofounder of the Cleveland Clinic. His contributions to the field of stress research are often overlooked given the long shadow cast by Cannon.

Stress Comes of Age

Between 1910 and 1936, the laboratories of two pioneering physician-scientists, Walter Bradford Cannon of Harvard Medical School and Hans Selye of McGill University, established the early foundation for the field of stress research. This foundation initially comprised two distinct physiological pillars, the sympathetic-adrenal medullary system and the hypothalamic-pituitary adrenocortical system, reflecting the research emphases of Cannon and Selye, respectively. How did the publications of these two influential biomedical pioneers set

the stage for contemporary research in adaptations to acute and chronic intermittent stressful stimulation?

Walter Bradford Cannon and the sympathetic-adrenal medullary system.
At the beginning of his tenure as a faculty member at Harvard Medical School,
Cannon (Figure 3.2) followed in the footsteps of his mentor and department
chair, Professor Henry P. Bowditch, and studied properties of the digestive
system (Benison & Barger, 1987). In particular, Cannon was one of the first
investigators to combine food mixed with the salts of heavy metals and the use of
newly discovered X-rays to visualize the digestive processes of cats in real time.
In foreshadowing the development of future research interests, Cannon mentioned at the end of one of his early publications that "[s]igns of emotion, such as
fear, distress, or rage, are accompanied by a total cessation of the movements of
both the large and small intestines" (Cannon, 1902, p. 75).

Beginning in 1910, Cannon moved into a new area of investigation that included studies of the adrenal medulla and the sympathetic nervous system in
laboratory animals. In addition to studying the physiology of the adrenal medulla, he broadened his focus to include psychological stimuli and emotional
responses that were often associated with sympathetic nervous system discharge
and adrenal medullary secretion (Cannon, 1919; Cannon & de la Paz, 1911).

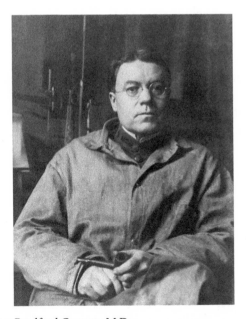

Figure 3.2. Walter Bradford Cannon, M.D.
This image is licensed under the Creative Commons Attribution 4.0 International License.

Homeostasis. As Cannon began his experiments on the adrenal medulla, he was aware of the writings from the late 1800s of the renowned French physiologist Claude Bernard, as well as discussions with his mentor, Professor Bowditch, who spent one year in Bernard's laboratory following graduation from Harvard Medical School. Bernard, as described earlier, advanced the theory that bodily systems cooperate to maintain a relatively constant internal environment, or *le milieu intérieur* (Bernard et al., 1974). These same bodily systems would also come together to direct a return to a constancy of *le milieu intérieur*, even after major disruptions to an organism. Thus, Bernard's view near the end of his life was that higher animals exist in a close and informed relationship with the external world, and the relative constancy of *le milieu intérieur* results from moment-to-moment adjustments in various physiological systems (Holmes, 1986).

Cannon expanded the list of major disruptions to an organism to include stressful stimuli. Cannon also built directly upon Bernard's theory by introducing the concept of *homeostasis*, with the central nervous system playing a critical role in directing the necessary adjustments in bodily systems to maintain a constancy of the internal environment. A key component of this homeostatic balance was central control of the sympathetic nerves and the adrenal medulla and the secretion of epinephrine (EPI).

Stressful stimuli. As noted by Mason (1975a), as early as 1914, Cannon employed the term *stress* in describing experiments on physiological responses to emotional stimuli (Cannon, 1914b). He continued to use the term *stress* as a means of describing the relationship between emotional and physical stimuli and the concomitant physiological responses in his laboratory experiments (e.g., Cannon, 1928). In a later paper (Cannon, 1935), he addressed the consequences of exceeding "critical stress levels," thereby overwhelming the homeostatic capacities of organisms and disrupting the internal environment. At the end of his career, he also referenced stress in discussions of industrial organizations and human communities (Cannon, 1932).

As Goldstein (2006) pointed out, Cannon was mistaken on several critical details relating to the function of the sympathetic nervous system and the adrenal medulla, but he was largely correct on the bigger picture. For example, Cannon (1940) argued that the sympathetic nervous system and the adrenal medulla were a single functional unit that employed the same chemical messenger, EPI. The chemical arsenal of the sympathetic nerves was expanded, Cannon thought, through the conversion of EPI into two other substances, sympathin E (excitation) and sympathin I (inhibition) (Cannon & Lissak, 1939; Cannon & Rosenblueth, 1933; Rosenblueth & Cannon, 1932). It was not until after World War II that von Euler (1948) provided definitive evidence that norepinephrine (NE) was the neurotransmitter released from sympathetic nerve endings, not EPI as Cannon had thought. It was later still that a host of investigators revealed the two broad classes of adrenergic receptors, alpha- and beta- and their subclasses (Ahles & Engelhardt, 2014; Pierce et al., 2002).

Service in the Great War. During his service as a medical officer in World War I, Cannon worked on a major clinical problem facing surgeons in army field hospitals in France: shock (Chambers & Buchman, 2001). Cannon's foundational belief was that shock represented a failure of homeostatic regulatory mechanisms. His initial hypothesis, based on earlier animal experiments in his laboratory at Harvard Medical School, was that shock was caused by adrenal exhaustion. He later dropped this hypothesis in favor of a toxic factor released into the circulation at the site of injury (Cannon, 1922). Eventually, he was forced to abandon his hypotheses and to accept that abnormal fluid sequestration was the primary cause of shock, based upon laboratory experiments conducted by Dr. Alfred Blalock of Vanderbilt University Hospital (Blalock, 1930). Interestingly, Cannon had a major influence on Blalock in spite of their opposing views on the nature of shock. In the end, they became close colleagues and friends (Chambers & Buchman, 2000).

Fight-or-flight response. Cannon was well aware that an increase in the activity of the sympathetic-adrenal medullary system would, at critical times, such as encounters with aggressive conspecifics or exposure to a predator, result in a loss of homeostatic balance. At such times, increased blood flow to the skeletal muscles, release of glucose from the liver, dilation of the bronchi to increase availability of oxygen, reduced blood flow to the skin and digestive system, and a host of other physiologic changes would address the immediate survival needs of an organism. Homeostasis could be re-established at a later time, possibly even at different set points, when the threat was eliminated and the survival of the organism was more certain (Cannon, 1914a, 1915, 1932).

In reflecting back in his autobiography about the importance of hunches, Cannon (1945, pp. 59–60) wrote the following:

> Another example I may cite was the interpretation of the significance of bodily changes which occur in great emotional excitement, such as fear and rage. These changes—the more rapid pulse, the deeper breathing, the increase of sugar in the blood, the secretion from the adrenal glands—were very diverse and seemed unrelated. Then, one wakeful night, after a considerable collection of these changes had been disclosed, the idea flashed through my mind that they could be nicely integrated if conceived as bodily preparations for supreme effort in flight or in fighting. Further investigation added to the collection and confirmed the general scheme suggested by the hunch.

Cannon and psychology. It is striking to note that Cannon, a classically trained physiologist, did not hesitate to weave psychological concepts into his work on the adrenal medulla and the control of EPI secretion. Several personal and professional relationships exposed Cannon to psychological theories and research. As an undergraduate at Harvard, he took a class from William James, a towering figure in American psychology. He was also close friends for many years with the noted experimental psychologist, Robert M. Yerkes, and their families were neighbors at their summer homes in New Hampshire for over three decades. In addition, Cannon maintained a close personal and professional relationship with the Russian Nobel Laureate, Ivan P. Pavlov, and hosted him during his two visits to the United States in 1923 and 1929 (Cannon, 1994; Fleming, 1984). Finally, he also published several important papers in behavioral science journals during his career (e.g. Cannon, 1927, 1942). His surprisingly broad embrace of scientific domains was captured in a letter to his friend and colleague, Dr. Carl Binger, a Harvard psychiatrist, in October 1934 (cited in *Psychosomatic Medicine, 19,* 180, 1957):

> I personally conceive of the well-grounded work of the psychologist and the psychiatrist as being related to one aspect, while the work of the physiologist is related to another aspect of the same unit. Therefore, I do not hesitate to use psychological terms along with physiological terms in descriptions. If the physiologist has observations which support or yield interpretation of the views of the psychologist or psychiatrist, why should they not be accepted and incorporated into the general scheme of things?

Cannon's openness to combining psychology and evolutionary biology with physiology through his experiments on homeostasis, the fight-or-flight response, stress, and emotions has ensured that his rich legacy continues to the present with contemporary researchers. This is in spite of the fact that many of his fundamental assumptions regarding the biology of the sympathetic nervous system and the adrenal medulla have not stood the test of time.

Cannon's concerns for a society under stress. At the end of his term as president of the American Association for the Advancement of Science (AAAS), Cannon delivered an address at the AAAS annual meeting in Philadelphia on December 27, 1940. Some of the ideas contained in his presidential address first appeared in an epilogue, "Relations of Biological and Social Homeostasis," to his widely read book, *The Wisdom of the Body* (Cannon, 1932). Cannon (1941) expressed grave concern regarding the ongoing political, military, economic, and social disruptions in the United States, Europe, and other parts of the world. He had observed firsthand the suffering experienced by wounded soldiers in field hospitals in France during World War I, and by many people across all segments of society during the economic collapse of the Great Depression of the 1930s. Hitler and the Nazis had recently invaded many countries in Eastern and

Western Europe and were continuing their air assaults on the United Kingdom, with the Soviet Union in the crosshairs. What principles could be identified to sustain nations during such times of ongoing upheaval and conflict?

Cannon drew on his four decades of experiments on homeostasis in laboratory animals to make a case for analogous homeostatic processes that may also operate at the level of societies, the so-called organic analogy (Cross & Albury, 1987). He suggested (Cannon, 1941, p. 4) that "[i]t may be that our bodies, which are the culmination of ages of experience, have learned secrets of management that are worthy of our study." For example, he noted that community-level, corporate, and governmental organizations constantly face the challenges of internal as well as external perturbations. As a starting point, he presented the example of the complex web for production and distribution of essential items for consumption by members of society, with an emphasis on "continuity of service." Although he was a liberal Republican in his political beliefs, he went on to argue that governmental agencies must be available to intervene and dampen the peaks and valleys of production and consumption and to ensure that the basic needs of all members of society are met. However, he also warned that societal efforts at promoting stability for each member should not come at the expense of individual liberty or creative expression (Cannon, 1941; Fleming, 1984). These are ideas that the United States and other countries continue to grapple with and that resonate with many today.

Hans Selye and the hypothalamic-pituitary-adrenocortical axis. Hans Selye (Figure 3.3), a junior faculty member at McGill University, made his entry into the

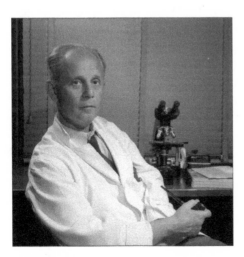

Figure 3.3. Hans Selye, 1956.

Photograph by Chris Lund. National Film Board of Canada, Library and Archives Canada (PA-116671).

field of stress research in a relatively modest way. On July 4, 1936, he published a brief letter to the editor in the prestigious international journal, *Nature*, in which he summarized a series of experiments on laboratory rats exposed to a variety of "nocuous agents" (Fink, 2016; Neylan, 1998). The nocuous agents included an unrelated series of challenges, including cold, surgical injury, spinal shock, muscular exercise, or sub-lethal doses of a variety of drugs or tissue extracts. He concluded that the rats developed a consistent triad of symptoms in three stages that was largely independent of the nocuous agent employed. He labeled this triad the "general adaptation syndrome." In a prelude to his publication in *Nature*, Selye reported on a series of experiments in laboratory rats that examined the effects of fasting, surgical shock, injury, restraint, cold exposure, or administration of drugs (e.g., morphine, atropine, formaldehyde, or adrenaline) on involution of the thymus and adrenal hypertrophy. These effects tended to diminish with continued or repeated exposure to the same stimulus (Selye, 1936a).

General adaptation syndrome (GAS). The three phases of physiological and pathological changes that Selye incorporated into the GAS included the following:

- *Alarm phase*: occurred within 6–48 hours following exposure to a nocuous stimulus and was attended by decreases in the weights of the thymus, spleen, lymph glands, and liver; reduced fatty tissue; loss of muscle tone; decrease in body temperature; and gastrointestinal erosions.
- *Adaptation phase*: occurred from 48 hours until 1–3 months after the beginning of repetitive exposure to a nocuous stimulus; the adrenals were greatly enlarged, body growth ceased, there was atrophy of the gonads, cessation of lactation, and enhanced production of thyrotropic and adrenotropic factors from the pituitary. Animals adapted to the deleterious effects of the nocuous stimulus but were more susceptible than controls to the deleterious effects of another stressor.
- *Exhaustion phase*: depending on the severity of and continued exposure to the nocuous agent, animals died at some unspecified point (usually within 3 months) with symptoms similar to those observed during the alarm phase. Selye hypothesized that animals died because they had exhausted their stores of "adaptation energy," though he was never able to define or measure adaptive energy (Figure 3.4).

As Selye recounted in his autobiography, *The Stress of Life* (Selye, 1978), his initial experiments with laboratory rats involved injections of ovarian and placental extracts, as he hoped to identify a new female hormone by using the triad of responses as a bioassay. The bioassay included: (i) adrenocortical hypertrophy, (ii) atrophy of the thymus and spleen, and (iii) gastric ulceration. Much to his

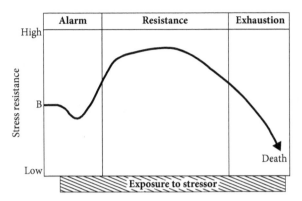

Figure 3.4. As originally presented by Selye (1946), the general adaptation syndrome (GAS) included three distinct stages when an animal or human is exposed to chronic stress: (i) the initial alarm reaction that occurs after stressor onset at baseline (B); (ii) the resistance stage, which includes a time when adaptive mechanisms counter the adverse impact of the stressor; and (iii) the stage of exhaustion, when the individual is no longer capable of mounting adaptive responses to the stressor. In some instances, death may occur.

dismay, Selye also observed this same triad of responses following injections of other tissue extracts, as well as formalin, a painful irritant to tissues. Exposure of rats to cold also resulted in the same triad of responses, and that finding prompted Selye to set aside his initial disappointment in not discovering a new hormone and to tackle this new opportunity to explore the "stress syndrome" and its potential relevance to diseases in humans.

Remarkably, Selye's 74-line letter to the editor of *Nature* contained no descriptions of experimental procedures, no quantitative data, no photomicrographs, and no references (Selye, 1936b). Yet, it is still frequently cited in publications today and has stimulated tens of thousands of experiments on stress and its role in disease processes since its publication. The field of stress research continues to be influenced by this initial report and the subsequent voluminous publication record of Selye over the next 46 years until his death in 1982 (e.g., Selye, 1946, 1951, 1955, 1973, 1975).

Being the first to propose a new theory doesn't ensure that one's views will hold up over time. Such is the case with Selye's initial report in 1936 and many of his publications that followed. He very quickly became convinced that the GAS, or stress syndrome, represented a major new approach to human disease for clinical medicine, and he was tireless in promoting this view. Due in large part to his promotional efforts, the word "stress" was added to the lexicon of many of the world's languages (Selye, 1978).

The early years. Hans Selye was born in Vienna in 1907 to a well-placed family. His father, Hugo, was a surgeon and the family estate was in Komárom, part of the Austro-Hungarian Empire. Following the end of World War I and the collapse of the Austro-Hungarian Empire, Komárom became part of the newly created Czechoslovakia. Beginning in 1924, Selye attended the German University of Prague, where he graduated with an M.D. in 1929 that included one year of study each in Paris and Rome. Following medical training, he completed a Ph.D. in organic chemistry while conducting research in the Institute for General and Experimental Pathology. Next, he spent one year at The Johns Hopkins University School of Medicine with support from a Rockefeller Foundation research fellowship. The ambience in Baltimore was not to his liking, so Selye transferred his fellowship to McGill University in Montreal to work in the laboratory of the distinguished biochemist, Professor James B. Collip. At the end of his fellowship, he returned to Prague for a brief period, but then traveled back to McGill at the invitation of Professor Collip, first as a lecturer and then as an assistant professor in the Department of Biochemistry (Selye, 1977).

The meteoric rise to prominence of Selye and his concept of stress is a case study in strategic risk-taking, effective marketing, and networking on a global scale. And all of this occurred before the advent of television, email, the internet, and social media platforms. Selye was promoted to associate professor at McGill in 1941, and he was able to enlist the support of Nobel Laureate Sir Frederick Banting, the co-discoverer of insulin, in securing initial research funding for his laboratory from the National Research Council of Canada (Viner, 1999).

Founding an institute. In 1945, Selye was recruited to the University of Montreal as professor and founding director of the Institute of Experimental Medicine and Surgery. In this institute of his creation, Selye sought to have an outsized influence on stress research throughout the world. His work ethic was second to none, and included being in the institute at least 12 hours per day, seven days per week, including holidays, unless he was traveling to give lectures. He was also intimately involved in the planning and execution of experiments and frequently checked the health of his animals and conducted autopsies at the end of the experiments (Szabo et al., 2012).

Publish or perish. Throughout his career, but especially at the institute, he published empirical and review articles in scientific journals at an astounding rate. As a case in point, over the course of his career, he published more than 1,700 articles and 32 single-author books and monographs. This output included an 800-page monograph (Selye, 1950), and a series of compilations, *Annual Report on Stress*, that were published from 1951 to 1955. Permit me to point out the obvious—no desktop or laptop computers! He also established a comprehensive library to catalog all published research on stress, and shared this vast store of information, numbering more than 100,000 publications, with scientists and the public at large. Later in his career, he published general reviews on his theory of stress in journals sponsored by a range of medical specialties and allied health professions (Szabo et al., 2012; Viner, 1999).

Attracting the best and brightest. Given this level of research activity, it is not surprising that Selye's institute was a bustling place. Over the course of his career, he trained 40 Ph.D. students and welcomed to his laboratory postdoctoral fellows and visiting scientists from around the world. He hit the proverbial jackpot with his first Ph.D. student, Roger Guillemin, who received the Nobel Prize for Physiology or Medicine in 1977 for his work on hypothalamic releasing factors. Guillemin, a senior medical student in Lyon, first encountered Selye when he presented a series of lectures in Paris (in French) in the spring of 1948 to overflow crowds. Guillemin has mentioned how dynamic and passionate Selye was about the topic of stress and diseases of adaptation. He approached Selye after one of his lectures and asked if there might be an opening in his laboratory. By the end of the year, Guillemin was in Montreal completing a thesis for his M.D. degree and working toward his Ph.D. in physiology under the direction of Selye. Although he quickly diverged in significant ways from Selye's more classical approach to experimentation, Guillemin still credits Selye with introducing him to a career in experimental medicine (Guillemin, 1985).

Guillemin's reaction to Selye's lectures was not unusual. Selye maintained an active travel schedule for much of his career, and these lectures provided him with an opportunity to enlist broad support for his theories relating to stress and diseases of adaptation. He was also fluent in at least five languages, which optimized his impact as a speaker and visitor to universities throughout the world. Many of his trainees and visiting scientists first encountered Selye during one of his lecture tours, and were later encouraged to join him in Montreal.

When only the Nobel Prize will suffice. Many of Selye's other students and trainees have been fiercely loyal to him prior to and following his death. Some have argued that he should have been honored with the Nobel Prize for his discoveries in steroid biochemistry and the physiology of stress. Selye was apparently nominated for the Nobel Prize on multiple occasions between 1949 and 1953 (Jackson, 2013, 2014b), and his best chance may have been in 1950 when the Nobel Prize for Physiology or Medicine was awarded to two chemists, Edward Kendall and Tadeus Reichstein, and a physician, Dr. Philip Hench, for their studies of cortisone and its use in the treatment of rheumatoid arthritis. Not only have some of his trainees expressed the opinion that Selye would have been a more appropriate recipient of the Prize than Hench, they have even taken exception to the fact that Hench's Nobel lecture and companion manuscript failed to cite any of Selye's relevant experimental work on anti-inflammatory effects of glucocorticoids during the 1940s (Szabo et al., 2012).

The rainmaker. A large laboratory requires significant financial resources for salaries, equipment, and supplies. Selye was incredibly successful at securing grant support for his institute at the University of Montreal. In 1953 alone, Selye received more than $103,000 in external grant support for his institute, which represented more than 55% of the total amount for external research funding for the entire Faculty of Medicine. My best guess is that medical school deans in the 1950s were just as focused on levels of external grant funding as medical school deans are today. This level of success in external funding gave Selye tremendous leverage with his dean and others in the university administration. At the peak of his career, he had two entire floors of the School of Medicine dedicated to his institute, with almost 100 staff members and 10–15 students at any given time (Jackson, 2013).

Blowing smoke. Selye's legacy has been tarnished with the release of tobacco industry documents revealing that he received considerable research support from tobacco industry sources and that he provided information from his laboratory that was used to further legal arguments and public relations efforts by the tobacco industry (Petticrew & Lee, 2011). Selye was also open to guidance from lawyers representing tobacco industry interests in terms of how he would approach writing a paper on the topic of smoking and stress. Note that Selye did smoke a pipe, but not cigarettes (see Figure 3.3). Selye also did not make public his consulting efforts with the tobacco industry or law firms retained by the tobacco industry.

Selye did receive substantial research support for his laboratory from the Council for Tobacco Research and Canadian tobacco industry sources beginning in 1969 and continuing until 1975. He testified before the Health Committee of the Canadian House of Commons on June 12, 1969, and shared his views against anti-smoking legislation. He was also a key attendee at a tobacco industry-supported conference held in the French Antilles in January 1972. I am confident that the weather at that time of year was much more favorable in San Martin that it was in Montreal. Selye's contribution to the published proceedings of this conference was edited extensively by tobacco industry insiders, and the volume was utilized in tobacco industry promotions for more than 20 years.

Petticrew and Lee (2011) have carefully reviewed documents in the Legacy Tobacco Documents Library available at the University of California, San Francisco, that related directly to Selye's involvement with the tobacco industry. Their careful review and analysis call into question the ethical standards that guided Selye's involvement with the tobacco industry and his willingness to allow his international reputation as a scientist to be subverted for the benefit of an industry that continues to market a product that damages the health of individuals throughout the world. This case study provides additional support for requirements relating to full disclosure of any support received by a researcher from industry sources, especially those with a vested interest in the research that is reported. This is true for medical researchers in general and researchers in psychiatry-related areas in particular (Bekelman et al., 2003; Fava, 2007).

Criticisms of the general adaptation syndrome. From the time he was a medical student in Prague, Selye was subjected to criticisms of his nascent theory of a syndrome of simply being sick, initially from his professors, and later from his colleagues and senior scientists whom he admired. At the beginning of his clinical training in medical school, Selye was struck by the constellation of symptoms that was common to many diseases (e.g., coated tongues, swollen glands, generalized body aches, reduced appetite), while his medical school professors were more interested in symptoms that distinguished one disease from another, leading to a differential diagnosis (Selye, 1978; Viner, 1999).

When Selye began his studies on endocrine responses to injections of tissue extracts or formalin, he made the connection between those early observations of sick patients as a medical student and a possible physiological basis for the symptoms that were common across several diseases. These nonspecific responses of the GAS could provide a new approach for medical science in designing strategies for the prevention of disease, and he was single-minded in pushing for that new approach for the remainder of his career.

Let's begin with Selye's definition of stress—"the nonspecific response of the body to any demand." Given this broad definition, virtually anything could be viewed as a stressor, from getting out of bed in the morning to confronting a robber in a dark alley to spilling coffee on your new suit on the drive to work to surviving the horrors of an extended tour of duty in a combat zone. To address some of these earlier criticisms, Selye made the following adjustments in his theory:

- With exposure to stress, the demand could be pleasant or unpleasant and could result in happiness or sadness. The pleasant demands were defined as *eustress* and the unpleasant demands were defined as *distress*. The biological changes were similar between eustress and distress, but the damage to bodily systems was much greater with distress.
- Stress always expressed itself in a nonspecific syndrome and the whole body had to be involved.
- Conditioning factors were introduced to explain why individuals differed in their responses to the same stressor. These included genetic differences, differences in prior experiences, and dietary differences. However, if one stripped away those conditioning factors, the constellation of nonspecific responses remained (Taché & Selye, 1985).

Cannon had concerns. Interestingly, Walter B. Cannon was one of the first senior scientists to criticize Selye's formulation of stress during a visit to present a lecture at McGill University, probably in the early 1940s. Selye's account of their meeting was presented in a later publication (Selye, 1978, pp. 280–281):

> Cannon was my first critic . . . I felt quite frustrated at not being able to convince the Great Old Man of the important role played by the pituitary and the adrenal cortex in my stress syndrome. He gave me excellent reasons why he did not think these glands could help resistance and adaptation in general and even why it would seem unlikely that a general adaptation syndrome could exist. But there was no trace of aggressiveness in his criticisms, no sting that could have blurred my vision to the point of refusing to listen.

In spite of Cannon's lack of enthusiasm for Selye's theory of stress, Selye did include the following tribute to Cannon following his death in 1945 on the title page of a featured review on the GAS that appeared in the *Journal of Clinical Endocrinology* in 1946: "Dedicated to the memory of that great Student of homeostasis, whose life [ref] and work [ref] have been the author's greatest inspiration." It is interesting to note that Cannon's name is not mentioned in the tribute, and the only way one can determine the subject of the tribute is to consult the reference list at the end of the article.

On the occasion of his publication of the first monograph describing experiments relating to the GAS (Selye, 1950), *The Lancet* included a review of the book, described as "Selye's gospel," with comments on the author and his body of work at that still-early point in his career. The reviewer stated (anonymous, 1951, p. 279), "Selye's *Stress* must be read by anyone who seriously professes to follow the most important trend of medicine at the opening of the second half of the 20th century." The reviewer expressed skepticism of Selye's theories until they were carefully evaluated and subjected to experimental verification.

Back and forth. The distinguished psychiatrist John W. Mason published a two-part critique of Selye's theories of stress and diseases of adaptation in 1975 that were spread over the first two issues of a new publication, the *Journal of Human Stress*. In the first article (Mason, 1975a), he pointed to several major concerns: (i) Selye's description of stress as a physiological response within the organism that is elicited by noxious stimuli, or stressors; (ii) Selye's statement that stress is elicited by any of a number of different stimuli but that the physiological stress response is nonspecific, or similar across the different stimuli; and (iii) the conclusion that the field of stress research had evolved as two separate camps, one primarily concerned with physical and endocrine stimuli, with the other focused more on psychosocial stimuli. Mason argued that findings from psychosocial aspects of the stress response made clear the many interacting variables that determined how a given individual would respond to a stressful stimulus. These variables included genetics, previous experiences, and behavioral predispositions. Thus, while Selye argued for a consistent and nonspecific response to stressful stimuli, Mason presented strong evidence in favor of more nuanced and heterogeneous patterns of responses to stressful stimuli. Was there a path forward such that these two disparate approaches to stress research could be integrated (Mason, 1975a)?

In the second part of his analysis, Mason (1975b) emphasized that some of Selye's stressors (e.g., exposure to heat or cold, forced exercise, restraint, injection of formalin, etc.) also included a strong measure of emotional distress, fear, and pain. This inadvertent inclusion by Selye of stressors that had psychological as well as physiological dimensions raised additional concerns about the nonspecific nature of the stress response. But Selye's research depended upon indirect measures of endocrine activity, including tissue weights and histological analyses. At the time the experiments were conducted, there were no methods to permit a direct assessment of endocrine activity by measurement of circulating hormone levels.

With the advent of sensitive and specific methods for the measurement of circulating steroid and peptide hormones beginning in the 1950s and continuing into the 1960s, it was possible to test directly some of these hypotheses about responses to psychological versus physiological stressors and the doctrine of nonspecificity. In Mason's own laboratory research, direct measures of circulating hormones revealed highly specific patterns of adrenocortical responses to various stressful stimuli in rhesus monkeys, and these and other findings raised serious concerns about the validity of the doctrine of nonspecificity (Mason, 1971).

In response to Mason's two-part critique, Selye, not surprisingly, mounted a spirited defense of his positions by responding to each of Mason's major concerns. He explained his initial reluctance to use the term *stress* and why he ultimately employed this term and encouraged its usage in all languages that lacked an appropriate descriptor. He paid homage to Walter B. Cannon and also asserted that his collection of more than 100,000 publications was predominantly supportive of his description of the GAS and the nonspecific nature of the response to stressful stimulation. He addressed the confusion created by the use of the terms *stress* and *stressor* over the years. He also invoked the importance of "conditioning factors" such as genotype, age, sex, prior exposure to stress, and so on, to explain why animals exposed to the same stressors might develop different patterns of pathology. Selye also pointed out that exposure to stress resulted in nonspecific effects as well as specific effects. This latter assertion continues to create confusion among researchers and did not adequately address several of Mason's specific concerns. Selye concluded with a strong statement of support for continued use of the term *stress* in the experimental and medical literature (Selye, 1975). In the end, it appeared to me that Mason's arguments carried the day and have guided researchers for more than 40 years.

A long list of concerns. Other investigators, including Ader (1980), Elliott and Eisdorfer (1982), and Engel (1985), pointed out the lack of crisply defined concepts related to stress, such that no definition has yet been advanced that is embraced by a majority of researchers (Le Moal, 2007; Levine, 2005; Levine & Ursin, 1991). Munck et al. (1984) also found Selye's concept of diseases of adaptation lacking in several respects, noting that this conception was largely dismissed beginning in the 1960s. In addition, they pointed out the extremely artificial (i.e., non-physiological) experimental conditions employed by Selye to demonstrate pathological changes in laboratory animals. Finally, they indicated that Selye's central thesis that hyperactivity of the adrenal cortex during prolonged stress would exacerbate the symptoms of rheumatoid arthritis, a particular disease of adaptation, was completely rejected with the discovery of the anti-inflammatory properties of cortisol.

As an alternative to the work of Selye and in recognition of newer experimental findings, Munck et al. (1984) argued that stress-induced increases in circulating glucocorticoids actually protect against the body's normal responses to stress. In this way, glucocorticoids acted as a buffer against further tissue damage and an even greater disruption of homeostatic balance. More recently, Frank et al. (2013) have introduced the notion that glucocorticoids, in addition to their anti-inflammatory actions, may also sensitize microglia in brain to produce an enhanced pro-inflammatory response to later infection or injury after an immediate danger has passed.

The circular reasoning undergirding the GAS has also been a continuing source of concern for many researchers. For example, the only way one could distinguish between distress and eustress was to assess tissue damage and morbidity. If tissue damage occurred, it was a distress response, but if no damage occurred, then it was a eustress response (Goldstein, 2006). Mason (1971, 1975a, 1975b) argued that all of the stressors originally employed by Selye caused fear and anxiety in the laboratory rats that were studied, and it was not surprising that the pattern of GAS responses was similar across treatment groups. Indeed, Selye did not incorporate central nervous system responses to emotional stimuli in his studies, and yet, emotions are especially salient in studies of human stress and disease. Finally, Selye's singular focus for the GAS was the hypothalamic-pituitary-adrenocortical system, to the general exclusion of all other stress-responsive neural and endocrine systems (Chrousos, 2009; Le Moal, 2007; McEwen, 2002a, 2000b, 2007; Natelson, 1983).

Clarifications are needed. Based upon the results of a workshop organized by Drs. Jaap Koolhaas and Eberhard Fuchs and held in Göttingen, Germany, in

2009, more restricted definitions of the terms *stress* and *stressor* were advanced to avoid confusion in those instances where activation of neural and endocrine systems is required to support the metabolic demands of ongoing behaviors. Further, these investigators argued that controllability and predictability must be factored into any experimental design relating to the physiological and behavioral responses of animals or humans to stressful stimulation. They suggested that the use of the term *stress* should be restricted to instances where the specific environmental demands imposed exceed an organism's ability to adapt. Simply documenting that a neuroendocrine response had occurred did not justify labeling the provocation as stressful. Finally, the authors concluded that employing ecologically relevant stressors would enhance the validity of experimental findings in the field of stress research (Koolhaas et al., 2011, 2017). Ecological validity of stressors will be discussed later, in Chapter 6, as part of an evaluation of animal models of mental disorders.

A laboratory test of the doctrine of nonspecificity. A critical aspect of Selye's definition of stress was its nonspecific nature. Selye conceded that other neural and endocrine changes could occur during exposure to various stressors; however, he argued there would always remain a nonspecific component of stress after deletion of the stressor-specific elements from the total stress response.

Pacak et al. (1998) subjected the "doctrine of nonspecificity" to an exhaustive test by comparing neuroendocrine response profiles of laboratory rats across a range of different stressors and stressor intensities. In their initial paper, the authors (Pacak et al., 1998) argued that Selye's theory of nonspecific responses was impossible to disprove without two simplifying assumptions. The first simplification was that, regardless of the stressor, the ratio of the intensity-related increment in response for neurohormone X to the intensity-related increment in response for neurohormone Y is a constant. The second assumption was that the magnitudes of both the specific and nonspecific components of the various neurohormones vary directly across the whole range of stressor intensities (Pacak et al., 1998).

The stressors employed in their experiments included the following: handling and subcutaneous (s.c.) or intravenous (i.v.) injection of 0.9% saline; i.v. administration of insulin in doses of 0.3, 1.0, or 3.0 IU/kg body weight; 1.0% or 4.0% formaldehyde solution injected s.c. in the right hind leg; removal of arterial blood from an indwelling catheter equal to 10% or 25% of total estimated blood volume; cold exposure for 3 hours at 4°C or −3°C; or immobilization for 2 hours. Blood samples were collected before and at timed intervals during and after exposure of rats to one of the stressors. Plasma levels of NE, EPI, and adrenocorticotropin (ACTH) were quantified, and each measure was expressed as an integrated area under the curve (AUC) measure for each animal to reflect the amplitude of the response to a given stressor.

The data for ACTH and EPI responses to hemorrhage and to a formalin injection appeared to fulfill the two assumptions required to test the doctrine of nonspecificity. The findings indicated that the ratio of the EPI responses to the more severe versus the less severe hemorrhage were smaller than the ratio of the EPI responses to the more severe versus the less severe formalin injection. In contrast, the ratio of the plasma ACTH responses for the more severe versus the less severe hemorrhage were much greater than the ratio of the plasma ACTH responses to the more severe versus the less severe formalin injection (Figure 3.5). Thus, the results of this study clearly refuted Selye's doctrine of nonspecificity if one accepts the two qualifying assumptions.

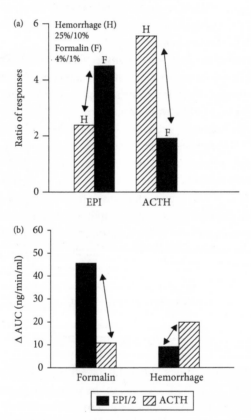

Figure 3.5. Tests of Selye's Doctrine of Nonspecificity. A: ratios (greater stress/less stress) of responses of plasma levels of EPI and ACTH for hemorrhage (H) and formalin (F). B: Increments in area under curve (ΔAUC) for plasma EPI and ACTH for formalin and hemorrhage. The Doctrine of Nonspecificity predicts that the arrows should be parallel to each other and of the same length.
Adapted from Pacak et al. (1998) with modifications.

Pacak and Palkovits (2001) expanded upon these initial findings by collecting data on related neural and endocrine responses to the five stressors described in the preceding. The additional measures included: plasma corticosterone, NE release in the paraventricular nucleus of the hypothalamus as measured by microdialysis, and activation of the immediate early gene, *c-fos*, by quantifying Fos immunoreactivity in 34 discrete brain areas. In combining the results of these two exhaustive studies, there was strong support for the existence of distinct stressor-specific neural and endocrine signatures. This series of experiments represents one of the few direct attempts to test Selye's doctrine, and clearly the doctrine of nonspecificity came up short.

Allostasis and Allostatic Load

A new view of stress. Given the many concerns about the conceptual framework of stress or lack thereof as promulgated by Selye, a new formulation was proposed by McEwen and Stellar (1993), who built upon the earlier work of Sterling and Eyer (1981, 1988). Animals and humans, from the lowest ranking to the most exalted, experience episodes of stress throughout their lives. In humans, these stressful episodes may occur during a daily regimen of exercise, a bout of illness, an interview for a job, or while driving a car on a busy highway. In these four examples of daily stressors and many others, the affected individual responds to each challenge based upon his or her genotype, developmental experiences, prior knowledge of the stressor, and real-time perception of the stressor. During these daily challenges, individuals must activate neural and endocrine systems to a sufficient degree to maintain homeostatic balance, sustain them during exposure to the particular challenge, and then promptly terminate the physiological responses when the challenge has been eliminated.

Unfortunately, this ideal pattern of onset, maintenance, and offset may be altered in such a way that a given neuroendocrine system remains up-regulated for an extended period of time after exposure to a stressor, or the level and frequency of stressful stimulation is much higher than expected. In these instances, the very bodily systems that aid in maintaining homeostatic balance may actually lead over time to damage of target tissues (McEwen, 1998, 2012). For example, activation of the sympathetic-adrenal medullary system is highly adaptive when an animal is exposed to an acute, socially threatening situation (i.e., fight-or-flight response). If these threats to one's rank or station in life occur frequently and over long periods of time, then the sympathetic-adrenal medullary system may actually promote an elevation in resting blood pressure and pathophysiological changes to cardiac and vascular tissues, leading to the development of atherosclerosis or hypertension.

Allostasis. Sterling and Eyer (1981, 1988) introduced the term *allostasis* (literally, stability through change) to capture the highly variable nature of stress-responsive bodily systems as they adjust their patterns of activity over the course of a day to maintain homeostatic balance. Rather than a strict constancy of the internal environment, Sterling and Eyers argued that homeostatic systems frequently adjust within defined ranges of activity to maintain some semblance of homeostatic balance. They also linked disregulation of these homeostatic systems to the development of pathology. Interestingly, allostasis builds a conceptual bridge between Cannon's work on homeostasis and Selye's work on diseases of adaptation.

Allostatic load. McEwen and Stellar (1993) extended the concept of allostasis by introducing the term *allostatic load* to reflect the damage to an organism that is exposed to frequent episodes of stressful stimulation over an extended period of time. One critical element of allostatic load is an inability of an organism to habituate to chronic intermittent stress, with an associated down-regulation of stress-responsive systems.

McEwen and Wingfield (2003) have placed the concepts of allostasis and allostatic load into an ecological and evolutionary framework. In doing so, they proposed two types of allostatic overload. Type 1 allostatic overload accompanies periods when energy demands exceed energy supplies and there is a direct threat to the survival of an organism. The organism enters into survival mode, such that allostatic load decreases and positive energy balance is re-established. In contrast, Type 2 allostatic overload may occur in a time of positive energy balance, but ongoing social conflict and other forms of social disruption may result in a constant pressure on allostasis. Escape from Type 2 allostatic overload is not possible; rather, affected individuals must learn to alter their patterns of behavior so as to adjust to the prevailing social system. If alterations in behavior do not occur, allostatic overload may lead to elevations in homeostatic mediators and accompanying physiological changes, which may lead eventually to pathological changes and/or death.

Effector systems. Another perspective has been advanced by Goldstein and Kopin (2007), who argued for a systems-level approach to the study of stress and allostatic processes. Following exposure to a stressor, highly specific patterns of effector responses are activated to close negative feedback loops. Effector systems include the hypothalamic-pituitary-adrenocortical axis, the sympathetic nervous system, the adrenal medulla, the renin-angiotensin-aldosterone system, the immune system, and others. They suggested that one must simultaneously track multiple effector systems to understand fully their interactions in the coordinated response of an organism to stressful stimulation.

Summary

Humans have thought about how to live a life of balance and harmony for at least the past three millennia. A major challenge to a healthy and balanced life involves exposure to stressors throughout the life span. An early conceptual breakthrough in this emerging field of science came in the mid-19th century with research of the renowned French physiologist Claude Bernard. Bernard introduced the concept of the fixity of *le milieu intérieur*. Later, the American physiologist Walter B. Cannon built upon Bernard's work and introduced the concept of homeostasis. But it was Hans Selye who introduced the concept of stress and advocated for its importance in the etiology of many chronic diseases. Although Selye's concepts and definitions left something to be desired, the term *stress* has endured for more than three-quarters of a century, and much of the credit for the staying power of stress in the biological and medical sciences is due to Selye's tireless efforts over the course of his career.

A major focus of this volume is on the role played by stressful life experiences in the onset and course of mental disorders. As we will see, many investigators have emphasized a dynamic interaction between an individual with a susceptible genotype and stressful experiences over the course of the life span in shaping the phenotype associated with a given mental disorder. A recent trend in research with animal models has been the use of stressors that are ecologically valid to the test animal. That is, the stressor is one that has relevance to laboratory animals under study and that activates homeostatic systems that have evolved to enhance the survival of animals exposed to similar stressors. The interconnected legacies of Bernard, Cannon, and Selye will serve as a thread that connects much that follows in this exciting body of research.

4

Stress Effector Systems

Brain circuits are essential in coordinating the physiological and behavioral responses of animals and humans exposed to stressful stimulation (McEwen, 2007). Stressful experiences, ranging from minor disturbances to life-threatening emergencies, are detected and processed by specialized brain areas and compared to prior experiences with the same or related stressors. The range of homeostatic physiological adjustments that must be made following exposure to various stressors requires neural, hormonal, and immune effector systems that are ultimately directed by stress-sensitive brain circuitry. This chapter will introduce the three primary stress-responsive effector systems that are essential in responses to internal as well as environmental perturbations. They include the sympathetic-adrenal medullary system, the hypothalamic-pituitary-adrenocortical (HPA) axis, and elements of the innate immune system. Chapter 5 will concentrate on brain circuits that are responsive to stressful stimuli, some of which are involved in regulating the three stress effector systems. These two chapters will introduce the key components of stress-responsive neural, endocrine, and immune systems that are thought to play critical roles in the pathophysiology of mental disorders.

The dynamic interplay between the brain and the periphery is reflected in the fact that some of the key signaling molecules and their associated receptors are found in peripheral tissues as well as in brain neurons and glial cells. In addition, feedback loops exist between brain and periphery such that some peripherally released lipophilic hormones cross the blood-brain barrier and access receptors in brain areas. Other signaling molecules that are water soluble or are too large to cross the blood-brain barrier may utilize afferent neural pathways into the brainstem to provide feedback on their levels of activity. For purposes of organization, this chapter will focus almost exclusively on the peripheral effector systems. In the next chapter and those that follow, some of these same signaling molecules will be discussed in relation to their central mechanisms of action.

The Sympathetic-Adrenal Medullary System

Prior to delving into the structural components of the sympathetic-adrenal medullary (SAM) system, I will provide an overview of catecholamine (CA) biosynthesis, describe the process of CA inactivation, and present the types of CA receptors.

Catecholamine Biosynthesis

A brief overview of CA biosynthesis is included in Figure 4.1. The precursor for CA biosynthesis is the amino acid tyrosine, which is derived from the diet or from hydroxylation of the amino acid phenylalanine in the liver. Tyrosine is taken up into catecholaminergic nerve terminals in the brain and periphery as well as chromaffin cells of the adrenal medulla and is converted into dihydroxyphenylalanine (DOPA) by the actions of the soluble cytoplasmic enzyme, tyrosine hydroxylase (TH). The conversion of tyrosine to DOPA is the rate-limiting enzyme in CA biosynthesis, and TH activity is in turn regulated

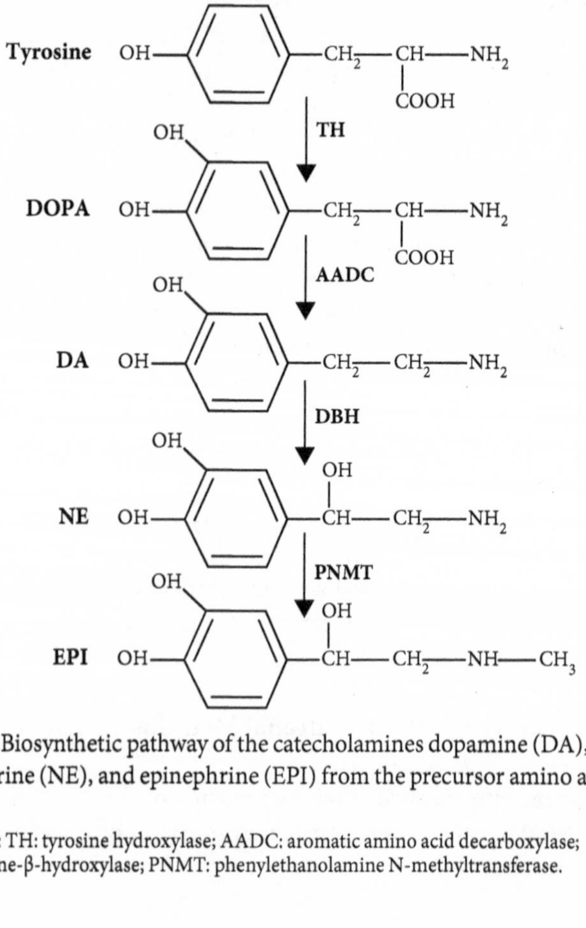

Figure 4.1. Biosynthetic pathway of the catecholamines dopamine (DA), norepinephrine (NE), and epinephrine (EPI) from the precursor amino acid, tyrosine.

Abbreviations: TH: tyrosine hydroxylase; AADC: aromatic amino acid decarboxylase; DBH: dopamine-β-hydroxylase; PNMT: phenylethanolamine N-methyltransferase.

by several processes, including feedback inhibition by CAs. DOPA is converted into dopamine (DA) by aromatic amino acid decarboxylase in the cytoplasm, and then DA is taken up into storage vesicles and converted into norepinephrine (NE) by the enzyme dopamine-β-hydroxylase (DBH). The uptake of DA into storage vesicles is carried out by vesicular monoamine transporters (VMAT-1 and -2), with VMAT-1 being the neuroendocrine form and VMAT-2 being localized to neurons. NE functions as a neurotransmitter in its own right, or it may be converted into epinephrine (EPI) by the enzyme, phenylethanolamine-N-methyltransferase (PNMT), which employs S-adenosyl-methionine as a co-factor. PNMT catalyzes the formation of EPI in chromaffin cells of the adrenal medulla; however, it is also present in some brain neurons as well as extra-adrenal chromaffin tissues in the periphery (Kvetnansky et al., 2009).

Catecholaminergic Receptors

This section will discuss two types of CA receptors, adrenergic receptors (ARs) and dopamine (DA) receptors. Both types of receptors are subsumed under the G protein-coupled family of cell surface receptors and mediate the effects of NE, EPI, and DA on target cells in the periphery as well as the brain.

   Adrenergic receptors. ARs include nine distinct gene products: three α_1 receptor subtypes (α_{1a}, α_{1b}, α_{1d}), three α_2 receptor subtypes (α_{2a}, α_{2b}, α_{2c}), and three β receptor subtypes (β_1, β_2, β_3). G protein-coupled receptors have seven transmembrane domains, with an extracellular N-terminus and an intracellular C-terminus (Table 4.1). These receptors are coupled to G proteins, which are heterotrimers consisting of α, β, and γ subunits. G proteins vary based upon their α-subunits, which include G_s (stimulatory G protein for adenylyl cyclase), G_i and G_o (inhibitory G proteins of adenylyl cyclase), and G_q and G_{11} (G proteins that couple α-ARs to phospholipase C). Activation of G protein-coupled receptors by NE or EPI results in the dissociation of guanine dinucleotide (GDP) from the α-subunit of the AR, allowing binding of GTP to the G protein. Intracellular effects of AR-activated α-subunits include adenylyl cyclase, phospholipase C, and ion channels. The α-subunits are inactivated by hydrolysis of bound GTP to yield GDP and phosphate, followed by reassociation of the α-subunit with the β-γ subunit (Biaggioni & Robertson, 2018; Cotecchia, 2010; Wachter & Gilbert, 2012).

   The number of ARs and their level of responsiveness are not static features; rather, they may vary over a significant range on target cells. A prominent characteristic of ARs is that even when levels of NE and EPI remain elevated for prolonged periods, such as during exposure to a stressful stimulus, there is a diminution of the target cell response that occurs as quickly as a few minutes after the onset of stimulation. The rapid decrease in responsiveness of ARs to

Table 4.1 Classes of Catecholamine Receptors (α-Adrenergic, β-Adrenergic, and Dopaminergic), and Their Associated G Proteins, Second Messenger Responses, and Selected Peripheral Tissues with Physiological Responses

Receptor Type	G Protein	Second Messenger Response	Tissue	Response
Adrenergic				
α_1	G_q	↑↑↑ IP3, ↑↑↑ DAG	Blood vessels of skin, kidney, GI system	Vasoconstriction
α_2	G_i	↓↓↓ cAMP	Presynaptic nerve terminals	↑↑↑ NE release
β_1	G_s	↑↑↑ cAMP	Heart	↑↑↑ HR and stroke volume
			Kidney	↑↑↑ Renin release
			Stomach	↑↑↑ Ghrelin release
β_2	G_s	↑↑↑ cAMP	GI tract	↓↓↓ Motility
			Adipocytes	↑↑↑ Lipolysis
			Skeletal muscle	Vasodilation
β_3	G_s	↑↑↑ cAMP	Adipocytes	↑↑↑ Lipolysis
Dopaminergic				
D1-class	G_s	↑↑↑ cAMP	Renal tubules	↑↑↑ Natriuresis
D2-class	G_i	↓↓↓ cAMP	Zona glomerulosa	↓↓↓ Aldosterone secretion

Abbreviations: IP3: inositol triphosphate; DAG: diaceylglycerol; cAMP: cyclic adenosyl monophosphate; HR: heart rate; GI: gastrointestinal. Refer to the text for additional details.

stimulation by sustained elevations in NE, EPI, or various sympathomimetic drugs has been termed *desensitization* (Hausdorff et al., 1990; Strittmatter et al., 1977), and is mediated by several pathways, including phosphorylation of ARs by one of seven G protein-coupled receptor kinases (GRKs). Phosphorylation of ARs enhances their affinity for β-arrestins, which can lead to internalization of ARs. One should keep in mind that β-arrestins can also stimulate G protein-independent intracellular signaling pathways (Rajagopal et al., 2010). β_3-ARs tend to be more resistant to desensitization than other subtypes of ARs.

Short-term desensitization has been viewed as two separate processes. Homologous desensitization involves loss of responsiveness exclusively of the receptors that have been exposed to sustained activation by an agonist. In contrast, heterologous desensitization occurs when desensitization of one receptor by its agonist also leads to desensitization of another type of receptor that does not bind that agonist. Long-term desensitization appears to involve decreases in the number of receptors through sequestration as well as reductions in replacement of receptors (Hausdorff et al., 1990).

Dopaminergic receptors. DA receptors are found in the periphery as well as the central nervous system. There are two classes of DA receptors, encompassing five subtypes. The D1-class of receptors includes D1 and D5 receptors, while the D2-class includes the D2, D3, and D4 subtypes (Table 4.1). DA receptors are also subject to desensitization when there are sustained elevations in DA levels in the vicinity of target cells.

With respect to their role in peripheral stress responses, DA receptors are found in the smooth muscle cells lining blood vessels, nephrons of the kidney, and cells of the zona glomerulosa of the adrenal cortex. In addition, presynaptic DA2 autoreceptors can inhibit release of DA from nerve terminals. DA receptors will be discussed in greater detail later in this volume regarding their involvement in the etiology of several mental disorders (Beaulieu & Gainetdinov, 2011).

Inactivation of Catecholamines

Following release from a nerve terminal, CAs are rapidly inactivated by a variety of degradative processes. Principal among them is reuptake of the CA into the presynaptic nerve terminal (Uptake 1), an energy-dependent process mediated by the NE transporter protein (NET) or the DA transporter protein (DAT). Approximately 90% of locally released NE and DA are taken back up into their presynaptic terminals, where they may be repackaged into storage vesicles and subsequently released following depolarization of the neuronal membrane. NET and DAT display selectivity in which CAs they will transport back into the presynaptic terminal, with the former being much more selective for NE versus EPI, and the latter being much more selective for DA than NE or EPI.

CAs are also subject to enzymatic inactivation by monoamine oxidase (MAO) in the cytoplasm of nerve terminals and by catechol-O-methyltransferase (COMT) in non-neuronal effector cells in the periphery. Non-neuronal cells take up CAs by Uptake 2, an energy-dependent process with lower specificity and affinity for CAs than Uptake 1 but with a higher maximum rate of uptake. Uptake 2 also favors EPI over NE. Uptake 2 sites in the periphery include the kidney, liver, and lungs, and they are inhibited by high levels of corticosterone (CORT) (Kvetnansky et al., 2009).

Sympathetic Nerves

The cell bodies of preganglionic sympathetic nerves are located in the intermediolateral columns of the thoracic and lumbar segments of the spinal cord. They receive direct input from medullary, pontine, and hypothalamic nuclei, as will be discussed in Chapter 5. The axons of some preganglionic sympathetic nerves exit the spinal cord ipsilaterally to make synaptic contact with postganglionic sympathetic cell bodies in the paravertebral chain. The paravertebral ganglia are interconnected to form a chain on either side of the spinal cord, usually with one pair of ganglia per segment. Exceptions to this general rule are the superior cervical ganglia at the rostral end of the sympathetic chain and the stellate ganglia at the rostral end of the thoracic segments. The superior cervical ganglia innervate many blood vessels and tissues of the head (e.g., salivary and mucosal glands, pineal gland, blood vessels), while the stellate ganglia project to tissues and organs in the thoracic cavity and the neck and arms. Other preganglionic nerves bypass the sympathetic chain and project within the splanchnic nerves to the prevertebral ganglia that innervate the abdominal and pelvic viscera, including the adrenal medulla.

Preganglionic sympathetic neurons generate action potentials in postganglionic sympathetic nerves by releasing acetylcholine onto nicotinic receptors located on the dendrites. A postganglionic neuron tends to relay the stimulatory inputs from one to several preganglionic neurons, and they often arise from the same spinal segment. A postganglionic axon forms multiple neuroeffector junctions with its target cells (Jänig & McLachlan, 2013).

Adrenal Medulla

Chromaffin cell complexity. In many respects, the adrenal medulla resembles a sympathetic ganglion that contains postganglionic cell bodies lacking axons. The secretory cells of the adrenal medulla are referred to as chromaffin cells. They secrete NE or EPI into the circulation in response to release of acetylcholine from sympathetic preganglionic fibers of the splanchnic nerve, followed by stimulation of nicotinic acetylcholine receptors. Secretory cells within the adrenal medulla include EPI-containing and NE-containing cells, with the former differing from the latter by the presence of PNMT. Chromaffin granules contain water, various proteins, adenosine triphosphate (ATP), lipids, and either NE or EPI. The most prominent protein is chromogranin A, which is formed from the Golgi apparatus and enclosed with the other constituents by a single vesicular membrane. The release of CAs, together with other compounds from adrenal chromaffin cells, occurs via exocytosis. For more than half a century, studies of chromaffin cells maintained in culture have added greatly to methodological developments in neurobiology and have enriched our understanding of mechanisms underlying stimulus-secretion coupling (Borges et al., 2018).

Chromogranin A is not simply a victim of exocytotic release from the chromaffin cell after serving its purpose of facilitating the storage of CAs. Instead, chromogranin A functions as a prohormone, giving rise to several important polypeptides, including pancreastatin, vasostatin I and II, catestatin, and serpinin. These peptides play important roles in regulating glucose and calcium homeostasis, endothelial permeability, angiogenesis, immune responses to pathogens, and myocardial contractility (Helle et al., 2018).

Until relatively recently, secretory activity of the adrenal medulla was viewed as a relatively straightforward process, reflecting Cannon's original concept of the fight-or-flight response. Stressful stimuli or internal disruptions to homeostasis (e.g., decrease in blood glucose) → increased central stimulation of sympathetic preganglionic cell bodies → increased firing of sympathetic preganglionic fibers in the splanchnic nerves → release of acetylcholine onto ionotropic nicotinic receptors on adrenal medullary chromaffin cells → depolarization of chromaffin cells and release of NE and EPI. More recent studies have revealed a much more complex and highly regulated process for release of CAs and other signaling molecules from the adrenal medulla. For example, chromaffin cells express metabotropic muscarinic receptors as well as nicotinic receptors for acetylcholine, and both play a role in CA release. Second, exocytotic release of CAs is accompanied by the simultaneous release of DBH, ATP, chromogranin A, and a host of signaling peptides, including NPY, galanin, adrenomedullin, vasoactive intestinal peptide (VIP), beta-endorphin, the enkephalins, and others. Third, chromaffin cells express the serotonin transporter molecule and 5-HT_{1A} receptors, even though they lack the ability to synthesize serotonin. The serotonin transporter and 5-HT_{1A} signaling have been shown to dampen the EPI response to acute stressors (Brindley et al., 2016). Finally, splanchnic preganglionic nerve terminals also release a peptide during periods of sustained stimulation that appears to play a critical role in the regulation of chromaffin cell secretory activity.

A new stimulus for chromaffin cells. Pituitary adenylate cyclase-activating polypeptide (PACAP) is composed of 38 amino acids and was originally isolated from ovine hypothalamus by Miyata et al. (1989) based upon its ability to stimulate adenylate cyclase in anterior pituitary cell cultures. Although it shared considerable homology with VIP, PACAP was 1,000 times more potent than VIP in stimulating adenylate cyclase. In spite of its name (which is unfortunately limiting), PACAP is found in many other brain areas as well as in peripheral tissues. Of particular note, PACAP is co-localized with acetylcholine in preganglionic nerve terminals that innervate adrenal medullary chromaffin cells.

In two reviews regarding control of CA release from adrenal chromaffin cells, Eiden and his coworkers (Eiden & Jiang, 2018; Smith & Eiden, 2012) have made a compelling case for dual neurotransmission to allow for differential control of CA secretion during basal levels of activity versus periods of sustained high levels of splanchnic stimulation. Acetylcholine release from small synaptic vesicles in preganglionic terminals appears to regulate basal levels of CA secretion from the adrenal medulla. However, during periods of sustained high-intensity stimulation of the adrenal medulla by presynaptic inputs, there is a rapid desensitization of chromaffin cell responsiveness to the effects of acetylcholine on a timescale of seconds to minutes in spite of continued depolarizations of the sympathetic preganglionic terminals. With sustained stimulation, large dense core vesicles containing PACAP are recruited in addition to the acetylcholine-containing small synaptic vesicles. PACAP acts on PAC1 receptors (a G protein-coupled receptor) located on the outer membrane of chromaffin cells to stimulate sustained release of EPI and NE, as well as enhanced levels of biosynthetic enzyme capacity, to ensure replenishment of CA stores that have been released.

PACAP signaling also regulates the expression of an impressive group of additional signaling molecules, including peptide hormones, neuropeptides, growth factors, cytokines, and enzymes responsible for hormone processing or the activation of extracellular enzymatic or hormonal cascades. Many of these signaling molecules appeared to be released from chromaffin cells into blood during exposure to intensely stressful stimuli, providing an additional role for PACAP in the integration of various peripheral stress-responsive biological systems (Ait-Ali et al., 2010).

Plasma Catecholamines and Sympathetic-Adrenal Medullary Activity

Blood sampling and measurement. The pioneering experiments of Cannon (1914a, 1914b, 1915) and Cannon and de la Paz (1911) on EPI secretion from the adrenal medulla depended upon bioassays for the quantification of circulating EPI. It was not until the mid-1970s that analytical methods were developed that made possible the routine measurement of picogram quantities of NE and EPI in plasma samples of unrestrained laboratory rats (Peuler & Johnson, 1977). In the 1990s, newer analytical methods permitted measurement of plasma CAs and their metabolites by high-performance liquid chromatography (HPLC) with electrochemical detection (Holmes et al., 1994).

Because of the remarkable sensitivity of the sympathetic-adrenal medullary system of laboratory rats to handling, restraint, and venipuncture necessary for the collection of blood samples, methods were developed for the placement of indwelling catheters in arteries or veins of laboratory rats (Chiueh & Kopin, 1978; Paulose & Dakshinamurti, 1987; Popper et al., 1977; Steffens, 1969). Indwelling, chronic catheters provided researchers with the advantage of obtaining multiple blood samples from freely behaving animals in the absence of handling or other disturbances. Remote sampling of blood via an indwelling arterial or venous catheter is an absolute requirement for obtaining accurate baseline measures of circulating NE and EPI in freely behaving laboratory rats and tracking responses to stressful stimulation (Chiueh & Kopin, 1978; Kvetnansky et al., 1978).

Studies with laboratory mice present an even greater challenge given their smaller size compared to laboratory rats. However, Grouzmann et al. (2003) reported that blood samples (0.25 ml) obtained from chronic carotid artery catheters resulted in basal plasma levels of NE and EPI that were comparable to basal levels reported in laboratory rats. Following exposure of mice to acute cold water immersion stress, levels of both CAs were elevated significantly above basal levels.

Circulating NE is derived from two principal sources. The primary neurotransmitter of postganglionic sympathetic nerves is NE. Sympathetic nerves innervate most of the tissues of the body (e.g., heart, blood vessels, spleen, intestines, etc.), where NE is released from sympathetic nerve endings and binds to adrenergic receptors on target cells. Some of the locally released NE (5%–20% depending on the morphology of the neuroeffector junction) leaks away unmetabolized and enters the circulation. NE is also released from the adrenal medulla directly into the circulation upon stimulation of adrenal medullary chromaffin cells by sympathetic preganglionic nerves that release acetylcholine (Goldstein et al., 1983). Figure 4.2 provides an overview of the organization of the sympathetic-adrenal medullary system.

Yamaguchi and Kopin (1979) employed the pithed rat preparation to study the release of peripheral CAs when the spinal cord was stimulated electrically. During sustained electrical stimulation of the spinal cord, plasma levels of NE peaked later than levels of EPI (approximately a 3-minute delay) given that EPI is released directly into the circulation from the adrenal medulla, whereas NE that is released from sympathetic nerve terminals must diffuse away from the neuroeffector junction before it enters the circulation. These investigators also reported that 25%–40% of the circulating NE during direct stimulation of sympathetic outflow was derived from the adrenal medulla. Kvetnansky et al. (1979) found that approximately 30% of the NE in blood was derived from the adrenal medulla during the early stages of immobilization stress. After one hour of immobilization stress, there was a change-over, such that nearly 100% of the circulating NE was derived from sympathetic nerves.

Finally, McCarty and Kopin (1979) reported that the intensity of stressful stimulation affected the release of NE from the adrenal medulla. Under basal conditions, the adrenal medulla contributed a negligible amount of NE in the

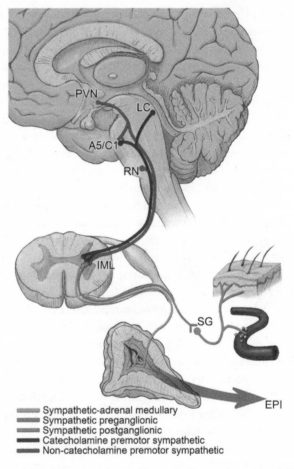

Sympathetic-adrenal medullary
Sympathetic preganglionic
Sympathetic postganglionic
Catecholamine premotor sympathetic
Non-catecholamine premotor sympathetic

Figure 4.2. Neural pathways regulating the sympathetic-adrenal medullary system response to stress. Depicted in this illustration are sympathetic postganglionic projections to skin and a section of a blood vessel, where norepinephrine is released from nerve terminals (blue dots), and sympathetic preganglionic projections to the adrenal medulla, where epinephrine (EPI) is released into the circulation from chromaffin cells (see also Plate 2).

Abbreviations: PVN: paraventricular nucleus of the hypothalamus; LC: locus coeruleus; A5/C1: A5 noradrenergic and C1 adrenergic neuronal cell groups; RN: raphe nuclei; IML: intermediolateral column of the spinal cord; SG: sympathetic ganglion; EPI: epinephrine.

Adapted from McCarty (2016) and used with permission.

circulation; under mildly stressful conditions (handling and transfer to a strange environment), the percentage of NE from the adrenal medulla increased to 30%; and following an intense stressor (5 minutes of intermittent footshock), the percentage of NE from the adrenal medulla was 45%.

Using in vivo microdialysis of the adrenal medulla of laboratory rats, Kuzmin et al. (1995) studied the effects on CA secretion of acute immobilization stress for 60 minutes. Adrenal medullary dialysate was collected before, during, and after immobilization and later analyzed for content of NE and EPI. Their results indicated that under basal conditions, EPI/NE in dialysate was 3.7 ± 0.4 pmol/ml, which was similar to the ratio of the two CAs in adrenal medullary tissue. There were dramatic increases in levels of both CAs after 15 minutes of immobilization, but the ratio of EPI/NE remained approximately 4.0. In contrast, 2-deoxy-D-glucose (2-DG, 500 mg/kg, i.v.) elicited a relatively selective increase in dialysate levels of EPI, while levels of NE remained constant. EPI/NE peaked at approximately 10.0 one hour after injection of 2-DG (Kuzmin et al., 1995). In an earlier study that combined adrenal medullary microdialysis and measurement of circulating CAs, Kuzmin et al. (1990) reported that plasma NE from the adrenal medulla of laboratory rats increased from 9% under basal conditions to 50% during hemorrhage.

Circulating EPI. In contrast to the complex origin of circulating NE, the origin of circulating EPI is much more direct. In laboratory rats, most if not all of the circulating EPI is derived from the adrenal medulla under basal conditions and during and following stressful stimulation (Kvetnansky et al., 1979; McCarty & Kopin, 1979; Yamaguchi & Kopin, 1979). Extra-adrenal sources of the EPI-synthesizing enzyme, PNMT, and measurable tissue levels of EPI have been reported by several laboratories, but these peripheral tissues do not appear to contribute in a significant manner to circulating EPI levels in laboratory rats. For example, EPI has been quantified in cardiac tissue (Caramona & Soares da Silva, 1985) and PNMT mRNA levels have been detected in several tissues, including skin (Pullar et al., 2006), spleen (Andreassi et al., 1998; Warthan et al., 2002), thymus (Andreassi et al., 1998; Warthan et al., 2002), cardiac tissue (Goncalvesova et al., 2004; Krizanova et al., 2001; Kvetnansky et al, 2006), and sympathetic ganglia (Kubovcakova et al., 2006; Kvetnansky et al., 2006).

Clearance of CAs from blood. The rate of removal of CAs from blood is relatively rapid, with a half-life of just over one minute (Yamaguchi & Kopin, 1979; Goldstein et al., 1983). Plasma levels of NE and EPI have a significant capacity to increase above basal levels, and the increments in plasma levels of NE and EPI increase monotonically with increasing intensities of acutely stressful stimulation. In contrast, plasma levels of CORT do not have as great a dynamic range of response and do not track well with graded increases in intensity of acutely stressful stimulation (De Boer et al, 1990; Natelson et al., 1981, 1987). Finally, plasma levels of NE and EPI peak sooner and return toward baseline levels more rapidly than CORT following a brief period of stressful stimulation (De Boer et al., 1989). In addition, circulating CORT dampens the release of NE from sympathetic nerve endings during stressful stimulation, probably by acting at central sites that regulate sympathetic outflow (Kvetnansky et al., 1993).

One study has examined the genetic determinants of plasma levels of NE during various phases of an acute session of immobilization stress (Klimeš et al., 2005). These investigators identified two genomic regions on chromosome 10 in rats that contained quantitative trait loci (QTL) that influenced the sympathetic nervous system response to acute immobilization. Their findings indicated that temporal phases of the response to an acute stressor may have specific genetic determinants that can be identified and studied experimentally. Sampling of blood from arterial or venous catheters was also important for capturing the differing time courses of adrenocorticotrophic hormone (ACTH) and CORT responses during and after stressful stimulation (Kearns & Spencer, 2013).

Other Circulating Markers of Stress

Neuropeptide Y (NPY). NPY is a 36-amino acid peptide that is found in the central nervous system as well as in the periphery (Allen et al., 1983; Reichmann & Holzer, 2016; Zukowska-Grojec et al., 1988). It was named due to its enrichment of tyrosine (one-letter abbreviation: Y), including a tyrosine amide at the C-terminal residue and a tyrosine at the N-terminal residue (Tatemoto et al., 1982). The physiological effects of this peptide in mammals, which include regulation of food intake, energy balance, cardiovascular function, circadian rhythms, stress responsiveness, and anxiety, result from activation of four distinct G protein-coupled receptors (Y1, Y2, Y4, and Y5) (Reichmann & Holzer, 2016; Silva et al., 2002).

In the periphery, NPY is a potent vasoconstrictor, is co-localized with NE in sympathetic nerves innervating the heart and vasculature, and is present in the adrenal medulla and the myenteric plexus of the gut. NPY is co-localized with NE in large dense core granules of sympathetic nerve terminals, but it is not found in the more numerous and readily releasable pool of small dense core vesicles. In humans and in laboratory rodents, NPY is co-released with NE during sustained periods of stressful stimulation, such as occurs during prolonged exposure to stress, particularly cold exposure (Kuo & Zukowska, 2007). In addition, NPY is released into the circulation from the adrenal medulla and from platelets. Given its stimulation of smooth muscle proliferation and vascular hypertrophy, NPY may serve as a link between intensely stressful stimulation and subsequent vascular remodeling (Zukowska-Grojec, 1995).

In chronically catheterized laboratory rats, plasma NPY levels increased in an intensity-dependent manner during footshock stress and during graded hemorrhage, but not during immobilization stress. A modified cold pressor test, with rats standing in 1-cm deep cold water, was an especially potent stimulus for NPY release into plasma, especially if exposure was prolonged and if platelet aggregation was inhibited by intravenous administration of heparin (Kuo & Zukowska, 2007; Zukowska-Grojec, 1995; Zukowska-Grojec et al., 1988).

In summary, plasma levels of NPY reflect sympathetic-adrenal medullary activity during intense and prolonged exposure to stressful stimulation. In addition, increased levels of circulating CAs during exposure to intense stressors appear to increase the sensitivity of blood vessels to the effects of NPY. Testosterone appears to enhance and estrogens depress the release and biological effects of peripheral NPY. Taken together, the findings detailed in the preceding indicate that NPY signaling in the periphery is a critical component of the physiological response to stressors (Kuo & Zukowska, 2007).

Plasma ghrelin as a marker of chronic stress. Ghrelin, a 28-amino acid peptide that is aceylated at the serine-3 position, is well known for its effects on stimulation of growth hormone release and food intake and regulation of energy balance. It is produced in cells of the gastrointestinal tract as well as in discrete areas of the brain (Nojima et al., 1999). Approximately 75% of circulating ghrelin is derived from the stomach, with most of the remainder secreted from the proximal small intestine. Ghrelin exerts its biological effects by binding to growth hormone secretagogue receptors (GHSR1a), a G protein-coupled receptor that occurs in many peripheral tissues, including the anterior pituitary, as well as in discrete nuclei of the hypothalamus, hippocampus, and amygdala (Yin et al., 2014). This circulating peptide hormone is unusual in that it readily penetrates the blood-brain barrier. Ghrelin secretion is mediated in part by release of NE from sympathetic nerve terminals, but not by EPI release from the adrenal medulla (Mundinger et al., 2006).

Meyer et al. (2014) reported that plasma levels of acylated ghrelin (AG) were increased significantly in laboratory rats 24 hours after the last of 14 consecutive days of immobilization stress (4 hours per day) or swim stress (1 hour per day) relative to handled controls. In contrast, plasma levels of AG were not increased relative to handled controls in animals exposed to a single session of immobilization stress. In addition, adrenalectomy prior to chronic stress exposure actually enhanced the effects of chronic restraint stress on plasma levels of AG. These investigators concluded that plasma AG may represent a peripheral hormonal pathway that does not require an intact adrenal cortex and is activated following chronic intermittent stress exposure. A subsequent experiment revealed that plasma AG levels remained elevated for up to 130 days following the last of 14 daily immobilization stress exposures (Yousufzai et al., 2018).

These findings point to circulating levels of AG as a novel index of chronic stress exposure. AG is also unusual in that it can readily penetrate the blood-brain barrier, where it potentially serves as a signal to brain circuits regarding long-term stress effects in the periphery.

Summary

Processes relating to central and peripheral CA synthesis, release, and inactivation, as well as signaling through G protein-coupled receptors on effector cells, are tightly regulated through multiple feedback mechanisms. Studies of sympathetic-adrenal medullary responses to stress in conscious, freely behaving laboratory animals were hampered initially because of the extremely low basal levels of NE and EPI in blood and the extreme sensitivity of the sympathetic nerves and the adrenal medulla to mild handling and restraint associated with many blood collection procedures. Radioenzymatic assays and later HPLC analytical methods solved the former problem, while use of chronic arterial or venous catheters for remote blood sampling solved the latter problem. Plasma levels of NE reflect patterns of activation of sympathetic outflow, although some NE is also released from the adrenal medulla during stressful stimulation. Plasma levels of EPI provide an accurate index of adrenal medullary secretion. Both CAs are cleared rapidly from the circulation and respond monotonically to increasing intensities of stressors.

Because plasma CAs and related peptides have been measured in laboratory rats and in humans, the potential for translational and reverse translational studies of sympathetic-adrenal medullary responses to stress are quite favorable. Measures of plasma CAs may be especially valuable in rat models of mental disorders and in patients with mental disorders to track the involvement of acute stress responsiveness on behavioral phenotypes and treatment effectiveness. Repeated blood sampling in laboratory mice over a brief period of time, while highly desirable, is very challenging given the limited blood volume of mice.

Hypothalamic-Pituitary-Adrenocortical (HPA) Axis

Measures of HPA axis activity have figured prominently in studies of several mental disorders in humans, as well as in experiments with animal models of these disorders. In particular, HPA axis dysregulation appears to be an important feature of schizophrenia, major depressive disorder, and post-traumatic stress disorder. Measures of cortisol and ACTH have provided insights into distinguishing subgroups of patients that may share a common pathophysiology, as well as in tracking responses to therapy and the probability of recurrence of symptoms (Bradley & Dinan, 2010; Mehta & Binder, 2012; Pariante & Lightman, 2008; Walker et al., 2013).

As a prelude to considering the involvement of the HPA axis in various animal models of mental disorders, the following subsection will provide an overview of the organization, regulation, and peripheral and central biological effects of adrenal corticosteroids. This information will then be applied to animal models of mental disorders beginning in Chapter 8.

Overview of the Hypothalamic-Pituitary-Adrenocortical Axis

Components of the HPA axis. There are three principal components to the HPA axis:

1. *Hypothalamic paraventricular nucleus (PVN)*: The median parvocellular portion of the PVN of the hypothalamus contains the cell bodies of neurosecretory neurons that project to the median eminence and synthesize corticotropin-releasing factor (CRF) as well as arginine vasopressin (AVP). CRF is a 41-amino acid peptide, and its amino acid sequence is identical in mice, rats, and humans (Vale et al., 1981). AVP is a posterior pituitary hormone that causes vasoconstriction and regulates water resorption by kidney tubules. Note that the nomenclature for CRF and related peptides and their receptors (as opposed to corticotropin-releasing hormone [CRH]) throughout this book is consistent with published recommendations as approved by the International Union of Pharmacology (Hauger et al., 2003).

2. *Anterior pituitary gland*: CRF and AVP are co-secreted by PVN neurosecretory neurons and enter the pituitary portal circulation, where they are transported to the anterior pituitary and act synergistically to stimulate release of ACTH from storage vesicles in anterior pituitary corticotropes. Corticotropes comprise approximately 10% of anterior pituitary cells. CRF acts on CRF-1 receptors and AVP stimulates AVP V1b receptors. Experiments in conscious rats established that CRF stimulation of ACTH secretion was markedly potentiated by simultaneous i.v. administration of AVP (Rivier & Vale, 1983). ACTH is a 39-amino acid peptide that is one of several biologically active peptides that is cleaved post-translationally from the larger 260-amino acid proopiomelanocortin (POMC), a protein synthesized in corticotropes. Others include β-lipotropin, beta-endorphin, and various melanocyte stimulating hormones (Lowry, 2016).

3. *Adrenal cortex*: The adrenal cortex is composed of three distinct layers, and each specializes in producing one or several steroid hormones (Figure 4.3). The three layers include the outer zona glomerulosa, the middle zona fasciculata, and the inner zona reticularis.
   - The zona glomerulosa is composed of cells that synthesize and secrete aldosterone, a mineralocorticoid hormone whose principal actions are to regulate blood pressure and stimulate increased resorption of sodium

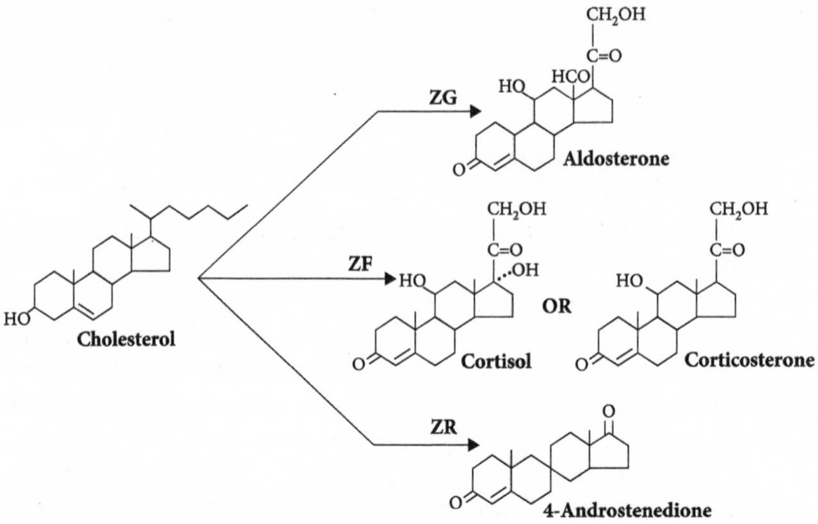

Figure 4.3. Biosynthesis of steroid hormones in the adrenal cortex from the precursor molecule, cholesterol. Aldosterone is the primary hormone synthesized in the outer zona glomerulosa (ZG); cortisol or corticosterone is synthesized in the middle layer, the zona fasciculata (ZF). Androgens, including 4-androstenedione, are synthesized in the inner zona reticularis (ZR).

and increased excretion of potassium from the distal convoluted tubules and collecting ducts of the kidneys.

- The middle zona fasciculata synthesizes and secretes glucocorticoids. These cells contain melanocortin (MC) 2 receptors that bind to ACTH from the circulation. A member of the melanocortin family of G protein-coupled receptors, MC-2 receptors require the presence of the MC-2 accessory protein to bind ACTH, which results in a G_s-mediated increase in intracellular levels of cyclic adenosyl monophosphate (cAMP) and activation of protein kinase A (PKA). Activation of PKA induces rapid synthesis of CORT via nongenomic mechanisms that involve post-transcriptional modification of steroidogenic proteins, including phosphorylation of hormone-sensitive lipase, a protein that increases intracellular cholesterol, the precursor of steroid hormones within the cell, and phosphorylation of steroidogenic acute regulatory protein (StAR) (Arakane et al., 1997), which facilitates the transport of cholesterol inside the mitochondria where a number of enzymatic reactions lead to glucocorticoid synthesis. Mobilization of cholesterol and its transfer from the outer to the inner mitochondrial membrane are considered the rate-limiting steps in steroidogenesis.
- The inner zona reticularis synthesizes and secretes a variety of androgenic steroids, including dehydroepiandrosterone and androstenedione.

Figure 4.4 presents an overview of the organization of the HPA axis.

Receptors for glucocorticoids. Two intracellular receptors for endogenous glucocorticoids have been isolated and characterized, including the mineralocorticoid receptor (MR) and the glucocorticoid receptor (GR). The former is the primary receptor for the mineralocorticoid, aldosterone, while the latter is the primary receptor for glucocorticoids. MRs and GRs in their unbound form are found primarily in the cytoplasm of cells in the periphery and the brain, where they form complexes with other proteins, including heat shock proteins. Receptor activation occurs when the MR or GR receptor binds its ligand, dissociates from the multi-protein complex, forms homodimers or heterodimers, and reveals its nuclear localization domain. The activated forms of MR and GR are translocated to the nucleus, where they bind to a palindromic

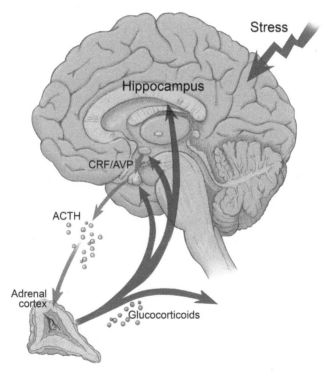

Figure 4.4. Influence of stress on the HPA axis, illustrating negative feedback effects of circulating glucocorticoids at the level of the anterior pituitary, the paraventricular nucleus of the hypothalamus (PVN), and higher brain centers (e.g., hippocampus) (see also Plate 3).

Abbreviations: CRF: corticotropin releasing factor; AVP: arginine vasopressin; ACTH: adrenocorticotropic hormone.

Adapted from McCarty (2016) and used with permission.

15 DNA base pair consensus sequence (glucocorticoid response element, GRE), often located in the vicinity of the promoter region of target genes that are activated or repressed (de Kloet et al., 2005). There is a significant time delay of at least an hour between translocation of MRs/GRs to the nucleus and the resulting genomic effects that occur in the target cells. These changes in the function of target cells can persist for several hours to multiple days (Spencer & Deak, 2017).

With few exceptions, GRs are found in cells throughout the body, whereas MRs are much more restricted in their distribution, with especially high concentrations in the collecting ducts of the kidney and the hippocampus. In brain, MRs have a 10-fold greater affinity for CORT than GRs (Reul & de Kloet, 1985), and this difference has important ramifications that will be discussed in detail in the next chapter.

Regulation of glucocorticoid synthesis and release. Synthesis and secretion of glucocorticoids is stimulated by ACTH binding to MC-2 receptors, which is followed by sequential, enzyme-mediated processing of cholesterol into cortisol or corticosterone (CORT serves as an abbreviation for either), as well as factors affecting growth of and blood flow to the adrenal cortex. CORT is highly lipid soluble; thus, it cannot be stored in vesicles but is synthesized as needed and diffuses passively into the blood draining from the adrenal cortex and through the adrenal medulla into the general circulation. There is a delay of approximately 3–5 minutes between elevations in ACTH in blood and synthesis of CORT, followed by entry of newly synthesized CORT into the circulation.

Rapid feedback in the PVN. Classic experiments by Dallman et al. (1987) revealed that HPA axis activity is tightly regulated under basal conditions and during and after periods of stressful stimulation. They described three distinct time domains for CORT-induced negative feedback: (i) a rapid, nongenomic effect, which unfolded in seconds to minutes; (ii) an intermediate effect that occurred within 3 hours, involving genomic and nongenomic effects; and (iii) a genomic effect that required at least several hours to occur. Elevations in circulating CORT engage in negative feedback at the level of the PVN and the anterior pituitary to inhibit further secretion of CRF and ACTH, respectively. In addition, CORT binds to GRs in the hippocampus to further inhibit HPA axis activity. Additional information about the role of the hippocampus in negative feedback regulation will be presented in Chapter 5. Negative feedback at the level of the PVN and the anterior pituitary appears to involve nongenomic effects of CORT on membrane-associated GRs given the rapid nature of the inhibition (on the order of minutes). Membrane-associated GRs are a lower affinity and lower density class of GRs that share homology with the higher affinity and more abundant intracellular GRs (Nahar et al., 2016). In contrast, negative feedback at the level of the hippocampus is much slower to take effect (on the order of hours) and involves binding of CORT with GRs, leading to downstream effects involving nuclear transcription and protein synthesis.

In a series of experiments, Evanson et al. (2010) demonstrated that rapid negative feedback effects on ACTH and CORT release following restraint stress in laboratory rats could be inhibited by infusion of a synthetic glucocorticoid, dexamethasone (DEX), into the PVN. DEX-induced inhibition of HPA activity was blocked by co-infusion of an endocannabinoid CB1 receptor antagonist. The same effects were observed if DEX was covalently bound to bovine serum albumin, blocking entry of DEX into PVN cells. In addition, exposure of rats to restraint stress increased hypothalamic levels of an endogenous endocannabinoid, 2-arachidonoyl glycerol, providing further support for a role for endocannabinoid signaling in fast feedback inhibition of the HPA axis. These results were consistent with glucocorticoid-mediated fast feedback inhibition of the HPA axis at the level of the PVN involving stimulation of membrane-bound GRs and G protein signaling, which resulted in enhanced endocannabinoid synthesis in PVN neurons. Endocannabinoids then traveled retrogradely to bind to CB-1 receptors to inhibit glutamate release from presynaptic excitatory synapses (Tasker & Herman, 2011).

An added layer of complexity was introduced when Nahar et al. (2015) reported that the rapid nongenomic actions of glucocorticoids on fast feedback inhibition of PVN neurons were dependent upon the presence of nuclear GRs. They deduced that nuclear GRs played a role in transducing the rapid effects of membrane-bound GRs, were involved in the signaling cascade, or regulated a component of the signaling cascade.

Rapid feedback in the anterior pituitary. Anterior pituitary corticotropes are a site for CORT-induced rapid feedback inhibition of ACTH secretion. Several mechanisms have been described to account for these rapid nongenomic feedback effects of CORT. Corticotropes maintained in vitro display electrically excitable properties and fire single action potentials as well as CRF-induced bursts in firing. In addition, AVP stimulates an increase in the frequency of action potentials. The bursting pattern of firing in corticotropes is dependent upon activation of large-conductance calcium- and voltage-activated potassium (BK) channels. Bursting results in greater increases in intracellular Ca^{++} than single action potentials and contributes to CRF/AVP-induced stimulation of ACTH secretion (Tagliavini et al., 2016). In a series of in vitro experiments, Duncan et al. (2016) reported that pretreatment of corticotropes with CORT reduced spontaneous spiking activity and prevented the transition from spiking to bursting following treatment with CRF/AVP. Recordings from corticotropes obtained from BK knockout mice revealed that CORT also inhibited excitability of corticotropes through BK-independent mechanisms.

The release of ACTH from corticotrope cells is also regulated by the activation of Annexin 1 (ANX-A1), a protein produced in non-endocrine folliculostellate cells in the pituitary and secreted to act on endocrine cells via binding to its putative receptor, the formyl peptide receptor, a family of G protein-coupled receptors found in many cell types. In corticotropes, ANX-A1 inhibits CRF-stimulated ACTH secretion from storage vesicles, presumably by a mechanism downstream of cAMP and Ca^{++} influx that involves local reorganization of the actin cytoskeleton (Buckingham et al., 2006). CORT can inhibit ACTH secretion by promoting ANX-A1 translocation from the cytoplasm to the outer surface of the plasma membrane, a process dependent upon activation of protein kinase C. CORT also regulates ANX-A1 expression. However, while CORT-induced translocation of ANX-A1 to the outer plasma membrane occurs rapidly and involves post-translational modification of the protein, CORT-induced ANX-A1 expression is much slower to occur. It is nevertheless important for replenishing the stored ANX-A1 in the cytoplasm that is depleted after CORT-induced membrane translocation (Buckingham & Flower, 2017).

Stress hyporesponsive period. A special feature of early postnatal development of the HPA axis in laboratory rats is the stress hyporesponsive period that is evident at PND 2 and extends well into the second week of postnatal life. During this time, the HPA axis maintains a low level of basal CORT secretion, but otherwise is largely nonresponsive to stressful stimuli (surgical stress, handling, ether stress, thermal challenge). During this stage in postnatal development, there is very little CRF present in the median eminence and there is reduced content of ACTH in the anterior pituitary; however, there is an enhanced negative feedback effect of CORT at the level of the anterior pituitary. Thus, the HPA axis over this 12–13-day period maintains stable but low levels of circulating CORT, presumably to ensure proper neuronal development in CORT-sensitive brain areas (Sapolsky & Meaney, 1986).

Corticosteroid-binding globulin (CBG). Several excellent reviews of steroid-binding proteins have appeared (Hammond, 2016; Henley & Lightman, 2011; Henley et al., 2016; Meyer et al., 2016). Most of the CORT secreted from the adrenal gland is bound to carrier proteins, with 80%–90% bound to CBG and 10%–15% to albumin. The remaining 5% exists in an unbound or free form and may diffuse across plasma or neuronal membranes and bind to cytosolic MRs or GRs. CBG, which is primarily synthesized by hepatocytes, has one steroid binding site per molecule, and binds insoluble CORT molecules with high affinity but low capacity. Two conformational states of circulating CBG occur: a high-affinity form (65%–70%) that is converted irreversibly to a low-affinity form (30%–35%) with subsequent release of free CORT. In contrast, circulating albumin, which is the most abundant circulating protein, binds CORT with low affinity but high capacity. According to the "free hormone hypothesis" advanced by Mendel (1989), steroid hormones that are bound to circulating proteins are considered biologically inactive, and provide a reservoir of inactive circulating hormone as well as regulate the amount of free hormone available for diffusion into cells. During exposure to various stressors, CBG expression and levels in the circulation decrease, with a concomitant increase in levels of unbound CORT.

Henley and Lightman (2011) summarized evidence that CBG functions as much more than a simple carrier protein. In one study, Petersen et al. (2006) used $cbg^{(-/-)}$ null mice and wild-type controls to explore the role of CBG in the actions of CORT under basal conditions and following exposure to lipopolysaccharide (LPS)-induced septic shock. As expected, $cbg^{(-/-)}$ null mice displayed a lack of CORT binding activity in serum. In addition, mice lacking CBG had reduced blood levels of total CORT but a 10-fold increase in unbound levels of CORT and a doubling of circulating levels of ACTH; $cbg^{(-/-)}$ null mice were more susceptible to the deleterious effects of LPS-induced septic shock and exhibited higher levels of inflammatory cytokines and a higher mortality rate. The inability of $cbg^{(-/-)}$ null mice to inhibit ACTH secretion through negative feedback and down-regulate levels of inflammatory cytokines cannot be explained by reductions in unbound levels of CORT. Rather, Petersen et al. (2006) argued that CBG is much more than a mere CORT transporter protein and may play an active role in bioavailability, targeted delivery, and/or signal transduction of CORT in target cells. These and many other findings led Willnow and Nykjaer (2010) to propose that, under some conditions, CORT bound to CBG may enter some target cells by receptor-mediated endocytosis, followed by internalization and discharge of free CORT followed by recycling of receptors. This carrier-mediated process is similar to the uptake of cholesterol-containing lipoprotein molecules from the circulation. Such a process of receptor-mediated endocytosis of CBG-CORT complexes would represent a departure from predictions of the free hormone hypothesis.

CBG has been detected in various areas of the brain, including several hypothalamic nuclei, the bed nucleus of the stria terminalis, periaqueductal gray, cerebellum, hippocampus, and ependymal cells. In addition, it is present in the median eminence and the posterior pituitary. It is possible that CBG may regulate the bioavailability of CORT within some brain neurons and glia. CBG may be especially important in regulating the HPA axis (Henley & Lightman, 2011).

One gland, two rhythms. In nocturnal laboratory rats and mice, basal plasma levels of ACTH and CORT exhibit a distinct circadian rhythm of approximately 24 hours, with a peak in levels occurring at the onset of the active phase with lights-off and a return to lower levels over the last several hours of the active period. In many laboratories, vivarium lights are regulated on a 12-hour light:12-hour dark photoperiod, with lights on at 06:00 hours. Superimposed on this circadian rhythm of ACTH and CORT secretion is a series of ultradian pulses that occur about every 60 minutes.

Ultradian rhythms. The ultradian rhythm of CORT secretion under basal conditions occurs independently of hypothalamic control of the anterior pituitary, and instead depends on dynamic interactions between pituitary corticotropes and CORT-synthesizing cells in the adrenal zona glomerulosa. An ultradian pulse is initiated with positive feed-forward stimulation by ACTH of adrenal synthesis and secretion of CORT. This is followed by negative feedback regulation of ACTH secretion from corticotropes by circulating CORT. This feedback loop of ACTH stimulation followed by CORT inhibition has built-in time delays that produce the ultradian rhythm of CORT secretion. There is a delay in the response of adrenal zona glomerulosa cells to a pulse of ACTH due to the fact that CORT must be synthesized and released on demand. CORT cannot be stored within vesicles of the adrenal cortex because of its lipophilic nature—it would simply diffuse out of the vesicles and adrenocortical cells. Thus, time is required for de novo synthesis of CORT following a pulse of ACTH. In contrast, nongenomic fast negative feedback by CORT involving membrane binding sites on pituitary corticotropes occurs without significant delay. Finally, ultradian rhythms of ACTH and CORT were maintained with a constant infusion of a low dose but not a high dose of CRF. These results confirmed predictions based upon mathematical modeling of HPA axis activity (Gjerstad et al., 2018).

In an earlier set of experiments, Walker, Spiga, et al. (2015) explored the role of intra-adrenal inhibition of CORT synthesis in ultradian rhythms of adrenocortical secretion. Such a mechanism of intra-adrenal inhibition would make possible the rapid synthesis and release of glucocorticoids while also buffering against uncontrolled release of CORT following a stress-induced surge in ACTH. Intra-adrenal feedback of CORT synthesis and secretion is rapidly antagonized by ACTH, presumably via activation of MC2Rs, effectively disinhibiting the system and enabling a rapid early response to another pulse of ACTH. These and other feedback mechanisms allow the HPA axis to strike a balance between reactivity and regulation. There is an obvious need for the HPA axis to respond to stressful stimuli, but that response must be measured to avoid excessive levels of CORT exerting a prolonged negative feedback inhibition at the level of the anterior pituitary, the PVN, and the hippocampus (Walker, Spiga, et al., 2015).

In spite of these concerns, CORT ultradian rhythms can influence the magnitude of the CORT response to an acute stressor. If exposure to an acute stressor occurs during the increasing phase of an ultradian pulse, the CORT response is greater than if the acute stressor occurs during the falling phase (Windle et al., 1998).

Circadian rhythms. The mechanisms underlying circadian rhythms in CORT secretion have been studied extensively in laboratory strains of mice and rats. The trough of plasma CORT during the inactive (light) phase of the day-night cycle is 0–5µg/100ml, while the peak in plasma CORT during the active (dark) phase is 15–20µg/100ml (Spencer & Deak, 2017). The suprachiasmatic nuclei (SCN) located in the ventral hypothalamus generate self-sustaining rhythms by both genetic and neural mechanisms and are considered the master clock of the mammalian brain (Reppert & Weaver, 2002). The SCN entrains its phase to environmental cues, especially ambient light, and then synchronizes oscillators in other brain regions and in peripheral tissues to coordinate circadian rhythms in body temperature, metabolic activity, hormone secretion, and locomotor activity. One such peripheral tissue is the adrenal cortex, where clock gene expression appears to be independent of stress-induced ACTH secretion but can be entrained by SCN control of sympathetic drive to the adrenal cortex through the splanchnic nerve.

Although basal levels of circulating CORT vary considerably over the course of a 24-hour period, the maximum levels of CORT measured following exposure to an acute stressor tend to be fairly consistent. The dynamic range of a CORT response to stimulation by ACTH is somewhat limited due to constraints on maximum rates of synthesis and release of CORT that can be achieved within the adrenal cortex. In spite of this constraint, the magnitude of the CORT response does vary reliably with stressor intensity, but only within a limited range (Natelson et al., 1987; Spencer & Deak, 2017).

Two excellent reviews (Kalsbeek et al., 2012; Son et al., 2018) have summarized results from experiments on the functional significance of adrenal cortical innervation for daily rhythms in CORT secretion. For example, direct electrical stimulation of the splanchnic nerve increased adrenal cortical sensitivity to ACTH. In addition, trans-neuronal retrograde viral tracing experiments from the adrenal gland have revealed through second-order labeling a direct input from neurons of the PVN to spinal preganglionic sympathetic neurons, and third-order labeling in SCN neurons (Buijs et al., 1999).

The functional significance of these multi-synaptic connections linking the SCN and PVN with the adrenal cortex for the daily rhythm in adrenal CORT release was revealed by using adrenal microdialysis combined with splanchnic denervation. The SCN appears to employ two mechanisms to regulate the daily rise in plasma CORT. One mechanism involves activation of parvocellular PVN neurons and release of CRF and AVP, and the other operates through increased firing of the splanchnic innervation to the adrenal cortex, which in turn enhances the sensitivity of adrenal zona glomerulosa cells to circulating ACTH.

The adrenal cortex also has its own complement of functional circadian clock genes that display cell-autonomous and self-sustaining characteristics. Adrenal cortical clock gene expression appears to be independent of stress-induced ACTH secretion, but it can be entrained by increased splanchnic input to the adrenal cortex. Approximately 240 genes in the adrenal cortex displayed circadian rhythms in rates of transcription. The rhythmic secretion of CORT and its capacity to phase-shift peripheral clocks in other tissues (e.g., liver, kidney, heart) suggest that CORT serves as a link between the SCN master clock and other peripheral oscillators. However, other humoral signals appear to play a role in the entrainment of oscillations in peripheral tissues given that some rhythms in gene transcription rates persist in liver cells that lack GRs (Balsalobre et al., 2000).

Given that the adrenal medulla also receives input via the splanchnic nerve, it is possible that chromaffin cells, through their secretory products and close proximity, might influence adrenal cortical rhythms in gene expression and sensitivity to ACTH. Circadian analyses of the rates of expression of core clock genes in the adrenal gland show differences in expression levels and in cycling between the adrenal medulla and different layers of the adrenal cortex. Such expression differences of core clock genes might lead to tissue-specific changes in clock-controlled gene expression (Dickmeis, 2009).

Uncoupling from the SCN. Although the normal circadian rhythm of CORT is determined by the entrainment of the SCN to the light-dark cycle, the circadian phase of CORT secretion from the adrenal cortex can be uncoupled from the SCN if animals are given restricted daily access to food (Spencer & Deak, 2017). For example, if laboratory rats and mice are given access to food each day only in the first few hours after lights are turned on, they engage in less feeding, and their circadian rhythm of CORT secretion shifts, with peak levels occurring at the new anticipated time of daily food availability (Girotti et al., 2009). These findings suggest that the circadian rhythm of CORT secretion is not controlled exclusively by the SCN, but that a separate central neural system, the food-entrainable oscillator, may also play a role in diurnal CORT secretion (Blum et al., 2012).

The odd couple. The adrenal cortex and the adrenal medulla are distinctly different tissues. The adrenal cortex is derived from intermediate mesodermal cells, whereas the adrenal medulla develops from neural crest cells migrating from sympathetic ganglia. The adrenal cortex secretes a variety of steroid hormones under control of various circulating hormones, whereas the adrenal medulla releases its primary hormone, EPI, following direct stimulation by sympathetic preganglionic neurons. Steroid hormones are highly lipophilic, whereas EPI is water-soluble.

In spite of these and other differences between cells of the adrenal cortex and the adrenal medulla, these two tissues come together in many species, including laboratory rodents and humans, to form a single gland with an outer cortex and an inner medulla, all encased in a fibrous capsule. The boundary between chromaffin cells and cortical cells is not distinct; rather, clusters of chromaffin cells penetrate into the three cortical layers, and islets of cortical cells are found within the medulla surrounded by chromaffin cells. These close associations between cells of the cortex and the medulla open up numerous possibilities for intra-adrenal routes of communication (Ceccato et al., 2018).

The adrenal cortex and the adrenal medulla receive blood flow well in excess of levels required for nutrient delivery. This elevation in blood flow appears to ensure the prompt entry of adrenal hormones into the circulation. Blood flow to the adrenal medulla increases during sustained elevations in CA secretion, whereas increases in adrenocortical secretory activity are not accompanied by increases in blood flow (Breslow, 1992).

Chromaffin cells experience very high concentrations of glucocorticoids because of the proximity of the zona glomerulosa to the adrenal medulla. A series of classic experiments by Wurtman and Axelrod (1965) demonstrated that adrenal glucocorticoids were required to maintain normal levels of PNMT in chromaffin cells. In hypophysectomized rats, low doses of ACTH were sufficient to stimulate adrenal cortical synthesis of glucocorticoids and restore adrenal medullary PNMT to control levels. In contrast, replacement doses of glucocorticoids required to maintain adrenal medullary PNMT levels in hypophysectomized rats were approximately 100–300 times higher than doses required to re-establish basal circulating levels of glucocorticoids. The explanation for this dramatic difference in doses of glucocorticoids was the unusually high levels of glucocorticoids found in the adrenal medulla due to its proximity to the adrenal cortex (for a review, see Wurtman, 2002).

What aspects of intra-adrenal blood flow explain these unusually high levels of glucocorticoids bathing the chromaffin cells of the adrenal medulla? The results of several studies of blood flow within the adrenal gland have revealed that the adrenal arteries form a subcapsular plexus from which two types of arteries arise: short arteries that supply the cortex and longer arteries that pass through the cortex to supply the medulla. Usually a single vein exits the gland and drains into the inferior vena cava (right adrenal) or the left renal vein (left adrenal). There does not appear to be an adrenal portal system to drain blood directly from the cortex to the medulla and deliver the very high levels of glucocorticoids (Kikuta & Murakami, 1982; Sparrow & Coupland, 1987). Einer-Jensen and Carter (1995) proposed that local transfer of glucocorticoids from adrenal cortical cells to medullary arteries traversing the cortex is the mechanism which ensures that uniformly high levels of glucocorticoids are delivered to the adrenal medulla to support the synthesis and activity of PNMT.

Intra-adrenal communication is not a one-way street leading from cortex to medulla; rather, it involves a dynamic two-way communication between cortex and medulla. For example, the secretory products of chromaffin cells appear to exert a paracrine effect on the function of adrenocortical cells. These paracrine messengers include CAs as well as the plethora of peptides released from chromaffin cells. Co-culture systems have been developed to explore paracrine interactions between various cell types. Two cell types are grown in co-culture, but are separated by a semipermeable membrane that permits exchange of paracrine factors. Adrenocortical cells exhibited a 10-fold increase in glucocorticoid synthesis when co-cultured with chromaffin cells, compared to adrenocortical cells cultured alone (Ehrhart-Bornstein et al., 1998; Schinner & Bornstein, 2005).

Summary

The HPA axis has been closely associated with physiological responses to stressful stimulation since the original report by Selye (1936b) regarding the general adaptation syndrome. The traditional view of the HPA axis has emphasized CRF stimulation of ACTH secretion from the anterior pituitary, followed by stimulation of synthesis and secretion of CORT from the adrenal cortex. CORT provides negative feedback to the pituitary and PVN to inhibit continued HPA axis activation. More recent studies have unmasked the subtle yet important modulatory factors that can affect CORT secretion independently of circulating ACTH. These include peptides and other substances released from adrenal medullary chromaffin cells, interleukin-10, circadian processes controlled by the intrinsic adrenal clock, and sympathetic nerve terminals that provide direct neural input to the adrenal cortex. The HPA axis plays a pivotal role in a range of physiological processes in the periphery and through CORT signaling in brain areas, and it regulates behavioral and neural responses to stressful stimuli. Later in this volume, we will see how the HPA axis has been linked to symptoms associated with a number of mental disorders.

The Immune System

Dealing with Pathogens and Confronting Danger

If an infectious agent is successful in gaining entry into the body by breaching the skin or the mucous membranes of the digestive, reproductive, or respiratory systems, then a rapid response is necessary to recognize and eliminate the invading bacterium or virus. Two components of the immune system fulfill this function: the innate immune system and the adaptive immune system. The rapidly mobilized innate immune system has evolved to detect and eliminate invading pathogens based upon their molecular differences from host cells. Components of the innate immune system can also call into play the adaptive immune system, which is highly specific in attacking an invading pathogen but requires 4–5 days to become fully mobilized. In the subsections that follow, we will delve into the ways that stressful stimuli can activate the immune system, especially the innate immune system, in the absence of an infection or a non-penetrating injury. The consequences of stress-induced immune activation have far-reaching implications for the pathophysiology of several mental disorders, as we will see in later chapters.

In many ways, the immune system is the new kid on the block when considering neural and humoral responses to stressful stimuli. After all, the prevailing view for many decades was that the immune system protected the body from invading pathogens and was largely self-regulating and concerned about distinctions between "self" and "non-self." It made little sense for the components of the immune system to also be subject to the stresses and strains of daily life. However, a radically different view of the fundamental purpose of the immune system emerged that suggests it has evolved to detect damage and protect against danger. In doing so, it interacts with a network of other bodily tissues, including the brain (Matzinger, 1994, 2002).

In his well-crafted and comprehensive review of interactions between the central nervous system and the immune system, Dantzer (2018) pointed to early efforts in the 1920s by investigators at the Institut Pasteur in Paris to alter immune function in guinea pigs exposed to Pavlovian conditioning (Metalnikov & Chorine, 1926). This line of research was given new life by Ader and Cohen (1975), who reintroduced the phenomenon of conditioned immunosuppression. If the activity of the immune system was subject to conditioning, then it quickly followed that brain areas must be involved. Several key reports in the 1970s and 1980s provided compelling evidence of interactions between the central nervous system, the endocrine system, and the immune system, including pioneering studies by Besedovsky et al. (1979, 1981, 1983, 1986). Other studies provided clear evidence of direct innervation of immune cells of the spleen, bone marrow, lymphatic tissue, and thymus by postganglionic sympathetic nerves (Madden & Felton, 1995).

In their influential review, Elenkov et al. (2000) described the presence of sympathetic noradrenergic nerve fibers in various lymphoid organs, the release of NE from the sympathetic nerve terminals in these organs, and the expression of adrenergic receptors on lymphoid cells, which are able to respond functionally to stimulation. The varicose axon terminals of sympathetic nerves do not make synaptic contact with immune cells. Rather, NE released from sympathetic nerve terminal diffuses a considerable distance from its site of release and exerts its effects non-synaptically. In the following subsections, we will explore the various interconnections between the nervous system, hormonal systems, and immune cells and their critical involvement in responses to stressors.

Immune System Responses to Danger

The innate immune system has evolved in multicellular organisms to recognize, contain, and eliminate invading pathogens. The basis for recognition of invading pathogens is tied to pathogen-associated molecular patterns (PAMPS), highly conserved molecules (e.g., proteins, carbohydrates, and double-stranded RNAs) that are unique to pathogens and are not found in the host body. An example of a PAMP is LPS, an endotoxin that is a prominent component of the outer membrane of gram-negative bacteria. Molecules like LPS are detected by soluble or membrane-associated pattern recognition receptors (PRRs) (Janeway, 1989). One family of PRRs, the toll-like receptors (TLRs), are expressed on the outer plasma membrane of neutrophils, macrophages, and dendritic cells, and when activated stimulate inflammatory and antimicrobial innate immune responses. This cascade of intracellular changes involves activation of the transcription factors nuclear factor κB (NFκB) and interferon-regulated factors (IRFs). Among the multiple genes that may be transcribed are the antiviral interferons; the proinflammatory cytokines interleukin-1β (IL-1β), IL-6, and IL-12; tumor necrosis factor-α (TNF-α); and various chemokines, all of which can serve as chemoattractants and direct immune cells to the site of an infection (Akdis et al., 2016). The first interleukin, leukocyte pyrogen or IL-1, was first reported by Dinarello et al. (1977), and this seminal discovery has been followed by many additions to the list of ILs since that time.

A second family of receptors, the nucleotide binding oligomerization domain (NOD)-like receptors (NLRs), are cytoplasmic receptors that recognize microbial products and danger-associated molecular patterns within the cell. Upon activation, NLRs activate multiple downstream signaling pathways that promote inflammatory responses, inflammasome assembly, activation of the NF-κB pathway, and transcriptional activity (Motta et al., 2015).

In instances of non-penetrating injuries to the body, damage to bodily tissues can result in cell death and the release of molecules that are normally safely tucked away inside cell membranes, an example of sterile inflammation (Chen & Nuñez, 2010). Examples include extracellular heat shock protein-72 (Hsp-72), uric acid crystals, high mobility group box 1 (HMGB-1), IL-1α, IL-33, IL-16, and ATP. These and other molecules, referred to as damage-associated molecular patterns (DAMPs) or alarmins, are bound by PRRs and the damaged cells can be eliminated by phagocytosis.

It may come as a surprise that members of the IL-1 cytokine family (e.g., Il-1α, IL-1β, IL-18, IL-33, etc.) could function as DAMPs. However, Martin (2016) has made a compelling case that IL-1 family members serve as key players in necrosis-related sterile inflammation and can also amplify the inflammatory response to PAMPs released during infection-related tissue damage. In contrast, with programmed cell death through apoptosis, IL-1-related DAMPs are not released because the plasma membrane is able to retain cytoplasmic proteins until the dying cell is engulfed by macrophages.

More recently, Rider et al. (2017) suggested that some alarmins could serve a dual purpose in cells that are not necrotic or have loss of integrity of the plasma membrane. In such instances, these molecules, now referred to as stressorins, may reflect cellular stress resulting from DNA damage, heat shock, or oxidative stress. Stressorins, including HMGB1, IL-1α, IL-33, and IL-16, share structural and sequence similarities, do not require receptor stimulation or de novo synthesis, and likely sense intracellular damage through post-translational modifications. Similar to cytokines, but in contrast with alarmins, they are most likely actively secreted by somatic cells but require no additional processing by specific innate immune cell proteases and signal in a manner similar to alarmins (Rider et al., 2017).

In addition, immune cells can recruit other cells to engage with the invading pathogens by secreting two diverse classes of proteins, cytokines and chemokines. The sentinel function is carried out by macrophages and dendritic cells, immune cells that are found throughout the body and are constantly sampling the local tissue environment in search of invading pathogens. When PAMPs or DAMPs are detected and PRRs are activated, specific genes in the macrophages are induced and the cells change into an activated state. For inflammasome-independent cytokines, such as IL-6 and IL-10, activation of NFκB results in inflammatory gene transcription, translation, protein synthesis, and cytokine release. Refer to Table 4.2 for a summary of the immune signaling molecules that are discussed in this section.

Inflammasomes and Inflammation

For inflammasome-dependent pathways, there is a more complex two-step process that results in release of the proinflammatory cytokines, IL-1β and IL-18. First described by Martinon et al. (2002), inflammasomes are intracellular multi-protein platforms that function as sensors of DAMPs or PAMPs, and activators of pro-inflammatory caspases, which lead to the cleavage of pro-inflammatory cytokines and the subsequent release of proinflammatory cytokines. Several distinct inflammasomes have been characterized, and they generally consist of a cytosolic sensor, an adaptor protein, and an effector caspase, typically caspase-1. Considerable attention has been directed at nucleotide-binding oligomerization domain, leucine-rich repeat and pyrin domain protein 3 (NLRP3), a stress-responsive inflammasome that plays a key role in peripheral and brain inflammatory responses. Activation of PRRs leads to NLRP3 gene transcription, translation, and protein production. Once the cell is "primed" with NLRP3 protein, a second activation signal (including a broad range of PAMPs and DAMPs) is required for NLRP3 to interact with ACS (adaptor protein apoptosis-associated

Table 4.2 Selected Proinflammatory and Anti-inflammatory Cytokines and Their Receptors, Cells of Origin, Target Cells, and Selected Functions

Cytokine	Receptors	Sources	Target cells	Function
IL-1β	IL-1 type 1 R IL-1 type 2 R	Macrophages, monocytes lymphocytes, etc.	T cells, fibroblasts, and epithelial and endothelial cells	Mediates sickness behaviors; HPA axis activation; lymphocyte, macrophage, and neutrophil activation; stimulates IL-6 synthesis (proinflammatory)
IL-4	IL-4R type 1 IL-4R type 2	T cells, basophils, mast cells, eosinophils	T cells and B cells	Anti-inflammatory effects through inhibition of IL-1β, IL-6, and TNF-α; stimulates B and T cell proliferation
IL-6	IL-6R	Macrophages, T cells	Monocytes, macrophages, T cells, B cells, etc.	Mediates the acute phase response, promotes fever, can down-regulate inflammation by inhibiting TNF-α and IL-1 (usually proinflammatory)
IL-10	IL-10R1/IL-10R2 complex	Macrophages, T cells, monocytes, dendritic cells	Macrophages, T cells, monocytes, dendritic cells, etc.	Anti-inflammatory effects through inhibition of IL-1β, IL-6, and TNF-α; stimulates B cell production and antibody production
TNF-α	TNFR1, TNFR2	Macrophages, NK cells	Macrophages, T cells, B cells, NK cells, mast cells, etc.	Proinflammatory mediator of fever and reduced appetite associated with sickness behavior; stimulates the HPA axis; high levels can lead to septic shock; also plays a role in anti-inflammatory processes

speck-like protein containing a caspase recruitment domain), which then recruits procaspase-1 through its caspase recruitment domain. This assembly of proteins is considered the inflammasome, and once formed, it triggers the cleavage of procaspase 1 to active caspase-1 (a protease enzyme). Caspase-1 then cleaves pro-IL-1β and pro-IL-18 into mature IL-1β and IL-18, respectively, followed by their secretion from the cell (Rathinam et al., 2012).

Subsequent secretion of proinflammatory cytokines and chemokines increases vascular permeability locally and permits the infiltration of neutrophils and circulating protein molecules (acute phase proteins such as C-reactive protein) that can further aid in eliminating the invading pathogen. These changes result in local swelling, redness, tenderness, and heat, components of the classic localized inflammatory response that many of us experience after a splinter penetrates the skin or when an ingrown toenail flares up.

In many instances, this rapid and relatively indiscriminate targeting of PAMPs is sufficient to beat back an invading pathogen. However, the potential for rapid proliferation by many bacterial pathogens, which can undergo cell divisions approximately every 20 minutes, occasionally overwhelms the innate immune response. At this point, the phylogenetically more recently evolved adaptive immune system springs into action. The adaptive immune system is limited to the jawed vertebrates. Although it is slower to attain full capacity, it has the ability to single out a specific pathogen based upon antigens present on the outer cell membrane. Importantly, the adaptive immune system becomes more effective with each exposure to a given pathogen, and some of its cells retain a memory of the antigen associated with a given pathogen. Cells of the adaptive immune system also benefit from signaling molecules released from cells associated with the innate immune response, receiving information relating to the location of the challenge and when to terminate the response.

Neural and Hormonal Influences on the Immune System

Innate immune cells such as macrophages and monocytes express β_2, α_1, and α_2 adrenergic receptors. Release of NE from sympathetic nerves and EPI from the adrenal medulla stimulates β_2ARs, which results in alterations in the transcription of immune response genes in the nucleus. This typically leads to enhanced synthesis of the proinflammatory cytokines IL-1β, IL-6, and TNF-α but suppression of type 1 interferon genes, which exert potent anti-viral effects (Cole et al., 1998; Cole et al., 2010). Beyond their effects on innate immune functioning, NE and EPI gain access to the critical tissue microenvironments where immune response gene regulation occurs, including primary and secondary lymphoid organs, the musculoskeletal system, and most of the important organs and tissues in the periphery. These wide-ranging effects of the sympathetic-adrenal medullary system on immune function can occur during periods of stressful stimulation and emphasize further the importance of the central nervous system as a modulator of immune activity (Irwin & Cole, 2011).

Another important regulator of innate immunity is the HPA axis and the release of CORT from the adrenal cortex (Figure 4.5). When CORT binds to its

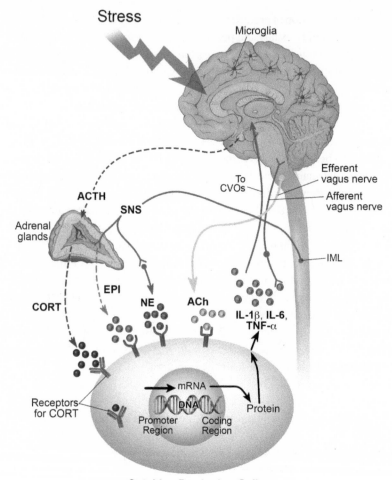

Cytokine Producing Cells

Figure 4.5. Stress stimulates the release of cytokines in the periphery. Cytokine-producing cells have receptors for glucocorticoids (CORT, blue dots), NE (red dots), EPI (orange dots), and acetylcholine (ACh, yellow dots). There are outer membrane receptors for CORT, NE, EPI, and ACh as well as cytoplasmic receptors for CORT. The proinflammatory cytokines IL-1β, IL-6, and TNF-α (green dots) can provide feedback to brain areas by binding to receptors on afferent vagal nerve fibers or by entry into brain at the circumventricular organs that lack a fully-formed blood-brain barrier. One consequence of cytokine signaling to brain is the activation of brain microglia (see also Plate 4).

GR and is translocated to the nucleus of immune cells, it can directly inhibit proinflammatory gene expression. In addition, GR binding of CORT can enhance transcription of some anti-inflammatory genes and short-circuit the activity of some proinflammatory transcription factors (Irwin & Cole, 2011). Cytokines also regulate the activity of the HPA axis and the release of EPI from the adrenal medulla, introducing another layer of complexity in the interactions between the immune system and the adrenal gland (Jenkins et al., 2016; Turnbull & Rivier, 1999).

Under certain conditions, CORT and other glucocorticoids may exert proinflammatory effects. The proinflammatory effect of glucocorticoids may reflect inhibition of the synthesis and release of anti-inflammatory factors. Alternatively, the proinflammatory effect could result from enhanced synthesis and release of proinflammatory mediators. In the first instance, DEX administered 24 hours prior to LPS enhanced the proinflammatory cytokine response in the placenta. In the second example, the effect was dose-dependent; physiological levels of CORT can be proinflammatory in some circumstances, whereas high or pharmacological levels of CORT can have anti-inflammatory effects (Dantzer, 2018).

Proinflammatory effects of CORT are also observed following stress-induced activation of the HPA axis. If laboratory rats are pre-exposed to an acute stressor or to repeated stressful stimulation, it results in a sensitized response to subsequent administration of LPS. The sensitized effect has been demonstrated in peripheral immune cells as well as in microglia from the hippocampus. In the hippocampus, exposure to stress leads to release of the DAMP, HMGB1, from microglia, followed by activation of PRRs and the NLRP3 inflammasome (Frank et al., 2007; Frank et al., 2015; Weber et al., 2015).

An Evolutionary Bias in Immune Responses to Stress

Sterile inflammation occurs when a non-penetrating injury to the body (e.g., closed head trauma) results in a proinflammatory response, with innate immune cells attracted to the site of damage to deal with necrotic tissue. But how does one explain a robust sterile inflammatory response when an undergraduate volunteer is brought into a laboratory and is asked to prepare a speech with little lead time and deliver it to a skeptical group of evaluators (Allen et al., 2014)?

In two superb review articles (Miller & Raison, 2016; Slavich & Irwin, 2014), complementary arguments were advanced to explain why social stressors precipitate a proinflammatory response. Slavich and Irwin (2014) described a well-honed anticipatory response of the innate immune system prior to an injury that could result in tissue damage and a high likelihood of infection. By mobilizing immune cells to possible sites of infection, an organism would increase the probability of post-injury wound healing and recovery. For most of our evolutionary history as a species, humans have confronted potential sources of danger from predators or from hostile conspecifics. The anticipatory immune responses that served us so well for thousands of years have now carried over to modern humans who confront a range of non-lethal social stressors related to social conflict and isolation, rejection by a loved one, loss of a job, and so on. Repeated exposure to social adversity results in an up-regulation of proinflammatory innate immune response genes and a down-regulation of anti-viral innate immune response genes. These transcriptional effects are tied to sympathetic-adrenal medullary and CORT responses to repeated stressors. Slavich and Irwin (2014) have termed this anticipatory response the *conserved transcriptional response to adversity*.

Miller and Raison (2016) argued that modern humans continue to carry with them an evolutionary bias in how the innate immune syste responds to stressors. The prevailing dangers confronting early humans were associated with hunting for food, being hunted by predators, or direct competition with conspecifics for social status. They recalled that early humans evolved in a pathogen-rich environment, so any wound was a possible life-or-death situation. They suggested that those individuals who responded to threatening social or environmental cues with an anticipatory activation of the innate immune system would have higher survival rates. Such a system would not place a high penalty on false alarms, such as when the threats did not materialize. Fast-forward to modern humans, and we retain the capacity of non-threatening social stressors to activate the innate immune system.

In both of these reviews, the authors emphasize the deleterious effects of the evolutionary bias toward activation of the immune system by social stressors. In particular, they made strong connections between immune activation and the onset of anxiety disorders and major depressive disorder. These and other connections to immune activation will be discussed more fully in later chapters.

Summary

The innate immune system is excellent at multitasking. Its well-established role as a rapid-responding first line of defense against invading pathogens has been studied in detail. More recently, the innate immune system has been shown to respond to threats of danger with robust proinflammatory activation. Peripheral immune cells are able to respond to several other stress-effector systems because the cells express receptors for CORT, CAs, and a host of peptides and other signaling molecule. Access to this extensive network of neural, hormonal, and neuroendocrine systems positions macrophages and dendritic cells to respond effectively to a variety of danger signals. When the innate immune system is kept in a hyper-reactive state for extended periods of time, there are dire consequences. These dire consequences will surface again in later chapters dealing with mental disorders.

Conclusions

The sympathetic-adrenal medullary system, the HPA axis, and the innate immune system have coevolved to serve as front-line defenders in periods of acute versus chronic intermittent exposure to stressors. Some of the stress effector systems have evolved for rapid responses, such as the emergency functions of the adrenal medulla in fight-or-flight situations, while others are slower to engage, such as the HPA axis, but exert long-term changes in brain circuits and behavior through alterations in transcriptional activity. Finally, the innate immune system has evolved the capacity to anticipate dangerous or threatening social situations and preemptively spring into action. These three stress effectors systems are also highly integrated, with each influencing and being influenced by the others. This exquisite level of integration is all in the service of maintaining the homeostatic balance of laboratory animals and humans as they deal with what are at times unpredictable and potentially dangerous circumstances. Ultimately, there is a high cost to pay if these stress effector systems are maintained on high alert for extended periods of time, and bodily systems are unable to re-establish a reasonable homeostatic set-point. More on that later.

5

Stress-Sensitive Brain Circuits

In this chapter, we will use Chapter 4 as a guide to explore stress-responsive brain circuits involved in regulation of sympathetic-adrenal medullary outflow. From there, we will explore brain circuits that regulate the HPA axis. Finally, we will consider how brain circuits respond to and engage in immune activation during sterile inflammation and the release of proinflammatory cytokines. Three major methodological advances will also be highlighted: optogenetic and chemogenetic control of neuronal activity and behavior in laboratory animals and the generation of new animal models by using genome-editing tools.

Brain Circuits Involved in Control
of Sympathetic-Adrenal Medullary Activity

Darwin and Emotional Expression

Saper (2002), in his review of central control of the autonomic nervous system, explicitly connected Darwin's work on emotional expressions in animals and humans (Darwin, 1872) with later work by Cannon (1929) on the physiological underpinnings of emotions, including an emphasis on the critical role played by the brain. Although he was limited to observational studies, Darwin quickly appreciated that observable changes related to autonomic responses, such as changes in heart rate, respiration, redness of the face, sweating, and piloerection, were part and parcel of emotional expressions. These important observational studies have served as the foundation of research on emotions for nearly 150 years.

Regions involved in central control of the autonomic nervous system must match ongoing homeostatic demands of individuals with their moment-to-moment responses to external and internal stressful stimuli. To respond effectively in the face of these critical demands, some brainstem autonomic centers receive visceral sensory information and monitor critical variables in blood, while forebrain centers are involved in regulating behavioral responses associated with feeding, drinking, thermoregulation, circadian rhythms, cardiovascular regulation, energy mobilization, immune system function, and emotional responses relating to threats from conspecifics or predators. Given the many critical functions subserved by the autonomic nervous system, it is not surprising that the various brain areas that control autonomic activity are widely distributed along the neuraxis and are highly redundant and interconnected to allow for differentiation and fine control of autonomic stimulation to the many peripheral organs and tissues that receive neural inputs (Morrison, 2001; Saper & Stornetta, 2015).

Fight-or-Flight

Early conceptions of the sympathetic nervous system, including in publications from Walter B. Cannon's laboratory, emphasized global responses to homeostatic challenges and situations that generated a fight-or-flight response. Contemporary views on the regulation of sympathetic outflow emphasize the exquisite central control over sympathetic preganglionic outflow to various target tissues that matches with the nature and intensity of the various challenges, be they physiological or behavioral. The fight-or-flight response is now viewed as just one option among many patterns of sympathetic activation that can be achieved with input from several descending brain pathways (Morrison, 2001; Saper, 2002).

Central Autonomic Network

The concept of a central autonomic network that controls peripheral autonomic activity through several interconnected areas distributed from brainstem to forebrain has been an important organizing principle in this wide-ranging field of research (Loewy, 1991). This network of brain areas exerts moment-to-moment control of visceral function and homeostatic balance in the face of internal or external challenges. The central autonomic network is organized in three closely interconnected regions: spinal, brainstem, and forebrain. Spinal parasympathetic and sympathetic preganglionic neurons display stimulus-specific patterns of responses to various internal and external provocations and are influenced by descending brainstem and forebrain projections. The lower brainstem is involved in reflex control of the circulation, respiration, and gastrointestinal function. The upper brainstem integrates autonomic activity with pain pathways and behavioral responses to stressors. Hypothalamic areas are crucial for integrating autonomic and endocrine responses to homeostatic challenges and adaptation, whereas limbic areas, including cortical areas and the amygdala, integrate emotional and stress-related autonomic responses. A selective overview of these interconnected brain areas, with an emphasis on sympathetic premotor neurons, is presented in Figure 5.1, and each is described in more detail in the sections that follow.

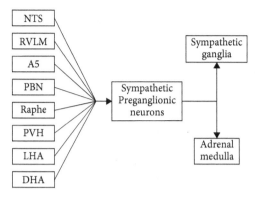

Figure 5.1. Compilation of eight brain areas that send direct monosynaptic projections to sympathetic preganglionic cell bodies in the intermediolateral column of the thoracic and lumbar segments of the spinal cord. Sympathetic preganglionic neurons project from the spinal cord to sympathetic postganglionic neurons within sympathetic ganglia or to chromaffin cells in the adrenal medulla.

Abbreviations: NTS: nucleus tracti solitarii; RVLM: rostral ventrolateral medulla; A5: noradrenergic cell group located in the ventrolateral portion of the pons; PBN: parabrachial nuclei; raphe: raphe nuclei located in the brainstem; PVH: paraventricular nucleus of the hypothalamus; LHA: lateral hypothalamic area; DHA: dorsal hypothalamic area.

Many of the experiments on descending projections to preganglionic sympathetic neurons have been motivated by a deeper understanding of how the brain regulates basal blood pressure. An abundance of evidence suggests that the most important neurotransmitters involved in fast-acting synaptic input to sympathetic preganglionic neurons are glutamate and γ-amino butyric acid (GABA), and to a lesser extent glycine. In addition, a variety of peptide and catecholamine neurotransmitters also co-occur in these synaptic terminals and may modulate the effects of excitatory (glutamate) and inhibitory (GABA and glycine) inputs to the sympathetic preganglionic cells (Llewellyn-Smith, 2009).

Brainstem and midbrain areas. Several descending projections to sympathetic preganglionic neurons in the intermediolateral cell column of the thoracic spinal cord from the brainstem have been described, including the rostral ventrolateral medulla (RVLM) and the ventrolateral portion of the nucleus tracti solitarii (NTS) (Guyenet, 2006). The RVLM includes the C1 neuronal cell group of EPI-synthesizing neurons, which sends descending projections to sympathetic and parasympathetic preganglionic neurons as well ascending projections to the PVN and other hypothalamic, thalamic, and basal forebrain nuclei. In addition, axon collaterals arising from C1 neurons communicate with other brainstem nuclei, including the NTS, dorsal motor nucleus of the vagus, parabrachial nucleus, the locus coeruleus, and periaqueductal gray (PAG).

Although C1 neurons have the enzymatic machinery necessary to synthesize catecholamines, it appears that their primary signaling pathway is through release of glutamate from nerve terminals. C1 neurons have been advanced as a key site within the brainstem that responds to a variety of extreme physical and physiological stressors such as pain, hemorrhage, hypoxia, hypoglycemia, and immune activation (Guyenet et al., 2013; Stornetta & Guyenet, 2018). Using an optogenetic approach (refer to the end of this chapter for details), Abbott et al. (2009) injected a lentivirus into the RVLM that expressed a channelrhrodopsin (ChR2) paired with a catecholaminergic neuron-preferring promoter. The ChR2-expressing neurons were non-GABAergic and non-glycinergic and more than half were catecholaminergic. Photo-stimulation of these transfected neurons resulted in significant increases in blood pressure and sympathetic nerve discharge, confirming that C1 neurons function to enhance sympathetic activity.

The NTS is the primary brain area for reflex regulation of the circulation. The caudal portion of the NTS receives input from peripheral baroreceptors, volume receptors, and chemoreceptors. NTS neurons send projections to the intermediolateral column of the spinal cord, where they influence sympathetic outflow to the adrenal medulla and other peripheral sympathetic target tissues (Mtui et al., 1993). Pontine A5 noradrenergic neurons send a dense projection to the intermediolateral column in thoracic spinal cord (Clark & Proudfit, 1993). These neurons appear to play an important role in pain perception, but may also stimulate sympathetic outflow to peripheral tissues. In addition, the Kölliker-Fuse subnucleus of the parabrachial complex sends a direct projection to sympathetic preganglionic neurons (Tucker & Saper, 1985).

Campos et al. (2018) studied calcitonin gene-related peptide (CGRP)-expressing neurons in the external lateral parabrachial nucleus. Their results were consistent with this discrete population of neurons responding to a wide range of visceral sensory disturbances (e.g., increased CO_2 levels, painful stimuli, gastric distention) and influencing adaptive behaviors to mitigate against these harmful disruptions.

The PAG appears to be well-positioned to be a source for pattern generation relating to external and internal threats to homeostasis given its extensive afferent inputs from the forebrain and its efferent pathways to the thalamus, hypothalamus, locus coeruleus, parabrachial nucleus, and other areas. Such threats include fight-or-flight encounters with a conspecific or a predator, painful stimuli related to wounding or injuries, and significant blood loss. Each threat requires coordinated activation/inhibition of brainstem, spinal, autonomic, and behavioral activities to yield individualized patterns of physiological and behavioral responses to counteract the disruptions in homeostatic balance (Benarroch, 2012; Saper & Stornetta, 2015).

The nucleus raphe pallidus mediates tachycardia and hyperthermia in response to acute exposure to audiogenic stress (95 dB for 30 minutes/day × 3 days). Injections of the GABA$_A$-receptor agonist muscimol into the raphe pallidus diminished the tachycardia and hyperthermia associated with acute exposure to audiogenic stress. Muscimol-treated rats did not differ from vehicle-injected controls during a fourth drug-free exposure to audiogenic stress or to exposure to a novel stressor, restraint, several days later. These findings clearly implicate the nucleus raphe pallidus in mediating the autonomic responses to acute audiogenic stress but not in the development of habituation to repeated exposure to audiogenic stress (Nyhuis et al., 2016).

Hypothalamus. Identification of brain areas that control sympathetic outflow has been facilitated by trans-neuronal tract-tracing experiments using the pseudorabies virus. Using this tracer, several laboratories have demonstrated that neurons from the PVN and the lateral hypothalamic area project directly to sympathetic preganglionic neurons in the thoracic spinal cord. Each neuron in these descending pathways from the hypothalamic nuclei projects to only one branch of the autonomic nervous system, either sympathetic or parasympathetic, but not both. In addition, a similar segregation occurs within the suprachiasmatic nucleus, such that circadian variations in autonomic activity can be regulated. This functional separation within the hypothalamus reflects the anatomical separation of the preganglionic cell bodies of the two branches of the autonomic nervous system at the level of the spinal cord. These studies also revealed that hypothalamic nuclei are involved in regulation of sympathetic outflow to a variety of peripheral target tissues (Buijs, 2013; Buijs et al., 2003).

In a report from Ranson et al. (1998), descending projections from the PVN (primarily the medial parvocellular subnucleus) were visualized using an anterograde tracer, and sympathetic preganglionic cells in the intermediolateral area of the spinal cord were labeled with a retrograde tracer injected into the stellate ganglion. Their findings indicated that PVN terminals apparently made synaptic contact with the dendrites and soma of sympathetic preganglionic neurons. In addition, PVN neurons also projected to the NTS, parabrachial nuclei, the dorsal motor nucleus of the vagus, and the raphe nuclei. Further studies revealed that a significant proportion of these spinally projecting PVN neurons were oxytocinergic. Physiological experiments demonstrated that these oxytocinergic PVN neurons excited cardiac sympathetic preganglionic neurons controlling heart rate (Yang, Han, & Coote, 2009). Additional studies indicate that direct PVN inputs to parasympathetic preganglionic neurons influence vagal activity in the heart, liver, and pancreas (Dampney, 2011).

The dorsomedial hypothalamus (DMH) also appears to have significant impact on sympathetic nervous system responses to acute stressors. Stress-induced activation of DMH neurons results in increases in arterial pressure and elevations in sympathetic input to the heart, blood vessels, and brown adipose tissue. Given that the DMH does not project directly to sympathetic preganglionic neurons in the spinal cord, this hypothalamic area must act through other clusters of sympathetic premotor neurons. Several groups have demonstrated descending projections from the DMH to the RVLM (sympathetic vasomotor responses) and the raphe pallidus (sympathetic drive to the heart) that mediate these stress-related effects (Fontes et al., 2011; Horiuchi et al., 2006).

Additional hypothalamic nuclei with direct projections to sympathetic preganglionic neurons include the dorsal hypothalamic area, lateral hypothalamic area, perifornical area, and the retrochiasmatic nucleus. Neurons of the lateral hypothalamic area are similar to the PVN in that they also project to parasympathetic preganglionic neurons (Saper et al., 1976).

Forebrain areas. Many experiments have identified the central nucleus of the amygdala as an important brain area in the regulation of cardiovascular responses to fear- and anxiety-provoking situations. Projections from the central nucleus of the amygdala to the parabrachial nucleus, the NTS, the RVLM, and the dorsal motor nucleus of the vagus suggest that this stress-sensitive area of the limbic system can exert indirect influences on sympathetically and parasympathetically mediated blood pressure responses to stressful stimulation. There are reciprocal ascending projections from some of these brainstem areas to the central nucleus of the amygdala, pointing to a critical and ongoing exchange of information relating to levels of environmental stress and required adjustments in the cardiovascular system (Saha, 2005; Veening et al., 1984).

The insular cortex is the primary interoceptive cortical area and integrates sensory information relating to visceral function, pain, and temperature. The insular cortex also influences spinal autonomic outflow through a projection to the lateral hypothalamus. In addition, the ventral anterior cingulate cortex, through its extensive interconnections with the amygdala, hypothalamus, and brain stem, modulates peripheral autonomic activity.

The medial prefrontal cortex (mPFC) is well-positioned to influence sympathetic outflow during stress given its projections to the NTS, posterior hypothalamus, central nucleus of the amygdala, parabrachial nucleus, and RVLM. Experiments that have employed lesions, local administration of neurotransmitter agonists or antagonists, or direct electrical stimulation of subregions of the mPFC suggest that the prelimbic subregion inhibits sympathetic outflow but increases parasympathetic activity. In contrast, the infralimbic subregion enhances sympathetic outflow during exposure to acute stress. Although the hippocampus has no direct projections to brainstem autonomic nuclei, it does send nerve terminals to NTS-projecting regions of the mPFC, including the infralimbic cortex, suggesting that hippocampal actions on autonomic function might involve this ascending projection to the mPFC (McKlveen et al., 2015; Ulrich-Lai & Herman, 2009).

Another pathway of interest from the infralimbic cortex is its projection to the BNST and then to autonomic cell groups within the PVN. In a series of experiments, Radley et al. (2006) revealed that neurons in the infralimbic cortex exerted tonic inhibitory control over PVN neurons that projected to brainstem and spinal autonomic centers in response to acute restraint stress. These findings suggest that the infralimbic cortex may stimulate autonomic outflow through a descending pathway to the brainstem but inhibit autonomic outflow during acute stress through a pathway to BNST and then to autonomic cell groups within the PVN.

Central command and control. In a classic experiment using double-virus trans-neuronal labeling of stellate sympathetic preganglionic neurons innervating the heart and chromaffin cells of the adrenal medulla, Jansen et al. (1995) reported that several areas in the brainstem and hypothalamus were labeled with one or both viruses. In the brainstem, these areas included the RVLM, the rostral ventromedial medulla, and the caudal raphe nuclei (magnus, pallidus, and obscurus). In the midbrain, neurons in the caudal ventrolateral PAG were labeled, and in the hypothalamus labeled neurons were noted in the PVN, periformical area, and lateral hypothalamic area. These investigators concluded that double-labeled neurons in the hypothalamus, midbrain, and brainstem could serve as central "command neurons" that would simultaneously activate sympathetic outflow to multiple target tissues during exposure to severely threatening situations such as those occurring during the flight-or-flight response.

Dampney (2011) presented a more expansive view of hypothalamic command neurons such that they could direct the patterned activities of somatomotor, autonomic, and endocrine outputs during highly stereotyped behaviors. Using the fight-or-flight response as an example, hypothalamic command neurons would receive input from peripheral sensory receptors and other brain areas involved in regulation of emotions and project to the PVN to stimulate ACTH release, project to sympathetic preganglionic neurons to stimulate increased heart rate or release of EPI from the adrenal medulla, and project to motor cortex and striatum to activate specific patterns of behavior related to defensive actions.

Experimental evidence in support of this broader view of command neurons was presented by Krout et al. (2003), based upon results of double-virus tract tracing experiments in laboratory rats. In the first experiment, a retrograde neuronal tracer was injected into the lateral parafascicular thalamic nucleus, which projects to motor cortex and to striatum. A second retrograde trans-neuronal tracer was injected into the stellate ganglion, which provides sympathetic input to the heart. They demonstrated double-labeling of cholinergic neurons of the pedunculopontine tegmental nucleus (PPN). In a second experiment, one trans-neuronal tracer was injected into primary motor cortex and the other into the stellate ganglion. Double-labeled neurons were detected in the lateral hypo-thalamic area (LHA), where 50% of the neurons contained orexin, and in the PPN, where 95% of neurons were cholinergic. Other double-labeled neurons were found in areas of cortex, hypothalamus, and brainstem. The double-labeled neurons in the PPN and the LHA likely affect motor activity and sympathetic drive to the heart through multisynaptic connections.

Summary

This section has provided a brief and highly selective overview of the central reg-ulation of the sympathetic nervous system. A great deal depends on the constant flow of visceral sensory input to these autonomic brain circuits, the distribution of this information to multiple locations in the brainstem, midbrain, and fore-brain, followed by the production of patterned outflow of sympathetic premotor cell groups to the preganglionic neurons in the intermediolateral cell group of the thoracic and lumbar spinal segments. These patterns of sympathetic out-flow can range from the equivalent of a five-alarm fire during the fight-or-flight response to more modest levels of activation in response to changing levels of arousal or to moment-to-moment changes in blood pressure. As we will see in subsequent chapters, the sympathetic nervous system and the adrenal medulla are remarkably tuned to levels of stressful stimulation, and the magnitude of the responses can habituate with repeated exposure to the same stressor or show facilitation when a novel stressor is presented following habituation to a prior stressor (McCarty, 2016).

Brain Circuits Involved in Control of the HPA Axis

A major milestone in research on stress and the brain was the demonstration of binding sites for ^{3}H-corticosterone in the hippocampal pyramidal cells of CA1–3 and the granule cells of the dentate gyrus of laboratory rats (Gerlach & McEwen, 1972). This finding from the laboratory of Dr. Bruce McEwen at the Rockefeller University forged a critical link between the secretory activity of the adrenal cortex and genomic effects within a brain area associated with learning and memory and sensitivity to acute and chronic stressors. It also stimulated continuing investigations of genomic effects of glucocorticoids on nerve cells in many areas of the brain (Joëls & Baram, 2009).

PVN Afferents

Herman and his colleagues have produced several excellent overviews of the axonal inputs to CRF-containing neurons in the PVN and their responsiveness to stressful stimuli (Herman, 2013; Herman et al., 2003; McKlveen et al., 2015; Myers et al., 2017; Ulrich-Lai & Herman, 2009). In addition to these PVN afferents, there are additional brain areas that feed into the PVN through these directly projecting pathways. An overview of brain areas that project directly to the PVN is included in Figure 5.2.

Brainstem and midbrain areas. Several brain areas are involved in regulation of the HPA axis. A brief description of relevant areas follows.

NTS. CRF-containing neurosecretory neurons within the PVN receive a dense catecholaminergic projection from the A2/C2 adrenergic cell groups in the vicinity of the NTS. These NE- and EPI-containing cells groups appear to exert a stimulatory effect on CRF release by signaling through α_1 adrenergic receptors. Microdialysis studies have provided clear evidence of enhanced NE release in the PVN following exposure to different stressors (Pacak et al., 1995). This NTS

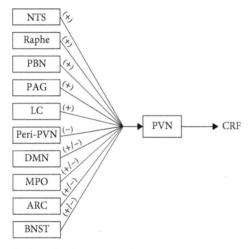

Figure 5.2. Compilation of 10 brain areas that send direct monosynaptic excitatory (+) and/or inhibitory (–) projections to the parvocellular portion of the hypothalamic paraventricular nucleus (PVN). Parvocellular neurons release CRF at the level of the median eminence, where it is conveyed to anterior pituitary corticotropes that release ACTH.

Abbreviations: NTS: nucleus tracti solitarii; raphe: raphe nuclei located in the brainstem; PBN: parabrachial nuclei; PAG: periaqueductal gray; LC: locus coeruleus; peri-PVN: GABAergic neurons located in close proximity to PVN parvocellular neurons; DMN: dorsomedial nucleus of the hypothalamus; MPO: medial preoptic area; ARC: arcuate nucleus; BNST: bed nucleus of the stria terminalis.

pathway conveys critical information regarding disruptions to homeostasis in the periphery, including LiCl-induced illness, hypovolemia, hypoxia, hypotension, and immune activation. In addition, increasing CORT levels appear to block the stimulatory effects of NE in the PVN (Herman et al., 2003; Myers et al., 2017).

Herman (2018) reviewed the effects of NTS neurons that contain NE or EPI on CRF neurons in the PVN. NE released from nerve terminals in the PVN act via α_1 adrenergic receptors on CRF-containing neurons or through presynaptic activation of glutamate release to stimulate the HPA axis during exposure to acute stress.

Raphe nuclei. There is a modest serotonin (5-HT) input directly to CRF-containing neurons in the PVN that originates from the dorsal and to a lesser extent the median raphe nuclei. Release of 5-HT from these nerve terminals appears to signal through $5HT_{1A}$ receptors to stimulate CRF release. Projections from the dorsal and medial raphe nuclei also innervate areas surrounding the PVN and this matter will be discussed in the following subsections (Herman et al., 2003; Myers et al., 2017).

PAG. Several subdivisions of the PAG send direct projections to CRF-containing neurons in the PVN, and these subdivisions may support stressor-specific neural and behavioral responses. Some of these inputs appear to be stimulatory and involve glutamate signaling. In particular, a variety of stressors stimulates enhanced neuronal activity in the dorsolateral PAG, including audiogenic stress, swim stress, restraint stress, and exposure to a predator (Herman et al., 2003; Myers et al., 2017).

Parabrachial nuclei. Several parabrachial nuclei send direct projections to the PVN. These terminals appear to be mostly glutamatergic, suggesting a stimulatory role for these inputs on CRF secretion. The parabrachial nuclei are activated by stressors as diverse as LiCl-induced illness and restraint stress and serve as a key brain area for integration of autonomic and neuroendocrine responses (Herman et al., 2003; Myers et al., 2017).

Locus coeruleus (LC). The LC (A6 noradrenergic cell group) contains the greatest concentration of NE-expressing neurons in the brain. Although the LC provides a dense innervation of the hippocampus and cerebral cortex, it provides relatively few nerve terminals in the vicinity of CRF cell bodies in the PVN. LC input to the PVN appears to be more important during exposure to an acute stressor versus exposure to chronic intermittent stressors (Herman et al., 2003; Myers et al., 2017).

Hypothalamus. Several hypothalamic nuclei and cell groups provide significant innervation of the CRF-containing neurons within the parvocellular portion of the PVN. The majority of these synaptic inputs contain GABA and appear to be inhibitory in nature. These projections will be discussed in greater detail in the following subsections.

Peri-PVN zone. The PVN is surrounded by stress-sensitive GABAergic neurons that express subunits for glutamate receptors. When these neurons are activated by other brain areas through a glutamate signaling pathway, they release GABA onto PVN neurons, thereby inhibiting release of CRF. The suprachiasmatic nucleus inhibits CORT secretion through input to these peri-PVN neurons (Herman et al., 2003).

Dorsomedial nucleus. This nucleus appears to provide a mix of stimulatory and inhibitory inputs to parvocellular PVN neurons. There is a wealth of anatomical and physiological evidence to support stimulatory glutamatergic inputs from the dorsomedial nucleus to the PVN. There is also evidence of neurons in dorsomedial nucleus that provide inhibitory GABA inputs to PVN neurons (Herman et al., 2003).

Medial preoptic area (MPO). The MPO resembles the dorsomedial nucleus in providing excitatory and inhibitory inputs to the PVN depending on the cell type and subarea being considered. For example, stimulation of the medial portion of the nucleus activates GABAergic neurons that decreased CRF release. In contrast, stimulation of more laterally placed cell groups increased firing rates of parvocellular neurons. The lateral regions of the medial preoptic area contain intermingled GABA and glutamate neurons, and this finding explains in part the stimulatory versus inhibitory effects of MPO inputs to the PVN. Neurons in the MPO also express receptors for androgens, estrogen, and progesterone, and may serve as an interface between gonadal hormones and regulation of the HPA axis. It should be noted that parvocellular PVN neurons do not express receptors for gonadal steroids; thus, the sensitivity of the HPA axis to gonadal steroids must be conveyed by afferent projections into the PVN (Herman et al., 2003).

Arcuate nucleus. Projections from the arcuate nucleus to the PVN may convey information relevant to states of energy homeostasis. Arcuate nucleus neurons are responsive to circulating glucose, leptin, and insulin and stimulate as well as inhibit food intake depending on the pattern of activation of neuronal cell groups. Several experiments suggest that the HPA axis is activated by negative as well as positive energy balance, suggesting that both types of deviations from a homeostatic set point are interpreted as stressful stimuli (Herman et al., 2003).

Bed nucleus of the stria terminalis (BNST). The BNST is a complex limbic forebrain structure now considered part of the extended amygdala (Alheid & Heimer, 1988), and it includes 20 cell groups arranged along an anterior-to-posterior axis. Cell groups of the BNST play a major role in regulating the HPA axis via projections to CRF-containing neurons in the PVN. A majority of these inputs, especially from the anterior portions of the BNST, appear to be GABA-containing inhibitory nerve terminals that affect basal secretory activity as well as stress-induced activation of the HPA axis. Another type of influence is exerted by the fusiform nucleus of the BNST, which contains CRF-positive neurons that project to CRF-containing PVN neurons. Local release of CRF in the PVN activated the HPA axis, with increases in circulating CORT. The impact of BNST cell groups on stress responsiveness is dependent upon the frequency and repetition of the stressors. For example, lesions of the anteroventral BNST reduced HPA responses to an acute stressor, but potentiated HPA responses to a chronic unpredictable stress paradigm. The posterior-medial BNST appears to play a role in dampening sensitization of the HPA axis after prolonged exposure to stressful stimulation. Neurons in the posterior-medial subdivisions of the BNST express androgen and estrogen receptors, and studies have indicated that androgen-expressing neurons project to the PVN and appear to stimulate HPA axis activity (Crestani et al., 2013).

Radley and Sawchenko (2015) have studied the contributions of the anterior portion of the BNST on enhanced HPA responses following two weeks of chronic variable stress (sensitization) versus dampened HPA responses following two weeks of chronic intermittent restraint stress (habituation). Sensitization of HPA responses was accompanied by reduced activation of Fos and reduced expression of glutamic acid decarboxylase (GAD) in GABA neurons in the anterior BNST. In contrast, habituation of HPA responses was associated with consistent levels of activation of Fos and increased GAD expression in GABA neurons in the anterior BNST.

The posterior BNST exhibits abnormal expression of CRF_2 receptors associated with PTSD-like behavioral symptoms. The pBNST sends dense inhibitory projections to several stress-sensitive brain regions, including the LC, medial amygdala, and PVN. These circuits may be involved in coordinating the neuroendocrine, autonomic, and behavioral responses to stress. Optogenetic activation of CRF_2-positive neurons in the pBNST resulted in decreased anxiety-like behavior, reduced HPA axis responses, and decreased fear memory for the stressor (Henckens et al., 2017).

The BNST is also a critical part of a stress-sensitive circuit involving the hippocampus → BNST → PVN that is sexually dimorphic and involved in fear states of long duration as well as extended responses to stress. The BNST may also play an important role in mood and anxiety disorders (Lebow & Chen, 2016).

Indirect Pathways Affecting the PVN

Several brain areas, including the hippocampus and the prefrontal cortex, have long been associated with regulation of the HPA axis. Yet these and other brain areas lack direct projections to parvocellular PVN neurons and must exert their effects on the HPA axis through other areas that have direct projections to the

PVN. These indirect-projecting brain areas will be discussed in the following subsections.

Hippocampus. The hippocampus has long been known to play an important role in negative feedback regulation of the HPA axis (e.g., Gerlach & McEwen, 1972). It is somewhat surprising, therefore, that this critical target for circulating CORT does not send a direct projection to the PVN. Several experimental strategies have been employed to demonstrate that hippocampal neurons inhibit HPA axis activity under basal conditions and terminate HPA responses to acute psychogenic stressors (e.g., restraint stress, exposure to a strange environment, audiogenic stress) but not to reactive stressors (hypoxia or ether exposure). A circumscribed set of neurons in the ventral subiculum appears to play a major role in inhibiting HPA responses to psychogenic stressors through projections to the BNST, the peri-PVN zone, the MPO, and the dorsomedial hypothalamic nucleus.

Prefrontal cortex (PFC). The prelimbic prefrontal cortex (plPFC) sends glutamatergic projections to the anterior portion of the BNST. The infralimbic prefrontal cortex (ilPFC) sends direct projections to many brain areas, including the NTS, multiple subregions of the BNST, the dorsomedial nucleus of the hypothalamus, the posterior hypothalamus, and the MPO (Wood et al., 2019). In response to acute stress, the plPFC plays an inhibitory role in regulating the activity of the HPA axis, and this effect appears to be mediated by GRs. In contrast, the ilPFC was shown by Radley et al. (2006) to exert a stimulatory effect on PVN neuroendocrine neurons during acute exposure of laboratory rats to restraint stress. The ilPFC also exerts a negative feedback effect on the HPA axis during chronic exposure to stressful stimulation (McKlveen et al., 2015).

Exposure to chronic variable stress (CVS) does not result in habituation of HPA axis responses. Following exposure of rats to CVS, a stress-responsive circuit was identified that encompassed cortical, hypothalamic, and brainstem nuclei, including the NTS, posterior hypothalamic nucleus, and the mPFC (Flak et al., 2012).

Amygdala. Widespread activation of the amygdala stimulates HPA axis activity. To gain greater anatomical precision, studies have focused on the contributions of the central, basolateral, and medial subnuclei during exposure of laboratory animals to various stressor paradigms.

Central nucleus of the amygdala. The central nucleus appears to stimulate CRF synthesis and release from parvocellular PVN neurons when laboratory animals are exposed to various reactive stressors such as immune activation following a peripheral IL-1β injection, hemorrhage, and visceral illness following administration of lithium chloride (LiCl). In contrast, psychogenic stimuli such as novelty, restraint, footshock, or air-puff startle result in a minimal increase in neuronal activation. To further differentiate between responses to reactive versus psychogenic stressors, conditioning experiments have revealed that neuronal activation in the central nucleus can be conditioned by administration of LiCl but not by fearful experiences. The central nucleus sends efferent projections to the NTS, lateral parabrachial nucleus, and some subgroups of the BNST. The projection from the central nucleus involves GABAergic neurons making synaptic contact with postsynaptic GABAergic neurons in the BNST. Thus, the central nucleus → BNST → PVN pathway appears to utilize sequential GABAergic inhibitory inputs such that activation of CRF-containing neurons occurs by disinhibition.

Medial nucleus of the amygdala. The medial nucleus also exerts a stimulatory effect on the HPA axis. Neurons of the medial nucleus are much more responsive to psychogenic stressors such as restraint stress, exposure to a novel environment, and fear conditioning, but are much less responsive to reactive stressors such as ether stress, hypovolemia, and immune activation. Neurons in the medial nucleus of the amygdala project to several brain areas that project to the PVN, including several subregions of the BNST, the MPO, the anterior hypothalamus, and the peri-PVN zone. Many of these areas that project to the PVN involve GABAergic neurons. In addition, central nucleus efferents also express GAD and appear to employ GABA as an inhibitory neurotransmitter. Similar to the central nucleus but not overlapping with it, the medial nucleus appears to activate PVN neurons by a process of disinhibition.

Basolateral nucleus of the amygdala. The anterior portion of the basolateral nucleus sends prominent projections to the central and medial nuclei of the amygdala, whereas the posterior portion of this nucleus sends some efferent projections to the BNST and select hypothalamic nuclei. The basolateral nucleus plays a critical role in integrating the effects of stress on the HPA axis and memory for stressful experiences. During a chronic stress protocol, the basolateral nucleus was activated by novel stressors, pointing to a role in HPA axis sensitization (Herman et al., 2003).

Lateral septum. Ventrolateral septal neurons do not project directly to the PVN, but do innervate the peri-PVN zone and other PVN-projecting hypothalamic nuclei, including the anterior hypothalamus, medial preoptic area, and the lateral hypothalamus. The vast majority of neurons in this portion of the septal complex express GABAergic markers, thus suggesting an inhibitory influence on PVN-projecting cell groups. As these PVN-projecting cell groups contain glutamatergic as well as GABAergic neurons, the lateral septum is well positioned to modulate HPA axis activity through stimulatory as well as inhibitory inputs to the PVN (Herman et al., 2003).

In laboratory rats with highly selective excitotoxic lesions of the lateral septum, Singewald et al. (2011) reported that lesioned rats had enhanced plasma ACTH and CORT responses to acute swim stress, as well as a more passive coping style characterized by more floating and reduced active escape behavior. Intraseptal GR receptor blockade modulated the behavioral responses, but not the HPA responses to swim stress. Intraseptal administration of a 5-HT$_{1A}$ receptor antagonist resulted in enhanced and extended ACTH and CORT responses to swim stress. In contrast, a 5-HT$_{1A}$ receptor agonist dampened HPA responses to swim stress and decreased passive coping behaviors. These findings strongly point to a role for the lateral septum in promoting active stress coping behaviors and inhibition of HPA axis activation that are mediated in part by intra-septal 5-HT$_{1A}$ signaling.

Thalamus. Several thalamic nuclei are stress responsive, as indicated by post-stressor induction of the immediate early gene, *c-fos*. Of these, the posterior portion of the paraventricular nucleus of the thalamus (pPVT) appears to be a critical relay for regulating HPA responses to chronic intermittent exposure to stressors. In particular, the pPVT is activated by a novel stressor in animals previously exposed to a homotypic stressor each day for several days. This stressor paradigm resulted in enhanced HPA axis responses to the novel stressor, a process known as facilitation. Lesions of the pPVT have been shown to block habituation to repeated presentation of the same stressor as well as facilitation to a novel stressor (Bhatnagar & Dallman, 1998; Bhatnagar et al., 2002).

The pPVT is well-positioned anatomically to play an important role in habituation and facilitation of HPA, behavioral, and possibly autonomic responses to chronic intermittent stress (Hsu et al., 2014). The neural inputs to the rat pPVT have been studied using tract-tracing techniques, and include prelimbic, infralimbic, and insular cortical areas; the hippocampal subiculum; the dorsomedial nucleus, suprachiasmatic nucleus, arcuate nucleus, and the lateral hypothalamic area of the hypothalamus; PAG; parabrachial nucleus; entorhinal cortex; zona incerta; amygdala; and the BNST. Brain areas receiving projections from the pPVT include the infralimbic cortex, dorsal agranular insular cortex, entorhinal cortex, shell of the nucleus accumbens, central nucleus of the amygdala, basolateral nucleus of the amygdala, BNST, and the suprachiasmatic nucleus. As summarized by Hsu et al. (2014), the pPVT, by virtue of its afferent and efferent projections, receives information related to stressful stimuli, circadian rhythms, and memory processes while influencing HPA responses to stress, mood, motivation, reward, and drug-seeking behavior. PVT neurons also influence neuronal activity patterns in the medial PFC and may influence depression-like behaviors (Kato et al., 2019).

Finally, the pPVT has been advanced as a central processing hub for stressful stimuli. Beas et al. (2018) examined the effect of a locus coeruleus → PVT dopaminergic projection that plays a critical role in responsivity to stress. Approximately 80% of PVT neurons express D2 receptors, and DA signaling is important during exposure to stressors. Stress-induced release of DA from locus coeruleus nerve terminals disinhibits pPVT glutamatergic neurons that project to the nucleus accumbens to enhance adaptive physiological and behavioral responses.

Suprachiasmatic nucleus. This hypothalamic nucleus sends projections to GABAergic neurons in the peri-PVN region and dorsomedial hypothalamus. In addition to its circadian influences, the suprachiasmatic nucleus has inhibitory actions on CORT responses to novelty stress (Herman et al., 2003).

Stress-Induced Synaptic Plasticity in the PVN

Synaptic relationships in the PVN. Our challenge in this section is to understand how brain areas influence CRF release from hypophysiotropic neurons of the medial parvocellular division of the hypothalamic PVN. At the synaptic level, anatomical studies have demonstrated that CRF cell bodies are innervated by glutamatergic and GABAergic axon terminals that mediate fast synaptic transmission in the PVN for regulation of HPA axis activity (Decavel et al., 1992; van den Pol et al., 1990). Monoaminergic and peptidergic neurotransmitters are also present as co-transmitters with GABA or glutamate and exert a slower acting neuromodulatory role on PVN neurons. Both asymmetrical (glutamatergic) and symmetrical (GABAergic) synapses are present in the PVN. Quantitative electron microscopic studies have demonstrated that approximately half of all synapses onto CRF-synthesizing neurons are GABAergic, and the remaining ones are asymmetrical and presumably glutamatergic. These findings have been confirmed by in vivo studies in laboratory mice and rats. For example, microinjections of glutamate into the PVN stimulated increased activity of the HPA axis, whereas administration of an ionotropic glutamate receptor antagonist before exposure to stress blunted the HPA stress response. In contrast, GABAergic signaling has been shown to dampen baseline HPA activity. Microinjections of a $GABA_A$ receptor antagonist under basal conditions resulted in significant activation of PVN neurons, pointing to a release from tonic inhibitory influences of GABA, a phenomenon known as disinhibition. It appears that the activity of CRF neurons is regulated at any given time by a dynamic balance between stimulatory glutamate and inhibitory GABA inputs (Bains et al., 2015).

Exposure to a single stressor such as immobilization or restraint causes an activation of HPA activity and induces long-term priming of the HPA axis to a subsequent novel stressor (Armario et al., 2008). Kuzmiski et al. (2010) explored the synaptic mechanisms of this priming effect and suggested that it was explained in part by short-term potentiation of glutamate synapses in the PVN. Associated with this short-term potentiation of glutamate synapses was a CRF-dependent depression of postsynaptic NMDA receptors, which prevented the vesicular release of an inhibitory retrograde messenger that under basal conditions prevents multivesicular release of glutamate during short-term potentiation. Glutamatergic synapses exhibited a capacity for multivesicular release for up to 72 hours after a single acute stressor. Glutamate synapses in the PVN also appear to be increased following chronic intermittent exposure to stressors, and there are associated effects on HPA axis activity under basal conditions and following subsequent exposure to a stressor (Bains et al., 2015).

Using in vivo optical recordings in freely behaving mice, J.S. Kim et al. (2019) reported that CRF neurons in the PVN displayed rapid activation in response to the stress of white noise (85dB for 5 minutes), with a average return to low basal levels of activity within 4 minutes after noise offset. The response to a second burst of white noise 30 or 120 minutes after the initial burst of white noise revealed rapid habituation of the CRF neuronal response. Habituation of the CRF neuronal response was extinguished after 3 weeks without white noise exposure. In addition, habituation did not generalize between white noise and footshock stressors. Importantly, these investigators did not observe an effect of CORT feedback on CRF neuronal responses to stress or on habituation of the response to repeated exposure to the noise stressor. However, CRF did inhibit tonic activity of CRF neurons under basal conditions. These novel findings challenge traditional notions of how CORT negative feedback operates at the level of the PVN under basla conditions as well as during and after exposure to an acute stressor (J.S. Kim et al., 2019).

The power of inhibition. Under basal conditions, tonic inhibition of CRF-containing neurons in the PVN appears to restrain HPA axis activity. This tonic inhibition is mediated by GABA release that can occur spontaneously or following generation of action potentials and involves stimulation of post-synaptic $GABA_A$ receptors. In stress-naive animals, GABAergic synapses on PVN neurons fail to exhibit long-term plasticity. However, after exposure to an acute stressor, both long-term potentiation (LTP) and long-term depression (LTD) can be induced at GABAergic synapses. Whether these synapses exhibit LTP or LTD is not a consequence of the stressor protocol employed; instead, it is a function of when brain slices were prepared for in vitro recordings following the stressor. LTP was induced only if slices were prepared immediately after a stressor, but LTD could be induced only in slices prepared 90 minutes after the end of the stressor. These temporal windows for opposing forms of plasticity are explained by two different neuromodulators, NE and CORT, which exhibit different time courses for action in the PVN. Specifically, NE, which is released at the onset of a stressor, is essential for LTP through activation of β-adrenergic receptors → activation of protein kinase A → upregulation and activation of dormant mGluR1s on PVN neurons. In contrast, LTD requires CORT acting on cytosolic GRs in PVN neurons. The activation of GRs inhibits an intracellular regulator of G protein-coupled receptor signaling, which amplifies mGluR5 signaling and culminates in the liberation of the opioid peptide enkephalin from somato-dendritic vesicles. Enkephalin acts as a retrograde signal and inhibits the release of GABA from presynaptic nerve terminals (Bains et al., 2015).

Glutamatergic synapses are a key target for several neuromodulators that regulate HPA axis activity. For example, NE, which stimulates the HPA axis during stress, acts on α_1-adrenergic receptors to increase the frequency of spontaneous glutamatergic synaptic currents in PVN neurons. The stimulatory effects of NE on HPA activity were blocked by intra-PVN microinjections of glutamate receptor antagonists, providing further evidence for NE inputs to the PVN acting through glutamate signaling.

Endocannabinoids (eCBs). The eCBs appear to exert a negative impact on HPA axis responses; eCBs are released from postsynaptic cells and act on CB1-type receptors on presynaptic terminals to inhibit release of neurotransmitters, including glutamate and GABA. PVN neurons produce eCBs in an activity-dependent fashion. The release of these molecules at glutamatergic synapses produces depolarization-induced suppression of excitation. Although the contribution of this eCB-mediated, activity-dependent modulation of glutamate transmission to HPA axis activity remains to be determined, one possibility is that it dampens excitatory synaptic input during times of high PVN activity. In hypothalamic slices, application of CORT or its synthetic analog, DEX, stimulates the rapid synthesis of eCBs and inhibits glutamate release from presynaptic terminals through a putative membrane receptor that acts through a G protein-coupled signaling pathway (Bains et al., 2015).

In experiments with laboratory rats, acute administration of a CB1 receptor antagonist (AM251, 1.0 or 2.0 mg/kg) resulted in elevations in basal plasma levels of CORT and enhanced CORT responses to acute noise stress (95 dB for 30 minutes). In contrast, AM251 did not result in increased basal levels of ACTH but, at the higher dose, did potentiate noise stress-induced increases in ACTH. The exact site(s) of action of eCBs in modulating HPA axis response to stressful stimulation awaits further experimentation (Newsom et al., 2020).

CRF Neuronal Responses to Stress Influence Behavior

In an elegant series of experiments in freely behaving mice, J. Kim et al. (2019) demonstrated that CRF neurons in the PVN are exquisitely sensitive to aversive as well as appetitive stimuli. Using in vivo calcium imaging, these investigators demonstrated that CRF neurons in the PVN were activated immediately after exposure to aversive stimuli, including a forced swim test, tail suspension, simulation of an avian predator above the cage, or an i.p. injection of LiCl. In contrast, CRF neurons in the PVN were inhibited following exposure of mice to appetitive stimuli, including presentation of food or a mouse pup using females only.

Optogenetic activation or inhibition of CRF neuronal activity in the PVN was sufficient to induce a conditioned place preference or a conditioned place aversion, respectively, following conditioning trials over a 4-day period. In addition, conditioned place preference (food present) or conditioned place aversion (LiCl injection) could be partially overridden by optogentic control of CRF neuronal activity. Taken together, these findings point to a critical role for CRF neurons in the PVN in encoding the positive and negative valences of various stimuli (Kim et al., 2019).

CRF, Urocortins, and Their Receptors

We have already established that CRF plays a crucial role as a hypothalamic releasing factor that converts stress-related signals that impinge on the PVN into ACTH release from anterior pituitary corticotropes, which in turn stimulates the synthesis and secretion of CORT from the adrenal cortex. In addition, CRF is involved in sympathetic-adrenal medullary and behavioral adaptations to stressful stimulation and plays an etiologic role in several mental disorders.

A large family. However, CRF is but one member of a family of closely related and highly conserved peptides that includes urocortin 1 (Ucn1), Ucn2 (stresscopin-related peptide), and Ucn3 (stresscopin). The Ucns are related to urotensin-1 found in fish and sauvagine found in amphibians. These four peptides contain 38–41 amino acids, share 26%–54% sequence homology, and bind to two distinct G protein-coupled receptors, CRF_1 and CRF_2. CRF_1 and CRF_2 are coded by different genes, share 70% sequence homology, and have distinct distributions in brain areas and peripheral tissues (Bale & Vale, 2004; Dautzenberg & Hauger, 2002; Henckens et al., 2016; Hsu & Hsueh, 2001).

CRF is found in high concentrations in the PVN, central nucleus of the amygdala, and brainstem regions involved in autonomic regulation. Ucn1 is expressed in high concentrations in cell bodies of the centrally projecting portion of the Edinger-Westphal nucleus in the midbrain as well as in several peripheral tissues (Kozicz et al., 2011; Vaughn et al., 1995). Ucn1-positive neurons have been implicated in termination of the stress response and in the effects of rewarding stimuli and drugs of abuse as well as in regulation of feeding behavior, with a pattern of activation that is complementary to the HPA axis. Ucn1 binds to both types of CRF receptors and has been shown to stimulate the secretion of ACTH in vivo and in vitro. Deficits in terminating the stress response have implicated disruptions in regulation of Ucn1 in the pathogenesis of anxiety disorders and depression (Kozicz, 2007; Weninger et al., 2000).

Ucn2 is expressed in the PVN, supraoptic nucleus, arcuate nucleus, the LC, motor nuclei of the brainstem, and the ventral horn of the spinal cord (Reyes et al., 2001), whereas Ucn3 is expressed in the median preoptic nucleus, posterior part of the BNST, anterior and lateral hypothalamic areas, the peri-PVN zone, and the medial nucleus of the amygdala (Lewis et al., 2001). Both Ucn2 and Ucn3 have high affinity for CRF_2 but not CRF_1 receptors. In addition, both peptides are expressed in several peripheral tissues (Table 5.1). Experiments with a triple knockout mouse strain lacking the three urocortin genes revealed a role for brain urocortin signaling in recovery from exposure to stressors (Neufeld-Cohen et al., 2010).

CRF binding protein. An addition modulatory element for CRF and Ucn1 signaling is the presence of CRF binding protein (CRF-BP), a 37-kDa N-linked glycoprotein found in brain and peripheral tissues (Potter et al., 1992). In humans, CRF-BP has been detected in the liver and in blood, where it inactivates CRF, especially during pregnancy when CRF levels are elevated significantly and could stimulate ACTH release from the anterior pituitary. CRF-BP is expressed in high levels in the cerebral cortex, dentate gyrus, olfactory bulb, amygdala, BNST, raphe nuclei, and dispersed cell groups in the brainstem reticular formation. CRF and CRF-BP are co-localized in some but certainly not all of these brain areas. In the anterior pituitary, CRF-BP was co-localized with ACTH in a majority of corticotropes that were visualized. Thus, CRF-BP may have actions independent of CRF in some brain areas, but in others where they are co-localized, it could modulate the effects of CRF by intracellular and intercellular mechanisms. Experiments with transgenic mice that overexpressed CRF-BP or were genetically depleted of CRF-BP (CRF-BP KO mice) failed to reveal dramatic alterations in basal activity or stress-induced responsiveness of the HPA axis (Bale & Vale, 2004).

Table 5.1 Characteristics of the Members of the Family of Corticotropin-Releasing Factor (CRF)-Related Peptides, Including Urocortins (Ucns) 1, 2, and 3

	rCRF	Ucn1	Ucn2	Ucn3
Number of amino acids	41	41	38	38
Homology with human CRF	100%	43%	34%	26%
Preferred receptor	CRF_1	$CRF_{1/2}$	CRF_2	CRF_2
Binding to CRF-BP	Yes	Yes	No	No

Abbreviations: rCRF: rat CRF; CRF-BP: CRF binding protein.

Summary

Understanding how brain areas regulate the activity of the HPA axis has been an active area of investigation since the 1970s. A portion of a single chapter cannot possibly do justice to the wealth of information that has been generated. However, as summarized in the preceding, several key brainstem, midbrain, and forebrain structures play essential roles in regulating the activity of the CRF-containing neurons in the PVN through excitatory and inhibitory inputs. In addition, other brain areas send projections to some of these primary brain regulatory areas, further adding to the complexity of neural information reaching parvocellular neurons within the PVN.

A major goal of research on the HPA axis has been to understand how homeostatic and psychological stressors are transduced by specific brain areas such that neural information conveyed to CRF neurons in the PVN alters HPA axis activity from a basal state to an appropriate level of activation that matches with the nature of the stressor and the prior experience of the individual animal or human. There are also continuing investigations using animal models or human patients that relate to how stressful stimulation can result in inappropriate patterns of activation of the HPA axis in various mental disorders. These dysfunctional HPA patterns of activity may result from altered inputs from key brain areas or from synaptic changes at the level of the CRF neurosecretory neurons within the PVN.

The family of CRF-related peptides and their receptors and CRF-BP were also discussed. CRF, Ucn1, Ucn2, and Ucn3 are found in discrete areas of the brain where they serve as neurotransmitters and neuromodulators that govern physiological and behavioral responses to stressful stimulation and other forms of homeostatic challenge.

Stress Effects on Structural Remodeling of Neurons

Focus on the Hippocampus

Deleterious effects of CORT. Exposure of laboratory animals to acute and chronic stressors can reversibly alter parameters of structural integrity of neurons in select brain areas. Interest in this research area grew out of early experiments that demonstrated the susceptibility of the hippocampus to the damaging effects of high levels of CORT, whether delivered exogenously or associated with the effects of CORT over the life course (Aus der Muhlen & Ockenfels, 1969; Sapolsky, 1992). Additional support for focusing special attention on the hippocampus was explained by the demonstration of binding sites for CORT and sex hormones in this brain area. Thus, the hippocampus provided a gateway into this important area of research that has broadened as new aspects of brain function have been revealed, including neurogenesis and epigenetic changes in gene expression. In the sections that follow, emphasis will be placed on structural changes in neurons in three areas of the brain: hippocampus, amygdala, and prefrontal cortex. These areas make up a prominent stress-responsive brain circuitry and exert significant effects on memory processes, decision-making, emotional responsiveness, and executive functioning (McEwen et al., 2016).

Deleterious effects of stress. One of the first studies to document structural changes in the brain following sustained high levels of stress took advantage of an unfortunate situation. Eight vervet monkeys (*Chlorocebus aethiops*) housed in a Kenyan primate center died spontaneously between 1984 and 1986. At autopsy, these monkeys (4 ♂s and 4 ♀s) were found to have multiple gastric ulcers, a high frequency of bite wounds, and hyperplastic adrenal cortices. Six of the eight members of the experimental group appeared to have been victims of sustained social stress from being low-ranking individuals in captive breeding groups, and all died spontaneously. Only one of six control animals (3 ♂s, 3 ♀s) came from a social group and all were euthanized at the end of specific experimental protocols. The results revealed significant hippocampal degeneration at the light-microscopic and ultra-structural levels, but with minimal damage outside of the hippocampus. There was no evidence of hippocampal structural alterations in control monkeys (Uno et al., 1989).

Sex hormones and the hippocampus. A much more subtle and reversible form of hippocampal plasticity was reported by Woolley et al. (1990) that required no experimental manipulations. Adult female rats were followed over the course of the 4–5-day estrous cycle to determine if the structure of hippocampal neurons displayed alterations that were reflective of changes in circulating levels of estrogen and progesterone. In the 24-hour period between late proestrus and late estrus, there was a 30% decrease in apical dendritic spine density in CA1 hippocampal pyramidal cells. Over the next several days, spine density returned to proestrus levels. No changes were observed in CA3 pyramidal cells or in the dentate gyrus over the same time period.

Building on this finding of hippocampal plasticity over the course of the estrus cycle, Woolley et al. (1990) reported that injections of CORT (10 mg/day × 21 days) in laboratory rats resulted in decreased numbers of apical dendritic branch points and decreased total apical dendritic length in CA3 pyramidal cells compared to sham-injected or uninjected controls. No changes were observed in CA1 neurons or in granule cells of the dentate gyrus. In a follow-up study, laboratory rats that were exposed to chronic intermittent restraint stress (6 hours/day × 21 days) exhibited significant decreases in total dendritic length and in the number of branch points in the apical dendrites but not the basal dendrites of CA3 pyramidal cells (Watanabe et al., 1992b).

Excitatory amino acids. CA3 pyramidal neurons receive mossy fiber afferents from the dentate gyrus that release excitatory amino acids, which may play a role in the dendritic changes following repeated daily administration of CORT or repeated daily exposure to restraint stress. Daily administration of the antiepileptic drug phenytoin or the antidepressant tianeptine prevented the atrophy of CA3 apical dendrites following chronic daily CORT or restraint stress, but did not prevent other CORT-induced alterations in adrenal hypertrophy or reduced size of the thymus. These results were consistent with blockade of the effects of excitatory amino acids released from the mossy fiber inputs to hippocampal CA3 neurons (Watanabe et al., 1992ac).

Magariños and McEwen (1995) reported on the contributions of CORT and excitatory amino acids in the loss of apical dendrites from CA3 pyramidal neurons following repeated daily bouts of restraint stress. Blockade of CORT synthesis with cyanoketone prevented stress-induced dendritic atrophy. Similarly, the NMDA receptor antagonist, CGP 43487, blocked stress-induced dendritic atrophy. These findings indicated that dendritic atrophy precipitated by daily bouts of restraint stress for 21 days required CORT secretion and signaling at NMDA receptors. In a comparison of the ultrastructural changes in mossy fiber-CA3 synapses of control and chronically restraint-stressed rats, Magariños et al. (1997) reported that mossy fiber synaptic terminals of control rats were filled with small, clear vesicles. In contrast, synaptic terminals from chronically stressed rats displayed a repositioning of vesicles, with densely packed clusters near active zones. In addition, the energy-generating capacity of mitochondria was enhanced in the synaptic terminals of chronically stressed rats. These findings were consistent with a chronic stress-related increase in the efficiency of mossy fiber synapses and enhanced release of excitatory amino acids that in turn caused dendritic retraction in CA3 neurons.

Joëls et al. (2004) related the effects of chronic unpredictable stress for three weeks on regulation of the HPA axis. Following chronic unpredictable stress, GABAergic inhibitory input to CRH-containing PVN neurons was reduced while glutamatergic input to dentate granule cells was enhanced. Chronic exposure to stress also reduced synaptic plasticity in the dentate gyrus and the CA1 region of the hippocampus. Finally, there were reduced responses of CA1 neurons to serotonin. These neural and endocrine alterations following chronic unpredictable stress could increase the expression of depression-like behaviors in susceptible individuals.

Karst et al. (2005) described connections between elevated levels of circulating CORT, activation of membrane-associated MRs, and rapid increases in the frequency of miniature excitatory postsynaptic potentials in CA1 pyramidal neurons and reduced paired-pulse facilitation, pointing to CORT-induced enhancement of the probability of glutamate release. Activation of a membrane-associated MR would permit changes in neuronal activity within minutes after stress-induced increases in secretion of CORT from the adrenal cortex. In addition, CORT could bind to cytosolic MRs and GRs and activate gene-mediated signaling pathways that have a much slower onset (Joëls & Baram, 2009).

Further experimental evidence was presented by Christian et al. (2011) in favor of a critical role for NMDA receptor signaling in dendritic retraction following chronic immobilization stress for 10 days in laboratory mice. These investigators employed transgenic mice with selective deletion of NMDA receptors from CA3 pyramidal neurons and compared them to non-mutant C57BL/6 littermates. Control mice displayed significantly increased HPA activity and retraction of short-shaft dendrites of CA3 pyramidal neurons, but not of long-shaft dendrites of CA3 pyramidal neurons. Dendritic reorganization of short-shaft neurons occurred throughout the longitudinal axis of the hippocampus and also included a retraction of dendrites in dorsal CA1 pyramidal neurons. In mutant mice, there was a strikingly different pattern of results, with no evidence of dendritic retraction in hippocampal pyramidal neurons in CA1 or in CA3. Mutant mice did exhibit HPA axis activation and behavioral changes consistent with exposure to chronic intermittent stress.

A further consideration for probing the relationship between stress-induced CORT secretion and dendritic retraction in the hippocampus is the nature of inputs to CA3 neurons. Input from entorhinal cortex to the dentate gyrus divides further through connections between the dentate gyrus and CA3 pyramidal neurons. On average, one granule cell innervates 12 CA3 neurons, and each CA3 neuron sends axon collaterals to about 50 neighboring CA3 neurons, as well as about 25 inhibitory cells. This network of interconnected neurons leads to a 600-fold amplification of excitation, as well as a 300-fold amplification of inhibition. The downside to this high degree of interconnectedness is the susceptibility to damage from excitatory amino acids. Some of these reversible alterations in hippocampal dendritic structure also occur quite naturally, such as during the estrus cycle, hibernation, or exposure to chronic intermittent stress.

Chronic Stress and the Amygdala

Vyas et al. (2002) were struck by the laser-like focus of many investigators on stress-induced structural changes in hippocampal neurons to the exclusion of other brain areas involved in the neural circuitry of stress. The amygdala, another key limbic structure involved in physiological and behavioral responses to stress, was the subject of their elegant study. This group of investigators also employed two models of chronic stress using laboratory rats: immobilization stress (2 hours/day × 10 days) and chronic unpredictable stress (2 stressors/day at random from a group of 8 stressors × 10 days). Exposure to chronic immobilization resulted in dendritic retraction in hippocampal CA3 pyramidal neurons, a finding consistent with previous reports. A remarkably different pattern of results was noted for pyramidal and stellate neurons in the basolateral nucleus of the amygdala (BLA), where there was increased dendritic branching in responses to chronic immobilization. Finally, chronically immobilized rats made fewer entries and spent less time in the open arms of an elevated plus-maze (EPM), indicating increased levels of anxiety-like behavior.

Mitra et al. (2005) compared the effects of acute versus chronic immobilization stress (2 hours per day for 1 or 10 days) on patterns of spine formation in the BLA of laboratory rats. Chronic stress resulted in a significant increase in spine density on primary and secondary dendritic branches of spiny neurons in the BLA. In contrast, acute immobilization stress failed to alter spine density or dendritic arborization when measured 24 hours later. However, exposure to this acute stressor did produce a delayed increase in spine density on primary dendrites in the BLA 10 days later. There was also a delayed development of anxiety-like behaviors in the EPM in acutely stressed rats.

In a later study, Bennur et al. (2007) examined the role of the serine protease, tissue-plasminogen activator (tPA), which plays a key role in spine plasticity and stress-induced increases in anxiety-like behaviors. They exposed wild-type C57BL/6 mice (tPA$^{+/+}$) and tPA knockout mice (tPA$^{-/-}$) to chronic restraint stress (6 hours/day × 21 days) or to an unstressed control condition, and then examined structural alterations in the medial (MeA) and BLA nuclei of the amygdala. In tPA$^{+/+}$ mice, chronic restraint stress resulted in significant reductions in spine density in medium spiny stellate neurons in the MeA but enhanced spine density in the BLA. In contrast, tPA$^{-/-}$ mice exhibited an attenuation of the reduction in spine density in the MeA, but the stress-induced increase in spine density in the BLA was unaffected. Taken together, the results of these studies provided a new perspective on the effects of acute versus chronic stress on synaptic plasticity that emphasizes the differential impact of stressors on specific brain areas and the site-specific effects of molecular mediators. There was also evidence for a strong temporal element related to changes in spine density. These findings may be especially relevant for mental disorders that are characterized by high levels of fear and anxiety (Bennur et al., 2007; Vyas et al., 2002).

Chronic Stress and the PFC

The PFC is another critical component of the stress circuitry of the forebrain (McKlveen et al., 2019). Indeed, it is a brain area that displays remarkable sensitivity to acutely stressful stimuli (Arnsten, 2009). The results of a variety of behavioral paradigms have clearly demonstrated the deleterious effects of stress on functioning in the PFC. For example, rats exposed to inescapable shock displayed impairments in a Y-maze task that were traced back to deficits in selective attention. Exposure of rats to an acute but relatively mild stressor resulted in impairments in accuracy of responding to a PFC-dependent spatial working memory task and often produced a perseverative pattern of responses. In contrast, stressed and control rats did not differ in a spatial discrimination task that was not dependent on the PFC. These and other findings clearly indicate that acute exposure to uncontrollable stressors impairs performance in PFC-mediated behavioral tasks and diverts behavioral control to more primitive brain circuitry, including the amygdala and hippocampus.

A lingering question concerned why the PFC was so quick to disengage from ongoing modulation of behavior soon after animals were exposed to an acute uncontrollable stressor. Arnsten (2009, 2015), in two superb review articles, described the roles played by NE and DA within the PFC of animals under basal conditions and following exposure to acute stress. Under normal, low-stress but alert conditions, basal levels of NE released in the PFC stimulate high-affinity α_{2A}-adrenergic receptors, and neural activity related to working memory is optimized. If stress levels are increased acutely, NE release in the PFC is increased and lower affinity receptors are engaged, including α_1 and β_1 adrenergic receptors. Under these conditions, PFC neuronal function and cognitive performance are impaired. There is an inverted U relationship between NE release in the PFC and cognitive performance such that very low or very high levels of NE release are associated with poor cognitive performance. Results from experiments with laboratory mice and rats, rhesus monkeys, and humans, using a variety of approaches, are consistent with this inverted U relationship (Arnsten, 2009, 2015).

A similar inverted U relationship exits for acute stressors, DA release in the PFC, and cognitive performance. Optimal levels of DA in the PFC act at D1 receptors to facilitate cognitive performance. Higher levels of DA release following exposure to acute stressors appear to act at D2 receptors, with associated decreases in cognitive performance. Another contributor to stress-induced elevations in CA levels in the PFC may be impairments in CA metabolism by glial cells due to blockade of CA uptake by elevated levels of CORT. These findings have been synthesized by Arnsten (2009) to indicate that optimal levels of NE signaling increase the "signal" associated with performing cognitive tasks, whereas optimal levels of DA signaling reduced the "noise" associated with performing cognitive tasks. As the role of the PFC in cognition is compromised by exposure to stressors, other subcortical areas such as the amygdala thrive under stressful conditions and switch the brain from a state of higher-order processing to a state of reflexive and more emotion-laden processing (Arnsten, 2015).

Another series of experiments with laboratory rats using in vivo and in vitro approaches revealed that CORT acts on MR and GR receptors on glutamate nerve terminals in the PFC to enhance the readily releasable pool of vesicles and increase depolarization-induced glutamate release following acute footshock stress. This action of CORT was rapid and did not involve genomic actions of the hormone. The authors concluded that CORT was necessary but not sufficient for this overall effect as other (genomic) factors appeared to contribute to the enhanced depolarization-induced release of glutamate (Treccani et al., 2014).

Cerqueira et al. (2007) were interested in how chronic stress might influence interconnections between the hippocampus and the PFC. They exposed laboratory rats to chronic unpredictable stress for 4 weeks and compared them to handled control rats. Their results revealed that chronic stress dramatically impaired working memory and behavioral flexibility. They further examined the neural correlates of these behavioral changes in chronically stressed animals. The hippocampus sends neural projections to the mPFC, forming glutamatergic synapses on pyramidal cells and interneurons. In control rats, high-frequency electrical stimulation of the CA1-subiculum area resulted in long-lasting increases in the amplitude of the postsynaptic potential in the ipsilateral PFC. In contrast, chronically stressed rats displayed a significant impairment in long-term potentiation in the PFC. In stressed animals, layers I and II but not layers III–VI were reduced in size, but the numbers of neurons in these two cortical layers were not affected.

Radley et al. (2008) examined the effects of chronic restraint stress (6 hours/ day × 21 days) on dendritic spine morphology in the medial PFC (mPFC) in laboratory rats. Sample sizes included 8,091 spines for unstressed controls and 8,987 spines for chronically stressed rats. They observed a significant impact of chronic stress on reductions in average dendritic spine volume and surface area, and both changes were more evident in the distal portions of the apical dendrites. There was also a prominent alteration in stressed animals that was characterized by a decrease in large spines and an increase in smaller spines. These investigators suggested that chronic exposure to stress compromised the ability of dendritic spines to mature and stabilize, and these changes may have consequences for neuronal activity and synaptic transmission.

Employing a different experimental approach, Casabai et al. (2018) exposed laboratory rats to 9 weeks of chronic mild stress, while a second group of rats served as undisturbed controls. Beginning on the fourth week of chronic mild stress, these rats displayed a significant reduction in sucrose consumption compared to controls. This behavioral change reflected a depression-like behavioral phenotype. Their ultrastructural analyses of the ilPFC revealed that chronic stress was associated with a significant reduction in the total number of synapses and myelinated axons in the deeper cortical layers of the ilPFC. In addition, the lengths of synaptic membranes were increased in chronically stressed rats, perhaps to compensate in part for the decrease in total number of synapses. Finally, chronic stress reduced the numbers of symmetrical and non-symmetrical synapses in the deep layers of the ilPFC. These results suggest that PFC pyramidal neurons from chronically stressed rats have significant reductions in intra- and inter-cortical connectivity.

What Does Sex Have to Do with It?

As will become obvious in later chapters in this book, most experiments with animal models of various mental disorders have utilized males and actively excluded females. This state of affairs has constrained an ability to understand why there are prominent sex differences in the prevalence, severity, and response to treatments of mental disorders in humans, with females more likely to develop mental disorders with an adult onset and males more likely to exhibit disorders with a developmental onset. It has become apparent that gonadal steroids play a major role in how the brain changes in response to acute versus chronic stressors. In recognition of this shortcoming in research designs, the US National Institutes of Health issued a policy directive requiring that all grant proposals must consider sex as a biological variable in the description of proposed experiments (Clayton & Collins, 2014). Similar policy changes have also been enacted in Canada and the European Union.

Framing the challenge. In their timely perspective, Joel and McCarthy (2017) suggested a multidimensional framework for the classification of sex differences: (i) persistent versus transient across the life span, (ii) context-independent versus context-dependent, (iii) dimorphic versus continuous, and (iv) a direct versus an indirect effect of sex. Rarely have experiments taken a broad-based approach such as this to understand sex differences in neural aspects of behavior. Joel and McCarthy further reported that their combined studies of human brains have revealed that significant variability in the degree of maleness versus femaleness of specific brain measures was much more typical than internal consistency in the degree of maleness-femaleness across different brain measures. Going forward, they urged inclusion of some female subjects and analyses that include sex as a biological variable. However, studies need not be powered to specifically detect sex differences; rather, they should be sufficiently powered to determine if sex is a contributing variable. There is also a compelling need for development of behavioral phenotyping strategies that work equally well with male and female subjects.

Several excellent reviews have described how males and females differ in the pathways activated by acute versus chronic stress that impact neuronal structure and function in several brain areas (McEwen, 2010; McEwen et al., 2016). I will present several examples of these important sex differences in neural and behavioral responses to stress, and the interested reader is encouraged to consult the many excellent review articles on this topic for additional details.

Sex-stress interactions. Shansky et al. (2010) explored the effects of estrogen (E) on the mPFC → BLA circuit in ovariectomized (OVX) and OVX + E female rats exposed to immobilization stress for 2 hours per day for 10 days or left undisturbed. Neurons in the mPFC, some of which projected to the BLA and were confirmed by injecting a retrograde tracer in the BLA, were then analyzed for apical dendritic length and spine density. There was no evidence of dendritic remodeling in mPFC neurons that were unlabeled (i.e., did not project to the BLA) in unstressed OVX + vehicle and OVX + E females. In BLA-projecting neurons, chronic immobilization stress did not alter dendritic length in OVX + vehicle females. In contrast, chronically stressed OVX + E females displayed increased dendritic branching that was limited to intermediate branches and an increase in spine density in all mPFC neurons in OVX + vehicle females and an increase in spine density in OVX + E females that was limited to BLA-projecting neurons. For purposes of comparison, an earlier report from this group of investigators noted that chronic stress caused a retraction of apical dendrites in unlabeled mPFC neurons but had no effect in BLA-projecting neurons. There were no changes in spine density in either population of mPFC neurons (Shansky et al., 2009). These results suggest that E impacts the mPFC → BLA pathway in ways that make it more sensitive to the effects of chronic stress.

The locus coeruleus (LC) is the major NE-containing nucleus of the brain, and it is more sensitive to the effects of stressors and to the stress-related neurohormone, CRF, in female compared to male rats. In a comprehensive study of the cellular anatomy of LC neurons, Bangasser et al. (2011) reported that the LC dendritic field was larger and denser in females compared to males. Analyses of individually labeled LC neurons confirmed a greater level of complexity of LC dendrites in females compared to males. One consequence of these structural differences is that LC neurons in females may receive and process greater amounts of afferent input in the peri-LC area. This would include limbic projections to the LC that relay emotionally relevant information, possibly translating into greater emotional responses to stressful stimuli in females versus males. Depending on the level of arousal generated by ascending projections from LC neurons, these structural differences could be adaptive in stressful environments; alternatively, they could place females at greater risk of developing some psychiatric disorders such as depression (Bangasser et al., 2011).

Wei et al. (2014) compared the effects of repeated restraint stress (2 hours/day × 7 days) on temporal order recognition memory (TORM) in adolescent and adult male and female laboratory rats. TORM is influenced to a significant degree by the mPFC, a brain area especially sensitive to stress. Chronically stressed male rats did not show a preference for the novel object in a two-choice TORM task, but control males did. In contrast, control and repeatedly stressed female rats displayed significant preferences for the novel object in the two-choice TORM task, indicating no impact of stress on this memory task in females. Electrophysiological studies in mPFC pyramidal neurons revealed that chronic stress reduced glutamatergic neurotransmission and glutamate receptor expression in males, but not in females. To examine the protective effects of E on cognitive and electrophysiological responses to chronic stress, these investigators administered an E antagonist to females each day prior to restraint stress. Blockade of E receptors rendered females susceptible to the effects of chronic stress on the TORM task and in measures of glutamatergic transmission in the mPFC. In contrast, if E was administered to male rats prior to each restraint stress, it protected these males against the decrements in the TORM task and in measures of glutamatergic transmission. Additional experiments revealed that blockade of aromatase, an enzyme involved in the synthesis of E, also unmasked the deleterious effects of stress on mPFC electrophysiology and performance in the TORM task in stressed females. Aromatase activity was much higher in the PFC of females compared to males. Taken together, these results suggest that E protects against the detrimental effects of repeated stress, mediated in part by CORT, on glutamatergic transmission and cognition, and that E levels appear to explain the greater resilience to chronic stress observed in females.

Summary. The three studies highlighted here are emblematic of what is possible if females are included in studies that address behavioral, neural, and molecular effects of chronic stress. There is much catching up to do to understand how sex hormones impact specific brain circuits that are relevant for understanding the etiology of psychiatric disorders in humans. Excluding female animals from preclinical experiments because they are "too variable" is an excuse whose time has passed.

Immune-Sensitive Circuits in the Central Nervous System

Cytokines are large hydrophilic molecules that face challenges in breeching the tight junctions of the cells that form the blood-brain barrier and entering brain areas. In spite of these issues, circulating proinflammatory cytokines and peripheral immune cells have several direct and indirect ways to communicate with the central nervous system (Quan & Banks, 2007).

Over, Under, Around, and Through

One pathway for circulating cytokines to signal the brain involves stimulation of primary afferent neurons in vagal sensory ganglia by proinflammatory cytokines during thoracic and abdominal visceral infections. During instances of infections in the oral cavity, the trigeminal nerves are engaged. Stimulation of vagal afferent activity may involve direct interaction of cytokines with their respective receptors on vagal sensory nerve fibers, or indirect interaction through stimulation of chemosensory glomus cells embedded in vagal paraganglia. Because vagal paraganglia are supplied by blood and lymph vessels, it is likely that vagal afferents also respond to alterations in proinflammatory cytokines in blood and lymph (Goehler et al., 2000; Maier & Watkins, 1998).

In a second humoral pathway, toll-like receptors (TLRs) on macrophage-like cells residing in the circumventricular organs and the choroid plexus respond to circulating PAMPs by producing proinflammatory cytokines. The circumventricular organs, which occur in the midline in close proximity to the 3rd and 4th ventricles, include the subfornical organ, the organum vasculosum of the lamina terminalis (OVLT), the area postrema, the pineal gland, the posterior pituitary gland, the median eminence, and the subcomissural organ. These structures lack a fully formed blood-brain barrier and serve as limited ports of entry from peripheral circulation into the brain (i.e., subfornical organ, OVLT, area postrema), as well as locations for secretion of substances from the brain into the circulation (Kiecker, 2018). As the circumventricular organs are highly vascularized and contain fenestrated capillaries, cytokines in blood can pass through the circumventricular organs and enter the brain by a process of volume diffusion via cerebrospinal fluid (CSF) (Vitkovic et al., 2000).

The choroid plexus is present in all four brain ventricles and produces CSF. Epithelial cells of the choroid plexus surround the fenestrated capillaries that deliver blood from the periphery and form the blood-CSF barrier, which is considerably more permeable than the blood-brain barrier. Although there is a barrier for blood-borne substances to cross into the CSF, some signaling molecules and immune cells are capable of gaining entry into the CSF (Kiecker, 2018; Praetorius & Damkier, 2017). Marques et al. (2007) demonstrated in mice that the expression of genes in choroid plexus epithelial cells was affected by LPS-induced peripheral inflammation. In particular, mRNA levels of IL-1β and TNF-α were rapidly induced. These results were taken as evidence that choroid plexus cells could transduce immune signals from the periphery to the brain. In a broader synthesis of available data, Schwartz and Baruch (2014) proposed that the choroid plexus is well situated to serve as a neuro-immune interface that is capable of integrating signals from brain parenchymal cells with signals from blood-borne immune cells. At times of localized brain inflammation, the choroid plexus can be induced to permit entry into the brain of peripheral leukocytes that can serve anti-inflammatory functions and restore inflamed tissues to a normal state.

Another mechanism of communication from the periphery into the brain involves extracellular vesicles released into CSF from epithelial cells of the choroid plexus. Under basal conditions, choroid plexus epithelial cells secrete exosomes from cytoplasmic multivesicular bodies into CSF. Systemic inflammation activates the exosome secretory process, resulting in enhanced release of inhibitory RNA-containing exosomes into the CSF. These extracellular vesicles readily cross the ependymal cell layer lining the ventricles and are taken up by astrocytes and microglia, where they convey a pro-inflammatory signal (Balusu et al., 2016).

A third pathway involves saturable transport systems to convey a limited number of classes of cytokines from the blood into the brain. These transport systems have been described for IL-1α, IL-1β, IL-6, and TNF-α. The amount of cytokines in blood that enter the brain is modest, but compares favorably with some water-soluble compounds. These transport rates were affected by genotype, age, time of day, and brain area studied (Banks et al., 1995). Finally, a fourth pathway involves stimulation of IL-1 receptors located on perivascular macrophages and endothelial cells of brain venules. Activation of these IL-1 receptors by circulating cytokines results in the local production of prostaglandin E2 and precipitates neurally mediated febrile and metabolic alterations in response to peripheral immune activation (Irwin & Cole, 2011).

Engagement of the various immune-to-brain communication pathways ultimately leads to the production of proinflammatory cytokines by microglial cells (refer back to Figure 4.5). This process involves activation of rapid afferent neural pathways, as well as a slower transfer of peripheral immune status into the brain. Activation of the neural pathway probably sensitizes target brain structures for the production and action of cytokines that are transported across the circumventricular organs and the choroid plexus into the brain. In this way, the immune-protected status of the brain is maintained, but critical information on levels of inflammation in the periphery is still conveyed in several creative ways (Dantzer et al., 2008).

Not So Privileged

There is a long history to the concept of "immune privilege" of the central nervous system (Medawar, 1946). After all, the brain exhibits very low rates of generation of new neurons in adulthood, thus rendering it susceptible to the damaging effects of infiltrating peripheral immune cells. Galea et al. (2007) argued that immune privilege does not imply the total absence of immune system components but, rather, their highly regulated access. They suggested that immune privilege was limited to brain parenchyma, whereas peripheral immune access to the ventricles, choroid plexus, meninges, and circumventricular organs was similar in scope to peripheral tissues. The brain parenchymal cells are bathed in CSF produced by the choroid plexus, and CSF in the ventricles is continuous with CSF in the subarachnoid space between the inner meninges and the outer meninges. Louveau et al. (2015) described functional lymphatic vessels lining the dural sinuses that exhibited molecular signatures matching with lymphatic endothelial cells and that connected to deep cervical lymph nodes. These meningeal lymphatic vessels form a network that provides for clearance of macromolecules and immune cells from the brain. This network of meningeal vessels provides a means by which antigens contained in interstitial fluid that drains from areas within the blood-brain barrier could stimulate an innate immune response in the periphery. Note that the blood-meningeal barrier is more permissive than the blood-brain barrier to entry of immune cells and allows them to circulate within the meninges under normal conditions (Louveau et al., 2017).

Systemic infections in laboratory animals or humans are often accompanied by a fever and changes in behavior that reflect a general malaise. These changes in behavior include decreased activity, lack of interest in social interactions, diminished consumption of food and water, hippocampal-dependent changes in cognition, alterations in pain sensitivity, and increases in slow wave sleep. Peripheral or intraventricular administration of the proinflammatory cytokines IL-1β or TNF-α to laboratory animals induces a spectrum of sickness behaviors in a dose- and time-dependent fashion. Administration of another proinflammatory cytokine, IL-6, does not induce the sickness phenotype but does induce fever. However, IL-6 does appear to contribute to the upregulation of IL-1β and TNK-α in the brain (Dantzer et al., 2008). From an adaptive standpoint, the counter-measures to contend with a peripheral infection reflect reductions in energy expenditures associated with normal daily activities in favor of increased energy expenditures to elevate body temperature and reduce heat loss. Cytokine-induced elevations in body temperature enhance the production of immune cells and inhibit the further proliferation of bacterial or viral pathogens (Dantzer, 2001).

Microglia Rise to the Top

Residents of the brain. Microglia constitute approximately 5%–10% of total brain cells and serve as the brain's resident phagocytes. While they resemble macrophages and dendritic cells in the periphery, they do not share a common lineage. Microglia are derived from erythromyeloid cells of the yolk sac and migrate to the central nervous system very early in embryonic development. In contrast, peripheral monocytes and macrophages are derived from hematopoietic stem cells and are replaced in bone marrow, with new cells delivered through the circulation to areas of need. Microglia are also distinct from other glial cells and neurons, which arise from neuroectoderm. There is an interesting juxtaposition with respect to these phagocytic cell types, with perivascular, meningeal, and choroid plexus macrophages positioned on the outside of the blood-brain barrier looking in, and microglia interspersed among the brain parenchyma looking out from behind the relative protection of the blood-brain barrier (Li & Barres, 2018).

Under normal conditions, microglia represent a self-reproducing population of immunological sentinels within the brain parenchyma. Far from enjoying a leisurely "resting state," microglia observed in vivo engage in constant surveillance of the local environment by extending protrusions to make contact with astrocytes, neuronal cell bodies, and blood vessels. Tissue debris and metabolic byproducts can also be engulfed by these ever-changing extensions, which sample the total extracellular space and brain parenchyma several times per day.

Microglia also react rapidly following brain injury. A highly localized disruption of the blood-brain barrier induced by a laser-focused lesion of a brain capillary resulted in an immediate microglial response that was matched to the extent of damage. In these cases, microglia served a shielding function by walling off the damaged area. A similar response could be mounted if pathogens were detected in the brain (Li & Barres, 2018; Nimmerjahn et al., 2005).

Microglia also stand out in being long-lived based upon a series of experiments by Füger et al. (2017). In laboratory mice, individual microglia were genetically labeled and visualized using multiphoton microscopy, which involved monitoring biweekly for the first 6 months, followed by monthly observations for as long as the labeled cells persisted. The results of this study revealed that neocortical microglia had a median life span of greater than 15 months, with approximately 50% of the microglia surviving for the entire 26–28-month life span of C57BL/6 mice.

Primed to respond. Microglia become more responsive to proinflammatory stimuli with increasing age, a process referred to as microglia priming. Microglial priming involves an enhanced and prolonged response to homeostatic disturbances that is much stronger than in naïve microglia. Primed microglia also undergo structural changes, with enlarged soma and retracted dendritic arbors, and respond vigorously to the presence of proinflammatory cytokines (Wolf et al., 2017).

These findings were of great relevance when a team of researchers examined mechanisms of immune memory and the possible engagement of brain microglia (Wendeln et al., 2018). Mice were given injections of a low dose of LPS (500 µg/kg) once per day for 1 day or for 4 consecutive days. Three hours following the first LPS injection, there was an increase in circulating cytokine levels, but only modest increases in brain cytokines. After the second injection, circulating levels of proinflammatory cytokines were reduced compared to their levels after the first LPS injection, indicating peripheral immune tolerance. Contrary to these changes, brain cytokines were increased after 2 LPS injections, indicating a brain-specific training effect induced by the first LPS challenge. After 4 LPS injections, proinflammatory cytokines were no longer elevated in the brain, indicating immune tolerance. Associated with these training and tolerance effects was differential epigenetic reprogramming of brain-resident microglia that persisted for at least 6 months and reflected a form of innate immune memory. These changes were not driven by direct LPS effects in the brain, partial breakdown of the blood-brain barrier, or by penetration of peripheral immune cells into the brain. Taken together, these findings suggest that immune memory in brain microglia might affect the severity of any neurological insults that occur with an inflammatory component (Wendeln et al., 2018).

Stress sensors in the brain. Frank et al. (2019) reviewed the extensive evidence in support of the view that microglia subserve the function of neuroimmune sensors of stress. Microglia also express receptors for signaling molecules associated with peripheral stress responses, including CORT, NE, and EPI. In addition, microglia also secrete an array of proinflammatory and anti-inflammatory cytokines under appropriate conditions. Exposure to stressful stimuli also impacts microglial function by release of DAMPs in the brain, resulting in a proinflammatory response. In the case of peripheral administration of LPS, a bacterial PAMP that does not cross the blood-brain barrier, the peripheral immune stimulus is conveyed into the brain indirectly, as noted earlier, resulting in microglial activation. Activated microglia may be especially well prepared to respond to further signs of danger to the organism through alterations in molecular, circuit-level, and behavioral alterations (Frank et al., 2019).

Within the brain, microglia are maintained in a surveillance mode by the actions of several signaling pathways, including the CD200–CD200R axis (Cluster of Differentiation). CD200 is a membrane glycoprotein that is widely expressed by neurons, endothelial cells, and oligodendrocytes in the brain, while CD200R is an important inhibitory receptor present on microglia. Exposure to the acute stress of tail shock (100 shocks at 1.6 mA) reduced CD200R expression in subregions of the hippocampus and amygdala and in isolated hippocampal microglia. In contrast, there were parallel increases in expression of CAAT/Enhancer Binding Protein-β, a transcriptional suppressor of CD200R. Intra-cisternal administration of a soluble fragment of CD200 prior to tail shock blocked microglial priming as well as the release of the alarmin, high mobility group box-1 (HMGB1), in the hippocampus. These findings indicate that acute stressors disrupt immune regulatory mechanisms that normally constrain microglial priming (Frank et al., 2018).

Applying the brakes. Much of the foregoing discussion dealt with processes relating to priming of microglial proinflammatory response to PAMPs (associated with pathogens) and DAMPs (associated with tissue damage) through activation of pattern recognition receptors (PRRs). This initial microglial response provides for neuronal repair and recovery. However, if left unchecked, microglial inflammatory responses may lead to continued production of proinflammatory mediators, recruitment of peripheral immune cells to the brain, and possibly the development of various brain pathologies. Such changes may also lead to secondary damage and sluggish neuronal repair processes (Lobo-Silva et al., 2016).

IL-10 is one of several anti-inflammatory cytokines that counters damage done by excessive and unchecked levels of inflammation. Stimulation of IL-10 receptors results in decreased proinflammatory cytokine gene expression by microglia, decreased antigen presentation to T cells, and prevention of apoptosis. Anti-inflammatory cytokines, including IL-10, IL-13, and IL-4, also promote the differentiation of primed microglia into an anti-inflammatory phenotype that is neuroprotective and participates in resolution of the localized inflammation, phagocytic removal of any tissue debris, and repair of damaged tissue. Thus, a dynamic balance must be struck between the proinflammatory and anti-inflammatory phenotypes of microglial cells to ensure that homeostatic challenges are addressed quickly and then promptly resolved (Lobo-Silva et al., 2016).

Summary

A complex relationship exists between the brain and the peripheral immune system. The idea that the brain is immune-privileged has been superseded by experiments that have emphasized an ongoing and active dialogue between the brain parenchyma, the choroid plexus and CSF, and the lymphatic vessels that drain the meninges. Microglia are the resident macrophages of the brain, and they are especially sensitive to acute and chronic stressors. In addition, microglia can recruit peripheral immune cells to the brain. Several anti-inflammatory cytokines play a critical role in dampening the proinflammatory phenotype of primed microglia and preventing damage to healthy neurons and glial cells. Dysregulation of neuron-glial signaling pathways by stressful stimulation in early life, adolescence, or adulthood may play an important role in the development of mental disorders, as will be discussed in later chapters of this book (Calcia et al., 2016; Wohleb, 2016).

Control of Brain Circuits by Optogenetic and Chemogenetic Approaches

Let There Be Light

Advances in the study of neural circuits that control normal and abnormal patterns of behavior in laboratory mice have been enhanced by the powerful combination of genetic manipulations of defined populations of nerve cells and regulation of their activity by precisely controlled optical input. These optogenetic techniques typically include three critical components: (i) microbial opsin genes, with each gene coding for a specific protein that displays light-induced changes in electrical current across a cellular membrane; (ii) methods for eliciting specific opsin gene expression of sufficient intensity in cells of interest within targeted areas of the brain; and (iii) techniques for placement of light sources of specific wavelengths and intensities to control neuronal activity in targeted areas of the brain in freely behaving laboratory animals. The various technical advances that were required finally came together beginning about 2009, and since that time there has been a surge of peer-reviewed papers centering on optogenetic techniques to manipulate the activity of neuronal circuits and behavior (Deisseroth, 2015). Refer to Figure 5.3 for an overview of this remarkable technology.

Three microbial opsins were originally employed in optogenetics research, including the following:

- Bacteriorhodopsins pump protons out of cells and exert inhibitory effects by hyperpolarization of the neuronal membrane.
- Halorhodopsins (HRs) pump Cl^- into the cell and exert inhibitory effects by hyperpolarizing the neuronal membrane. HRs respond maximally to yellow (589 nm) light.
- Channelrhodopsins (ChRs) permit positively charged ions (e.g., Na^+) to flow through the opsin pore, resulting in depolarization of the neuronal membrane. ChR1 responds to green (535 nm) and yellow (589 nm) wavelengths of light, while ChR2 responds to blue (470 nm) light.

These opsins use all-*trans* retinal as the chromophore, which is present in mammalian brain tissue in sufficient quantities; thus, no additional chemical cofactors are required.

From this initial starting point, targeted manipulations of the opsin channel pore of channelrhodopsin resulted in the creation of inhibitory Cl^- conducting channels. Other target manipulations or discoveries of naturally occurring variants of the opsin molecules have made possible faster kinetics, greater

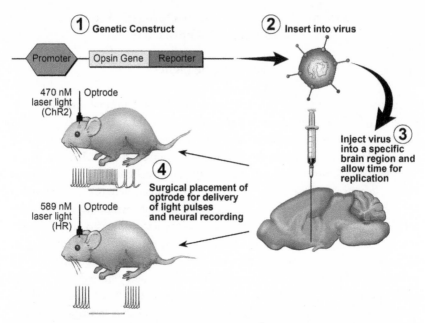

Figure 5.3. Optogenetic control of neuronal activity in freely behaving laboratory mice. 1. Pairing of a bacterial opsin gene with a promoter sequence that conveys neuronal specificity together with a reporter that identifies those neurons that express the opsin gene. 2. Insertion of the construct into a virus, typically an adreno-associated virus. 3. Stereotaxically-guided injection of the virus into a brain area of interest, with several weeks allowed for uptake and replication of the DNA construct. 4. Surgical placement of an optrode that permits delivery of controlled fiber optic light pulses in proximity to the brain area under study as well as direct recordings of neuronal activity. Two simple examples are presented: use of channelrhodopsin-2 (ChR2) paired with blue light at 470 nM to stimulate neuronal activity and use of halorhodopsin (HR) paired with yellow light at 589 nM to inhibit neuronal activity. Additional details are provided in the text (see also Plate 5).

stability, altered ion conductances, and shifted color-response properties (Deisseroth, 2015). Because of the spectral separation of ChR2 and HR, simultaneous insertion of these two opsins allows bidirectional controls of neuronal activity (Zhang, Gardinaru, et al., 2010).

Targeted delivery of the opsin gene to a specific population of neurons was a critical step in the development of optogenetics. Typically, the opsin gene is paired with a promoter sequence that conveys specificity for a particular type of neuron. An example would be a neuron that contains the enzyme tyrosine hydroxylase and employs DA as its neurotransmitter. In addition, a florescent protein marker such as enhanced yellow florescent protein is included to facilitate anatomical localization of the inserted opsin gene. The resulting material is inserted into a viral vector, either a lentivirus or an adeno-associated virus (AAV), with stereotaxic delivery of the viral vector into a localized brain area of interest. The viral vector is taken up by neurons and glial cells in the area surrounding the site of injection, but only those dopamine neurons specified by the promoter sequence will respond to light pulses. Functional levels of opsin gene expression are usually reached within 2–3 weeks after injection into cell bodies, but may take as long as 6 weeks to reach functional levels of expression if injections are in distal axon terminals (Deisseroth, 2015).

Transgenic mice provide opportunities to limit gene expression to defined subsets of neurons. To express opsin genes in subsets of neurons, one can employ short transgene cassettes carrying recombinant promoters or bacterial artificial chromosome (BAC)-based transgenic constructs. Several transgenic mouse lines carrying ChR2 together with the Thy-1 promoter have been generated without observable behavioral or reproductive defects. In addition, more than 290 cell-specific Cre-driver transgenic mouse lines have been made available by individual laboratories and the Gene Expression Nervous System Atlas (GENSAT) project at the US National Institute of Mental Health (Gong et al., 2007). These conditional AAV expression vectors carry transgene cassettes that are activated only in the presence of Cre, and the use of strong ubiquitous promoters to drive the Cre-activated transgene selectively amplifies opsin gene expression levels only in the neurons and glial cells of interest in the brain and spinal cord.

A significant challenge that remained was the nature of the light source required for activation of the opsin molecule that was inserted into brain neurons of freely behaving laboratory mice. The nontrivial hurdles that had to be cleared related to control of local heat generation (LED light sources generated too much heat) and precision delivery of light of a specific wavelength into areas remote from the surface of the brain; additionally, the light source had to be sufficiently powered to overcome light scattering and absorption from chemical constituents of the local cellular environment. These challenges were overcome with the development of optogenetic interfaces based upon laser diode-coupled fiber optics that permitted millisecond time-scale control over neuronal activity. The laser diode light source could be programmed to activate opsin channels with brief pulses of light separated by specified inter-pulse intervals. Eventually, the development of specialized dual-function optrodes made possible delivery of light pulses and the simultaneous collection of electrophysiological measures of neuronal activity (Dufour & De Koninck, 2015).

Optogenetic approaches have been successfully employed to study a range of animal models of psychiatric disorders. Some of these experiments will be presented beginning in Chapter 8. In addition, optogenetic strategies may be on the distant horizon for clinical uses in humans with a variety of medical problems, including psychiatric diagnoses. We will return to this issue in Chapter 16.

A DREADDed Approach

Chemogenetic methods utilize small molecules to activate, inhibit, or modulate neuronal activity in identified neurons (for reviews, see English & Roth, 2015; Roth, 2016; Sternson & Roth, 2014; Urban & Roth, 2015; Zhu & Roth, 2015). In many ways, this methodology resembles optogenetics, but without light as a controlling stimulus. The focus of chemogenetics has been to develop highly engineered G protein-coupled receptors (GPCRs) that will not bind endogenous ligands but will bind pharmacologically inactive small molecules. Initial efforts in the laboratory of Dr. Bryan Roth at the University of North Carolina at Chapel Hill involved subjecting an engineered human M3-muscarinic receptor to directed molecular evolution in yeast cells. The yeast cells were grown in a culture medium that contained clozapine N-oxide (CNO), a compound that readily penetrates the blood-brain barrier, exhibits favorable pharmacokinetics in laboratory animals and humans, and is inactive at naturally occurring GPCRs. During screening, only those yeast cells that expressed a mutant M3-muscarinic receptor that could be activated by CNO survived. After several cycles of selection, yeast cells with an M3-muscarinic receptor containing two mutations were isolated and found to exhibit activation by CNO in the nanomolar range, display no response to the presence of the endogeneous ligand acetylcholine, and lack biological activity in the absence of a ligand (i.e., no constitutive activity). This M3 receptor and CNO were the first designer receptor exclusively activated by designer drugs (DREADD) (Armbruster et al., 2007). In addition, the two amino acid substitutions associated with the mutations noted earlier (Y149C and A239G) could also be employed with the other muscarinic receptors (M1, M2, M4, and M5) to generate a family of DREADD-based receptors, with each family member displaying activation by CNO. To address the problem of CNO being back-metabolized into clozapine in some species, including humans (Gomez et al., 2017), another chemical actuator was identified that activates the muscarinic DREADDs. Perlapine, an FDA-approved antihistamine, is very safe, easily penetrates the blood-brain barrier, and has a >10,000-fold selectivity for the hM3Dq over the hM3 (Chen et al., 2015). With the development of a new DREADD involving the human κ opioid receptor (KOR) and referred to as KOR-DREADD (KORD), it is now possible to co-express hM3Dq and KORD within the same population of neurons to achieve excitation as well as inhibition of neuronal activity in the same animal (Vardy et al., 2015). A summary of DREADDs that have been developed to excite, inhibit, or modulate neuronal activity is presented in Table 5.2.

The challenges in employing DREADDs to excite or inhibit neurons in the brain are similar to those that were confronted by developers of optogenetics. Once a designer receptor is chosen, it must be inserted into a delivery system, dispatched to a specific brain area of interest, and expressed in specific cell types. To achieve a high level of spatial and cellular specificity, the gene for the designer receptor is typically paired with a gene promoter sequence that confers cell-type specificity. For example, pairing a designer receptor with the calmodulin-dependent protein kinase IIα promoter would result in specificity for excitatory glutamatergic cortical pyramidal neurons. DREADDs are typically expressed using an adeno-associated virus (AAV), although other options for delivery systems have been utilized. The AAV viral genome is replaced with DNA that contains the DREADD sequence under study. Once the DREADD-containing DNA sequence is packaged into the AAV capsid, it can be micro-injected directly into a dysfunctional brain region, where the capsid-containing DNA is introduced into neurons and incorporated into host DNA.

In studies of specific neural circuits, it would be highly desirable to deliver designer receptors to neurons that project to a specific brain region. One approach that has been taken to achieve this goal involves the use of canine adenovirus, a viral delivery system that is taken up into nerve terminals and retrogradely transported back to the cell bodies. An attractive feature of this virus is that it

Table 5.2 Designer Receptors Exclusively Activated by Designer Drugs (DREADDs)

	Designer Receptors				
	hM3Dq	hM4Di	GsD	Rq (R165L)	KORD
Designer drug	CNO	CNO	CNO	CNO	Salvinorin B
Signaling pathway	Ga_q	Ga_i	Ga_s	β-arrestin	Ga_i
Second messenger response	↑ Ca^{++}	↓ cAMP	↑ cAMP	β-arrestin translocation	↓ cAMP
Change in neuronal activity	Burst firing	Inhibition	Modulation	β-arrestin signaling	Inhibition

Abbreviations: cAMP: cyclic adenosine monophosphate; CNO: clozapine-N-oxide; GsD: Gas-coupled DREADD; hM3Dq: Gαq-coupled DREADD; hM4Di: Gαi-coupled DREADD; KORD: DREADD based on the κ opioid receptor.

generates minimal immunogenicity. Canine adenovirus has been employed to deliver Cre recombinase (capable of flipping DNA sequences flanked by precisely oriented loxP nucleotide sequence pairs) into nerve terminals in the PFC, where it was transported back to the cell bodies of the PFC-projecting neurons. Next, administration of loxP-flanked DREADDs into the dorsal raphe nucleus provided the measure of specificity, such that only PFC-projecting neurons that acquired Cre recombinase from the canine adenovirus could successfully flip and express the DREADD. Using this approach provides researchers with a technique to target in a highly precise way a set of neurons that projects to a discrete brain region (Junyent & Kremer, 2015).

In a more recent development in this rapidly moving research area, Magnus et al. (2019) recognized from the start the need to develop highly potent and selective agonists for chemogenetic systems that would have direct applications in clinical settings. Their starting point was to select a designer receptor (α7 nicotinic acetylcholine receptor [α7nAChR]) consisting of a receptor domain and an ion channel domain that would respond favorably to a drug currently approved by the US Food and Drug Administration. They searched for a drug that readily penetrated the blood-brain barrier, had an extended half-life in humans, and was well tolerated with minimal side effects, finally settling on varenicline, an antismoking medication. The next step in this process was to genetically engineer the designer receptor to enhance its sensitivity to varenicline. Using in vivo and in vitro experimental approaches, this team of researchers confirmed that extremely low doses of verenicline or a molecular variation could excite or inhibit neurons in the sub-nanomolar range, depending on the type of ligand-gated ion channel fused to the α7nAChR. This exciting new development could accelerate testing of this modified DREADD approach in clinical settings, including in the evolution of targeted therapies for mental disorders.

A CRISPR Approach to Animal Models

GWAS have consistently reported that several mental disorders are characterized by the presence of multiple risk genes, each with a small impact on the resulting phenotype. Based upon these findings, several animal models have been developed that include manipulations of a single risk gene using knockout or knockin experimental approaches. While these studies have provided valuable insights and will be featured in later chapters, they leave open the question of how multiple risk genes act in concert to achieve a dysfunctional behavioral phenotype.

One experimental strategy to develop animal models of a given mental disorder is through changes in multiple risk genes through the use of CRISPR-Cas9 genome-editing tools (Clustered Regularly Interspaced Short Palindromic

Repeats; CRISPR-associated proteins) (Heidenreich & Zhang, 2016). Site-specific nucleases, such as Cas proteins, enable relatively precise genetic modifications by inducing double-stranded DNA to break at targeted locations in the genome. A homology-directed repair pathway provides for a precise recombination event between a homologous DNA donor template and the damaged DNA site, resulting in accurate correction of the double-stranded DNA break. Using this technique, one can introduce specific mutations or transgenes into the genome. Site specificity for Cas9 is provided by a guide-RNA sequence (CRISPR RNA [crRNA]) that is associated with a *trans*-activating crRNA (tracrRNA) that forms Watson–Crick base pairs with the complementary DNA target sequence, resulting in a site-specific double-stranded DNA break. A simple two-component system has been successfully engineered for expression in eukaryotic cells and can achieve DNA cleavage at any genomic locus of interest. The use of in vivo gene editing provides an opportunity to genetically modify neuronal circuits and model pathophysiological changes through gene knockouts or epigenetic modifications without resorting to germline-modified mutant strains. Cas proteins can be delivered to specific areas of the brain using AAVs as the delivery vehicle, although the limited capacity of this virus is a potential problem (Heidenreich & Zhang, 2016). Li et al. (2018) described several promising alternative vehicles for delivery of CRISPR-Cas, including lipid- and polymer-based nanocarriers.

Two early reports demonstrate the promise of CRISPR-Cas9 genome-editing technology. Rutkowski et al. (2019) developed a mouse model of the 3q29 deletion, which confers significant risk for several mental disorders, including autism and schizophrenia. They reported that heterozygous (HZ) deletion of the syntenic interval on chromosome 16 of C57BL/6 mice reduced the transcription of 20 of 21 genes in this segment by approximately 50%. Relative to controls, HZ mice displayed disruptions in social behavior, cognition, and acoustic startle response; sensitivity to amphetamine; and reductions in body weight; and some of these alterations were sex-specific. These encouraging findings provide clear support for the value of CRISPR-Cas in contributing to the development of powerful new animal models for the study of mental disorders.

Tu et al. (2019) used CRISPR-Cas9 genome editing to generate a cynomolgous monkey (*Macaca fascicularis*) model of autism spectrum disorder (ASD) by disrupting the postsynaptic scaffold gene, *SHANK3*, with a two-base pair deletion in exon 12. The affected monkey displayed many of the classic signs of ASD, including repetitive behaviors, disruptions in social behaviors, and delayed vocalizations. This proof-of-concept study in a nonhuman primate species is encouraging and foreshadows expanded use of genome-editing technology in a range of mammalian animal models of mental disorders. Although CRISPR-Cas9 genome editing represents a major step forward in achieving targeted alterations in DNA, it is not without limitations. A significant refinement in this technique was recently reported by Anzalone et al. (2019). Prime editing provides for more precise editing of DNA by insertion of new genetic information into a specified DNA sequence. A prime editing guide RNA serves the dual purpose of specifying the target site on DNA and encoding the desired edit. This new and improved approach to DNA editing holds great promise for the development of animal models of mental disorders that incorporate multiple risk genes.

Summary

Optogenetic, chemogenetic, and genome-editing techniques represent sub-stantial new additions to the neuroscience toolbox that permit highly specific manipulations of identified brain circuits or risk genes involved in regulating behavioral responses to stress in animal models of mental disorders and their appropriate controls. Each technique affords specific benefits and presents some limitations. Sternson and Roth (2014) suggested that chemogenetic approaches have several compelling advantages over optogenetics, including the following:

- The designer drug (e.g., CNO or varenicline) can be administered via the drinking water or injected peripherally, and each is distributed widely in the brain.
- The designer drug can exert a sustained effect on neuronal activation, inhi-bition, or modulation that persists from minutes to hours.
- Activation of a DREADD does not require specialized and expensive equipment.
- From a translational perspective, the most frequently employed designer drugs have been safely administered to humans and they would not present difficulties if these techniques are adapted for clinical use.

In spite of these advantages of chemogenetic approaches, a major disadvantage remains. Optogenetic techniques provide precise temporal control over neu-ronal activation and inhibition, although delivery systems for designer drugs are under development that would address in large measure the issue of temporal control.

Results to date have showcased the power of these two techniques to dissect circuit-level control of behavioral and physiological processes in laboratory ani-mals. For example, chemogenetic and optogenetic techniques were employed to study the effects of cholecystokinin (CCK) neuronal projections from the NTS → PBN and NTS → PVN on regulation of food intake in mice (Roman et al., 2017). Vetere et al. (2017) employed chemogenetic silencing of 21 nodes within a larger network of 84 previously identified brain regions to understand the circuit-level control of fear memory consolidation in mice. Giardino et al. (2018) tackled the challenging problem of teasing apart the effects of parallel projections of orexin-positive neurons in the lateral hypothalamus (LH) that influenced negative versus positive emotional states. Combining chemogenetic and optogenetic approaches, these investigators described two non-overlapping GABAergic projections from the BNST → LH that have opposite effects on emotional state in freely behaving mice. Finally, Muir et al. (2019) presented a valuable review of studies of animal models of depression using optogenetic and chemogenetic techniques. These findings will be discussed in detail in Chapters 12 and 13.

Finally, harnessing the power of genome-editing tools to generate novel animal models of human mental disorders that reproduce alterations in multiple risk genes could be a game-changer. If these newly developed models have behavioral phenotypes that match well with specific human mental disorders, it would open up opportunities to explore circuit-level changes in the brain downstream of the genetic changes. In addition, these newer animal models would provide an excellent platform for testing new drug therapies. This is an area of research that bears watching over the coming years.

Summary

In this chapter, I have presented a brief overview of the critical brain areas that regulate as well as respond to changes in the sympathetic-adrenal medullary system, the HPA axis, and the immune system. These stress-responsive brain areas play essential roles in maintaining homeostatic balance in the face of a constantly changing environment, both internal and external. As we will see in later chapters, these same stress-responsive brain areas contribute in important ways to the onset and maintenance of symptoms of various psychiatric disorders and the responses to various treatments. With the impressive advances in knowledge from employing chemogenetic and optogenetic tools for studying these stress-responsive brain circuits, new targets have been identified for the future development of highly personalized pharmacological treatments to counteract circuit-level disturbances in these debilitating psychiatric disorders.

6

Animal Models in Psychiatry

Over 2,500 years ago, animals were first studied as a means of increasing knowledge of human anatomy and physiology. These early efforts were largely observational, and it was not until well after the birth of the Renaissance that experiments using animals led to a deeper understanding of human anatomy and physiology. For example, in the 17th century, William Harvey's comparative studies of the heart and vascular system in a range of species from eels to birds to mammals led to his foundational writings on the heart and circulatory system of humans (Ericsson et al., 2013).

In the late 18th century, the English physician Edward Jenner observed that people infected with cowpox did not develop smallpox. His experimental studies revealed that people inoculated with cowpox virus were resistant to later challenge with the smallpox virus. In France in the 19th century, Pasteur's animal experiments with the rabies virus led to the development of an effective vaccine against rabies.

In the more recent past, advances in many areas of clinical medicine, including infectious diseases, gene regulation, cardiovascular physiology, cancer biology, anesthesia, embryology, toxicology, metabolism, and nervous system structure and function have been propelled forward by the use of animal models. It is important to note that some of these advances in medical knowledge have benefited from experiments with very simple organisms, including bacteria and their viruses, fruit flies, zebrafish, sea slugs, and the soil nematode, *Caenorhabditis elegans* (*C. elegans*) (Harding et al., 2010).

Evolutionary Connections between the Behaviors of Animals and Humans

Darwin Got It Right

A compelling case can be made that laboratory and field studies of a variety of animal species inform our understanding of human behaviors (Shapiro, 2010). Such a notion caused quite a stir following the publication of Charles Darwin's landmark treatise, *On the Origin of Species*, in which he laid out in great detail his theory of the evolution of species by natural selection (Darwin, 1859). Later, he summarized his work on the comparative study of emotional behaviors in animals and humans (Darwin, 1872). This volume, which was a major contribution to the field of psychology in the 19th century, established an evolutionary connection between emotional expressions in various animal species with those of humans. Darwin's analyses covered a wide range of emotions, including anger, disgust, fear, guilt, horror, pride, shame, and shyness.

Consider the far-ranging implications of the following quote from a third volume by Darwin (1871, p. 105):

> Nevertheless the difference in mind between man and the higher animals, great as it is, is certainly one of degree and not of kind. We have seen that the senses and intuitions, the various emotions and faculties, such as love, memory, attention, curiosity, imitation, reason, &.c, of which man boasts, may be found in an incipient, or even sometimes in a well-developed condition, in the lower animals.

This revolutionary view of the interrelationships between humans and other animals, including those based upon behavioral and psychological traits, remains at the heart of contemporary research with animal models of mental disorders (Kendler & Greenspan, 2006).

Animal Anthropologists

Let's fast-forward to the late 1950s, when ideas were first being entertained of learning about early human origins in Africa by studying nonhuman primates in habitats similar to those experienced by early hominids. One of the first scientists to embrace this approach was Professor Sherwood Washburn (1911–2000) of the University of Chicago. Washburn's interest in this area of research was stimulated during a trip to what was then Northern Rhodesia to attend the Pan African Conference in Prehistory. While there for several weeks, he had many opportunities to observe three baboon troops living in close proximity to his hotel, and was impressed with the scientific importance of conducting careful, long-term observations of baboon social groups (DeVore & Washburn, 1992).

Washburn, a noted physical anthropologist, recruited a new graduate student, Irven DeVore, to conduct the field studies of baboons, even though DeVore had no prior experience with baboons, fieldwork, or Africa. This sounds like a recipe for disaster if you are a graduate student, but their highly successful collaboration (Washburn & DeVore, 1961) represents one of the first attempts to study nonhuman primates in their natural habitats, and it set the stage for many other long-term behavioral studies, including those of Schaller (2010) with mountain gorillas, Goodall (2010) with chimpanzees, and Altmann (1979) with baboons.

The next great theoretical leap in this progression occurred with the publication of yet another landmark volume; this time, it was *Sociobiology: The New Synthesis*, by Edward O. Wilson (1975). In this remarkable volume, Wilson persuasively argued that complex social behaviors of animals, including humans, could be explained, at least in part, as an outcome of natural selection. Altruism, aggression, and parental care were among the behaviors he discussed. In the final chapter of his book, Wilson presented his ideas on sociobiological theory as they applied to humans. This final chapter also served as the basis for a subsequent book that expanded greatly the application of sociobiological concepts to human societies (Wilson, 1981). His theories relating to human social behavior were embraced by many, but there was also a vocal and well-placed group of detractors, some of whom were his Harvard University colleagues (see, for example, Lewontin, 1979). In the end, I think it is safe to say that Wilson's views on sociobiology have stood the test of time.

Pioneering Studies with Animal Models

Three landmark studies from the 20th century have had an enduring impact on how we use animal models to understand human psychopathology. In each instance, the results of these experiments are often presented in introductory textbooks of psychology, and continue to influence the instruction of current generations of undergraduates.

Pavlov Rings the Bell

The noted Russian physiologist Ivan P. Pavlov (1849–1936) received the Nobel Prize in Physiology or Medicine in 1904 for his basic studies on digestion. Later in his career, as many undergraduate students in "Introduction to Psychology" know all too well, he described classical conditioning by observing that dogs tested in his laboratory apparently learned to associate a cue (think a bell ringing) with feeding, as evidenced by salivation in anticipation of a meal. He showed that after a number of pairings of the cue with meal presentation, the cue alone could elicit salivation by a hungry dog.

McKinney (1988) credits Pavlov with conducting the first laboratory experiments with an "animal model" and with recognizing the importance of these serendipitous findings as a means for understanding human psychopathology. In his laboratory in St. Petersburg, dogs were trained to discriminate a circle from an ellipse for a food reward. As the ellipse was gradually rounded to look more and more like a circle (width/height ratio of 9:8), the discrimination of the dogs worsened and, after three weeks, completely broke down. Even when the dogs were later presented with discriminations that were previously easy for them, they displayed persistent disruptions in behavior. In addition, the dogs became highly agitated and resisted being taken from their pens for transfer into the experimental room for testing.

Pavlov labeled the behavioral patterns of his dogs as "experimental neurosis" and suggested parallels with human neuroses. He also discussed ways in which genetic and developmental factors influenced the onset of experimental neurosis in dogs. Finally, he utilized his findings from the laboratory to formulate a theory of schizophrenia in humans that stimulated considerable research in Russia and other countries (Pavlov, 1928, 1941).

Monkey Business in Madison

Harry F. Harlow (1905–1981) was one of the most influential and controversial psychologists of the 20th century. In the course of his career, he received many awards and honors, including election to the National Academy of Sciences and receipt of the National Medal of Science. He had a troubled personal life, drank alcohol to excess, and suffered from frequent periods of depression. His views on women were chauvinistic, to put it mildly. Yet, he was a devoted teacher and a supportive mentor of graduate students, including women, who worked in his laboratory. Many of his experiments with rhesus monkeys would not receive approval from an animal care committee today because of ethical concerns for the welfare of the animals. Yet, many of his methods for best practices in the husbandry of rhesus monkeys in the laboratory were adopted by veterinarians and researchers around the world (Bloom, 2002; Suomi & Leroy, 1982).

After completing his Ph.D. at Stanford University in 1930, Harlow joined the Department of Psychology at the University of Wisconsin, Madison. Because of a lack of laboratory space for his planned experiments with laboratory rats, Harlow began studying primates at the local zoo, and he later acquired space to house primates in an empty building close to campus. Upon completion of extensive renovations carried out by Harlow and his students, this building became one of the first primate research laboratories in the world. A number of years after settling into the building, Harlow established a breeding colony of rhesus monkeys (*Macaca mulatta*) that were used initially to study the development of learning sets (Harlow, 1949).

From their experiences of establishing a breeding colony and placing newborns in a nursery away from their mothers, Harlow and his students quickly appreciated that infant monkeys reared by human handlers in the nursery setting were quite different from infants reared by their mothers. The nursery-reared infants tended to be socially withdrawn, were often observed to cling to the cloth diapers that lined their cages, and they became highly agitated when the cloth diapers were removed for cleaning. These initial observations matched well with clinical reports of Spitz (1945) and Bowlby (1951) on the deleterious effects of impoverished institutional rearing on human infants.

In his presidential address at the 66th annual meeting of the American Psychological Association on August 31, 1958, in Washington, D.C., Harlow summarized his now-classic experiments on infant rhesus monkeys reared with surrogate mothers made of wire mesh with and without a soft cloth covering and with and without a source of milk. This paper was subsequently published in the *American Psychologist* (Harlow, 1958) and remains one of Harlow's most cited journal articles. These experiments were clearly informed by observations of institutionalized human infants, but Harlow and his students were able to probe more deeply into the critical nature of an infant monkey's ties to its mother. Strangely enough, Harlow maintained that the idea for surrogate mothers came to him during a 1957 Northwest Airlines champagne flight over Detroit. He "turned to look out the window and saw the cloth surrogate mother sitting in the seat beside him with all her bold and barren charms" (Harlow et al., 1971). How many glasses of champagne did it take for this insight to occur?

Infant monkeys strongly preferred a cloth-covered surrogate mother to a wire mesh surrogate mother, even when the wire mesh mother contained a milk bottle and nipple. Indeed, some infants would cling to the cloth-covered mother while they nursed from the bottle attached to a nearby wire mesh mother. Harlow termed this response "contact comfort" and dispelled the notion attributed to drive reduction theory that mothers were important only because they provided milk to their infants.

Following these initial studies, Harlow devoted considerable effort to investigations of normal and abnormal primate social development and to laying the groundwork for producing primate analogs of human depression. One such procedure employed by Harlow and his students to induce a syndrome of depressive behaviors was total social isolation for the first 6 months of life (Harlow & Suomi, 1974). They further employed this model system to explore the effects of social isolation rearing of infant females on their maternal behavior in adulthood (Arling & Harlow, 1967), and the effectiveness of engagement with normally reared younger peers (think monkey therapists) in ameliorating the effects of early social isolation (Harlow & Suomi, 1971). Later refinements in inducing depressive-like behaviors in rhesus monkeys involved separating infants from their mothers for fixed periods of time or rearing groups of four infants together from birth, followed by periods of separation (Harlow et al., 1971; McKinney et al., 1971).

Dog Days in Philadelphia

Many graduate students dream of making breakthroughs in their dissertation research that will influence their chosen areas of study for years to come. Needless to say, this is not a frequent outcome as graduate students progress toward the oral defense of their dissertations. However, one striking realization of this dream occurred at the University of Pennsylvania in the late 1960s. Martin E. P. Seligman and Steven F. Maier, while graduate students in the laboratories of Professors Richard Solomon and Henry Gleitman, respectively, joined forces to conduct experiments on dogs exposed to inescapable shocks, which led to the development of the "learned helplessness" model for depression in humans. Seligman, who has spent most of his illustrious career at the University of Pennsylvania, gradually moved away from animal research to focus on clinical psychology, and he is known now for his research and popular writings on "learned optimism," well-being, happiness, and positive psychology. In contrast, Maier has spent much of his remarkable career at the University of Colorado, where he is a noted authority on stress and interactions between the nervous and immune systems in controlling behavior.

A famous quote from Louis Pasteur, "Chance favors the prepared mind," is an apt description of how Seligman and Maier came to design their first experiments on what was to become known as "learned helplessness" (Maier & Seligman, 1976; Maier et al., 2000). In Solomon's laboratory at the time, two graduate students, J. Bruce Overmier and Russell C. Leaf, were launching a study to determine how Pavlovian fear conditioning might influence later avoidance learning. Employing dogs, the animal of choice in the Soloman laboratory at the time, their experimental design involved three phases. In the first, dogs were restrained in slings and received 64 electric shocks to their hind paws, with each shock preceded by a warning light. The next day, dogs were placed into a shuttlebox and trained to jump over a low barrier into an adjacent escape chamber by associating a warning tone with the delivery of an electric shock to the. The crucial third phase of the experiment involved using the light as a warning signal in avoidance testing. A possible outcome in this transfer of stimulus control design was that the light signal, which had never been associated with avoidance conditioning but was associated with footshock, would induce the dogs to jump over the barrier to escape the shock. Unfortunately, the dogs were unaware of the prevailing theory about stimulus control of avoidance, so they often failed to escape the electric shock, and simply huddled down and waited for the shocks to terminate. If, however, the order of training was reversed and avoidance conditioning occurred before classical conditioning, the animals learned both tasks and the experiment could be completed (Overmier & Leaf, 1965).

As is often the case, a deviation in results from prevailing theory could have been discounted as a bothersome artifact or recognized as something quite interesting. Seligman and Maier were convinced that the unexpected results were important and, in fact, resembled a state of helplessness. In an earlier experiment, Overmier and Seligman (1967) exposed dogs to escapable shocks or to identical shocks that were inescapable. Controls received no shocks. When tested later for escape and avoidance learning, controls and animals in the first group learned to avoid shock, while animals in the second group were unable to learn the escape response, an effect that persisted for several days. Note that the first two groups of animals received identical shocks. Follow-up experiments by Seligman and Maier (1967) demonstrated that an initial experience with escapable shock prevented the deleterious effects of inescapable shock on later avoidance learning.

Fifty years after their breakthrough experiments, Maier and Seligman (2016) provided an update of learned helplessness based in large measure on laboratory experiments that have revealed the neural circuitry involved in this phenomenon. Contrary to their original formulation, failure to escape is *not* a learned response; rather, it is an unlearned response to stressful events, with impaired locomotor activity mediated through serotonergic activity in the dorsal raphe nucleus. What is learned is control over stressful events, with detection of control by the medial prefrontal cortex, followed by inhibition of neurons in the dorsal raphe nucleus. They argued that this new and improved formulation was particularly relevant for the treatment of depression.

As an aside, both Maier and Seligman are self-professed dog lovers, and these experiments took a heavy toll on both of them. As soon as they graduated from the Solomon laboratory, they switched to studies with laboratory mice and rats and even humans, and their results matched well with their foundational studies using dogs (Maier & Seligman, 2016).

Animal Models in Psychiatry

What Is an Animal Model?

As we shift gears to begin our consideration of the place of animal models in contemporary psychiatric research, it is helpful to define exactly what we mean by an animal model. As a starting point for discussion, let's consider how the online edition of the *Oxford English Dictionary* defines an animal model:

> an experimental model, especially of a disease or pathological process, using animals in place of humans.

This definition of an animal model clearly favors research on disease processes, where clear parallels exist between animal models and humans. For example, studies of hypertension, diabetes, epilepsy, strokes, and cancers in a variety of animal models have clearly advanced our understanding of these pathologies in humans. If this definition of an animal model was the standard by which current journal editors held manuscripts submitted for publication that involved research with animal models of mental disorders, very few papers would be accepted.

An improvement over the standard dictionary definition of an animal model was introduced by van der Staay (2006, pp. 133–134). In combining elements from several sources to construct his definition, he suggested that

> an animal model with biological and/or clinical relevance in the behavioral neurosciences is a living organism used to study brain–behavior relations under controlled conditions, with the final goal to gain insight into, and to enable predictions about, these relations in humans and/or a species other than the one studied, or in the same species under conditions different from those under which the study was performed.

Based upon his studies of primate models of depression, McKinney (1984, 2001) offered several insights that have broad implications for investigations of animal models of mental disorders. Listed in the following is a highly edited version of those insights, which remain relevant today:

1. An animal model cannot be expected to replicate all salient aspects of a mental disorder found in humans.
2. Animal models represent experimental preparations that allow for highly focused experiments on neuropathological changes and their associations with behavioral changes that would be difficult or impossible to conduct in humans.
3. There is no single "gold standard" animal model for a given mental disorder in humans. Progress is made by comparing results from a range of different animal models.
4. Animal models afford an opportunity to study the main effects of individual neuropathological changes, as well as interactions among different neuropathological changes.

5. One must proceed with caution whenever engaging in cross-species comparisons. However, if one exercises an abundance of caution, an evolutionary and comparative approach promises to contribute to advances in our understanding of the etiology and treatment of human mental disorders.

Building a Model: Signs versus Symptoms

In medical diagnosis, *signs* are objective indicators of disease that are typically measured by physicians, but often go unnoticed by patients (e.g., blood pressure). In contrast, *symptoms* are subjective indicators of disease or dysfunction that are obvious to patients and that often lead them to schedule a medical consultation (King, 1968). Although there are distinct differences between signs and symptoms, these terms are frequently used interchangeably, including in discussions of mental disorders (e.g., Andreasen, 1995).

If the topic of this book were animal models of essential hypertension, our efforts would be focused on the development of animal models with elevated blood pressure. Similarly, if the main topic of this book were animal models of diabetes, we would be involved in developing animal models with elevated levels of glucose in blood. In both of these examples, elevated blood pressure and elevated levels of glucose in blood are signs that are critical for the diagnosis of hypertension and diabetes, respectively. In addition, establishing the parallels between these two chronic diseases in humans and their respective animal models is relatively straightforward compared to comparisons between patients with a mental disorder and animal models of that disorder.

As we will see in subsequent chapters, animal models of mental disorders are developed based upon diagnostic systems that are almost exclusively derived from self-reports of symptoms from patients. These symptoms occur in clusters such that some patients have overlapping symptoms, but no patient experiences all of the symptoms. With this much heterogeneity inherent in mental disorders, as was discussed in Chapter 1, is there any wonder that developing valid animal models is so fraught with difficulty?

Models Have Their Limits

Criticisms of using animal models. There is considerable controversy regarding the study of animal models as a means of understanding the etiology and treatment of human mental disorders. At one extreme, Akhtar (2015) has argued from an ethical perspective that the harms of animal experimentation far outweigh any possible benefits to humans or other animals. Greek et al. (2012) have called into question any use of animal models to make predictions about drug responses in humans given extremes in intra- and interspecies variability in genetic makeup and metabolism of drugs. A less extreme view has been presented by Levy (2012), who argues that a very high standard must be set to justify research on animals, especially when suffering and distress are involved. Finally, Garner (2014) has pointed out the substantial mismatch between the design of typical animal model research studies and human clinical trials as an explanation for the extremely high failure rate of experimental drugs in clinical trials (>90%). He advocates for a dramatic change in the way preclinical research is conducted.

Others openly acknowledge the challenges of working with animal model systems to understand human mental disorders, but are fully supportive of their continued use (Nestler & Hyman, 2010). Thus, research on animal models of mental disorders tends to operate on shaky ground as the connections between a given syndrome in an animal model and the clinical correlates of the corresponding mental disorder in humans are tenuous at best. After all, symptoms associated with mental disorders involve complex changes in mood, executive function, and cognition that may not have direct parallels in animal models. We are unlikely to encounter a laboratory mouse that ruminates, a zebrafish that hears voices, or a laboratory rat that is contemplating suicide. In addition, mental disorders often involve a complex array of genetic risk factors, each of which makes very modest contributions to the overall disease phenotype. Importantly, there are no universally accepted biomarkers for mental disorders that can be modeled in animals. There are also pitfalls in using drugs that are effective in treating subsets of patients with mental disorders as a means to evaluate the validity of an animal model. Finally, some drugs have limited efficacy in patients, and neural changes effected by these drugs in animals may not reflect the etiology of the mental disorder being studied in humans (Gass & Wotjak, 2013; Hyman, 2018).

This is the point at which one either gives up because the challenge is too difficult or develops an alternative strategy. It has become obvious that an animal model cannot reproduce all or even most of the characteristics of a human mental disorder. In contrast, a more encouraging experimental strategy is to focus on animal models that incorporate some of the specific symptoms that are characteristic of human mental disorders. An experimental focus on reducing complex symptoms into their components has led to the identification of endophenotypes, which represent links between downstream symptoms associated with disease phenotypes and the upstream effects of genes (Table 6.1). Given this relationship, it may be argued that endophenotypes are more closely linked to affected genes than complex symptoms that form the basis for current classifications of mental disorders. In contrast, biomarkers of disease may not be under strictly genetic control. Endophenotypes include biochemical,

Table 6.1 Characteristics of Endophenotypes in Humans

1. The endophenotype is associated with illness in the population.
2. The endophenotype is heritable.
3. The endophenotype is primarily state-independent, and is measurable in an individual with symptoms or when an individual is in remission.
4. Within families, endophenotypes and illness co-segregate.
5. The endophenotype of affected family members is found in non-affected family members at a higher rate than in the general population.

Adopted from Gottesman and Gould (2003).

neurophysiological, neuroanatomical, neuropsychological, and neuroendocrine measures, and they represent a promising approach for improving the utility of animal models of mental disorders (Gottesman & Gould, 2003; Gould & Gottesman, 2006).

Limitations of diagnostic systems. Animal models of mental disorders have for too long been tethered to two diagnostic systems that combine pathophysiologically distinct profiles into the same diagnostic category. These two systems, *DSM-5* (American Psychiatric Association, 2013) and *ICD-11* (World Health Organization, 2019), were described in greater detail in Chapter 1 and have provided value over the years in several ways. Inter-rater reliability is quite high with the *DSM* and *ICD* systems, as clinicians share a common diagnostic language. In addition, the diagnostic categories feed into many national health information data acquisition systems and allow for clinicians and hospitals to seek reimbursement for their services from national health plans or insurance companies.

Unfortunately, neither the *DSM* nor the *ICD* captures the importance of prenatal or postnatal stressors as risk factors for development of mental disorders, and there are no direct links between diagnostic categories and underlying pathology. In addition, many individuals with one *DSM* diagnosis have a high likelihood of being comorbid for a second *DSM* diagnosis over their life span. There is little wonder that investigators interested in the development of animal models of mental disorders have faced significant barriers over the years (Anderzhanova et al., 2017; Kaffman & Krystal, 2012; Syed & Nemeroff, 2017).

Interestingly, some have argued that the recently proposed RDoC system, an initiative of the US National Institute of Mental Health (NIMH), may actually enhance the quality of animal models and improve their ability to shed light on the etiology of mental disorders and facilitate the development of new therapies (Kaffman & Krystal, 2012). The RDoC system provides a more favorable environment for the development of animal models because it emphasizes a measurable endophenotype that is associated with a specific brain circuit. These connections between RDoC and findings from animal models will be discussed in detail in the chapters that follow.

Model Animals

The comparative approach. Another strategy advanced by Insel (2007) is to focus more on "model animals" rather than "animal models." He argues that model organisms should be chosen strategically to test a specific hypothesis. For example, prairie voles (*Microtus orchrogaster*) are unusual among mammalian species in being monogamous and forming male-female pair bonds. This species offers an excellent opportunity to study neural and hormonal systems involved in the formation and maintenance of pair bonds and in bi-parental care of the young (Insel & Young, 2001). In contrast, using laboratory mice and rats to address these issues would make little sense given that neither species forms pair bonds and males do not play an active role in care of the developing young.

Another example concerns predatory behavior. If one is interested in the development of predatory behavior, it does not make sense to study a species that is not a predator under natural conditions. Grasshopper mice (genus *Onychomys*) are the only predatory rodents in North America, and their predatory behavior in the laboratory and under natural conditions has been studied in some detail (Langley, 1987; McCarty, 1975, 1978). In contrast, experiments on the predatory behavior of laboratory rats have been conducted in spite of the fact that this species is not typically considered a natural predator (e.g., Tulogdi et al., 2015).

Worms and flies and fish—oh my! In this subsection, I will present three examples of simpler organisms that have been advanced recently as valid model systems for studying human mental disorders. At first blush, it is tempting to dismiss these models as wildly inappropriate for learning anything about human psychopathology. One species lives in the soil and eats bacteria, one flits about and feeds on over-ripe fruit, and one is found in ponds and streams in Southeast Asia. However, there is a strong belief that the evolutionarily conserved nature of many psychiatric risk genes and their downstream molecular effects are conserved to a greater or lesser extent across these three model species as well as in laboratory mice and humans (Table 6.2).

C. elegans. The free-living soil nematode, *C. elegans*, is approximately 1 mm long in adulthood, feeds on bacteria, and has a life span of 2–3 weeks. There are two sexes—self-fertilizing hermaphrodites and males. Hermaphrodites have 959 somatic cells, including 302 neurons that make approximately 5,000 synapses. The cell lineage, position, and morphology of each neuron have been described and the connections of neurons are highly conserved across individuals.

Table 6.2 A Comparison of Numbers of Genes and Neurons and Genetic Homology in Five Species, Including Humans (*Homo sapiens*), Mice (*Mus musculus*), Zebrafish (*Dario rerio*), Fruitflies (*Drosophilia melanogaster*), and Nematode Worms (*Caenorhabditis elegans*)

Species	Neurons	DNA Base Pairs	Genes	% homology
Humans	10^{11}	3.3×10^9	19,000	100%
Mice	7×10^6	2.8×10^9	23,000	75%–80%
Zebrafish	10^6		26,000	70%
Fruitflies	10^5	1.23×10^8	13,600	60%
Nematode worms	302	10^8	19,000	40%

Modified from a table that originally appeared in Stewart et al. (2014).

Neurotransmitters employed in synaptic transmission include serotonin, acetylcholine, glutamate, DA, and GABA (Burne et al., 2011).

C. *elegans* was the first multicellular organism to have its genome sequenced, which revealed 19,000 protein-coding genes. Approximately 40% of these genes are conserved across other organisms, including humans (The C. *elegans* Sequencing Consortium, 1999).

There is a surprisingly rich behavioral repertoire in C. *elegans*, and these behaviors can be quantified to link genetic manipulations to behavioral changes and to model features of human mental disorders. The worms have well-developed sensory capacities and can locate food sources, detect and escape from noxious substances, localize potential mates, and move toward areas with optimal concentrations of oxygen and favorable temperatures. In addition, worms are sensitive to the effects of various drugs, including nicotine, alcohol, and some antipsychotic drugs. Finally, one can demonstrate forms of associative and non-associative learning in C. *elegans* (Burne et al., 2011), and these tests of learning can be incorporated into studies that model behaviors in humans. Recent studies using C. *elegans* have examined molecular and behavioral aspects of ethanol abuse and extended these findings back to humans (Davies et al., 2003; Mathies et al., 2015). There is also great potential for high throughput screening of compounds of interest in psychiatry using C. *elegans*.

Fruit flies. Since the early years of the 20th century, the fruit fly, *Drosophila melanogaster*, has played a central role in the field of genetics research. Thomas Hunt Morgan (1866–1945) was one of the first scientists to study the genetics of wild-type and mutant fruit flies and in his laboratory, first at Columbia University and later at the California Institute of Technology. Research efforts with his students led to seminal findings that advanced our understanding of the nature of genes and chromosomes (Mukhergee, 2016).

Fruit flies are easy to maintain in the laboratory, with minimal space requirements and no specialized equipment needs. The life span of fruit flies is approximately 1 month. Females lay as many as 100 eggs per day, and as many as 2,000 eggs over the course of a lifetime. Fertilized eggs hatch within 12–15 hours and the resulting larvae feed and grow for about 4 days until pupation. The pupal stage lasts approximately 4 days, and then the adult fly emerges. There is a wealth of information on well-characterized morphological and behavioral mutants, and the behavioral repertoire of fruit flies is extensive. The genome has been sequenced and there are approximately 13,600 protein-coding genes (Adams et al., 2000).

The first report linking single genes with behavior resulted from experiments with fruit flies and was published more than 50 years ago by Seymour Benzer (1967). Since those early efforts, there have been many reports of single gene effects on behavior in fruit flies, including for circadian rhythms, courtship behaviors, learning and memory processes, selective attention, and sleep deficits (Burne et al., 2011).

Several strategies have been employed to study the genetic basis of mental disorders in humans using fruit flies as a model system. An example of a forward-genetic approach to identify genes of interest involved studies of mutant flies that were unable to retrieve memories of odors previously associated with mild electric shocks. These behavioral deficits led to the identification of the *dunce* gene, which plays a role in modulating synaptic plasticity through its effects on cyclic AMP signaling (Davis & Dauwalder, 1991). A reverse-genetic approach was taken by expressing a potential human disease gene that does not have a homolog in fruit flies, and assessing its effects on behavior. The disrupted-in-schizophrenia-1 (*DISC1*) gene has been identified as a potential contributor to several mental disorders in humans, including schizophrenia and bipolar disorder. In transgenic fruit flies expressing *DISC1*, there were significant deficits in measures of sleep homeostasis. This was a promising finding given that disturbances in sleep and circadian rhythms have been reported in several mental disorders (Sawamura et al., 2008).

Fruit flies have significant but as yet unmet potential for advancing knowledge of the mechanisms underlying some mental disorders (Furukubo-Tokunaga, 2009). For example, up to 75% of all human disease genes, including those identified by large-scale GWAS, have a reasonable match in the fruit fly genome. Why, then, hasn't this model animal been embraced to shed light on the causes of mental disorders? One possible explanation for this lack of progress is the dearth of suitable behavioral assays of attention and cognition available for use in fruit flies. A critical remaining need is for the development of sensitive behavioral tests of sensory filtering, arousal thresholds, and sleep processes, among other functions. Each of these behavioral measures matches well with characteristics observed in many mental disorders, and can be studied in fruit flies and related back to some of the many candidate genes identified through GWAS (van Alphen & van Swinderen, 2013).

Zebrafish. Zebrafish (*Danio rerio*) have recently taken their place on the list of model organisms for psychiatry research (Stewart et al., 2014; Stewart et al., 2015). Zebrafish have been a mainstay in genetic and developmental research for many years. At first glance, one might question the relevance of using fish to model human mental disorders, and many have. However, zebrafish afford many advantages as a model organism, and they are becoming an important component in the array of model systems available to researchers.

Zebrafish are found in shallow ponds and streams in Southeast Asia and are easily maintained in the laboratory. Following fertilization, precursors to all major organ systems are in place within 36 hours, and developing embryos are transparent. Hatching occurs 2 days after fertilization, and larvae actively seek out food and display avoidance behaviors as early as 3 days post-fertilization. Adulthood is attained at 90 days of age, and zebrafish can live up to 5 years in captivity (Kimmel et al., 1995). There are approximately 26,000 protein-coding genes in the zebrafish genome, and 70% of zebrafish genes have at least one human orthologue (Howe et al., 2013). Zebrafish are certainly well positioned to serve as an early stage model system to generate new targets for drug development and hypotheses for connections between nerve circuits and behavior that can be tested further in mammalian species.

A further advantage of using zebrafish in preclinical research projects is the battery of sensitive behavioral paradigms that has been developed, especially in the area of anxiety research. Using two cameras, one on the side of the tank and one above the tank, and video-tracking software, the three-dimensional responses of individual zebrafish and small groups to placement in a novel tank can be recorded and quantified. Anxiety-like behaviors included diving, immobility, erratic movements, and remaining close to the walls of the tank (thigmotaxis). A second test involved tracking the behavior of a group of zebrafish before and after removal of a partition that reveals a predatory leaf fish swimming in an adjacent tank. Exposure to a predator results in a tightening of the shoal (the group of fish) and coordinated movement of the shoal to the bottom of the tank and positioned as far away from the predator as possible.

Sophisticated tracking of social interactions between zebrafish allows for quantification of normal social behavior and deficits in these behaviors following genetic or environmental manipulations. In addition, startle responses to novel or unexpected stimuli (e.g., tapping on the tank, loud noise, bright light, vibrations) are highly stereotyped in zebrafish, and provide an effective behavioral assay for anxiolytic and anxiogenic drugs. And of particular relevance to the theme of this book, zebrafish have a robust HPA response to stressful stimulation, with significant increases in CORT released from the inter-renal gland.

Zebrafish also have many of the same neurotransmitter systems that occur in the brains of laboratory mice and humans. These include acetylcholine, NE, DA, serotonin, GABA, histamine, and glutamate. Interestingly, zebrafish express 122 G protein-coupled receptors for biogenic amine neurotransmitters, significantly more than in laboratory mice (57) or humans (44), and many of these receptors remain to be characterized. Because larval zebrafish develop externally and are transparent, their neural pathways can be visualized and manipulated with great precision during early development, and are amenable to high throughput screening techniques (Stewart et al., 2015).

Several human mental disorders have been modeled in zebrafish, including attention deficit hyperactivity disorder (Lange et al., 2012), aggression (Norton et al., 2011), autism spectrum disorders (Stewart et al., 2014), drug abuse (Mathur & Guo, 2010), alcoholism (Gerlai et al., 2000), and post-traumatic stress disorder (PTSD) (Caramillo et al., 2015). These and related studies highlight a critical role for zebrafish in unmasking the etiology of these devastating disorders in humans.

Who Ate My Cheese?

Mice: From pets to profits. For more than 100 years, laboratory strains of mice and rats have served as the dominant animal models used in biomedical and behavioral research. In the late 1800s, unusual mutant mice, including coat color variants, were of great interest to collectors, or "fanciers," in many parts of the world. Clarence C. Little (1888–1971) maintained close ties with mouse fanciers in the United States and was a major proponent of using mice in laboratory research while he was a student, and later a faculty member, at Harvard University. After serving as president of the University of Maine and then the University of Michigan, Little founded the Jackson Laboratories in Bar Harbor, Maine, which remains a major repository and supplier of genetically defined mouse strains for investigators throughout the world (Rader, 2004).

Laboratory rats. The laboratory rat was championed as a valuable animal model for studies in growth, neuroanatomy, and psychology by Henry H. Donaldson (1857–1938) and Adolf Meyer (1866–1950). Donaldson and Meyer were colleagues at Clark University and the Worcester Hospital for the Insane, respectively, when Meyer used laboratory rats in a neuroanatomy course he taught as an adjunct faculty member at Clark University. Later, Donaldson moved from Clark University to the University of Chicago, and Meyer was appointed the first Psychiatrist-in Chief of The Johns Hopkins Hospital in Baltimore, Maryland. While serving as a scientific advisor to the Wistar Institute of Anatomy and Biology in Philadelphia, Donaldson promoted the establishment of a standard strain of laboratory rats (i.e., the Wistar strain). At the same time, Meyer encouraged research with laboratory rats in his new department at Johns Hopkins. It is interesting to note that Meyer worked with a wide range of organisms during his years as a laboratory researcher, and never favored the laboratory rat as the optimal animal model. However, in a brief span of time, the laboratory rat became the standard for basic laboratory research in psychology, and this pattern continues to the present (Logan, 1999, 2005).

Until the late 1980s, laboratory rats were favored over laboratory mice in neuroscience research, including in studies with animal models of mental disorders. This imbalance shifted dramatically with the development of tools to manipulate the genome of mice, and there is now a slightly greater number of neuroscience publications each year that use mice rather than rats. However, with the advent of improved techniques for altering the genome of laboratory rats, this imbalance may disappear in the coming years (Ellenbroek & Youn, 2016; Rosenthal & Brown, 2007).

Ease of use. Anyone who has worked with laboratory rats and mice is keenly aware that mice are not simply petite rats. The two species differ substantially across many dimensions of special relevance to neuroscience research. These include responses to human handling, patterns of social behavior, responses to addictive drugs, levels of impulsivity, and cognitive function (Ellenbroek & Youn, 2016). As the playing field is leveled with respect to the size of the genetic toolboxes for each species, it is critical for researchers to select the optimal species/strain combination (rat versus mouse) and associated behavioral assessments in developing animal models of human mental disorders. Experience has shown that genetic mutants can be generated quickly, but the difficult task of quantifying the behavioral phenotypes of each mutant requires considerable effort (Chadman et al., 2009).

As noted earlier, laboratory mice and rats are easily maintained and bred in the laboratory. The time from fertilization until birth is approximately 3 weeks, and litters are usually culled to a standard number soon after birth (6–10 pups per litter depending on the investigator). Pups remain with the mother for approximately 3 weeks (the preweaning period), and are dependent upon her as the primary source of nutrition, warmth, and physical stimulation through licking and grooming until about postnatal day 10. At weaning, animals are usually housed in small groups until adulthood (>45 days of age) (McCarty, 2017).

The prenatal environment of mice can be modified in several ways. The most dramatic involves the transplantation of fertilized eggs to the uterus of a mother of a different strain or treatment group. In addition, pregnant dams can be exposed to stressful stimuli or injected with various biologically active agents that may affect the dam and her developing young. Postnatally, litters or individual pups can be cross-fostered to mothers of a different strain or treatment group as a way of altering the postnatal maternal environment (McCarty, 2017). These experimental approaches will be discussed in detail when specific animal models are highlighted in Chapters 7–14.

Without doubt, strains of laboratory mice and, to a lesser extent, rats have been the most frequently employed animal models in preclinical research on mental disorders (Cryan & Holmes, 2005). Compared to worms, fruit flies, and zebrafish, laboratory mice and rats have the distinct advantage of being mammals and of having a slightly greater genetic homology with humans compared to the other species. However, these advantages do not guarantee success in the area of model development.

The genome of the laboratory mouse has been sequenced and includes 2.8×10^9 base pairs and approximately 23,000 protein-coding genes. There is 75%–80% homology between the mouse genome and the human genome, and this similarity opens up possibilities for modifying disease gene homologs in mice to model their effects in humans (Stewart et al., 2014).

With the expansion of GWAS findings as applied to mental disorders, there is an increasing number of genetic targets to be pursued in mouse models. Mice are particularly relevant for these studies, as there are many well-characterized strains with single gene mutations, and for some the behavioral phenotypes have been studied in some detail (Tarantino & Bucan, 2000). In addition, mouse models afford investigators an opportunity to explore how gene x environment interactions at particular times during development contribute to alterations in behavioral phenotypes that persist into adulthood. Such experiments have the potential to unmask disease pathways of relevance to clinical researchers (Desbonnet et al., 2012; Kannan et al., 2013).

By employing a range of 509 standardized mouse phenotyping tests, the International Mouse Phenotyping Consortium (IMPC) has sought to develop a comprehensive genome- and phenome-wide database of all knockout (KO) mouse strains developed in laboratories around the world. Researchers have analyzed cohorts of male and female KO mice on an isogenic C57BL/6N background from embryonic stem-cell resources developed by IMPC and made up of targeted null mutations with reporter gene elements. In IMPC Data Release 5.0 on August 2, 2016, 3,328 genes were fully or partially phenotyped. This represented approximately 15% of the protein-coding genes in the mouse genome (Meehan et al., 2017). Some of the KO mice that have been phenotyped have contributed valuable information that is directly relevant to the study of animal models of mental disorders.

Optimizing animal models. A reasonable question to ask at this point is: why aren't studies with animal models leading to the development of more effective drugs for the treatment of mental disorders? A continuing concern is that current animal models have not been optimized to match with the pathophysiology of their respective human disorders. Several investigators (e.g., Agid et al., 2007) have suggested avenues for improvement of animal models, including the following:

1. Rather than depending exclusively on knockout or transgenic mice to model a given disorder, one could develop models that reflect genetic vulnerability (i.e., gene dosage) for a mental disorder and then pursue experiments on gene x environment interactions.
2. Combine the genetic or developmental predisposing element with an ethologically relevant triggering stimulus applied in adulthood.
3. Study the effects of drugs that mimic the symptoms of schizophrenia or study the mechanism of action of drugs known to be effective in the treatment of a mental disorder.
4. Employ a multidisciplinary team of investigators to identify the most relevant aspects of a human mental disorder to be studied in a preclinical animal model, and then examine the model from multiple perspectives.
5. Utilize a battery of behavioral tests to strengthen the assessment of an animal model.

A Darwinian Perspective on the Genetics of Behavior

Kendler and Greenspan (2006) combined their considerable expertise in psychiatric genetics and the neurobiological basis of behavior in laboratory mice and fruit flies, respectively, to consider six points of convergence connecting their two fields of inquiry. First, they noted that estimates of heritability of behavioral traits in animal models and mental disorders in humans vary over a wide range (typically 10%–50%). A second consistent feature of mental disorders and behavioral phenotypes in selected animal models (e.g., memory processes, geotaxis, aggressive behavior, olfaction, etc.) involved regulation by multiple genes, each with a modest effect on the phenotypic trait in question. Third, they reported that genetic risk factors in humans may not be uniquely associated with a single mental disorder. Rather, some risk factors have been found to influence several mental disorders, including, for example, one risk factor that influences major depression, generalized anxiety disorder, and phobia. Similarly, studies employing a host of animal models have found consistent evidence for pleiotropic effects of individual genes. That is, a single gene may impact many different behavioral phenotypes. Fourth, experiments with human populations and with animal models have provided strong evidence that genetic effects on behavior may be modified by manipulations of the environment. A fifth point of convergence involves genetic influences on exposure to specific types of physical and social environments in psychiatric patients and in various animal species. Finally, differential modification by sex of genetic risk factors in humans and genetic effects on behavior in animal models have been reported.

Although these points of convergence were not surprising, this detailed analysis concluded that patterns governing genetic influences on mental disorders and on defined behavioral phenotypes in animal models were strikingly similar. This conclusion is reassuring and argues for continued exploration of genetic influences on behavior in laboratory animals to inform studies in the genetics of mental disorders in humans (Kendler & Greenspan, 2006). These issues will be explored further in the chapters that follow.

Concerns about Replication of Experiments

The toolkit for genetic manipulations in laboratory mice is impressive (Behringer et al., 2014). However, a limiting factor confronting most researchers interested in animal models of mental disorders remains the development of sensitive and reproducible measures of behavioral phenotypes. Increasingly, basic researchers are turning to experienced clinicians for more detailed information about behavioral phenotypes in patients that can inform the development of novel behavioral phenotypes in mice and other model organisms (Baker, 2011).

Replication is a concern. Another concern deals with the issue of reproducibility of findings related to behavioral phenotypes within and across laboratories (Kafkafi et al., 2018). This is especially relevant when findings in one laboratory stimulate an extension of experiments in another laboratory. But what if a simple replication of findings isn't so simple after all?

Consider the following landmark study (Crabbe et al., 1999). Investigators in three laboratories—the Oregon Health Sciences University in Portland, Oregon; the University of Alberta in Edmonton, Alberta, Canada; and the State University of New York in Albany, New York—joined forces to compare males and females from six inbred mouse strains, one F_2 hybrid from a cross of two of the inbred strains, and one null mutant of a gene coding for a serotonin receptor subtype in six behavioral tests. Behavioral testing began at 77 days of age, and included mice shipped directly from the various suppliers or reared in each of the laboratories. Extraordinary efforts were taken to standardize all aspects of animal housing, light-dark cycle, type of food, design of test apparatus, order of testing, time of day for testing, and so on.

The results were striking in that significant differences in results of behavioral testing did occur across laboratories. In addition, the pattern of strain differences for a given behavioral test also varied across the three laboratories. Interestingly, test results were similar for animals that were shipped directly from the supplier versus animals that were reared in each laboratory.

Some of the results from the three laboratories tended to be more consistent. For example, genotype had a significant impact on all behaviors tested and accounted for 30%–80% of the total variance. In addition, some of the classic paired-strain behavioral differences were reproduced in this study, such as ethanol consumption. Finally, the more robust the impact of the mouse strain, the more likely it was that the results were consistent across the three sites. For genetic effects that were smaller in magnitude, the results tended to be more sensitive to unknown environmental effects (Crabbe et al., 1999).

In a major extension of this three-site study, Wahlsten et al. (2006) compared behavioral data from 40–50 years ago with behavioral data collected more recently to determine if mouse strain differences in behaviors were consistent over time and across laboratories. In measuring strain differences in ethanol preference in a two-bottle choice test (10% ethanol versus tap water), the consistency of results over a 30+ year period was striking, especially for the high alcohol preference of the C57BL/6J strain versus the pronounced aversion to ethanol for the DBA/2J strain. Similarly, strain differences in open field behavior were consistent over a 50-year period, with results from multi-strain comparisons pointing to the A/J strain as the least active and the C57BL/6J strain as the most active during open field testing.

In contrast to the consistent findings for strain differences in alcohol preference and open field activity, there were notable inconsistencies in measures of elevated plus-maze behaviors across mouse strains. These inconsistencies were taken as evidence of substantial influences of laboratory-specific environmental factors on this frequently employed behavioral measure of anxiety-like behavior (Wahlsten et al., 2006).

The strain of substrains. Another issue to be mindful of in the design of experiments is the phenotypic differences between various substrains of inbred laboratory mice. One of the inbred strains of mice employed in the studies described earlier, the C57BL/6J strain, is frequently employed in neuroscience research. It has also become a commonly used background strain for the generation of genetically engineered mice, as will be discussed in the chapters on animal models of various mental disorders.

As Matsuo et al. (2010) reported, the three most common substrains of the C57BL/6 inbred strain include the C57BL/6J originally developed by Little at the Jackson Laboratories in 1921; the C57BL/6N, maintained at the National Institutes of Health (NIH) since 1951; and the C57BL/6C, derived from the NIH breeding stock and maintained by the National Cancer Institute beginning in the 1970s. In comparing the behavioral profiles of several thousand mice of these three substrains, these investigators demonstrated a significant divergence of some but not all behavioral measures across the three substrains. Their results emphasize the importance of carefully selecting and documenting the particular substrain that is employed in each experiment. These concerns also apply to the "129" family of mouse substrains (Kiselycznyk & Holmes, 2011).

Criteria for Determining the Validity of Animal Models

In an important paper in the field of animal models in psychiatry, Willner (1986) proposed three criteria to assess the utility of an animal model for enhancing our understanding of a given mental disorder in humans. His analysis focused on learned helplessness as an animal model of major depression in humans, and the three criteria he proposed were predictive validity, face validity, and construct validity. For predictive validity, Willner emphasized the consistency of responses to pharmacological treatments between the learned helplessness model and major depressive disorder in humans. In face validity, Willner noted that drug effects in the animal model required chronic treatment to match with the human disorder, and that symptoms of the human disorder should have correlates in the animal model. Finally, Willner proposed that construct validity reflected similarities between behaviors in the animal model and features of interest in the human disorder, including a theoretical connection to the disorder in humans (Willner, 1986).

Willner's initial set of criteria has been modified, enhanced, and expanded by other investigators as new information has been generated and other animal models of human mental disorders have been studied (Nestler & Hyman, 2010; Stewart & Kalueff, 2015; van der Staay et al., 2009). In addition, Belzung and Lemoine (2011) have presented a multifactorial formulation of validity that is especially helpful; essential features of their conception are included in Table 6.3. They emphasized the importance of selecting an appropriate strain/species for study, of giving attention to the developmental trajectory of a given disorder and its triggering conditions, of attending to the mechanisms relating to the mental disorder to be modeled, of noting consistency of findings between the animal model and the human disorder with regard to biological and behavioral endpoints, and of comparing the efficacy of drugs in treating the symptoms of disease in the animal model and the disorder in humans.

The social environment has not been given the attention it deserves in basic research on physiological responses to stressful stimuli. In particular, Koohaas et al. (2017) have argued for a significant shift in focus toward appraisal of social

Table 6.3 Categories of Validity Relevant to the Assessment of Animal Models of Human Mental Disorders

Type of Validity	Description
Homological validity	Appropriateness of the **species** and **strain** of the animal model to study and aspect(s) the human disorder.
Pathogenic validity	Tendency of the animal model to display pathological processes that resemble those of the human disorder. These pathological processes include **early environmental factors** that render an organism vulnerable to develop the disorder later in life and **triggering factors** that impact a vulnerable or a control organism in adulthood and lead to the disorder.
Mechanistic validity	Similarity of the **mechanism of disease** in the animal model to the actual or hypothesized mechanism underlying the onset/maintenance of the human disorder. The mechanism may be behavioral or neurobiological in nature.
Face validity	Consistency of observations between the animal model and the human disorder, including **behaviors** and **biomarkers**.
Predictive validity	Effectiveness of the animal model in mirroring the **etiology of disease onset** and the **response to a therapeutic agent** (drug or other treatment) in the human disorder.

Note: Nine important components of these five criteria are highlighted and are critical in assessing the results of any experiments.

These criteria and their descriptions were adopted from a publication by Belzung and Lemoine (2011).

stressors and individual differences in the appraisal process that may contribute to a greater understanding of outcomes associated with vulnerability versus resilience. It is possible that a significant degree of individual variability of physiological responses to laboratory stressors may be explained by inter-individual differences in appraisal of the stressor, particularly a social stressor such as chronic social defeat.

The Power of (Reverse) Translational Research

The "bench-to-bedside" image of translational research implies a unidirectional process whereby discoveries in a laboratory setting using model systems are translated into new therapies for the benefit of patients (Woolf, 2008). Unfortunately, this is an overly simplistic portrayal of a complex, bidirectional process where studies of animal models in the laboratory are informed by clinical observations and results of experiments with patients (e.g. Kesby et al., 2018), a reverse translational strategy (Figure 6.1). Similarly, studies with animal models open the way for new approaches in clinical research, patient care, prevention strategies, and identification of new drug targets (Donaldson & Hen, 2015).

A particular focus of the chapters that follow is the impressive body of translational research that examines how environmental stressors interact with susceptible genotypes to produce alterations in endophenotypes that are especially relevant to psychiatric diseases (Driscoll & Barr, 2016). Mental disorders present a significant challenge to basic scientists who work with animal models because so many of the hallmark symptoms of mental disorders are part and parcel of what it means to be human. But there is a brighter side to this challenge. Stressful stimuli and the biological and behavioral responses that are provoked by them have been intertwined throughout much of the evolutionary history of complex multicellular organisms. In mammals, including mice, rats, monkeys, and humans, the neural circuits, endocrine systems, and behavioral patterns that animals and humans call into play to deal with acute or chronic exposure to stressors are highly conserved (Scharf & Schmidt, 2012).

Critical to the success of translational research approaches is the fact that some laboratory animals, as well as patients with mental disorders, do not mount

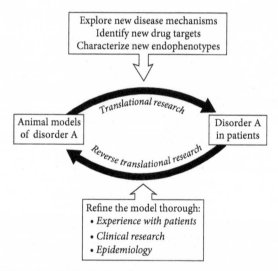

Figure 6.1. Bi-directional relationship between basic research studies with animal models and clinical research with humans. Translational research studies include experiments with animal models that inform the diagnosis, treatment, or prevention of mental disorders in humans. Reverse translational studies include clinical research findings or insights gleaned from clinical practice that lead to refinements in the design and execution of experiments with animal models.

adaptive responses when exposed to stressors. These maladaptive responses could take many forms, including exaggerated or diminished responses to an acute stressor, prolonged neural or endocrine activation following exposure to an acute stressor, or failure to habituate to repeated exposure to a low-intensity stressor. Indeed, some of the behavioral measures to assess the long-term effects of stress exposure on endophenotypes, including sensorimotor gating and fear conditioning and extinction, are strikingly consistent across experimental stress protocols with laboratory rodents and with humans (Hariri & Holmes, 2015).

No single animal model of a given mental disorder should be expected to capture all of the salient features of the disorder in patients. Indeed, the variability of individual patients who share a specific psychiatric diagnosis can vary widely. Thus, each animal model affords investigators an opportunity to consider the effects of a single risk gene or a specific environmental manipulation on a given set of behavioral endpoints. It is only when results from a variety of animal models are compiled and assimilated can one begin to assemble some of the underlying causes of behavioral or biological measures that contribute to disease etiology. These are important principles to keep in mind as we encounter specific experiments in later chapters of this volume (e.g., Bale et al., 2019; Monteggia et al., 2018).

Patience Is a Virtue

Gordon (2019) emphasized the long road from an initial basic science finding to the translation of that finding into a breakthrough for patients. One must have confidence in the power of basic research to generate research findings that will eventually inform drug discovery efforts, even if the payoff isn't for many decades. An example he cited was the development of a novel medication, brexanolone, that was approved by the US Food and Drug Administration on March 19, 2019, specifically for the treatment of postpartum depression. Brexanolone, or allopregnanolone, is a neuroactive steroid that was initially studied by Hans Selye (1941) as one of several metabolites of progesterone that was active in the brain, affecting sleep and producing anesthesia. Steven Paul and his collaborators became interested in neuroactive steroids beginning in the 1970s, and demonstrated a critical role for brain neuroactive steroids in adaptive responses to stressful stimulation. These protective effects of neuroactive steroids during stress were also demonstrated in lactating rats soon after birth and suggested that this class of compounds might be effective in treating postpartum depression. Further studies demonstrated that allopregnanolone acts as a modulator of $GABA_A$ receptors, where it enhances the inhibitory effects of GABA on neuronal activity (Zorumski et al., 2013). Clinical studies were then conducted and revealed that allopregnanolone levels decreased dramatically at the time of birth, possibly rendering some women at risk for the onset of post-partum depression (Gordon, 2019).

Summary

The end game for much of contemporary research on animal models of mental disorders has been to discover novel molecular targets to aid in the development of new psychotherapeutic agents. Indeed, the justification for much of neuroscience research funding in countries around the globe is that it will move us closer to solving the mysteries of disorders of the brain and behavior and stimulate the development of effective treatments. Given the extraordinarily high costs of mental disorders in developed and developing countries, as noted in Chapter 1, these research expenditures could yield important returns on investment. Only time will tell.

In the next series of chapters, I will build on this brief overview of animal models and describe in detail various model systems that encompass stressful stimulation and behavioral dysfunction, including those relevant for research in epigenetic mechanisms, schizophrenia, autism, bipolar disorder, anxiety disorders, depression, and post-traumatic stress disorder. Much of this body of translational research will involve studies with laboratory strains of mice and rats. However, I will also bring in findings from studies of simpler model organisms and from nonhuman primates as appropriate.

7

Stress, Development, and Epigenetics

Anthony J. Reading (1966, p. 440), in a journal article based upon his dissertation completed at The Johns Hopkins University, foreshadowed much of the exciting research on stress, development, and epigenetics that has occurred since the late 1990s, some of which will be featured in this chapter. He closed his paper on maternal effects on offspring behaviors in two inbred strains of laboratory mice by stating:

> it is possible to conceive of a self-perpetuating nongenetic system of transmission in which each generation of mothers influences the behavior of the succeeding generation in such a way that, in their turn as mothers, they exert the same influence on the generation that follows them.

The ideas advanced by Reading and others more than 50 years ago did not take root immediately, as there were no mechanisms that could explain how a nongenetic trans-generational system of transmission could operate from mothers to their offspring and on to succeeding generations. Keep in mind that Reading's paper was published just over a decade after Watson and Crick (1953) proposed the structure of DNA. This was also a period in which the tenets of modern genetics could not accommodate a mechanism(s) that would support a nongenetic mode of inheritance (Landman, 1991). Although a host of experiments with laboratory strains of mice and rats provided findings that were consistent with nongenetic transmission of phenotypic traits, mechanistic insights would not emerge until almost four decades later. More recently, experiments have revealed that stressful experiences of adult animals prior to mating can influence their offspring and extend for several generations later through epigenetic alterations encoded in germ cells. As we will see later in this volume, experiments like these have special relevance to research involving animal models of mental disorders (Nestler, 2016).

A Primer on Epigenetics

The term *epigenetics* was first introduced by Conrad H. Waddington (1905–1975) to capture, from an embryological perspective, the dynamic processes by which changes in the phenotype could occur without changes in the genotype (Waddington, 1942). Waddington's initial conceptualization of epigenetics ("all those events which lead to the unfolding of the genetic program for development") was considered by many to be too all-encompassing and at times confusing (Schuebel et al., 2016). Over time, however, the term *epigenetics* was retained, but the definition became more specific and the mechanisms underlying epigenetic changes were described in exquisite detail. There are three essential features of epigenetics that should be kept in mind for the remainder of this chapter. First, epigenetic changes do not involve a change in the sequence of bases in DNA. Second, epigenetic alterations tend to be readily reversible. Third, some epigenetic alterations may persist over the lifetime of an organism, and may even be transmitted to succeeding generations through epigenetic alterations in germ cells. Since 2000, there has been a remarkable uptick in the use of the term *epigenetics* in the scientific literature, including in experiments on chromatin modifications that alter gene transcription (Haig, 2012).

At the close of the last century (1999 to be specific), a symposium on epigenetic factors in psychiatric genetics was featured on the program of the 7th World Congress on Psychiatric Genetics (Petronis & Gottesman, 2000). The opening speaker for this symposium, Irving I. Gottesman, was one of the early champions of an epigenetic approach to schizophrenia through an influential book he coauthored with James Shields (Gottesman & Shields, 1982). The speakers in this symposium foreshadowed the explosive growth of interest in epigenetic contributions to psychiatric disorders that would occur in the first decade of the 21st century and that continues to the present.

A principal focus of this chapter is the study of early life epigenetic alterations during offspring development that are transmitted across generations (for reviews, see Franklin & Mansuy, 2009; Keller & Roth, 2016; Kundakovic & Champagne, 2015; Meaney & Szyf, 2005a; Roth & Sweatt, 2010). This is a vital area of inquiry given the overwhelming evidence that exposure to stressors early in life increases the risk for development of mental disorders in adolescence and early adulthood (Bolton et al., 2017; Entringer et al., 2015; Murgatroyd et al., 2010; Tsankova et al., 2007). As we will see, studies in animal models have provided critical insights into stress-induced epigenetic alterations that persist into adulthood and that may transmit risk to succeeding generations.

The purpose of this first section is to provide an overview of epigenetic alterations in DNA and histone proteins that affect gene transcriptional activity. Such epigenetic effects in the absence of changes in DNA base sequences may provide a mechanism to explain Reading's proposed nongenetic system of transmission of maternal effects on offspring behavior. In the subsections that follow, I will highlight three modes of epigenetic regulation of gene activity. They include post-translational modification of histones, methylation of DNA, and chromatin remodeling. Also included is a brief discussion of the effects of non-coding microRNAs (miRNAs).

Targeting Histones

A pretty package. With the emergence of a defined nucleus in eukaryotic organisms came the challenge of packaging the DNA containing the genetic code for that organism into the very small space provided by the nucleus. Consider the magnitude of the problem: 2.2 meters of linear DNA must be squeezed into a nucleus of a human cell that is approximately 10 μM in diameter. To accomplish this task, DNA forms complexes with several classes of specialized histone and nonhistone proteins to form chromatin. The fundamental unit of chromatin is the nucleosome, which consists of an octomeric disc of two copies each of four core histones (H2A, H2B, H3, and H4). DNA wraps around this octomer like thread around a spool, with 146 base pairs of DNA making slightly less than 2 turns around the histone disc. Fourteen relatively weak histone-DNA contacts provide positional stability of the DNA-nucleosome complex. After a short spacer segment of 10–50 base pairs of DNA, the next nucleosome forms, such that chromatin takes on the appearance of beads on a string. A fifth histone, H1, serves as a connector between successive nucleosomes. The long string of nucleosomes is further compacted into a secondary helical structure, a pipe-like solenoid array that is further condensed into loops of approximately 100,000 base pairs each. The N-terminal tails of the histone octomers protrude from the nucleosome cores and the turns of the DNA molecule, where they are subject to reversible post-translational modifications through methylation, acetylation, ubiquitination, or phosphorylation of specific amino acids (Figure 7.1). For the remainder of this chapter, I will limit discussions of histone modifications to methylation and acetylation.

The various post-translational modifications of histones have been referred to as the "histone code," and these alterations enhance to a significant degree the information capacity of the genetic code (Allis & Jenuwein, 2016; Jenuwein & Allis, 2001; Strahl & Allis, 2000). These post-translational modifications to histones do not act in isolation from other epigenetic changes, including DNA methylation; rather, they combine to form a complex network to encode responses to acute stressors, modify responses to future stressors, shape phenotypic characteristics, and influence risk for mental disorders (Klengel & Binder, 2015; Klengel et al., 2014; Sweatt & Taminga, 2016).

A natural tension arises between the need for condensation and effective storage of DNA versus the need for DNA to be accessible for transcription of genes and replication of DNA during cell division. When a portion of the DNA

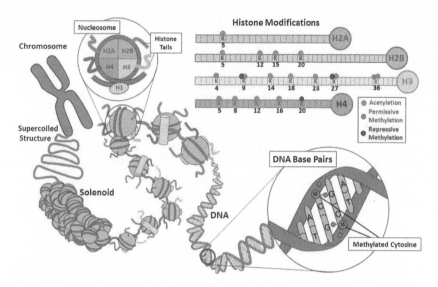

Figure 7.1. The dynamic (epi)genome: DNA methylation, histone post-translational modifications and chromatin structural organization. Within the nucleus of eukaryotic cells, chromosomes are composed of DNA coiled around an octamer of histone proteins to form nucleosomes, the basic repeating unit of chromatin. Histone H1 proteins stabilize the coupling, wrapping and stacking of nucleosomes into a 30 nm solenoid and higher order supercoiled chromatin fiber. The histone octamers are composed of four pairs of histone proteins (H2A, H2B, H3, and H4), which have globular domains and N-terminal tails that protrude from the nucleosome (H2A also has a C-terminal tail). Each histone tail can undergo numerous post-translational modifications. The most common forms of mammalian acetylation and methylation modifications of lysine (K) residues are shown. Additionally, mammalian DNA can be chemically modified by methylation and hydoxymethylation (M) of the 5' position of the cytosine base of 5'-cytosine-phosphodiester-guanine (CpG) dinucleotides. Chromatin structure directs the activity (expression) of genes: genes within tightly packed nucleosomes are silenced, whereas genes within relatively spaced nucleosomes are actively transcribed (expressed). The process of remodeling chromatin into domains of different transcriptional potentials is regulated by reciprocal changes of DNA methylation and histone modification in response to extrinsic cues and/or changes in intrinsic properties of cells (see also Plate 6).
Adapted from Weaver et al. (2017) and used with permission of Dr. Weaver.

molecule is tightly wound around a nucleosome core, the genes it contains are not readily accessible to the transcriptional machinery required for producing the corresponding mRNAs. This relatively inactive state of DNA is referred to as heterochromatin. Euchromatin represents a more relaxed chromatin state that is mediated by post-translational acetylation or phosphorylation of amino acid residues of histone tails, thereby reducing the affinity of histone octomers for DNA and increasing gene transcription (Allis & Jenuwein, 2016).

Writing, erasing, and reading. The amino acid residues of histone tails serve as targets for enzyme-catalyzed modifications that can alter gene transcription. The enzymes that catalyze these modifications may be thought of as writers and erasers of histone marks, some of which are transitory while others persist for longer periods of time. For example, histone acetylation is catalyzed by histone acetyltransferases (HATs, a writer family), whereas histone deacetylases (HDACs, a family of erasers) remove the acetyl group. In a similar way, histone methyltransferases (HMTs) catalyze the addition of a methyl group, while histone demethylases (HDNs) remove the methyl group. Readers enter the picture as proteins that bind to the modified histone tails, and effect increases or decreases in gene transcription.

Targeting DNA

Direct methylation of cytosine residues within DNA is catalyzed by DNA methyltransferases (DNMT3a and DNMT3b), and typically occurs at cytosine-phosphate-guanine (CpG) dinucleotides. During cell division and DNA replication, DNMT1 adds a methyl group to the unmethylated strand of hemi-methylated DNA. These highly stable epigenetic marks typically exert a repressive effect on gene transcription, but under some circumstances they may actually enhance gene transcription. DNA methylation appears to reduce gene transcription by several mechanisms. One mechanism involves the masking of DNA base sequences to prevent recognition by activating transcription factors. In addition, methylated DNA may bind to methyl-CpG-binding domain proteins, which recruit histone-modifying enzymes and chromatin remodeling complexes to further compact nucleosomes and inhibit gene expression.

Demethylation is a much more complex process than DNA methylation. Enzymatic oxidation of 5-methylcytosine by ten-eleven translocation proteins (TET1, TET2, and TET3) leads to the formation of 5-hydroxymethylcytosine, followed by 5-formylcytosine and then 5-carboxycytosine. Passive demethylation occurs during DNA replication, when DNMT1 is unable to recognize 5-hydroxymethylcytosine, resulting in the newly synthesized strand being unmethylated. In active demethylation, thymidine DNA glycosylase removes 5-formylcytosine or 5-carboxycytosine, activating base-excision repair activity and replacement with unmethylated cytosine (Scourzic et al., 2015).

Patterns of DNA methylation in neurons appear to be exquisitely sensitive to environmental stressors, and there is evidence that these epigenetic marks may be transmitted to the next generation. In support of these stressor-induced changes, activity of DNMT3a in the brain is the highest of the DNMT family of enzymes. In addition, high levels of oxidized forms of 5-methylcyctosine are found in the brain, indicating active removal of methyl marks from DNA (Bagot et al., 2014). We will discuss the consequences of DNA methylation later in this chapter.

Time to Remodel

Nucleosomes serve as an effective barrier to transcriptional activity. This is a problem if you happen to be the promoter region of a gene that is wrapped around a nucleosome. To address this issue, the relative positions of nucleosomes along the DNA molecule are dynamically regulated by a group of complexes known as regulators. These four families of ATP-dependent protein complexes slide, eject, or restructure nucleosomes, such that stretches of the DNA molecule are available in a carefully regulated manner for gene transcription as well as DNA replication and repair (Clapier & Cairns, 2009). Experiments on chromatin remodeling in animal models of psychiatric disorders and in clinical populations have appeared relatively recently, with a concentration of experiments in areas of drug and alcohol abuse and autism spectrum disorders (e.g., Moffat et al., 2019; Salery et al., 2017). This is an area of epigenetic research that will likely expand in the coming years.

Small RNAs Deliver a Big Punch

MicroRNAs (miRNAs) were initially discovered in experiments with developmental mutants in the nematode worm, *C. elegans* (Lee et al., 1993; Wightman et al., 1993); miRNAs are one of several classes of noncoding RNAs, so called because they do not code for protein products. Following transcription, the hairpin in the primary miRNA transcript is recognized and cleaved within the nucleus into a 70-nucleotide precursor. Following translocation to the cytoplasm, the hairpin is enzymatically removed to yield a 22-nucleotide duplex miRNA. Either strand of the duplex may function as an miRNA, with suffixes of 3P or 5P to indicate those strands derived from the 3' and 5' ends, respectively. Each strand is added to an RNA silencing complex that then binds to nucleotides 2–8 of the 3' untranslated region of an mRNA, resulting in either destabilization of the transcript or inhibition of protein synthesis (Mendell & Olson, 2012; Wright et al., 2018).

The primary role of miRNAs is in extra-nuclear regulation of gene expression by inhibiting the translation of recently transcribed mRNAs into protein products. This inhibitory effect is possible because each miRNA has a nucleotide sequence that binds to complementary sequences within mRNAs, thereby limiting access of the mRNA to the machinery of protein synthesis. Each miRNA may regulate the translation of several to hundreds of different mRNAs into proteins, and individual mRNAs may be inhibited by multiple miRNAs. These overlapping inhibitory signals represent a complex system for regulating the translation of individual mRNAs into proteins.

There has been considerable interest in examining potential roles for miRNAs in the pathophysiology of various mental disorders, including schizophrenia, bipolar disorder, major depressive disorder, and autism spectrum disorders. Some clinical studies have involved experiments with post-mortem brain samples, while others have utilized samples of peripheral blood. The former may reveal miRNAs for further study in animal models of the relevant disorders, while studies with peripheral blood mononuclear cells may be useful in identifying miRNAs that can serve as biomarkers of specific disorders, quantify responses to drug treatments, or aid in stratification of patients. There is certainly great interest in considering specific miRNAs as potential targets for new drugs to treat mental disorders. In this regard, there have been advances in the use of designer miRNAs or miRNA antagonists to treat cancer patients. A major challenge ahead will be in facilitating the successful delivery of these drugs to the brain. A novel aspect of miRNA therapeutics is that by targeting a single miRNA molecule, one gains access to a complex network of hundreds of involved genes. This may be a blessing or a curse, depending on the various genes involved and their composite downstream effects (Alural et al., 2017; Geaghan & Cairns, 2015; Wright et al., 2018).

Summary

To borrow from the title of a review article by Meaney and Szyf (2005b), laboratory animals and humans must live ". . . at the interface between a dynamic environment and a fixed genome." Having the benefit of constancy in the sequence of bases in DNA provides a dependable molecular code that has been honed over evolutionary time. However, epigenetic mechanisms such as those described in the preceding provide a hedge against rapid and unpredictable changes in the environment. In particular, stressful early life experiences can be "biologically embedded" in a developing organism and maintained into adulthood. It is also the case that stressful experiences in adulthood can be transmitted to succeeding generations through epigenetic changes in DNA or through the effects of miRNAs on the germline. Epigenetic alterations in gene expression provide a level of flexibility in shaping phenotypic characteristics while still maintaining the constancy of the genetic code (Weaver et al., 2017).

Epigenetics of Early Life Stress

Setting the Stage

Separation and handling. Building upon foundational studies by Seymour Levine (1925–2007) on the lasting effects of early handling and separation of litters of rat pups from their mothers (Levine, 1957, 1962), Denenberg and Whimby (1963) examined the trans-generational effects of neonatal handling on rats. Litters of rats were removed from their mothers for 3 minutes per day from postnatal days (PNDs) 1–20. Control litters were left undisturbed from birth to weaning. Female offspring of handled and control litters were mated in adulthood. Soon after birth, litters of the two female groups (handled and control) were assigned to one of three conditions: (i) litters remained with the natural mother, (ii) litters were in-fostered to a mother of the same group, or (ii) litters were cross-fostered to a mother of the opposite group. Offspring from these six groups (2 prior experiences of mothers × 3 rearing conditions) were weaned and weighed at 21 days of age and then tested in an open field arena beginning at 50 days of age. Body weights at weaning were greater for rats reared by mothers who were handled as neonates, and there was no effect of foster rearing. Results of the open field data were complicated by a significant effect of in-fostering per se on number of squares entered. However, the authors concluded that the prenatal and postnatal maternal environments mediated the changes in body weight at weaning and open field behavior in adulthood that were observed in mothers who were handled in infancy. In a follow-up series of experiments, Denenberg and Rosenberg (1967) revealed that handling of female rats in infancy affected the weaning weights and activity levels of animals into the F2 generation.

Consistent with these studies, Ressler (1962), using C57BL/10 and Balb/c inbred strains of mice, reported that differences in parental handling of pups were affected by the genotype of the mothers *and* the genotype of the pups. He concluded that differences in maternal behaviors between the two inbred strains may have reflected differences in the way the mothers were handled when they were pups, rather than genetic differences alone (Umemura et al., 2015).

Two other early reports focused on cross-generational transmission of information, and each relied upon cross-fostering to delineate prenatal versus postnatal maternal effects. Bronstein et al. (1975) demonstrated that weanling rats preferred the same diet as their biological mothers/foster mothers consumed, and Skolnick et al. (1980) found that early separation of rat pups from their mothers increased later susceptibility to stress-induced gastric lesions. These susceptibilities were transmitted to the offspring through effects of the uterine environment, with no impact of the postnatal maternal environment.

With the benefit of hindsight, the two studies by Denenberg and his students (Denenberg & Rosenberg, 1967; Denenberg & Whimby, 1963) could certainly be criticized today on methodological grounds and for the inconsistencies in their behavioral data. However, these studies remained important in that they foreshadowed a paradigm shift that would occur more than 25 years later. Early on, Levine (1957, 1962) and Ressler (1963), and later Denenberg (1999), suggested that the enduring effects of neonatal handling on rat pups might be explained by changes in mother-pup interactions. These suggestions were converted into testable hypotheses beginning in the 1990s.

A mother's love. A powerful and wide-ranging series of studies from the laboratory of Professor Michael Meaney at McGill University built upon these initial findings by focusing on the effects of neonatal handling on the behavior of rat mothers and their pups. In addition, Meaney and his colleagues expanded into the realm of epigenetic modifications by probing the neural, endocrine, and molecular changes that mediated the effects of alterations in maternal care on offspring physiological and behavioral measures (Meaney & Szyf, 2005a, 2005b).

Compared to control rat mothers with litters that were left undisturbed from birth to weaning, neonatal handling of rat litters resulted in increased frequency of licking and grooming of the pups by their mothers, as well as increases in arched-back nursing postures (LG-ABN). A wide range of rates of LG-ABN were apparent in a laboratory population of mother rats caring for their litters, and those mothers with high scores for LG-ABN resembled mothers whose litters were handled in infancy. Forging a link between early handling and naturally occurring differences in maternal behaviors was a critical insight provided by Meaney and his colleagues (Liu et al., 1997).

In a path-breaking series of experiments, Francis et al. (1999) reported that mothers with high rates of LG-ABN produced female offspring who, in adulthood, also had high LG-ABN scores when they gave birth to their own litters. In addition, female offspring of high LG-ABN mothers were less fearful when tested as adults in an open field arena. To determine how these behavioral traits were transmitted across generations, these investigators cross-fostered two pups per litter between high LG-ABN mothers and low LG-ABN mothers. To control for the process of cross-fostering per se, two pups per litter were in-fostered between litters of high LG-ABN mothers or between litters of low LG-ABN mothers. They found that pups born to low LG-ABN mothers but reared by high LG-ABN mothers resembled their foster mothers when they cared for their own litters. In addition, pups born to low LG-ABN mothers but reared by high LG-ABN foster mothers were less fearful in an open field arena. Complementary effects were reported for pups born to high LG-ABN mothers but reared by low LG-ABN mothers, with cross-fostered females having low LG-ABN scores and exhibiting greater fearfulness during an open field test. The behavioral and endocrine differences between offspring of high and low LG-ABN mothers showed a high degree of plasticity in response to manipulations of the post-weaning social environment (Champagne & Meaney, 2007).

The maternal environment also affected components of the HPA axis, including levels of glucocorticoid receptors (GRs) in the hippocampus and CRF mRNA levels in the hypothalamic paraventricular nucleus (PVN). Offspring of high LG-ABN mothers had higher levels of hippocampal GRs and lower levels of CRF mRNA in the PVN compared to offspring of low LG-ABN mothers. These results were consistent with lower levels of HPA stress reactivity in offspring of high LG-ABN mothers.

Maternal care and epigenetic changes. Subsequent studies from Meaney's laboratory examined the mechanisms responsible for the programming of offspring HPA responses. High levels of LG-ABN during the first week after birth altered cytosine methylation patterns of the exon 1_7 GR promoter within the area that binds the transcription factor, nerve growth factor-inducible protein A (NGFI-A). The 5' CpG dinucleotide of the NGFI-A sequence was always methylated in the offspring of low LG-ABN mothers, but was infrequently methylated in the offspring of high LG-ABN offspring. In contrast, the 3' CpG dinucleotide remained methylated in offspring of both types of mothers. These differences were apparent as early as PND 6 and were maintained well into adulthood. Importantly, cross-fostering of pups between high and low LG-ABN mothers resulted in pups that had the same methylation pattern as their foster mothers. Further, offspring of high LG-ABN mothers had greater levels of histone acetylation of the 1_7 GR promoter, allowing binding of NGFI-A to the promoter sequence. This led to increased expression of GR mRNA in the hippocampus and enhanced negative feedback of the HPA axis and reduced stress responses in offspring of high LG-ABN mothers (Weaver et al., 2004, 2007).

These epigenetic changes in gene expression may also be susceptible to changes in the dietary content of methyl donors. Such dietary changes could impact developing young during gestation and the preweaning period, adding an additional layer of complexity onto the dynamic interactions that occurred between genes and environment (McGowan et al., 2008).

Maternal care and estrogen signaling. Extensions of these results indicated that pups of high LG-ABN mothers also differed from pups of low LG-ABN mothers in having higher levels of mRNAs for estrogen receptor-α and -β in the medial preoptic nucleus of the hypothalamus. In addition, female offspring of high and low LG-ABN mothers differed in reproductive function and maternal sensitivity to newborn pups when tested in adulthood. Reciprocal cross-fostering of litters between high and low LG-ABN mothers reversed the differences in estrogen receptor-α and -β and oxytocin receptor mRNA levels, and partially reversed differences in reproductive development, confirming that patterns of maternal care were responsible in large measure for the neural and behavioral differences (Cameron et al., 2008; Champagne et al., 2006).

The impact of differences in maternal care on gene expression in offspring was far greater in magnitude than simply the genes for several steroid hormone receptors. In fact, based upon their experiments on the hippocampal transcriptome, Weaver et al. (2006) reported that more than 900 genes were differentially regulated by the maternal environment. More recent studies indicate that the epigenomic responses to differences in maternal care are not limited to single gene promoter regions, but include clusters of genes across broad regions of individual chromosomes (McGowan et al., 2011; Suderman et al., 2012).

In a timed-cross-fostering study, Peña et al. (2013) reciprocally cross-fostered litters between high and low LG-ABN mothers on PND 6 or 10 in an effort to delineate the critical windows of sensitivity for the effects of differences in maternal care on hormone receptor mRNA levels in the medial preoptic nucleus. The sensitive periods for the three receptor mRNAs were as follows: for estrogen receptor-α, birth to PND 10; for estrogen receptor-β, beyond PND 10; and for oxytocin, before PND 6.

Exposure to predator scent. Building on the studies by Meaney and his colleagues, McLeod et al. (2007) took advantage of the plasticity in maternal behaviors by exposing rat mothers and their litters to the odor of a cat or a control condition (rabbit odor or no odor) for 1 hour on the day of birth. Compared to control females, predator odor-exposed females licked and groomed their pups and were in arched back nursing postures more frequently during PNDs 1–5. Adult female offspring of predator odor-exposed and control females were bred and maternal behaviors were noted during PNDs 1–5 as well. Similar patterns of licking and grooming and arched back nursing postures were apparent, with female offspring of predator odor-exposed mothers having higher maternal behavior scores. Reciprocal cross-fostering of predator odor-exposed and control litters revealed that increases in LG-ABN of pups tracked with the postnatal maternal environment and not with the birth mother. In a final experiment, female offspring of predator odor-exposed mothers had increased levels of estrogen receptor-α and -β mRNAs in the medial preoptic nucleus of the hypothalamus compared to female offspring of control mothers.

Summary. Michael Meaney and his colleagues revolutionized the study of gene x maternal environment interactions and delineated some of the epigenetic mechanisms that underlie nongenomic transmission of information across generations. Building on earlier work by Levine, Denenberg, and others, Meaney's group demonstrated a causal link between pup responses to neonatal handling with changes in maternal behaviors directed toward the handled pups. These patterns of maternal behavior, including frequency of LG-ABN, were found to be normally distributed in breeding populations of laboratory rats and mice. If pups were reciprocally cross-fostered between high and low LG-ABN mothers, their HPA responses to stress and their behavioral responses to novelty matched with the phenotype of the foster mother that provided maternal care and not the phenotype of the biological mother. Remarkably, rates of maternal LG-ABN were transmitted to the next generation based upon the experiences of female pups with their mothers. Other experiments reported that inbred strains of laboratory mice and rats differed in their patterns of maternal behaviors, and in many instances, these strain differences were modified by cross-fostering. In extensive experiments on the epigenetic changes in pups that resulted from care provided by their mothers during the first 10 days of postnatal life, Meaney's laboratory stimulated a paradigm shift in behavioral neuroscience that continues to the present and that has important implications for investigations with human children and adults at risk of mental disorders.

Encoding and Transmitting Paternal Experiences

Natural Barriers Protecting the Germline

Primordial germ cells are segregated from somatic cells early in prenatal development, and undergo a genome-wide reduction in DNA methylation during migration to the gonadal ridge. After colonizing the embryonic gonad, mitotically arrested spermatogonia acquire the germ cell-specific epigenetic programming that permits them to undergo spermatogenesis in adulthood. As we will see in the following, all of these processes may be altered by stressors or environmental perturbations (e.g., diet, infection, toxins) that impact a male fetus during intrauterine development (Lane et al., 2014).

Puberty marks a stage at which developing sperm cells are sequestered within the relatively privileged micro-environments of the testis and epididymis. Formation of the blood-testis and blood-epididymis barriers protects developing germline cells as they progress from mitotic spermatogonia → meiotic spermatocytes → post-meiotic spermatids → fully differentiated spermatozoa. These development stages unfold within a fluid medium that is distinct in makeup from the surrounding interstitium. In the case of the epididymis, each of the three main segments—the caput, the corpus, and the cauda—maintains its own microenvironment that is finely tuned to the needs of the developing sperm. In the first two segments of the epididymis, extracellular vesicle (EV)–containing molecules play critical roles in supporting sperm motility and oocyte recognition. In the cauda, EVs release molecules that enhance sperm viability and maintain sperm cells in a quiescent state (Sullivan, 2013, 2015; Sullivan & Saez, 2013).

One potential barrier to the transmission of paternal experiences through epigenetic marks in sperm relates to the nuclear, cytoplasmic, and morphological changes that occur during spermatogenesis. Along the way, germ cell histones are exchanged in large part for protamines, and any epigenetic marks are lost in the process. Protamines are small, arginine-rich, highly basic nuclear proteins that allow denser packaging of DNA into the sperm head than would histones, and with this more compressed packaging of DNA comes a cessation of transcriptional activity. Cytoplasmic volume is also greatly reduced, and with it most of the existing RNA transcripts (Miller et al., 2010).

A Father's Influence

The nature of the message. In their thought-provoking review, Morgan et al. (2019) discussed potential mechanisms for germline transmission of nongenetic information from fathers to their offspring and beyond. They reasoned that such a process of information transfer from father to offspring would require three critical components:

- A vector to convey information from the father to the maternal reproductive tract and a future embryo. The most obvious vector is the sperm cell, but there are others.
- A molecular signal that could encode a paternal experience and transfer this molecular information to precipitate downstream responses.
- A target cell or tissue that could recognize the signal and effect a change in embryonic development or alterations in the maternal reproductive tract.

Notes in a bottle. Well, not quite, but extracellular vesicles (EVs, also referred to as microvesicles or exosomes) do appear capable of conveying molecular signals to maturing sperms cells, fertilized ova, and tissues of the female reproductive tract, thereby influencing fetal development (Morgan et al., 2019). EVs are composed of a lipid bilayer containing transmembrane proteins that encloses cytosolic proteins and RNAs. EVs may be formed and released by budding from the plasma membrane of cells of origin. In addition, EVs may arise within cells of origin, with secretion occurring when the membranous structures fuse with the inner cell membrane. Surface molecules on EVs bind to receptors on target cells, and at this point receptor-ligand interactions may occur, or the EV may be internalized into the cytoplasm of the target cell. Once liberated from the EV, the signaling molecules can alter the physiological state of the target cell (Tkach & Théry, 2016).

EVs and sperm. Sperm maturation in the epididymis has been identified recently as a likely point at which environment stimuli can alter sperm programming. In a methodologically sophisticated approach, Reilly et al. (2016) reported on significant changes in the composition of miRNAs contained in specialized EVs, called epididymosomes, along the length of the mouse epididymis from the caput → corpus → cauda. Epididymosomes are derived from epithelial cells lining the epididymis, and contain a complex cargo of proteins and lipids, as well as a complex blend of more than 350 miRNAs. Many of these miRNAs are in much higher concentrations within the epididymosomes compared to the surrounding epithelial cells. In addition, more than 50 miRNAs were found only in sperm and EVs within the epididymis, but not in the surrounding epithelial cells. The specific miRNAs contained within the epididymosomes also changed substantially along the length of the epididymis. Data were presented from an in vitro experiment involving co-incubation of caput epididymosomes and spermatozoa that revealed a transfer of five different miRNAs from epididymosomes to spermatozoa at a time when transcription was largely silent within the highly compacted sperm DNA. Epididymosomes may also deliver their miRNA cargo to the female reproductive tract and the fertilized oocyte, contributing an epigenetic memory trace of prior paternal stressful experiences to the developing embryo. Finally, an added layer of complexity involves modifications to transfer-RNA-derived small RNAs (tsRNAs) within spermatozoa as yet another type of epigenetic signal. Modifications to tsRNAs appear to increase RNA stability, which may increase the half-life of sperm tsRNA effects after fertilization and facilitate the transfer of paternally acquired traits to the developing embryo. In addition, tsRNA modifications could change the structure of tsRNAs and alter the specificity of their interactions with other molecules in the embryo (Chen et al., 2016; Morgan et al., 2019).

Fetal Origins of Mental Disorders

David J. P. Barker (1938–2013) conducted many influential epidemiological studies that confirmed a relationship between adverse aspects of the fetal and perinatal periods and the programming of chronic diseases such as cardiovascular disease, hypertension, and diabetes later in life (Barker, 1990, 1995). His corpus of research, which stimulated the emergence of a field of study referred to as "the developmental origins of health and disease," has had a major impact on international efforts to improve maternal and infant health. The underlying rationale behind the developmental origins of health and disease field of research is that the prenatal and early neonatal periods are developmental windows that are exquisitely sensitive to the enduring effects of perturbations in the environment (Bock et al., 2015; Weinstock, 2008, 2017). Particular attention has been directed to studies of prenatal programming of epigenetic changes in gene expression that contribute to increased risk for mental disorders later in life (Bale et al., 2010; Chan et al., 2018; Kim et al., 2015; O'Donnell & Meaney, 2017). As we will see in later chapters, the three-hit concept of vulnerability holds promise for understanding the effects of early life adversity on later development of mental disorders. The three hits include: (1) genetic predisposition, (2) prenatal or neonatal exposure to stressors, and (3) adolescent or adult exposure to stressors (Daskalakis et al., 2013).

Life at the Interface: The Placenta

The core function of the placenta and its membranes is to serve as an interface for exchanging nutrients and wastes between the embryonic and maternal circulations and to provide an environment supportive of growth of the embryo. Additional functions include production of hormones that regulate maternal hemodynamic and metabolic activities to ensure that the embryo remains viable. The relatively nonvascular decidua of maternal origin serves the additional purpose of being a physical barrier between maternal blood and the embryonic trophoblasts, thereby preventing premature mixing of potentially immunogenic elements (Bolon & Ward, 2015).

The morphology and gene expression of the mouse placenta is modified extensively during gestation in response to the embryo's evolving metabolic demands. Given that the fully formed placenta develops from maternal and embryonic cells, the sex of the developing embryo is an important consideration in studies that explore the impact of prenatal stress on the developing young. Another factor to keep in mind is the gestational age of embryos when pregnant females are exposed to stressors. Exposure of pregnant females to stressors during the first week of gestation can have dramatically different effects on offspring when they are adults, compared to stressors delivered during the final week of gestation (Bronson & Bale, 2016). These two issues will be discussed later in this chapter.

Development of the Placenta

Before the placenta is functional. Bolon and Ward (2015) have described in great detail the development of the mouse placenta. Following fertilization on embryonic day (ED) 0, the zygote goes through two successive cell divisions to arrive at the 4-cell stage by ED 2.0. Next, the embryo begins its regional

anatomical specialization at roughly the 8-cell stage, as it exits the distal ovi-
duct through the utero-tubal junction into the lumen of the uterus on ED 2.5.
Two days later, the mouse blastocyst consists of approximately 200 cells when
implantation in the uterine wall occurs on ED 4.5. Prior to implantation, the
uterine wall has been primed to support developing embryos through the changing concentrations of circulating maternal estrogen and progesterone, which
lead to decidualization of the endometrium. The embryo also participates in
controlling this decidual reaction, acting through the trophoblast giant cells
that form the outer layer of embryonic tissue that lies in close proximity to the
uterine wall. Major changes in the decidua-rich uterine wall that promote embryo attachment and survival include stromal cell expansion, enhanced angiogenesis and vascular permeability, and increased secretory capability of the
glandular epithelium. The decidual reaction provides support for the embryo
until formation of a functioning placenta. These changes are influenced by maternal immune cells, including uterine dendritic cells and uterine natural killer
(uNK) cells. Successful implantation also requires cooperation between maternal uterine tissue and the embryo.

The yolk sac is the first functional placental structure in the mouse beginning
at ED 8.5, and remains the only tissue supporting gas and nutrient exchange until
the definitive placenta begins to assemble (approximately ED 10.0–ED 10.5).
Gases move across the yolk sac by diffusion, but macromolecules are transferred
by the process of histiotrophic nutrition, whereby yolk sac phagocytes engulf
secretions from uterine glands and convey them to the embryo. The yolk sac vascular tree is established by ED 8.0–8.5, but continues to form branches until EDs
12–14, suggesting that the yolk sac continues to fill a histiotrophic role even after
the definitive placenta has taken over as the principal means of embryonic support (which occurs at approximately ED 12.5). The allantois, the precursor of the
umbilical cord, arises as a narrow bridge of mesoderm from the caudal end of
the embryo. As gestation progresses, the allantois projects toward the chorion,
and the fusion of these two organs at approximately ED 8.5 produces the chorio-
allantois. Completion of this connection is essential for creation of an efficient
system of gas and nutrient exchange later in gestation (Bolon & Ward, 2015).

Emergence of a functional placenta. The placenta is complete and fully functional by ED 12.5. To meet the growing metabolic demands of the embryo, the
placenta includes a greatly expanded interface for exchange of fluids, gases, and
macromolecules between the maternal and embryonic vascular compartments,
a process referred to as hemotrophic nutrition. The maximum weight of the placenta (~100 mg) is attained at ED 14.0–14.5, even though fetal weight doubles
from ED 15 until birth (Bolon & Ward, 2015).

Adamson et al. (2002) studied maternal and fetal circulation within the
mouse placenta by preparing plastic vascular casts and making serial histological

sections of implantation sites from ED 10.5 to ED 21. They observed that each radial artery carrying maternal blood into the mouse uterus formed 5–10 branches of dilated spiral arteries located within the metrial triangle.

Using diffusion-weighted and contrast-enhanced MRI techniques to study placental anatomy and physiology in laboratory mice at EDs 14.5 and 18.5, Solomon et al. (2014) reported that maternal blood moved through the spiral arteries to converge via trophoblast-lined canals into the placenta, where it diverged into pools within the intervillous spaces in the labyrinth (Figure 7.2). Fetal and maternal blood then traveled through the labyrinthic microcirculation in opposite directions. The close proximity of fetal vessels with the intervillous spaces ensures efficient exchange of gases, ions, and nutrients between the two circulatory systems. Within the labyrinth, layers of trophoblast cells of fetal origin line maternal blood vessels, serving as a protective barrier for the developing embryo.

The maternal blood constituted about 64% of the total placental volume, the fetal blood was about 24% of the total volume, and the various trophoblast components were about 12% of total volume. The behavior of fluid within the maternal blood pools of the placenta resembled freely diffusing water at 37°C. In contrast, fetal capillaries displayed a rapid flow of fluids to ensure adequate exchanges of nutrients. Finally, trophoblast cells, which experienced a large degree of exchange of water molecules between the fetal and maternal systems, had an apparent diffusion coefficient that was intermediate between the maternal and fetal compartments (Solomon et al., 2014).

Placental gene expression. The proper development of the placenta requires the carefully coordinated activity of many critical genes, including those coding for growth factors, transcription factors, extracellular matrix proteins, and proteins involved in cell signaling, to name a few. For each placental gene, up-regulation or down-regulation must occur within a carefully orchestrated cascade that ensures normal development of the embryo/fetus. Several functional groups of genes appear to be regulated at critical developmental stages, such as those involved in angiogenesis and cell cycle regulation on ED 10.5 compared to those involved in regulation of transcription and nuclear proteins at ED 17.5. Many of these gene regulatory pathways are affected by maternal hypoxia, maternal nutritional status, and levels of maternal stress (Gheorghe et al., 2010).

A wave of DNA demethylation occurs during cleavage of the fertilized ovum, followed by genome-wide de novo methylation after implantation. Although the male genome is widely demethylated soon after fertilization, the maternal genome is only partially demethylated. In the gastrulating embryo, the extent of DNA methylation is high, but it decreases in various tissues during the course of differentiation (Gheorghe et al., 2010).

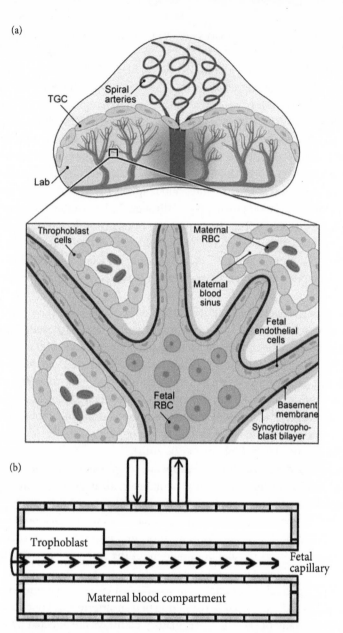

Figure 7.2. Schematic diagrams summarizing (A) the structure and main components of a mouse placenta and (B) the movement of fluids in each of these main compartments as visualized by diffusion MRI. Inset in A details the fetal–maternal–trophoblastic interactions in the labyrinth (Lab) area: fetal cells are surrounded by endothelial cells and membranes; fetal capillaries are surrounded by maternal blood sinuses, which conduct red blood cells (RBC) and are lined by trophoblast cells. Fluid exchanges between the fetal capillaries and the maternal blood pools are mediated by the trophoblasts, including the trophoblast giant cells (TGC) (see also Plate 7).

Placental Barrier to Maternal CORT

The HPA axis is activated when pregnant dams are exposed to stressors and circulating levels of CORT increase in maternal blood. Given that CORT is a highly lipophilic molecule, it would be expected to readily penetrate the blood-placental barrier. Under normal conditions, the placenta forms an effective barrier to limit passage of CORT from the maternal circulation to the developing embryo through the actions of the enzyme, 11β-hydroxysteroid dehydrogenase type 2 (11β-HSD-2), which converts adrenal glucocorticoids (cortisol in humans and corticosterone in rodents) into inactive metabolites (cortisone and 11β-dehydrocorticosterone, respectively) (O'Donnell et al., 2009; Welberg & Seckl, 2001). During pregnancy, if 11β-HSD-2 was inhibited by chronic administration of carbenoxolone or bypassed by administration of dexamethasone, a synthetic glucocorticoid not metabolized by 11β-HSD-2, the resulting offspring displayed significant alterations in HPA axis regulation and behavioral responses to stress (Shoener et al., 2006; Welberg et al., 2000).

To examine the effects of stress during the last week of pregnancy on placental expression of 11β-HSD2 in Long-Evans rats, Peña et al. (2012) exposed females to restraint stress for 1 hour per day during days 14–20 of pregnancy. Control females were left undisturbed in their home cages during days 14–20 of pregnancy. Females were sacrificed 1 hour after restraint stress on day 20 of pregnancy, and placental tissue samples were collected for later analyses. Exposure to prenatal stress was associated with a significant decrease in placental levels of 11β-HSD-2 mRNA, a significant increase in placental levels of mRNA for DNMT3α, and a significant increase in placental DNA methylation at CpG sites within the 11β-HSD-2 promoter. These findings demonstrate that the placental enzymatic barrier to glucocorticoids is vulnerable to stress during the third week of pregnancy in laboratory rats. The reduction in rates of 11β-HSD-2 transcription in the placenta may place developing embryos at risk of long-term changes in HPA axis regulation and behavioral responses to stress that would be expected to persist into adulthood.

In an earlier study by Mairesse et al. (2007), pregnant Sprague-Dawley rats were exposed to restraint stress (45 minutes × 3 times per day) for the final 11 days of gestation. They, too, reported decreased expression of 11β-HSD-2 in the placenta of stressed fetuses. In addition, they noted a significant decrease in expression of glucose transporter type 1 (GLUT1) in the placenta of stressed embryos. GLUT1 is the most highly expressed glucose transporter in the placenta and is essential for the facilitated diffusion of glucose from mother to fetus. The decrease in GLUT1 explains in part the reduction in body weights of prenatally stressed ED 21 fetuses, as well as their reduction in blood levels of glucose.

Prenatal Stress

There are several pathways by which maternal exposure to stress during pregnancy can affect the developing fetus. These maternal responses to stress include activation of the HPA axis, increased activity of the maternal sympathetic-adrenal medullary system and release of catecholamines, immune activation and increased cytokine levels, release of reactive oxygen species, and increased secretion/formation of serotonin and tryptophan. Rakers et al. (2017) have argued that prenatal stress effects on fetal development and physiological and behavioral measures later in life involve the synergistic effects of multiple stress-responsive pathways acting in concert.

Prenatal Stress—Pass It On

Hybrid mice (C57BL/6J x 129) were used in experiments by Morgan and Bale (2011) because of their robust stress responses and their previously characterized sex differences in key physiological and behavioral measures. F0 females were placed with males, and copulation was confirmed by the presence of a vaginal plug. Pregnant females were exposed to a variable stress paradigm (a different stressor each day for 7 days) on gestational days 1–7 (stress-group). The stressors that were employed were non-habituating and did not induce pain or adversely affect maternal health, gestation, litter size, or maternal behaviors toward the pups. F0 control females were not exposed to stressful stimuli. Previous reports from this laboratory noted that F1 male offspring of prenatally stressed females exhibited behavioral and physiological stress sensitivity and a dysmasculinized phenotype. The sensitive period for masculinization of the mouse brain by testosterone occurs during the last several days of gestation and extends into the first several days after birth. However, sexually dimorphic patterns of gene expression occur much earlier in gestation (Dewing et al., 2003).

A next step was to determine if these effects of prenatal stress on F1 males could be transmitted to their male offspring in the F2 generation. Whole brains were collected from F2 control and stress-group male and female pups on the day of birth, and expression of 93 genes involved in neural development was quantified. Seventeen genes differed significantly between F2 control males and females on the day of birth; in F2 stress-group males, expression of 13 of the 17 genes was more similar to control females than control males. Brains of F2 stress-group males also exhibited significant reductions in miR-322, miR-574, and miR-873, and again these values more closely resembled values in F2 control females. Administration of an aromatase inhibitor on PND 1 to block the conversion of testosterone to estrogen in neonatal mice resulted in dramatic changes in brain miRNA levels the next day. These results point to a critical role played by miRNAs in sexually dimorphic brain development.

F2 stress-group and control adult mice were subjected to a battery of behavioral and physiological tests. F2 stress-group males displayed significant reductions in anogenital distance and weight of testes and were immobile for more time in a tail suspension test compared to control males. F2 stress-group males and females did not differ from controls in performance on a spatial memory task or in plasma CORT responses to acute restraint stress. Taken together, these results indicate that prenatal stress of mothers during the first week of pregnancy may impinge on a sensitive period for development of sexually dimorphic patterns of gene expression and behavior, beginning neonatally and extending into adulthood. The transmission of prenatal stress effects through the male germline appears to involve alterations in the transcription of genes for miRNAs (Morgan & Bale, 2011).

High-risk male embryos. As noted earlier, male embryos are more susceptible to the deleterious effects of prenatal stress during the first week of gestation compared to female embryos. In addition, epidemiological and clinical studies have revealed that human males are at greater risk than females for several mental disorders, including schizophrenia, autism spectrum disorder, and attention deficit hyperactivity disorder. In each of these disorders, perturbations during gestation, such as exposure to stress or maternal infections, appear to place the developing fetus at increased risk of a diagnosis of mental illness later in life. The placenta is situated at the maternal-fetal interface and is likely to play an important role in conveying increased vulnerability to later disease onset in males versus females.

Placental inflammation. Bronson and Bale (2014) exposed pregnant hybrid mice (C57BL/6J x 129) to a variable stress paradigm (a different stressor each day for 7 days) on EDs 1–7. Control females were left undisturbed during this same time. Stressed and control females were sacrificed on ED 12.5, and placentae from male and female embryos were dissected free and frozen for later analysis of gene expression. Maternal stress increased expression of the proinflammatory cytokines IL-6 and IL-1β in placental samples from male but not female embryos. When offspring of prenatally stressed females were tested on PND 35, males but not females were more active, had more transitions from light to dark, and spent more time in the lighted portion of a light-dark box compared to controls. Expression of the gene coding for the D2 receptor in the nucleus accumbens was increased in males but not females.

To examine the involvement of placental inflammatory responses on later brain and behavioral changes, some control and prenatally stressed females received aspirin (acetylsalicylic acid, 162 mg/liter) in their drinking water during

EDs 1–7. Treatment with aspirin blocked the effects of prenatal stress on placental expression of IL-6 and postnatal behaviors in the light-dark box, while
partially restoring expression of the gene coding for the D2 receptor in the nucleus accumbens to control levels. These findings underscore the importance
of a stress-induced proinflammatory state in the placenta in programming the
changes in brain and behavior of male offspring tested on PND 35 (Bronson &
Bale, 2014).

Placental epigenetic effects. In three exciting reports from the Bale laboratory (Howerton & Bale, 2014; Howerton et al., 2013; Nugent et al., 2018), these
investigators were interested in the mechanisms relating to greater sensitivity
of male compared to female embryos to prenatal stress during the first week of
gestation. They started by utilizing a large-scale genomic screen at three times
during gestation (EDs 12.5,15.5, and 18.5) in a search for genes that differed in
expression between males and females and that were stress-responsive. They set-
tled on placental O-linked N-acetylglucosamine transferase (*Ogt*) as a molecular
marker of prenatal stress exposure in mice. *Ogt* codes for an X-linked enzyme
(OGT) that regulates more than 1,000 nuclear and cytosolic proteins involved
in chromatin remodeling through O-glycosylation of serine and threonine
residues. They reported that OGT mRNA and protein levels were dramatically
lower in placental tissue from male versus female embryos. In addition, the low
basal levels of placental OGT in males were reduced even further following prenatal stress. It is likely that *Ogt* escapes X-inactivation in placental trophoblasts,
thus providing females with two active copies of the gene versus one copy in
males. Chromatin immuno-precipitation (ChIP) assays were performed at the
Ogt locus with H3K4me3, a permissive chromatin mark indicative of transcriptional activation. A pattern of association with this activational mark was found
that was similar to the pattern detected for OGT mRNA and protein levels, with
a reduction for males and prenatal stress groups compared to control females. As
a further test of the importance of placental OGT in neural development of the
fetus, they utilized a transgenic mouse strain with targeted placental disruption
of *Ogt* and examined offspring for similarities to the prenatal stress phenotype.
Their results revealed that hypothalamic gene expression and the broad epigenetic miRNA environment in the neonatal brain of placental-specific hemizygous OGT mice was substantially altered compared to offspring of control
females (Howerton et al., 2013).

In an extension of this initial report, Howerton and Bale (2014) noted a reduction in expression of functional gene sets involved in endocrine and anti-
inflammatory signaling and an increase in those genes important in mitosis
and RNA/DNA replication and cell cycling. These results suggested that a reduction of OGT either transgenically or by prenatal stress could account for
dramatic changes in the endocrine function of the placenta and subsequent

disruptions in the relay of important signals to the developing fetus. They further reasoned that placentae from control females were fully differentiated and able to respond to environmental perturbations at ED 12.5, whereas placentae of prenatally stressed embryos and placentae with reduced OGT activity may still be progressing through a stage of rapid cellular proliferation. ChIP sequencing revealed reduced O-glycosylation at the 17β-hydroxysteroid dehydrogenase-3 (17β-HSD-3) locus in placentae of males exposed to prenatal stress. 17β-HSD-3 catalyzes the conversion of androstenedione to testosterone, and enzyme activity and testosterone levels were reduced and androstenedione levels were elevated in placentae of prenatally stressed male embryos.

When examined in adulthood, hemizygous OGT mice had 10%–20% reductions in body weights compared to WT littermates. Interestingly, these body weight differences were not apparent at weaning, suggesting that gonadal hormone changes at puberty may explain the body weight differences in adulthood. Male mice with reduced placental OGT also displayed HPA stress axis dysregulation, although the magnitude of the CORT response was less than for prenatally stressed male mice. In contrast, female hemizygous mice showed the opposite effect, with a blunted CORT response to acute stress (Howerton & Bale, 2014).

Nugent et al. (2018) tackled the question of how sex differences in placental OGT activity explain the greater impact of prenatal stress on male versus female offspring. Focusing on trophoblast cell-specific, actively translated mRNAs, they identified 4,560 genes with significant sex differences in expression on ED 12.5. The large number of sex differences in gene expression in this fetally derived placental cell type demonstrated a possible mechanism for establishing sex differences in trans-placental signaling and fetal development. Functional gene ontology analyses revealed two biological processes enriched in male trophoblasts relative to females, whereas 81 biological processes were enriched in female trophoblasts relative to males.

Sex-specific epigenetic programming in placental trophoblasts may underlie the greater vulnerability of male fetuses to developmental insults, including prenatal stressors. One possible mechanism for the greater vulnerability of male fetuses is through OGT regulation of the repressive epigenetic mark, H3K27me3. Male placentae have significantly lower levels of H3K27me3, resulting in altered hypothalamic programming of gene expression on ED 18.5 that was linked to prenatal stress exposure. These investigators concluded that placental OGT-mediated epigenomic programming promoted greater homogeneity in female trophoblast gene expression compared to males. When repressive transcriptional regulation was reduced in females, male-like transcriptional variability was induced, pointing to increased vulnerability to developmental insults (Nugent et al., 2018).

Epigenetic Transmission of Postnatal Stress Exposure

There is strong evidence that stressful experiences in adult males and females can be transmitted trans-generationally to their offspring through epigenetic alterations in DNA. The experimental strategies for exploring these preconception effects of stress differ when considering male and female parents, and these issues will be discussed in detail in the following (Blaze & Roth, 2015).

Stressed-Out Mothers

Sperm methylation codes for stress. To model early-life traumatic experiences, Franklin et al. (2010) exposed litters of C57BL/6 mice to unpredictable maternal separation (3 hours per day at different times during the dark cycle) combined with unpredictable maternal stress (restraint stress or cold swim stress) during the first 2 weeks of postnatal life (MS condition). Control (CON) litters were left undisturbed except for weekly cage cleanings. Following behavioral testing of mice in adulthood, MS and CON males were mated with primiparous C57BL/6 female mice to produce an F2 generation.

Maternal behaviors of MS mothers differed from CON mothers during the first postnatal week but not the second postnatal week. CON mothers displayed significantly more frequent LG/ABN episodes, and they were in the nest with their litters more frequently than MS mothers. There were no differences in these maternal behaviors in F2 females that were sired by F1 MS males.

F1 MS males displayed increased depression-like behaviors compared to CON males. F2 females but not F2 males that were sired by an F1 MS male displayed increased depression-like behaviors compared to CONs. F3 males but not females that were sired by an F2 male with a father who experienced MS displayed increased depression-like behaviors compared to CONs. Chronic treatment with desipramine for 14 days reversed the depressive-like behaviors in F2 MS females. In two tests involving exposure to unfamiliar environments, F1 MS males and F2 and F3 MS females exhibited shorter latencies to enter unfamiliar areas compared to appropriate CONs. These findings were interpreted as MS-induced deficits in behavioral control when mice were exposed to novel environments.

Franklin et al. (2010) reasoned that the behavioral changes that were observed in mice of the F1–F3 generations could be transmitted through epigenetic changes in the male germline. Using sperm from F1 MS males, they reported that DNA methylation was increased in the promoter regions of two candidate genes, the transcriptional regulator methyl CpG-binding protein 2 (MeCP2) and endocannabinoid receptor-1 (CB1). In another candidate gene coding for the CRF_2 receptor, DNA methylation was decreased in the promoter region. In two other candidate genes, monoamine oxidase A and serotonin receptor 1A ($5HT_{1A}$), there were no differences in methylation patterns. In sperm cells from F2 MS males, similar results were obtained, except that DNA methylation of the promoter region for CB1 was similar to CON males. Similar results were obtained for brain tissue samples from F2 MS females, with hyper-methylation of MeCP2 and CB1 but hypo-methylation of the gene for CRF_2 receptor. In all three instances, expression of mRNAs for MeCP2, CB1, and CRF_2 in brains of F2 MS females were decreased relative to F2 CON females.

These findings represent the first demonstration that postnatal stress in mice resulted in persistent alterations in behavior and germline methylation patterns across generations. Female mice displayed greater changes in depression-like behaviors, and this is consistent with the greater incidence of major depressive disorder in females versus males. Only five candidate genes were studied in this experiment, and it is likely that other genes were also affected by the maternal stress paradigm. In addition, each affected gene likely contributed modestly to the overall behavioral phenotype across generations (Franklin et al., 2010).

RNAs code for stress. A later study from this same laboratory employed the MS paradigm, but with a focus on the impact of small non-coding RNAs (sncRNAs) in sperm as potential vectors of these trans-generational effects on offspring (Gapp et al., 2014). F1 MS male C57BL/6J mice and their F2 MS off-spring exhibited alterations in several behavioral measures, including reduced latency to initially enter an open arm of the elevated plus-maze (EPM), increased time spent in a light-dark box, and increased time spent floating in a forced swim test. An examination of glucose regulation revealed that F1 MS males were similar to controls in serum levels of insulin and glucose. However, F2 MS males had significantly lower serum levels of insulin, as well as reduced levels of glucose under basal conditions and following acute restraint stress. Further studies suggested that F2 MS males displayed a metabolic pattern consistent with insulin hypersensitivity.

These investigators next examined content of sncRNAs in sperm samples from F1 MS males as a means of explaining the trans-generation effect of MS from the F1 to F2 generation. Several miRNAs (miR-375-3p, miR-375-5p, miR-200b-3p, miR-672-5p, and miR-466-5p) were up-regulated in F1 MS sperm samples, and their possible targets included regulation of DNA and RNA, epigenetic regulations, or RNA binding and processing. In addition, piRNA cluster 110 was significantly down-regulated in F1 MS sperm. miRNAs were also altered in the serum and hippocampus of F1 and F2 MS males, but not in the sperm of F2 MS males. miRNAs did not differ from controls in F3 MS animals even though there were behavioral differences. These investigators suggested that changes in miRNAs that initially occurred in sperm cells as a result of MS may be encoded by other nongenomic or epigenetic marks in F2 males, such as DNA methylation or histone post-translational modifications (Gapp et al., 2014).

A final experiment provided a test of the potential causal link between altered miRNAs in sperm and behavioral and physiological changes in succeeding generations. Purified total RNA samples from the sperm of MS-exposed F1 males were microinjected into the male pronucleus of wild-type fertilized mouse oocytes. Control fertilized oocytes received microinjections of total RNA samples from unstressed control male mice. The results were quite striking in that the resulting offspring that received microinjections of RNA from MS-exposed males displayed the behavioral, metabolic, and molecular disruptions that were observed in F1 MS males. These results provided strong evidence for a prominent role for sncRNAs in the trans-generational effects of early life exposure to stress (Gapp et al., 2014). A more recent report notes that behavioral alterations and glucose dysregulation affected MS mice up to the 4th generation, but depressive-like behaviors were apparent in F3 but not F2 and F4 MS males (van Steenwyk et al., 2018).

Stressed-Out Fathers

Stress and sperm miRNAs. In a study by Rodgers et al. (2013), hybrid male mice from a C57BL/6 x 129 cross were exposed to chronic variable stress for a 6-week period that encompassed adolescence and early adulthood (PNDs 28–70) or occurred exclusively in adulthood (PNDs 56–98). Controls were left undisturbed in their home cages. After stress exposure, males were housed individually with a female to permit time for recovery from stress exposure. Females were separated as soon as a copulation plug was detected (1–3 nights) to minimize any impact of the stressed male on later maternal behavior of the female toward her litter. Offspring of the three groups were later exposed to tests of HPA axis responsivity to acute stress or various behavioral measures. In addition, whole pituitary glands, left adrenal gland, and brain punches of the PVN and the BNST were collected, and microarray and gene set enrichment analyses were carried out. Finally, sperm samples were collected from males of the three groups and later analyzed for miRNA content.

The results indicated that male and female offspring of fathers stressed at either developmental stage exhibited significant reductions in plasma levels of CORT during and after acute restraint stress for 15 minutes. These decreases in HPA axis responsiveness did not appear to result from changes in central serotonin signaling. Offspring of stressed and control fathers did not differ on a battery of behavioral tests (tail suspension test, prepulse inhibition of the acoustic startle response, light-dark box activity, and maze learning). Expression of several key genes in the pituitary and adrenal gland involved in HPA axis responses to stress was not affected by paternal stress exposure. These included CRF_1 and POMC in the pituitary and melanocortin receptor-2 and 11β-HSD in the adrenal cortex. In the PVN and BNST, global pattern changes in transcription suggestive of epigenetic reprogramming were noted in offspring of stressed fathers. These changes included increased expression of CORT-responsive genes in the PVN. Exposure to chronic variable stress during both developmental stages resulted in significant increases in nine miRNAs in sperm samples relative to levels of the miRNAs in sperm samples from control males. These findings provide compelling evidence that exposure of males to stressful stimuli prior to mating can affect their first-generation offspring through epigenetic reprogramming in sperm cells. The alterations in HPA axis responsivity in offspring could prove to be adaptive, depending upon the nature of the environment in which they develop (Rodgers et al., 2013).

Using a different experimental approach, Short et al. (2018) reported that chronic CORT delivery in the drinking water of C57BL/6 male mice prior to mating affected anxiety-like and depression-like behaviors across multiple generations. Three miRNAs were elevated in sperm from CORT-treated mice, including miR-98, miR-144, and miR 190b, suggesting a mechanism for transmission of the effects of chronic CORT to succeeding generations.

Manipulating sperm miRNAs. In a stunning follow-up experiment, Rodgers et al. (2015) rigorously examined if sperm miRNA changes following stress, as described in the preceding, function post-fertilization to alter offspring HPA axis responsiveness to stress. A cocktail containing the nine miRNAs that were elevated in sperm samples of stress males as described earlier was microinjected into single-cell zygotes that were then implanted into CD-1 females. Offspring that received zygotic microinjections of the nine miRNAs displayed a remarkably similar pattern of HPA hypo-responsiveness to acute restraint stress compared to the offspring of stressed fathers in the previous experiments (Rodgers et al., 2013). The miRNAs from sperm stimulated the degradation of stored maternal mRNA transcripts in zygotes, thereby initiating a cascade of molecular events, including gene expression in the PVN, which resulted in altered HPA axis responses to acute stress (Rodgers et al., 2015).

Of mice and men. In related experiments, Dickson et al. (2018) examined the effects of chronic social instability stress (reconstituting social groups of 4 CD-1 outbred mice per cage twice per week for 7 weeks) beginning on PND 28 (Schmidt et al., 2007). There was a 5-fold reduction in levels of two miRNAs, miR-449a and miR-34c, in sperm from stressed males compared to unstressed controls. When stressed males were mated with control females, these two miRNAs, which are not found in oocytes, were decreased significantly in embryos at the 2-, 4-, and 8-cell stages, as well as the morula stage, compared to embryos that resulted from mating control males and control females. Finally, miR-449a and miR-34c levels were also dramatically reduced in sperm from off-spring produced by mating stressed males with control females. These results were extended to sperm samples collected from adult human males who varied in scores for adverse childhood experiences (ACEs). Remarkably, there were significant negative correlations between ACEs and sperm content of miR-449a and miR-34c. The consistency of these findings suggested that reduced sperm levels of miRNAs may contribute to the trans-generational transmission of adverse childhood experiences in humans and stressful experience in adolescence in mice (Dickson et al., 2018).

Defeated Fathers

Using the well-validated chronic social defeat stress (CSDS) paradigm (Krishnan et al., 2007), Dietz et al. (2011) bred groups of previously defeated and control C57BL/6J male mice with normal C57BL/6J female mice. CSDS was performed 30 days prior to mating. Offspring from these two groups were tested for levels of depression- and anxiety-like behaviors, and plasma CORT was measured under basal conditions and following acute stress. Other groups of male mice were mated prior to and following CSDS to further isolate the effects of social defeat on offspring behaviors. To indirectly assess the effects of epigenetic factors, sperm samples were collected from defeated and control fathers for in vitro fertilization (IVF), and resulting offspring were tested as described earlier.

Male and female offspring from defeated fathers displayed increased levels of depression-like (social avoidance following sub-maximal CSDS and forced swim and sucrose preference tests) and anxiety-like (novel arena and EPM) behaviors. In addition, male offspring of defeated fathers had elevated baseline levels of CORT. When offspring were produced by IVF, only one behavioral difference remained; male and female mice conceived with sperm from defeated fathers displayed significantly reduced latencies to immobility in the forced swim test. These investigators discounted epigenetic changes in the sperm of defeated fathers as an explanation for the behavioral changes in their offspring. Rather, they favored the view that the behavioral changes in the offspring of defeated fathers resulted from behavioral alterations in their mothers that were driven by their experiences with defeated male partners. Unfortunately, epigenetic changes in sperm were not measured directly in this experiment, and procedures related to collection and incubation of sperm cells for IVF could have erased some epigenetic marks (Dietz et al., 2011). These issues will surface again in the sections that follow.

What's That Smell?

Transmission of fear. The experiences of adult animals prior to mating may influence their future offspring, but in such instances the mode of transmission would involve trans-generational inheritance via alterations in the germline (Dias & Ressler, 2014a). To investigate the transmission of pre-mating stressful experiences to future generations, Dias and Ressler (2014b) trained adult male mice to associate an odor (acetophenone [ACET] or propanol [PROP]) with footshock in three consecutive daily training sessions. Control males did not undergo odor-shock pairings. Ten days later, control and previously shocked male mice were placed with adult females for 10 days, and then the males were removed. Females gave birth and their offspring (F1) were weaned and housed in groups until testing at 2 months of age.

F1 ACET males displayed enhanced behavioral sensitivity to ACET while F1 PROP males displayed enhanced behavioral sensitivity to PROP compared to F1 controls. These findings were striking in that these F1 males had never been exposed to these test odors previously. In addition, these enhanced odor sensitivities were transmitted to the F2 generation. Further studies using offspring from in vitro fertilization (to control for prenatal effects) and cross-fostering experiments (to control for postnatal maternal effects) confirmed that the transmission of enhanced sensitivity to an odor previously paired with electric shock in the F0 generation was transmitted through parental gametes. Further, ACET-specific olfactory sensory neurons were increased in number and size in brains of F1 ACET males that were odor-naïve. The sperm of F0 and F1 males had epigenetic alterations that were consistent with hypo-methylation of an olfactory receptor specific for ACET. The possibility that histones associated with this receptor were hyper-acetylated was also raised.

These findings are intriguing on several levels. First, the odor-shock pairings occurred well before F0 males mated with females. Second, the behavioral sensitivity to the odor associated with shock was apparent in the F1 and F2 generations, which had never been exposed to the odor. Third, cross-fostering and in vitro fertilization to control for postnatal and prenatal effects, respectively, were employed, and both conditions failed to alter the odor sensitivity of F1 and F2 offspring of F0 ACET males. Fourth, the experience of the odor-shock pairings in the F0 generation led to behavioral and anatomical changes in the F1 progeny. Fifth, the mechanism for this trans-generational transmission appears to have involved epigenetic changes in sperm that resulted from the odor-shock pairings.

Blocking transmission of fear. In a replication and extension of the previous study, Aoued et al. (2019) set out to interrupt the transmission of fear related to prior exposure to odor-shock pairings from F0 C57BL/6J male mice to their F1 male progeny. In this study, two odors were employed, acetophenone (ACET) and Lyral® (hydroxyisohexyl 3-cyclohexene carboxaldehyde). Lyral replaced PROP from the previous study. Three groups of adult male mice were generated for each test odor: (i) 5 odor presentations for 10 seconds each per day × 3 days; (ii) 5 odor presentations for 10 seconds each per day × 3 days, with each odor presentation followed by a single footshock (0.4 mA, 0.25 msec); and (iii) odor-shock pairings for 3 days as in (ii), followed by 3 days of extinction training in a different environment, with 30 odor presentations each day, but without footshocks. Twelve days after odor testing, males of the three groups were mated with naïve female mice, and F1 litters were weaned on PND 21. F1 males were tested in adulthood for odor-potentiated startle.

The results of these experiments replicated and extended the previous results reported by Dias and Ressler (2014b) in several important ways. Conditioned fear for either of two odors (ACET or Lyral) was passed from F0 fathers to their F1 adult offspring. An important control group included F0 male mice that were exposed to ACET but without shock pairings. Their F1 offspring did not show enhanced sensitivity to ACET compared to offspring of F0 males that were not exposed to ACET odors prior to mating. In addition, there was no cross-talk between odors after F0 male odor-shock pairings. That is, F1 animals sired by F0 males exposed to ACET-shock pairings were no more sensitive to Lyral than naïve controls. The reverse was also true. If F0 males received extinction training after odor-shock pairings, their F1 offspring did not display enhanced behavioral responses to the same test odor. At an anatomical level, odor-shock pairings in F0 male mice resulted in enhanced representation of M71 (ACET-responsive) or MOR23 (Lyral-responsive) odorant receptors in the olfactory system of F1 offspring. These anatomical changes in the olfactory system of F1 offspring were reversed if their F0 sires were exposed to extinction training prior to mating. Finally, evidence that the transmission of these behavioral and anatomical changes were transmitted through the germline was presented. F0 males that were exposed to odor-shock pairings displayed reduced methylation of the promoter regions for ACET-responsive odorant receptors (*Olfr151* and *Olfr160*) and a Lyral-responsive odorant receptor (*Olfr16*) in sperm samples. Importantly, these differences in gene methylation patterns of sperm samples were partially reversed by extinction training of F0 males.

These findings in laboratory mice provide encouragement for researchers and clinicians who are interested in the trans-generational impact of parental life stressors. If behavioral treatments could be designed and made available for teens and young adults who have undergone traumatic experiences, there is hope that the behavioral, anatomical, and molecular genetic alterations that are transmitted to the next generation could be prevented from appearing in the germline (Aoued et al., 2019).

Too Old to Mate?

Male fertility is maintained into advanced age, and requires that each cycle of cell division faithfully reproduces genetic and epigenetic information in newly synthesized DNA to maintain the integrity of the germline. However, aging has been associated with altered patterns of DNA methylation and an accumulation of de novo mutations in sperm cells of mammals. Milekic et al. (2015) addressed these issues in a study of 129SvEv/Tac mice. Three-month-old females were mated with either males of a similar age or males that were 12–14 months old (in human terms, 20 versus 45 years old). At 12 weeks of age, male offspring from young and old fathers underwent behavioral testing, and pooled sperm DNA samples were subjected to genome-wide methylation profiling. Their results indicated that offspring of older fathers exhibited reductions in exploratory behavior in an open field arena and reductions in acoustic startle responses and prepulse inhibition compared to offspring of young fathers. In addition, sperm DNA from older fathers displayed a significant loss of CpG methylation in regions associated with regulation of gene transcriptional activity. Similar analyses of DNA from brains of offspring sired by young and old fathers revealed CpG hypo-methylation at regions flanking transcription start sites. The authors concluded that age-related decreases in DNA methylation in sperm cells of older fathers appeared to underlie the changes in behavior and brain DNA hypo-methylation observed in their offspring (Milekic et al., 2015).

Summary

Building upon previous studies of early handling of litters of laboratory rats, Meaney and his coworkers revolutionized our understanding of gene x environment interactions and highlighted the importance of epigenetic changes as a mechanism to explain the nongenetic transmission of behavioral and neuroendocrine phenotypes across generations. Other lines of investigation have revealed that experiences of the father prior to mating may be transmitted to succeeding generations through alterations in the germline. A critical link in this transmission from father to offspring involved miRNAs associated with sperm cells and with EVs. The role of the placenta as a sex-specific and dynamic interface between a pregnant mother and her developing embryos has also been studied. Disruptions in placental physiology because of maternal stress exposure can alter the developmental programming of her embryos, and these changes may in turn be transmitted to future generations. Stress-induced changes in the male germline are reversible, which provides strong encouragement for the development of behavioral and pharmacological interventions in children exposed to early life stressors. Finally, there are encouraging signs that biomarkers of early life stress in children will be developed, and these advances will aid in the identification of at-risk children and provide a means for tracking their responses to treatments.

8

Stress and Schizophrenia

Siddhartha Mukherjee, a multi-talented physician-scientist and recipient of the Pulitzer Prize for General Non-Fiction in 2011 for his intimate portrait of cancer, *The Emperor of All Maladies*, was born into a Bengali family that experienced the multiple traumas associated with Partition, the cleaving of colonial India in 1947 into two separate countries, one with a Muslim majority (Pakistan) and one with a Hindu majority (India). Millions of people were displaced just prior to and following Partition, including Mukherjee's widowed paternal grandmother and her five sons, who moved from East Bengal to Calcutta in 1946. Two of the sons, Rajesh, the third-born, and Jagu, the fourth-born, developed mental illnesses (bipolar disorder and schizophrenia, respectively). In addition, the oldest son's first-born child, Moni, was also diagnosed with schizophrenia.

Consider this description of Jagu (Mukherjee, 2016, p. 3): "Jagu had been troubled from childhood. Socially awkward, withdrawn to everyone except my grandmother, he was unable to hold a job or live by himself. By 1975, deeper cognitive problems had emerged: he had visions, phantasms, and voices in his head that told him what to do. He made up conspiracy theories by the dozen. He often spoke to himself, with a particular obsession of reciting made-up train schedules."

Mukherjee (2016, p. 5) suggested that the trauma of moving from their ancestral village to Calcutta was a possible tipping point for Jagu. "In Calcutta, like a plant uprooted from its natural habitat, Jagu wilted and fell apart. He dropped out of college and parked himself permanently by one of the windows of the flat, looking blankly out at the world. His thoughts began to tangle, and his speech became incoherent." This unfortunately is a familiar pattern for any family member touched by the development of schizophrenia in a loved one.

Clinical Overview of Schizophrenia

Schizophrenia is an especially devastating mental illness, typically striking its victims just as they move from adolescence into adulthood. The global incidence of schizophrenia is approximately 1.0%, with males having a higher incidence and an earlier onset of symptoms than females. The disease is highly debilitating, with extraordinary costs incurred by individuals, families, and societies. The signs and symptoms of schizophrenia are highly diverse, and tend to cluster into three major categories: *positive symptoms*, including delusions, movements disorders, hallucinations, and disorders of thought; *negative symptoms*, including social withdrawal, a lack of pleasure in events of everyday life, and blunted affect; and *cognitive deficits*, including disruptions in memory and difficulties with staying focused and making decisions. The clustering of these signs and symptoms from one patient to the next may be non-overlapping, further complicating an already complex disease etiology (Andreasen, 1999; Kahn et al., 2015; Tandon et al., 2013). In addition, some of these symptoms may be shared by other diagnostic categories, including bipolar disorder, depression, and autism spectrum disorder. Finally, in spite of heroic attempts, there is still no biochemical, physiological, or imaging-based test available to aid in the diagnosis of schizophrenia (Arguello et al., 2010).

Migration and Madness

The forced migration of the Mukharjee family from East Bengal to Calcutta has been repeated many times before and after Partition. Recently, the civil war in Syria and instability in the countries of North Africa have motivated many families with young children, as well as young adults, to seek new lives in the countries of the European Union or in North America. Crossing the Mediterranean is the beginning of a perilous journey, and many of the migrants do not receive warm welcomes when they settle in their host countries. One consistent consequence of moving from a country of dark-skinned people to a country of light-skinned people is a significantly greater risk of schizophrenia in immigrants and their children compared to non-immigrants (relative risk = 4.8). These countries include the United States, Canada, Germany, The Netherlands, and Denmark. The *social defeat hypothesis* has been advanced to explain the elevated risk of schizophrenia in immigrants. The social defeat hypothesis makes a connection between a diathesis (risk genes) and the high levels of stress that attend migration and resettlement. Included in these stressors are the dangers of travel, the lack of familiar social support networks, discrimination, poverty, inadequate shelter, and language difficulties (Selten et al., 2013; Selten et al., 2017). The higher risk of schizophrenia in migrants may be mediated in part by enhanced DA signaling in the brain, especially in response to external stressors (Egerton et al., 2017).

The Evolutionary Paradox

Schizophrenia Keeps Hanging On

Schizophrenia is a disorder with high heritability (approximately 70%) that also has a relatively high prevalence of about 1% in the global population. However, schizophrenic patients, especially males, are much less likely to marry and have children, and they have shorter life spans compared to unaffected individuals. Thus, we must confront a genetically based disorder that results in decreased rates of reproduction, but that is maintained at a relatively high rate in the global population. One would expect that risk genes for schizophrenia would be under intense negative selection pressure, and would gradually be eliminated from the population over several generations. But the opposite is true—the prevalence of schizophrenia is remarkably consistent across racial and ethnic groups in countries around the world.

Huxley's Hypothesis

Sir Julian Huxley and his colleagues (Huxley et al., 1964) were among the first to tackle this evolutionary paradox and advance the idea that schizophrenia must confer selective advantages to affected individuals to offset the deleterious effects of the disease on reproductive fitness. They worked under the false assumption that schizophrenia was caused by a single dominant gene with low penetrance, such that only 25% of individuals with the gene actually developed schizophrenia. They proposed some physiological advantages for those who were carriers of the risk gene, including resistance to infections, fewer allergies, and elevated levels of hormones, including insulin. They further proposed that male and female carriers of the risk gene, and possibly females with schizophrenia, had higher than average rates of reproduction, thus counterbalancing the reduced rates of reproduction in males with schizophrenia. They concluded that these physiological and reproductive advantages of the schizophrenia risk gene offset the obvious disadvantages of those diagnosed with the disease, resulting in a stable prevalence of schizophrenia in the global population (Huxley et al., 1964).

The hypothesis that carriers of a putative schizophrenia risk gene have increased numbers of children to make up for the low reproductive rates of their clinically diagnosed siblings has been tested through the use of population-based studies in Finland and Sweden. These findings confirmed that schizophrenic patients do have reduced reproductive rates. However, siblings of schizophrenic patients did not differ from unaffected individuals in their rates of reproduction (Haukka et al., 2003; Power et al., 2013).

One End of the Distribution?

A very different view has emerged more recently that posits that schizophrenia is an unfortunate cost incurred on the balance sheet of human evolution. The positive selection pressure for genetic risk factors that favored higher order cognitive functions, including creativity, language, and social skills, were some of the same risk factors that predispose to schizophrenia. Thus, schizophrenia may represent one extreme of the normal variation in some of the traits that have made humans so successful from an evolutionary perspective (Crow, 2000; del Giudice, 2017; van Dongen & Boomsma, 2013).

Consistent with this view is the finding that risk genes for schizophrenia are more prevalent in genomic regions that are more likely to have undergone recent positive selection in humans (Srinivasan et al., 2016). This study made use of a proxy measure for evolutionary change, the Neanderthal Selective Sweep (NSS) score, with low NSS scores taken as an indicator of recent positive selection. Variants in brain-specific genes with low NSS scores were associated with greater risk for schizophrenia than brain-specific genes with high NSS scores. Further, this relationship was strongest for schizophrenia compared to other phenotypes. These authors concluded with the stunning suggestion "that the persistence of schizophrenia is related to the evolutionary process of becoming human" (Srinivasan et al., 2016, p. 284).

Many other explanations based in evolutionary theory have been proposed to bring clarity to this conundrum. For example, some have favored an explanation that involves balancing selection. Balancing selection occurs when multiple alleles are maintained in the gene pool of the population if the genotypes are under differing selection pressures or if the different selection pressures act upon a single allele under different circumstances. For example, schizophrenia or bipolar disorder may develop in some individuals with significant numbers of risk genes, but in their relatives, and even in unrelated individuals, some of these same risk genes may contribute to enhanced social skills and greater creativity (Keller & Visscher, 2015; Power et al., 2015). An alternative view is represented by variations on the mismatch hypothesis. These include the possibility that schizophrenia may have been a more adaptive phenotype in ancient times, it may have been a neutral phenotype in ancient times, or it may have persisted in the face of changes in environmental conditions (Daly et al., 2016; van Dongen & Boomsma, 2013).

Since the original hypotheses of Huxley et al. (1964), much has been learned about the genetic architecture of schizophrenia. In addition, some of the hypotheses advanced by Huxley and his colleagues have been disproven. Given the emphasis on dimensional approaches to mental disorders, it may very well be that schizophrenia is simply one extreme of the normal distribution of humans, and is the cost for the explosive development of neural, cognitive, and social adaptations over the past 150,000 years of the evolutionary history of *Homo sapiens*.

The Neurodevelopmental Hypothesis

In searching for the causes of schizophrenia, many investigators over time have embraced the neurodevelopmental hypothesis first proposed by Weinberger (1987). Weinberger's hypothesis was based upon three critical observations relating to schizophrenia: (i) onset of symptoms in late adolescence or early adulthood; (ii) the importance of stressful life events in onset and relapse; and (iii) the efficacy of neuroleptic drugs in treating schizophrenics. The first observation situates the onset of schizophrenic symptoms during a time of dynamic synaptic sculpting in highly evolved cortical areas of the brain, including the PFC. Stressful life events are a crucial aspect of the onset and recurrence of symptoms of schizophrenia, as detailed in Chapter 2. Finally, the efficacy of neuroleptics in treating the symptoms of schizophrenia brought the neurotransmitter DA into the spotlight, where it remains to the present (Weinberger, 1987).

Kesby et al. (2018) have issued a note of caution regarding studies of brain DA signaling in animal models of schizophrenia. They point out that clinical studies of patients with schizophrenia have revealed enhanced presynaptic DA function in the associative striatum, and not the limbic striatum as previously assumed. Unfortunately, many experiments with animal models employ measures of psychostimulant-induced increases in locomotor activity, a measure that involves increased DA activity in the limbic striatum.

These investigators suggested a strategy for modeling positive symptoms of schizophrenia in laboratory animals that reflect these more recent clinical results. By employing tasks involving attentional set-shifting and serial reversal learning in animal models, one can evaluate DAergic signaling in the associative striatum as opposed to the limbic striatum. This neuroanatomical mismatch between clinical and animal studies can be addressed in future studies and should be kept in mind in reviewing the studies described in the remainder of this chapter (Kesby et al., 2018).

Since Weinberger's seminal paper, new advances in research have brought the pathophysiology of schizophrenia into somewhat clearer focus (Rapoport et al., 2012). Several environmental stressors appear to play a substantial role in the etiology of schizophrenia, including maternal infections, complications during birth, early life adversity, life stressors during adolescence and adulthood, and drug use and abuse. These environmental stressors appear to interact with susceptible genotypes, leading to the onset of symptoms of schizophrenia beginning in late adolescence or early adulthood (Ayhan et al., 2016; Boksa & El-Kodor, 2003). In addition, Selemon and Zecevic (2015) have highlighted a connection between two critical periods in the development of the PFC and the later onset of schizophrenia. The first critical period in humans involves cell proliferation during the first trimester of gestation, and the second critical period occurs during adolescence, when pruning of excitatory synapses occurs. Both of these critical periods in PFC development are remarkably sensitive to environmental stressors, and these developmental processes have been investigated in great detail using a variety of animal models (e.g., Lu et al., 2011), as will be discussed in the following.

Attention, Please!

Based upon their careful clinical observations of 26 schizophrenic patients in the early stages of the disease, McGhie and Chapman (1961) hypothesized that these patients exhibited a dysfunction in selective and inhibitory aspects of attention. This seminal article has stimulated basic and clinical research on sensorimotor gating for more than six decades. What has become clear is that schizophrenic patients are overly sensitive to sensory stimulation, which in turn leads to cognitive fragmentation. In addition, schizophrenic patients show evidence of impairments in central nervous system inhibition, as reflected in measures of sensorimotor gating.

Among the many symptoms of schizophrenia, alterations in sensory motor gating lend themselves to study in animal models. Specifically, measures of prepulse inhibition (PPI) of the acoustic startle response and latent inhibition (LI) in laboratory animals provide an opportunity for basic researchers to probe potential neural underpinnings of endophenotypes related to schizophrenia in humans. The experimental paradigm for clinical studies has involved measures of the amplitude of reflex eye blink responses to a startling tone. If a weak prestimulus occurred 60–120 msec prior to the intense acoustic stimulus, there was a dramatic inhibition of the eye blink reflex amplitude and a shortening of startle latencies in healthy controls. In contrast, schizophrenic patients displayed less amplitude inhibition and reduced latency facilitation when the pre-stimulus occurred.

The neurobiological underpinnings of these sensorimotor gating deficits have been a subject of intense interest, and there is now a great appreciation for inter-individual differences in measures of sensorimotor gating. Measures of sensori-motor gating have been employed as an endophenotype in studies of risk genes for several psychiatric disorders, including schizophrenia. These measures may also be valuable as biomarkers to predict a favorable response to various thera-peutic interventions, including drugs and behavioral therapies (for reviews, see Braff & Geyer, 1990; Braff et al., 1992; Swerdlow et al., 2016).

Two tests that have frequently been included in experiments with animal models of schizophrenia include PPI of the acoustic startle response and LI. PPI as measured in laboratory rodents is especially valuable in that it compares fa-vorably to studies of sensorimotor gating deficits in schizophrenic patients. In laboratory mice and rats, PPI quantifies the ability of a weak acoustic stimulus preceding a high-intensity acoustic stimulus by 30–500 msec to inhibit or "gate" the startle response to the high-intensity stimulus (Figure 8.1A).

LI is also related to various gating theories of cognition in schizophrenia. The testing procedure involves repeated exposure of laboratory animals to a sensory stimulus, which slows the rate at which a test animal will acquire a stimulus-response association based upon that same stimulus (Figure 8.1B). Although deficits in LI have been reported in tests of schizophrenic patients, these deficits appear to be limited to acute episodes of illness (Powell & Geyer, 2007).

The Challenges of Modeling a Uniquely Human Disorder

In presenting a survey of the extensive literature on animal models of schizo-phrenia, several issues should be kept in mind. First, limitations of the current diagnostic systems present a challenge for any basic researcher who is inter-ested in developing an effective animal model. The inter-individual variability in symptoms from one patient to the next remains a significant hurdle. It is clear that current diagnostic systems in psychiatry have not yet seen the day when "nature is carved at its joints." That is, we have not achieved a partitioning of mental disorders into natural categories (Pickles & Angold, 2003). Second, re-cent GWAS have made clear that some risk genes are shared across several cur-rent diagnostic categories (e.g., schizophrenia and bipolar disorder), as are some endophenotypes (e.g., PPI). Finally, in spite of the fact that many symptoms of schizophrenia, such as hallucinations, delusions, and disordered thoughts, are impossible to model in animals, there has developed an expansive literature that has contributed to a somewhat clearer understanding of the etiology of this dev-astating disorder (Meyer & Feldon, 2010). In the sections that follow, I will at-tempt to provide the reader with a sampling of these exciting advances.

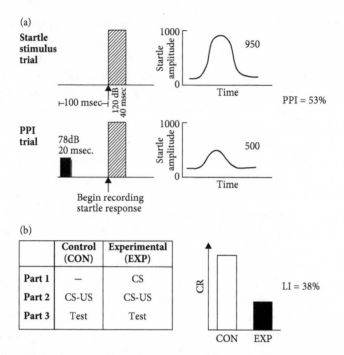

Figure 8.1. A: Pre-pulse inhibition (PPI) of the acoustic startle response (ASR). The top tracing reflects the startle response of a laboratory animal to an intense acoustic stimulus. The lower tracing reflects the startle response of a laboratory animal that was exposed to a lower-intensity acoustic stimulus prior to the intense acoustic stimulus. Note that the ASR is reduced by pre-exposure to the lower-intensity acoustic stimulus. B: Latent inhibition (LI) refers to the consistent finding that a familiar stimulus takes longer to acquire meaning than an unfamiliar stimulus within the context of a classical conditioning paradigm. If an animal has prior exposure to a conditioned stimulus (CS) such as a tone in Part 1, it will not exhibit as robust a conditioned response (CR) when the CS is later paired with an unconditioned stimulus (UCS) such as footshock in Part 2, with testing for strength of classical conditioning in Part 3.

Maternal Immune Activation

Epidemiological studies have suggested that risk of schizophrenia is elevated in offspring of mothers who experienced viral or bacterial infections during pregnancy (Brown and Derkits, 2010; Burgdorf et al., 2019; Debnath et al., 2015; Estes & McAllister, 2016; Lydholm et al., 2019). Building on this solid foundation of epidemiological studies, several laboratories have developed animal models to explore mechanisms that underlie this association. In their review of preclinical animal models of maternal immune activation, Gumusoglu and Stevens (2019) acknowledged the limitations posed by working with laboratory strains of mice and rats. However, they concluded that experiments with mice and rats are especially valuable in revealing molecular alterations during neural development of offspring that may be useful for the evolution of clinical interventions.

Two experimental models have received considerable attention, including timed administration during pregnancy of polyriboinositic-polyribocitidylic acid [poly(I:C)]or lipopolysaccharide (LPS) to pregnant laboratory animals, with subsequent testing and evaluation of their offspring. Poly(I:C) is a synthetic analog of double-stranded RNA that binds to toll-like receptor 3 and produces an acute phase response similar to a viral infection, with associated elevations in proinflammatory cytokines (Meyer et al., 2009). LPS is a component of the cell wall of gram negative bacteria and, after binding to toll-like receptor 4, stimulates an innate immune response similar to the response to a bacterial infection (Beutler & Rietschel, 2003). These two maternal immune activation models will be discussed separately in the following subsections.

Poly(I:C). Beginning in 2003, poly(I:C) was employed as a viral mimic in studies of laboratory mice and rats to simulate the features of a prenatal viral infection in humans, an established risk factor for later development of schizophrenia. Poly(I:C) offers several advantages to investigators over the use of viral pathogens in that it stimulates a nonspecific immune response, with elevations in various cytokines and type 1 interferons α and β, but without increases in antibodies or viral nucleic acids. In addition, the effects of poly(I:C) are time-limited, lasting no more than 48 hours. Thus, the drug can be administered such that it has an impact during a limited time in prenatal development. Finally, the intensity of the immune response can be controlled by administering graded doses of poly(I:C) (Meyer, 2014).

However, it is important to note the lack of consistency across studies in the dose of poly(I:C) employed, the route of administration, the gestational timing, and frequency of injections. In addition, poly(I:C) varies in molecular weight from lot to lot, even from the same supplier, and this can affect the magnitude of the maternal immune response (Careaga et al., 2017). With these concerns in mind, I have specified whenever possible the dosing parameters in the studies described in the following, as well as those reported in Chapter 9.

In an early foundational study, Zuckerman et al. (2003) examined the effects of prenatal immune activation on measures of LI, central DA responsiveness, and brain morphological changes. Pregnant Wistar rats received an injection of poly(I:C) (4.0 mg/kg, i.v.) on gestational day (GD) 15. Litters were weaned on PND 21 and testing was conducted on offspring on PND 35 (adolescence) or PND 90 (adulthood). LI was disrupted in poly(I:C)-treated male and female rats when tested in adulthood but not in adolescence, matching well with the pattern of change observed in schizophrenic patients. Administration of haloperidol or clozapine in adult animals reinstated LI when compared to offspring of saline-injected mothers.

Dose-response relationship. A critical feature of the poly(I:C) model that must be considered in the design of experiments is the relationship between prenatal dose of the viral mimic and the intensity of the immune response, which results in phenotypic changes in the offspring when tested in adulthood. In a comprehensive series of experiments, Meyer et al. (2005) conducted a dose-response study by injecting pregnant mice on GD 9 with varying doses (0, 2.5, 5.0 or 10.0 mg/kg, i.v.) of poly(I:C), and then subjected their adult offspring to a battery of tests to assess the extent to which they displayed a schizophrenia-like phenotype.

Poly(I:C) produced a dose-dependent increase in serum levels of IL-10 in non-pregnant female mice within 1 hour after injection, and levels remained significantly elevated relative to vehicle-injected controls for up to 6 hours. Fetal brain levels of IL-1β and IL-10 assayed 10 hours after a single injection of poly(I:C) to the mothers did not differ significantly from levels of vehicle-injected controls. However, at the highest dose of poly(I:C), the rate of spontaneous abortions was quite high.

When offspring were tested in adulthood, some but not all of the behavioral deficits exhibited a clear dose-dependent relationship across the three doses of poly(I:C) employed. Those that did included deficits in PPI, attenuation of the unconditioned stimulus pre-exposure effect, and an enhanced locomotor response to amphetamine, which were observed in mice subjected to prenatal administration of 5 or 10 mg/kg poly(I:C), but not to 2.5 mg/kg. In contrast, all three doses of poly(I:C) resulted in disruptions in LI, spatial working memory, and locomotor behaviors in an open field.

Timing of administration. The specific time during gestation when maternal immune activation occurs could also be a critical variable in determining the effects on developing fetuses (Meyer et al., 2008b). In one study, pregnant laboratory mice were injected with poly(I:C) (5.0 mg/kg, i.v.) or vehicle on GD 9 or GD 17. When tested in adulthood, mice exposed to maternal immune activation on GD 9 exhibited impaired PPI of the acoustic startle response and reductions in D1 receptors in the PFC. In contrast, exposure of mice to maternal immune activation on GD 17 resulted in working memory impairments, an enhanced locomotor response to an NMDA receptor antagonist, and reductions in NMDA receptor subunit-1 expression in the hippocampus. Several changes occurred in mice from both immune-challenged groups, including enhanced locomotor responses to amphetamine and reductions in Reelin- and parvalbumin (PV)-expressing interneurons in the PFC. These specific and common responses of offspring of mothers that received poly(I:C) at two different times during gestation may explain in part the complexity of different symptom clusters observed in schizophrenic patients.

PV interneurons. Oxidative stress-induced disruptions in the integrity of cortical PV interneurons have emerged as a pathological feature shared in common by several mental disorders, including schizophrenia, as well as in a range of animal models (Steullet et al., 2017). PV is a high-affinity calcium-binding protein that is expressed in interneurons whose inhibitory nerve terminals make synaptic contact onto the cell bodies and initial axonal segments of target neurons in the PFC and the hippocampus. These inhibitory neuronal circuits play a critical role in the development of attention, learning and memory, and social behaviors. Targeted disruption of PV-positive GABA neurons in the prefrontal cortex resulted in behavioral and neurophysiological alterations that were consistent with endophenotypes of schizophrenia (Woloszynowska-Fraser et al., 2017).

Strengths of the model. Several appealing features of the poly(I:C) prenatal maternal immune activation model are worth noting. First, offspring of poly(I:C)-treated dams display clear signs of a schizophrenia-like phenotype in adulthood but generally not in adolescence, matching well with the developmental course of the disease in humans. Second, the dose-dependent nature of the effects of the poly(I:C) model parallels epidemiological findings in humans, where only a small percentage of those individuals born to mothers who experienced infections during pregnancy will eventually develop symptoms of schizophrenia in early adulthood (Brown, 2011). In addition, the time-response studies point to an ability to expose a developing fetus to maternal immune activation at specific times during prenatal development. Finally, the dose-response studies described in the preceding point to the possibility of a sub-threshold or priming effect of prenatal maternal immune activation, such that vulnerabilities associated with modest neuro-developmental changes following maternal infection would require interaction with a susceptible genotype or a peri-adolescent environmental stressor to yield the full-blown symptoms of schizophrenia (Meyer & Feldon, 2012).

Maternal effects. In a comprehensive series of studies, Meyer and collaborators (Meyer et al., 2006; Meyer et al. 2008a; Richetto et al., 2013) injected pregnant mice with a viral mimic or vehicle on GD 9, and measured neurochemical and cognitive changes in their offspring in adolescence and adulthood. Exposure to a viral mimic during gestation activated the mother's immune system and increased cytokine levels in fetal brain tissue (Meyer et al., 2005). At birth, litters were fostered to vehicle-injected control mothers or to mothers that received the viral mimic. Cross-fostering viral mimic-exposed mice to vehicle-injected foster mothers did not alter the pattern of neural, cognitive, and behavioral changes that were evident in adulthood. However, cross-fostering offspring of vehicle-injected mothers to viral mimic-exposed foster mothers did lead to significant cognitive deficits, as well as neural and behavioral changes, when testing occurred in adulthood. Thus, immunological stress during pregnancy may affect maternal behaviors, such that being cared for by an immune-challenged mother may confer risk for adult psychopathology. However, placing prenatally immune-challenged offspring with a control foster mother did not protect against the development of neural and behavioral deficits in adulthood.

In another experiment, Willi et al. (2013) examined the relationship between altered regulation of glycogen synthase kinase 3β (GSK-3β) and protein kinase B (Akt) and their role in DAergic signaling and behavioral changes related to schizophrenia and bipolar disorder. They employed the prenatal poly(I:C) infection-based model using pregnant laboratory mice, as described earlier. Adult offspring of poly(I:C)-exposed mothers exhibited decreased total levels of AKT protein and reduced phosphorylation at AKT threonine residues in the mPFC. Prenatally immune-challenged offspring also exhibited increased GSK-3β protein expression and activation status in the mPFC. Acute pre-treatment with a selective GSK3β inhibitor (TDZD-8) reversed deficits in spontaneous alternation in a Y-maze and increased locomotor responses to a challenge dose of amphetamine.

Vulnerability to stress. Consistent with the suggestion of a priming effect of prenatal immune activation, Giovanoli et al. (2013) argued that stressful experiences during late adolescence might unmask vulnerability to psychopathology in laboratory mice previously exposed to a low-level prenatal immune challenge. Note that this argument was not based upon a gene x environment effect; rather, it presupposed a two-hit effect from this combination of environmental stressors. In an elegant test of this hypothesis, pregnant mice received a very low dose (1.0 mg/kg, i.v.) of poly(I:C) or vehicle on GD 9. Offspring born to poly(I:C) or vehicle-injected control mothers were weaned on PND 21, and then exposed to an assortment of stressors from PNDs 30 to 40. Testing of adult mice occurred from PNDs 70 to 100.

The results revealed several behavioral and neurobiological changes that were dependent upon the combination of a modest prenatal immune challenge and an adolescent stressor challenge. Specifically, there was a reduction in PPI of the acoustic startle reflex, enhanced locomotor responses to amphetamine and MK-801, and increased content of DA in the hippocampus. These behavioral and neurobiological alterations did not occur in mice exposed prenatally to poly(I:C) if the stressors were delayed until PNDs 50–60. Additional experiments with mice one day after the last of ten stressor sessions (i.e., PND 41) revealed that a prenatal immune challenge and adolescent stressor exposure combined to affect several neuroimmune parameters, including levels of activated microglia and hippocampal content of IL-1β, TNF-α, and prostaglandin E_2 in the hippocampus. These brain changes could not be explained by treatment effects on circulating levels of CORT or inflammatory cytokines. In addition, these neuroimmune alterations were not apparent in adult animals.

These findings are especially relevant for neuropathologies whose symptoms first appear in late adolescence or early adulthood, including schizophrenia. A low-level viral infection of the mother during gestation could sensitize her offspring to the later effects of environmental stressors during an especially vulnerable period in postnatal development, adolescence. These synergistic effects were particularly evident in behavioral and neuroimmune parameters that map well to the schizophrenic phenotype (Giovanoli et al., 2013).

Transgenerational effects. It is important to note that the effects of prenatal maternal immune activation with poly(I:C) can extend across multiple generations via trans-generational nongenetic inheritance (Weber-Stadlbauer et al., 2017). In this study, poly(I:C) (5.0 mg/kg, i.v.) or vehicle was administered to pregnant mice on GD 9, and their offspring (F1 generation) were tested in adulthood. As expected, F1 offspring exposed to maternal immune activation had deficits in social interactions and PPI, as well as enhanced fear responses compared to offspring of vehicle-injected controls. F2 offspring that were derived from mating poly(I:C)-exposed F1 males and females did not have deficits in PPI, but did display deficits in social behavior and enhanced fear responses as well as a novel behavioral change—increased despair in the forced swim test. Similar behavioral disruptions were observed in F2 offspring that resulted from a cross between an F1 poly(I:C)-exposed male and a control female and in F3 offspring that maintained the paternal lineage of poly(I:C) exposure.

Further experiments revealed striking changes in genome-wide transcriptional changes in the amygdala of poly(I:C) and control offspring from the F1 and F2 generations. Among the offspring of poly(I:C)-exposed offspring, there were 1,085 differentially regulated genes in the F1 generation, 2,883 differentially regulated genes in the F2 generation, and 1,132 differentially regulated genes that were common to both generations. Thus, prenatal immune activation may result in the transmission of similar as well as distinct phenotypic traits across generations. F2 and F3 offspring (including paternal as well as maternal lineages) may be especially valuable in experiments that employ a two-hit design, where trans-generationally transmitted vulnerabilities could be unmasked by exposure to stressors during early postnatal life, or in adolescence or early adulthood. These possibilities comport well with the complex patterns of disease risk in individuals with a family history of schizophrenia over several generations (Weber-Stadlbauer et al., 2017).

Consistency of findings. Boksa (2010), in her superb summary of the literature, presented an overview of behavioral and brain changes resulting from gestational administration of poly(I:C). Allowing for different doses and routes of administration of the viral mimetic, studies with mice versus rats, different ages when animals were tested, and differing testing protocols, the results were quite consistent. Compared to controls, offspring of poly(I:C)-treated dams consistently exhibited impairments in PPI and LI, enhanced locomotor activity following administration of amphetamine or MK801, decreased exploration during testing in an open field arena, and decreased social interaction. The findings described earlier from the study by Weber-Stadlbauer et al. (2017) fit well with this earlier summary of the literature. The reader is referred to this comprehensive summary for additional information on poly(I:C)-induced changes in neurotransmitter systems and molecular genetic parameters. More recent studies have examined the effects of the poly(I:C) model on expression of schizophrenia risk genes in brain areas of adolescent and adult rats (Hemmerle et al., 2015).

Non-human primate experiments. Given that the vast majority of prenatal maternal immune activation studies have involved experiments with laboratory strains of mice or rats, a next logical advance in this field of inquiry would be to adapt this model in a nonhuman primate species. In a series of studies (Bauman et al., 2014; Machado et al., 2015; Rose et al., 2017; Weir et al., 2015), researchers at the California National Primate Research Center and the University of California, Davis, utilized poly(I:C) to develop a maternal immune activation model using rhesus monkeys (*Macaca mulatta*). Poly(I:C) (0.25 mg/kg per i.v. dose) was administered to pregnant females in a series of three daily injections during the first trimester (GDs 43, 44, and 46) or during the second trimester (GDs 100, 101, and 103). After weaning at 6 months of age, poly(I:C)-exposed animals from both groups differed from controls in their patterns of attachment to their mothers.

Animals exposed to immune activation during the second trimester exhibited greater distress and self-soothing behaviors during an assessment of attachment behavior compared to controls and animals exposed to immune activation during the first trimester. These initial group differences in attachment behaviors also increased over 4 consecutive days of testing. As the animals matured out to 2 years of age, offspring from both groups of poly(I:C)-treated mothers differed from controls by displaying increases in repetitive behaviors and decreases in affiliative vocalizations. In first trimester-exposed monkeys, there was evidence of inappropriate approaching and remaining in close proximity to unfamiliar conspecifics. The authors concluded that the changes observed in monkeys born to mothers that received poly(I:C) injections during gestation extend findings in rodent models of maternal immune activation and may contribute to a deeper understanding of schizophrenia as well as autism (Bauman et al., 2014).

In a follow-up to the initial report, Machado et al. (2015) utilized noninvasive eye tracking and compared monkeys exposed to poly(I:C) during the first trimester with controls at 2.5 years of age in measures of social attention. Consistent with previous reports, the results revealed that poly(I:C)-exposed monkeys differed from controls when viewing pictures of monkeys' faces displaying a fear grimace facial expression. The poly(I:C)-treated monkeys took a longer time to fixate on the eyes, had fewer fixations directed at the eyes, and spent less time fixating on the eyes of the monkeys in the pictures compared to controls.

Two additional studies explored neuropathological and immune alterations in the maternal immune activation model in rhesus monkeys. In the first study, Weir et al. (2015) measured aspects of neuronal morphology in layer III pyramidal neurons in sections from the dorsolateral PFC from monkeys at 3.5 years of age. Pregnant females ($N = 4$) were injected with poly(I:C) on GDs 43, 44, 46, 47, 49, and 50, while control females received injections of saline on the same days ($N = 4$). Three doses of poly(I:C) were employed in this study (0.25, 0.5, or 1.0 mg/kg, i.v.), and sample sizes were 1, 2, and 1, respectively. Three hours after administration of poly(I:C), there were significant elevations in levels of IL-6, whereas in saline-treated females, levels of IL-6 did not increase or were minimally elevated. Poly(I:C)-exposed monkeys exhibited significant elevations in repetitive behaviors at 6 months of age compared to controls, confirming results from an earlier detailed behavioral study (Bauman et al., 2014). Measures of neuronal morphology revealed that apical dendrites of poly(I:C)-exposed monkeys were smaller in diameter, and there was a significantly larger number of oblique dendrites between the soma and the beginning of the selected section compared to similar measures in controls. This preliminary study with extremely limited sample sizes and three different doses of poly(I:C) was nonetheless encouraging of further explorations to gain a greater understanding of neuropathological changes in this nonhuman primate immune activation model of schizophrenia.

In a second study, poly(I:C) was administered to pregnant rhesus monkey females at the end of the first or second trimester, as described earlier (Bauman et al., 2014). Controls received saline injections or were left undisturbed. Blood samples were collected when offspring were 1 year old and again at 4 years of age to assess cellular immune function. Behavioral observations confirmed that poly(I:C)-exposed animals exhibited elevated levels of stereotyped and repetitive behaviors. At 1 year of age, poly(I:C)-exposed offspring had elevated production of IL-1β, IL-6, IL-12p40, and TNF-α under baseline conditions, and following stimulation of peripheral blood mononuclear cells in vitro with LPS or poly(I:C). At 4 years of age, poly(I:C)-exposed offspring maintained elevated levels of IL-1β, and there was also a pattern of increased production of the T-cell helper type-2 cytokines, IL-4 and IL-13. The increased levels of inflammatory cytokines under basal conditions and following stimulation were associated with the stereotyped and repetitive behaviors. Taken together, this series of experiments highlights the value of studying offspring of poly(I:C)-treated pregnant rhesus monkeys as a translational model of schizophrenia.

Lipopolysaccharide (LPS). Prenatal exposure to LPS also serves as a maternal immune activation model of schizophrenia (Wischhof et al., 2015). Pregnant Wistar rats were injected with LPS (100 μg/kg, i.p.) on GDs 15 and 16, while controls received injections of saline. At birth, LPS-treated and control pups were combined in equal numbers to form mixed litters that were placed with untreated foster mothers whose recently delivered litters had been removed. Cross-fostering eliminated any differences in maternal care or nutrition provided to the pups that were attributable to LPS administration. LPS and control male and female offspring were tested in adolescence and adulthood on several behavioral measures, and brain tissue sections were examined for PV expression and density of myelinated fibers.

The results from this study highlighted the differing responses of male versus female offspring exposed to maternal LPS-induced immune activation *in utero*, with females showing less pronounced cognitive impairments, less demyelination, and only a modest loss of PV-expressing cells. These findings match well with the much higher incidence of schizophrenia in male versus female patients, with a ratio of male to female of 1.4 (McGrath, 2005). Specifically, there were deficits in PPI on PNDs 45 and 90 in LPS-exposed male offspring and at PND 45 only in LPS-exposed female offspring. In contrast, LPS exposure did not affect the acoustic startle response in male or female offspring. For measures of locomotor activity and rearing in an open field arena, LPS-treated males and females did not differ. LPS-exposed males were more active and reared more frequently than control males on PNDs 33 and 60. LPS-exposed females were more active compared to control females on PNDs 33 and 60, and reared more frequently than control females on PND 33. In an object memory task, LPS-exposed males and females displayed deficits in working memory compared to appropriate controls, and the magnitude of the deficit was greater in LPS-exposed males than females. Male and female rats did not differ in their behavior on the elevated plus-maze (EPM), and there were no effects of LPS exposure prenatally on this behavioral measure.

Compared to controls, the number of PV immunoreactive cells was reduced significantly in LPS-exposed adult male rats in the mPFC, CA1 region of the hippocampus, and the lateral entorhinal cortex. In contrast, for LPS-exposed adult females, there was a significant decrease in PV-positive cells in the mPFC only. Finally, compared to controls, significant reductions in myelination were reported in LPS-exposed adult male rats in the mPFC, basolateral nucleus of the amygdala, CA1 region of the hippocampus, and the dentate gyrus. For LPS-treated adult female rats, there were significant reductions in myelination in the basolateral nucleus of the amygdala and the dentate gyrus, but these reductions, though significant, were reduced in magnitude compared to changes in the same brain areas of LPS-exposed males.

In this study, behavioral changes were observed in juvenile as well as adult males and females exposed prenatally to LPS, which did not match up with the delayed appearance of symptoms until very late adolescence or early adulthood in schizophrenic patients. However, a clear strength of this experiment was the greater impact of prenatal LPS exposure on males compared to females, which is in agreement with differences reported for schizophrenic patients (Wischhof et al., 2015).

The reader is encouraged to consult the excellent review by Boksa (2010) for a summary of behavioral alterations and changes in brain neurotransmitter systems and molecular parameters resulting from gestational exposure of laboratory mice and rats to LPS.

Prenatal Stress

Holloway et al. (2013) modeled schizophrenia-like changes in the brain by exposing pregnant mice to prenatal stress. They compared offspring of control mice with those whose mothers were exposed to a variable stress paradigm from GDs 9.5 to 15.5. Soon after birth, litters were assigned to one of the following groups: (i) control litters were in-fostered to control foster mothers; (ii) control litters were cross-fostered to prenatally stressed foster mothers; (iii) prenatally stressed litters were in-fostered to prenatally stressed foster mothers; and (iv) prenatally stressed litters were cross-fostered to control foster mothers. Exposure to prenatal stress resulted in increased expression of serotonin (5-HT_{2A}) receptors and decreased expression of metabotropic glutamate 2 receptors in frontal cortex of offspring in adulthood. Both neurotransmitter receptors have been implicated in the pathophysiology of schizophrenia. Cross-fostering had no impact on changes in expression of the two neurotransmitter receptors attributed to prenatal stress.

Matrisciano et al. (2012) utilized repeated restraint stress (30 minutes x 2 times per day) of female mice from GD 7 until delivery to precipitate a schizophrenia-like phenotype when male offspring were tested in adulthood. Compared to unstressed controls, prenatally stressed mice had reduced levels of social interaction, higher levels of activity in an open field arena, and decreases in PPI of the acoustic startle response. They also found that prenatally stressed mice had significant decreases in expression of metabotropic glutamate 2 (mGlu2) receptors, brain-derived neurotrophic factor (BDNF), and glutamic acid decarboxylase 67 in PFC on PNDs 1, 21, and 60, and decreases in mGlu3 receptor mRNAs in PFC on PNDs 1 and 21. Further, on PND 60, prenatally stressed mice had increased levels of type 1 DNA methyltransferase (DNMT1) and DNMT1 binding to the promoter region of the mGlu2/3 genes in the PFC compared to controls. Remarkably, all molecular and behavioral differences between prenatally stressed and control mice were eliminated in adulthood by administration of the mGlu2/3 agonist, LY379268 (0.5 mg/kg, i.p. twice each day for 5 days). Results from this study point to mGlu2/3 receptors as a novel drug target for the treatment of schizophrenia.

In a follow-up to this study, these investigators compared offspring of control and prenatally stressed mice in a battery of behavioral tests and in patterns of development of GABAergic neurons in the hippocampus and PFC (Matrisciano et al., 2013). The results of the behavioral test battery were again consistent with a schizophrenia-like behavioral phenotype, including hyperactivity, decreased social interactions, decrements in PPI of the acoustic startle response, increases in stereotyped behaviors, and decreases in contextual fear conditioning. Further investigations revealed that levels of DNMT 1 and 3a mRNAs in the PFC were elevated on PND 1, and decreased progressively out to PND 60. At each time point, however, levels of mRNAs for the two enzymes were significantly higher in prenatally stressed mice versus controls. Additionally, levels of mRNAs for the two enzymes in the hippocampus were significantly elevated in prenatally stressed mice on PNDs 7 and 60.

High levels of DNMT1 and 3a occurred in GABAergic neurons in the PFC and hippocampus of prenatally stressed mice, and in both brain areas, there were corresponding decreases in expression of reelin and glutamic acid decarboxylase 67 (GAD67) on PND 60. In prenatally stressed mice, there were also increased binding of DNMT1 and increased epigenetic changes in CpG-rich regions of the reelin and GAD67 promoters. Finally, treatment of prenatally stressed mice with a histone deacetylase inhibitor (valproic acid) or a DNA-demethylating agent (clozapine) normalized the behaviors of prenatally stressed mice.

Dong et al. (2015) also employed the prenatal restraint stress model to extend previous findings related to trophic factors and epigenetic changes in the brain. Adult male mice that were stressed prenatally exhibited significant increases in locomotor activity, expression of DNMT1, and ten-eleven-translocation hydroxylase 1 as well as decreases in social interaction and expression of BDNF transcripts in frontal cortex and hippocampus compared to unstressed controls. There was also clear evidence of epigenetic down-regulation in the expression of the BDNF gene. These findings are consistent with previous reports from this same laboratory on studies with post-mortem brains of schizophrenic patients, and suggest that epigenetic changes precipitated by prenatal stress may play a crucial role in the onset of symptoms of schizophrenia (Guidotti et al., 2014).

Koenig et al. (2005) explored the effects of a variable stress paradigm during the third week of gestation on female Sprague-Dawley rats. Control females were left undisturbed during pregnancy. Offspring of control and prenatally stressed mothers were tested in adulthood (PND 56). Compared to controls, prenatally stressed rats had persistent elevations in plasma CORT levels following acute re-straint stress, enhanced locomotor responses to amphetamine, diminished PPI, and disruption in sensory gating as reflected by recordings of auditory evoked potentials. Taken together, these changes induced by prenatal stress match well with many measures employed to validate animal models of schizophrenia.

Disruptions in Mother-Infant Contact

Maternal deprivation for 24 hours. Ellenbroek and Cools (2000) examined the effects of a single 24-hour period of maternal deprivation from PNDs 9 to 10 on PPI of the acoustic startle response and locomotor responses to apomorphine in adult animals. They further varied the genetic background of the animals tested by comparing Wistar, Fischer 344 (F-344), and Lewis strains of rats. In Wistar rats, they observed that maternal deprivation resulted in diminished PPI and a reduction in activity, coupled with an enhanced gnawing response to apomor-phine. They found that maternally deprived F-344 rats were similar to controls in basal startle amplitude and PPI, but apomorphine susceptibility was reduced compared to controls. Finally, in Lewis rats, maternal deprivation significantly reduced basal startle amplitude, but did not affect PPI or behavioral responses to apomorphine. The results with maternally deprived Wistar rats were con-sistent with a gene x environment interaction producing schizophrenia-like phe-notypic characteristics in adulthood (Ellenbroek & Cools, 2000; Ellenbroek & Riva, 2003).

Using the Ellenbroek and Cools (2000) maternal deprivation paradigm with Wistar rats, Rentesi et al. (2013) reported that maternally deprived rats tested in adulthood were more reactive following placement in a novel envi-ronment and were more responsive to d-amphetamine and apomorphine com-pared to controls. In addition, maternally deprived rats also had significant up-regulation of DAergic and serotonergic neurons in the amygdala and PFC and DAergic function only in the striatum. Finally, maternally deprived rats exhibited regionally specific changes in levels of D2 and 5-HT$_{2A}$ receptors as well as DARPP-32 protein levels. DARPP-32 is a protein localized to neurons that contain DA receptors, and it plays a key role in the integration of DAergic and glutamatergic signaling (Valjent et al., 2005). The authors concluded that rats that experienced maternal deprivation on PND 9 displayed a behavioral and neurobiological phenotype in adulthood that was an appropriate animal model for schizophrenia.

Additional experiments have revealed that maternal deprivation led to increased time spent in the open arms and more frequent open-arm entries during testing of adult males on an EPM. However, the responsiveness of the

HPA axis to stress in adult male and female rats was not affected by maternal deprivation (Llorente-Berzal et al., 2011).

An interesting experiment by Girardi et al. (2014) took a different approach in examining the consequences of maternal deprivation from PNDs 9–10 in Wistar rats, focusing on signs of schizophrenia-like phenotypic characteristics during the neonatal period and in adolescence. Plasma CORT levels were significantly higher in maternally deprived pups on PND 10 under resting conditions and 2 hours after a low-level stressor, a saline injection (0.3 ml, i.p.), compared to control pups that remained with their mothers.

Behavioral testing of animals from the four groups was conducted beginning on PND 45. Maternally deprived rats did not differ from controls in consumption of a 15% sucrose solution in a two-bottle preference test on two consecutive days. On the third day, with a 2.1% sucrose solution, unstressed controls and maternally deprived pups consumed less sucrose solution compared to pups of the two groups that received saline injections on PND 10. In the open field, rats of the four groups had comparable levels of activity; however, saline-injected controls and both groups of maternally deprived rats had fewer entries into the center squares compared to uninjected controls. For the EPM task, saline-injected controls and maternally deprived rats had fewer open-arm entries and spent less time in the open arms compared to their uninjected counterparts. Finally, maternally deprived rats spent less time in social investigation compared to controls, and the saline injection did not have an effect.

These results extend the impact of the maternal deprivation model to include early behavioral changes that map well to changes observed in pre-adolescence through early adulthood in individuals later diagnosed with schizophrenia. These changes included up-regulation of HPA responsiveness in neonates, reductions in social interaction, and increased anxiety as reflected in less time spent in the center squares of an open field arena (Girardi et al., 2014).

In their comprehensive review article, Marco et al. (2015) sounded a cautionary note regarding the complexity of the maternal deprivation model, and extended the impact of the model well beyond its utility as a means to gain insights into the etiology of schizophrenia. More broadly, the maternal deprivation paradigm provides an opportunity to examine brain processes that occur during a limited window of early postnatal development and that influence neural circuits that regulate a host of critical functions in adulthood. These include regulation of energy metabolism, immune function, nociception, and neuroendocrine and behavioral responses to stressors. The authors also pointed to the challenges faced by rat pups that are separated from their mothers for 24 hours during PNDs 9–10: absence of tactile stimulation provided by the mother; lack of milk from the mother, which leads to hypoglycemia and decreased levels of leptin; a potential decrease in maternal milk production after the pups were reunited with their mothers; and a decrease in body temperature of the pups while the mother was absent. Several mechanisms have emerged to explain in part the changes observed in maternally deprived pups when tested in adulthood, including a surge in CORT that occurs during maternal separation, a drop in leptin levels that may disrupt the development of hypothalamic nuclei involved in energy homeostasis, or a disruption in the development of brain endocannabinoid signaling, especially in the hippocampus and PFC. This array of changes precipitated by maternal deprivation must be considered as one relates behavioral or physiological changes in adulthood to a schizophrenia-like phenotype (Marco et al., 2015).

Brief repeated maternal deprivation. To minimize the negative effects of a 24-hour period of maternal deprivation, Novak et al. (2013) separated litters of Long-Evans rats from their mothers for 1 hour per day from PNDs 7 to 14. Control litters were left undisturbed with their mothers from birth until weaning. Some control and maternally deprived male rats were also subjected to immobilization stress for 30 minutes per day from PNDs 40 to 45. This constitutes a two-hit experimental design (maternal deprivation + immobilization) for this animal model of schizophrenia.

Focusing on DA signaling pathways in the striatum, these investigators found that maternal deprivation alone resulted in significant decreases in expression of D2 receptors and DA- and cAMP-regulated DARPP-32 on PND 18, but these differences were no longer apparent by PND 46. In rats exposed to maternal deprivation plus immobilization, there were significant increases in expression of D2 receptors and calcium/calmodulin-dependent protein kinase II (CaMKII) β subunit. These results are consistent with an additive effect of a neonatal stressor combined with a stressor applied during adolescence. Further, these molecular changes in the D2 signaling pathway in the striatum are consistent with changes reported for patients with schizophrenia.

Isolation Rearing after Weaning

As an alternative to drug-based animal models of schizophrenia, Geyer et al. (1993) examined the effects of social isolation beginning at 20 days of age (time of weaning) on PPI of the acoustic startle response in adult rats of two strains, Lister hooded rats and Sprague-Dawley rats. Rats were housed singly or in groups for at least 34 days prior to behavioral testing. Socially isolated rats of both strains exhibited significant decrements in PPI of the acoustic startle response compared to group-housed rats. Isolated Lister hooded rats but not Sprague-Dawley rats also had greater levels of locomotor activity over a 2-hour testing period compared to rats of the same strain maintained in social groups.

Finally, acute administration of the D2 receptor antagonist, raclopride (0.5 mg/kg), eliminated the deficit in PPI in isolated rats of the two strains, but did not affect responses in group-housed controls. These findings suggested that social isolation may alter the neural circuits responsible for PPI, and point to an up-regulation of DAergic systems as a critical component of these alterations. Thus, social isolation may provide a valuable animal model of schizophrenia given the similar changes in PPI in schizophrenic patients and socially isolated rats tested in adulthood. Weiss and Feldon (2001), in their review of the relevant literature, concluded that social deprivation immediately after weaning provides a robust and noninvasive model for stress-induced disruptions in PPI.

Stress during Adolescence

Choy and van den Buuse (2008) examined the effects of an early life stressor (maternal deprivation on PND 9) in combination with elevated CORT during adolescence on DAergic regulation of PPI in laboratory rats. CORT was delivered from 8 to 10 weeks of age by a subcutaneous pellet implanted at the nape of the neck to simulate a chronically stressful environment. Their primary finding in this study was that the combined effects of maternal deprivation plus CORT treatment resulted in an inhibition of DAergic regulation of PPI, possibly by desensitization of DA receptors or modulation of sensory gating in the nucleus accumbens.

In a series of refinements of this initial experimental approach, van den Buuse and his colleagues developed a protocol to examine gene x environment interactions in an animal model of schizophrenia. The general approach was to expose male and female laboratory mice to elevated levels of CORT (25–50 μg/ml in the drinking water) from 6 to 9 weeks of age to simulate chronic stress effects on the HPA axis. This technique is more targeted in its effects compared to subjecting animals to a chronic stress treatment that would produce a host of unrelated physiological changes, but it is not without its own drawbacks. The period 6–9 weeks of age was selected as it corresponds to late adolescence/early adulthood in laboratory mice (Hill et al., 2012), a time of elevated risk for the development of psychosis in humans. It is also important to include male and female animals in experiments of this type given the well-described sex differences in many aspects of schizophrenia (Wu et al., 2013).

In an initial experiment, Klug et al. (2012) examined the effects of CORT exposure during adolescence in male and female WT mice and in BDNF heterozygous (BDNF HT) mice. When tested in adulthood, male but not female BDNF HT mice that received CORT had significant memory impairments during Y-maze testing. There were no differences between groups in PPI or disruption of

PPI following administration of MK-801, an NMDA receptor antagonist. There was an increase in the startle response following administration of MK-801 in female BDNF HT mice, but not in male BDNF HT mice, that was independent of CORT administration. There were also significant alterations in various NMDA receptor subunits in the hippocampus of BDNF HT male but not female mice.

In a follow-up to the study by Klug et al. (2012), two experiments (Notaras et al., 2017; van den Buuse et al., 2018) determined the interactive effects of elevated CORT during adolescence and Val66Met polymorphisms in the gene coding for BDNF. A portion of the mouse BDNF gene sequence was replaced with the human sequence that contained the Val66Met polymorphism. Reduced levels of BDNF in the brains of schizophrenic patients have been reported, and the BDNF gene has been associated with an increased risk for several psychiatric disorders, including schizophrenia (Notaras et al., 2015ab; Weickert et al., 2003).

In the first experiment, Notaras et al. (2017) reported that mice with the Val-Met genotype had significant reductions in PPI compared to mice with the Met-Met and Val-Val genotypes. These differences were evident with or without CORT treatment. In addition, CORT treatment disrupted sensorimotor gating selectively in mice with the Val-Met genotype. Further, CORT treatment reduced startle reactivity of Val-Val male mice by 50%. These results favor the view that BDNF polymorphisms interact with levels of stressful stimulation, particularly during late adolescence, to modulate endophenotypes of schizophrenia.

In the second experiment, adult male and female mice (genotypes Val-Val, Val-Met, and Met-Met) were tested in adulthood for PPI. The main findings from this experiment revealed that apomorphine, a DA agonist, disrupted PPI in mice with the Val-Met and Met-Met genotypes, but had no effect in mice with the Val-Val genotype. Adolescent exposure to CORT had no impact on PPIs of Val-Met and Met-Met mice following administration of apomorphine. In contrast, CORT exposure diminished PPIs in Val-Val mice following acute administration of apomorphine. These results support the involvement of the Val66Met polymorphism in the development of schizophrenia (van den Buuse et al., 2018).

Adolescents who are at high risk of developing schizophrenia may also be more susceptible to the disruptive effects of stressors (Gomes & Grace, 2017a). To examine the underlying neural mechanisms responsible for the effects of stress in adolescence, Gomes and Grace (2017b) subjected adolescent laboratory rats (31–40 days of age) to restraint stress, footshock stress, or a combination of the two. Rats were assessed in adulthood (65–69 days of age) by tests in an EPM (anxiety), novel object recognition task (cognition), and locomotor response to amphetamine (DA system responsivity), and at 77 days of age, in vivo DA neuronal activity was measured in the ventral tegmental area (VTA). The three adolescent stress conditions each impaired body weight gain and increased anxiety-like responses in adult rats. Cognition was impaired by footshock and the combination of footshock plus restraint. Measures of DA neuronal responses were only affected by the combination of footshock plus restraint, with enhanced locomotor responses to amphetamine and an increased number of spontaneously active DA neurons in the lateral VTA.

Rats that had bilateral ibotenic acid lesions of the prelimbic PFC (plPFC) on PND 25 exhibited behavioral as well as DA system hyper-responsiveness to the effects of footshock stress during adolescence. These results indicate that schizophrenia-like changes in behavior and DA system hypersensitivity in adult animals can result from repeated exposure to intense stressors in adolescence. Alternatively, plPFC dysfunction enhanced the vulnerability of adolescent rats to a more modest level of stressor intensity. Thus, the plPFC may play a critical role in regulating the effects of stress during the period between adolescence and adulthood (Gomes & Grace, 2017b).

The MAM Model

The DNA methylating agent, methylazoxymethanol acetate (MAM), is a potent mitotoxin that produces dramatic disruptions in normal patterns of brain development if administered to pregnant laboratory rats prior to GD 16 (Nagata & Matsumoto, 1969). Professor Anthony Grace and his colleagues at the University of Pittsburgh have developed a gestational disruption animal model of schizophrenia that involves delaying administration of MAM to pregnant female rats until GD17 (Grace, 2017; Lodge & Grace, 2009; Moore et al., 2006). GD17 is a time during development when neurogenesis has peaked in most cortical regions of fetal brain and has peaked or halted in many subcortical regions. By delaying MAM administration (22 mg/kg) until GD17, subtle pathological changes in brain anatomy have been documented that are reminiscent of changes seen in post-mortem schizophrenic brains. These include a loss of PV-positive GABAergic interneurons, as well as reductions in thickness of the mPFC, hippocampus, and parahippocampal cortices, but without decreases in numbers of neurons in these areas. Behavioral changes in the MAM model that are consistent with a schizophrenia-like phenotype include deficits in PPI of the acoustic startle response, reversal learning, LI, and social interactions. In addition, adolescent MAM rats exhibited greater levels of anxiety-like behaviors when tested in an EPM. MAM rats tested in adulthood displayed hyper-responsivity to phencyclidine and amphetamine and had elevations in activity of DAergic neurons in the striatum and alterations in glutamatergic neurotransmission in the hippocampus. MAM rats also had a greater number of spontaneously firing ventral tegmental DA neurons. Inactivation of the ventral hippocampus in MAM rats normalized DA neuron population activity and the enhanced locomotor response to amphetamine. Taken together, the anatomical, neurophysiological, and behavioral changes observed in MAM rats provide a valuable animal model for studies of the etiology of schizophrenia (Du & Grace, 2013; Lodge & Grace, 2007, 2011; Modinos et al., 2015).

Stress responses. Compared to controls born to GD17 saline-injected mothers, MAM-treated rats displayed abnormal behavioral and neuroendocrine responses to acute versus repeated exposure to footshock stress (Zimmerman et al., 2013). Behavioral responses to 5 footshocks (1.0 mA, 2.0 seconds duration, every 60 seconds) were recorded at several ages between PNDs 22 and 54, and included measures of ultrasonic vocalizations (USVs, 22 kHz) and freezing behavior. Plasma CORT served as a measure of HPA activation following exposure to footshock stress (1.0 mA, 2.0 seconds duration, every 60 seconds for 10 minutes) on PNDs 31–40.

The results indicated that MAM rats emitted significantly more USVs, spent more time vocalizing, emitted USVs at a higher rate, and spent more time freezing after termination of footshock compared to saline controls. These differences were most evident at younger ages, and were diminished when testing occurred in adulthood. Adolescent MAM rats had blunted plasma CORT responses to a novel environment (handling and transfer to the footshock chamber but no footshocks delivered) and displayed no evidence of habituation by the tenth exposure. In contrast, saline controls exhibited a robust increase in plasma CORT in response to the novel environment, and a significant habituation of the CORT response by the tenth exposure to the novel environment.

The same pattern of responses was evident when MAM and control rats were exposed to footshock stress each day for 10 consecutive days (PNDs 31–40). MAM rats had blunted plasma CORT responses to footshock stress, and there was no evidence of habituation of the plasma CORT response to the tenth session of footshock stress. In contrast, saline controls exhibited a significantly greater plasma CORT response to footshock stress, and had a significant habituation of this response when exposed to footshock stress for the tenth time. These enhanced behavioral and blunted corticosterone responses to footshock stress in juvenile and adolescent MAM rats may render them more susceptible for developing a schizophrenia-like phenotype in adulthood (Gomes et al., 2016; Zimmerman et al., 2013).

Transgenerational effects. The MAM model is also of great interest because the schizophrenia-like phenotype that develops in offspring of MAM-treated dams may also be transmitted to a subset of the F2 and F3 generations, possibly through an epigenetic pathway (Perez et al., 2016). Analyses of differentially methylated regions revealed that one gene, the transcription factor *Sp5*, was hyper-methylated to a similar extent in F1 and F2 rats and may represent a heritable epigenetic alteration in MAM-treated rats. In addition, when compared to offspring of saline-injected controls, some F2 and F3 offspring of MAM-treated mothers displayed elevations in DA neuron population activity in the VTA, but not in firing rates or percentage of neurons with burst firing patterns. There was also a significant negative correlation between the population activity of DA neurons and PV expression in the ventral hippocampus in F2 rats. This effect was most evident for F2 offspring of crosses between a MAM-exposed father and a saline-treated mother. Tracking the F2 and F3 generations of MAM-treated mothers may provide an interesting approach for exploration of environmental influences on the development of schizophrenia-like phenotypic characteristics.

Stem cell treatment. In an exciting new experimental approach, Donegan et al. (2017) utilized two different stem cell–derived interneuron transplants injected into the ventral hippocampus of MAM-treated and control Sprague-Dawley rats on PNDs 40–45, with testing approximately 30 days later. One transplant was enriched with somatostatin (SST)-positive interneurons, while the other included an enriched population of PV-positive interneurons. These interneuron cell transplants became functionally integrated within the existing hippocampal circuitry and were especially effective in reversing deficits in negative and cognitive symptoms in the MAM model of schizophrenia.

Specifically, both types of hippocampal interneuron cell transplants reduced to control levels the elevations in hippocampal pyramidal cell firing rates and the number of spontaneously active DA neurons in the VTA in MAM-treated rats. In addition, PV-enriched cell transplants, but not SST-enriched cell transplants, reversed deficits in social interaction in MAM-treated rats. Both types of cell transplants eliminated MAM-related deficits in reversal learning, but only PV-enriched cell transplants normalized deficits in extra-dimensional set-shifting in MAM-treated rats.

Stem cell–derived interneuron transplants represent an intriguing new experimental approach to the treatment of schizophrenia. However, a host of issues must be addressed before this approach could be considered appropriate for clinical trials using schizophrenic patients. For example, would PV-enriched cell transplants be effective in humans if injected well after the onset of schizophrenic symptoms (i.e., adulthood)? Additionally, would these cell transplants continue to have positive effects over decades? The risks versus rewards of this neurosurgical procedure would also need to be critically evaluated by a range of interest groups (Donegan et al., 2017). Stay tuned!

Neonatal Hippocampal Lesions

Building upon clinical studies that implicated abnormal function of the hippocampus during development as a contributor to the onset of symptoms of schizophrenia in early adulthood, Drs. Barbara K. Lipska and Daniel R. Weinberger conducted an impressive series of experiments on the effects of neonatal disruption to the ventral hippocampus on adult patterns of behavior. One of their foundational experiments explored the effects of ibotenic acid lesions of the ventral hippocampus (Jarrard, 1989) on PND 7 in three strains of rats, Sprague-Dawley (SD), Fischer 344 (F344), and Lewis. PND 7 in laboratory rats corresponds to the middle of the second trimester of gestation in humans (Clancy et al., 2001), a time of high vulnerability for development of schizophrenia (Tseng et al., 2009). Rats of the three strains were tested in adolescence (PND 35) and adulthood (PND 56) for locomotor activity following exposure to a novel environment or administration of amphetamine (1.5 mg/kg, i.p.).

Strain differences. Compared to vehicle-injected controls, SD rats with lesions of the ventral hippocampus displayed increased spontaneous, amphetamine-induced, and swim stress–induced locomotor activity when tested in adulthood but not in adolescence. F344 rats with hippocampal lesions had enhanced spontaneous and amphetamine-induced locomotor activity compared to controls when tested in adolescence, and the difference was magnified further in adulthood. Lesions of the hippocampus did not affect spontaneous or amphetamine-induced locomotor activity at either age in Lewis rats (Lipska & Weinberger, 1995).

These studies clearly demonstrated an interaction between rat strain and a neonatal brain insult in influencing behavioral responses to stressors and to amphetamine. The authors suggested that previously documented differences in neuroendocrine responsivity to stress among these three strains (Dhabhar et al., 1993), and possibly DAergic responses to stress as well, could explain the divergent patterns of response to neonatal ventral hippocampal lesions.

An earlier study with SD rats revealed that ventral hippocampal lesions in adult animals (PND 42) did not result in hyperactivity following a saline injection compared to activity levels in sham-operated controls. Thus, the effects of neonatal ventral hippocampal lesions appeared to remain quiescent through adolescence, followed by exaggerated behavioral responses to a broad range of stressful stimuli in adult animals (Lipska et al., 1992; Lipska et al., 1993).

Lesion effects in adults. Additional experiments from several laboratories that employed adult rats following neonatal hippocampal lesions pointed to further behavioral, neuroendocrine, and neural changes that matched well with a schizophrenia-like phenotype. These included impairments in a working memory task, decreased habituation to repeated testing in an open field arena, deficits in social behavior, impairments in PPI and LI, and exaggerated decreases in PPI following treatment with apomorphine. In addition, neonatally lesioned rats displayed exaggerated ACTH responses to 2 minutes of auditory stress compared to sham-operated controls. In response to acute footshock stress, neo-natally lesioned animals exhibited continued elevations in plasma CORT over a 60-minute period, whereas sham-lesioned rats displayed peak plasma CORT levels at 20 minutes, with decreases after 60 minutes of stress. Another study demonstrated that neonatal VH lesions may alter the basal expression of BDNF in young adult animals. It also appeared that acute stress-related mechanisms involved in regulation of BDNF in the PFC in adulthood might be altered as a consequence of the neonatal lesion. Finally, evidence was presented that brain DA system responses to acute stressors and administration of amphetamine were attenuated relative to sham-operated controls. Taken together, these findings provided further support for the use of the neonatal hippocampal-lesioned rat as a model of schizophrenia-like phenotypic characteristics (Chambers & Lipska, 2011; Lipska, 2002; Lipska & Weinberger, 2000, 2002; Molteni et al., 2001; Tseng et al., 2009).

Tetrodotoxin model. Although there is evidence of subtle alterations in hippocampal function in schizophrenic patients, these changes do not result from a lesion per se (Harrison & Eastwood, 2001). To address concerns about the use of excitotoxic hippocampal lesions in neonatal rats to model aspects of the schizophrenia-like phenotype, Lipska et al. (2002) developed an experimental protocol for the temporary inactivation of the ventral hippocampus beginning on PND 7 with an infusion of the reversible blocker of voltage-gated sodium channels, tetrodotoxin (TTX). Controls were infused with artificial cerebrospinal fluid. When tested in a novel environment in adulthood, TTX-treated rats were more active and spent more time in the center of the novel environment following injections of saline, amphetamine, or MK-801 compared to controls. In contrast, measures of social behavior did not differ between rats of the two groups. It is important to note that these behavioral changes were reduced in magnitude compared to similar behaviors measured in rats with ibotenic acid lesions of the ventral hippocampus on PND 7. Thus, temporary disruption of the ventral hippocampus during a critical window of early postnatal development resulted in permanent changes in DA- and NMDA-related behaviors.

Additional experiments with TTX have focused on temporary inactivation of the entorhinal cortex, the ventral subiculum, or the PFC in laboratory rats on PND 8. When tested in adulthood, the three TTX-treated groups of rats, when compared to vehicle-injected controls, exhibited significant disruptions of LI that were accompanied by decreases in release of DA in the dorsal striatum and the core portion of the nucleus accumbens. These changes in LI and central DA disturbances in TTX-treated rats matched well with clinical observations of schizophrenic patients (for a review of these experiments, refer to Meyer & Louilot, 2014).

Models Based upon Selective Breeding

Apomorphine model. Ellenbroek and Cools (2002) provided an overview of their efforts to select outbred Wistar rats from their colony based upon naturally occurring differences in behavioral responses to apomorphine (APO, 1.5 mg/kg, s.c.), a DA agonist, as a way to gain a better understanding of schizophrenia. Their research was motivated in part by the extensive body of research that links alterations in brain DA systems with the onset and maintenance of schizophrenia (Belujon & Grace, 2015; Grace, 2016; Howes et al., 2016). Two lines of Wistar rats were developed after more than 20 generations of selective breeding, one with enhanced gnawing responses to APO (APO-SUS), and one with minimal gnawing responses to the drug (APO-UNSUS). With each generation, litters were screened and breeding pairs were selected from the two lines such that no brother-sister matings occurred. This approach to phenotypic selection maintained the genetic heterogeneity of the two lines, while enhancing the differences between lines in their responses to APO.

Although the two lines were selected based upon their behavioral responses to APO, a host of other anatomical, physiological, and behavioral differences between the lines emerged. For example, rats of the two lines differed in their behavioral responses to a novel environment, PPI, LI, behavioral responses to amphetamine, sucrose preferences, HPA responses to stressful stimulation, activity of brain DA systems, immune system reactivity, and sensitivity to vasodilators. Across a range of such measures, APO-SUS rats displayed consistent similarities with key features of schizophrenia (Ellenbroek & Cools, 2000; Ellenbroek et al., 1995).

In an early study of gene x environment interactions in the two lines, these investigators reported that APO-SUS litters reared by APO-UNSUS foster mothers had reduced behavioral responses to APO when tested in adulthood. Indeed, gnawing scores of cross-fostered APO-SUS rats were comparable to those of APO-UNSUS rats reared by their natural mothers. In contrast, cross-fostering of APO-UNSUS litters to APO-SUS foster mothers did not affect gnawing scores following administration of APO in adulthood (Ellenbroek et al., 2000).

In a follow-up to this original report, van Vugt et al. (2014) examined the effects of cross-fostering on patterns of maternal care and behavioral responses to APO in rats of the two strains. Compared to APO-UNSUS mothers, APO-SUS mothers displayed fewer episodes of non-arched back nursing, more self-grooming, and were absent from their litters more frequently. APO-SUS litters reared by APO-UNSUS foster mothers experienced significantly more non-arched back nursing episodes and significantly fewer arched back nursing episodes compared to APO-SUS litters reared by their natural mothers.

APO-UNSUS litters reared by APO-SUS foster mothers experienced significantly fewer non-arched back nursing episodes and their foster mothers were away from the nest and self-groomed more frequently compared to APO-UNSUS litters reared by their natural mothers.

These alterations in maternal behaviors of foster mothers were associated with changes in body weights and behaviors of the foster pups. Cross-fostered APO-UNSUS male pups had lower body weights at weaning compared to controls reared by their natural mothers. In contrast, cross-fostered APO-SUS pups (males and females) were heavier at weaning compared to controls reared by their natural mothers. Gnawing scores following administration of APO were reduced significantly in adulthood in cross-fostered APO-SUS rats, but were unchanged and remained very low in cross-fostered APO-UNSUS rats. These two studies provided clear evidence for an interaction between genotype and the pre-weaning maternal environment in determining the differences between lines in the behavioral responses to a DA agonist (Ellenbroek et al., 2000).

Three-hit model. Not to be outdone by those favoring a two-hit model of schizophrenia, Kekesi et al. (2015) presented a three-hit model of schizophrenia that encompassed the following elements: (i) selective breeding of Wistar rats based upon decreased pain sensitivity; (ii) social isolation from 4 to 7 weeks of age; and (iii) repeated daily administration of ketamine (30 mg/kg, i.p., 5 times/week, total of 15 injections) from 5 to 7 weeks of age. Outbred male and female Wistar rats served as controls in these experiments. Behavioral testing in adulthood revealed that selectively bred male but not female rats had lower pain sensitivity, whereas selectively bred females had increased acoustic startle and diminished PPI compared to males. Across several cognitive measures, selectively bred males had lower performance measures than females. In developing a composite risk score across all tests, these investigators found that selectively bred males displayed a higher schizophrenia-like phenotype than females. In addition, repeated administration of ketamine and social isolation did not add to the level of risk in selectively bred rats. Thus, the three-hit model was distilled down to a single factor—selective breeding based upon differences in pain sensitivity (Kekesi et al., 2015; Petrovszki et al., 2013). The more pronounced schizophrenia-like phenotype in male rats matched well with the higher incidence of schizophrenia observed clinically in males.

GABA. Zhang et al. (2010) sought to model in laboratory rats the decreased forebrain expression of glutamic acid decarboxylase (GAD), the rate-limiting step in biosynthesis of gamma amino butyric acid (GABA), in post-mortem brains of schizophrenic patients. They compared offspring of mothers that differed in their rates of LG-ABN in regulation of GAD1 in the hippocampus. Compared to offspring of high LG-ABN mothers, offspring of low LG-ABN mothers expressed lower levels of GAD1 mRNA, increased cytosine methylation, and decreased histone 3-lysine 9 acetylation of the GAD1 promoter in the hippocampus. These results indicated that early life experiences can alter the development of the GABA system, and these effects may be relevant to the etiology of schizophrenia.

Schizophrenia Risk Genes and Environmental Risk Factors

The complexity of schizophrenia as a neurodevelopmental disorder is daunting, with multiple risk genes, each with small effects, thought to interact with multiple environmental factors across multiple stages of development. This is especially true when one attempts to develop animal models that capture gene x environment interactions during various stages of development, which then contribute to a schizophrenia-like phenotype in adulthood (Ayhan et al., 2009; Jouroukhin et al., 2016; Karl & Arnold, 2014).

Included in the following are representative experiments that focused on four specific schizophrenia risk genes: Disrupted-in-Schizophrenia (*DISC-1*), neuregulin-1 (*NRG-1*), nuclear receptor related-1 protein (*Nurr-1*), and reelin. In these studies, laboratory mice with a specific manipulation of a schizophrenia risk gene were exposed to a high-risk environment (e.g., prenatal infection, exposure to stressful stimulation during adolescence, etc.), an experimental approach consistent with the two-hit model of schizophrenia etiology (Oliver, 2011). Adult animals with the schizophrenia risk genes were then compared to age-matched wild-type controls on various behavioral and neurochemical measures that comprised a schizophrenia-like phenotype (Moran et al., 2016).

Disrupted-in-Schizophrenia (*DISC-1*)

A misnomer? *DISC-1* was first identified in a large Scottish family and involved a balanced translocation t(1:11) (q42.1,q14.3) that co-segregated with schizophrenia, schizo-affective disorder, recurrent major depressive disorder, alcoholism, and conduct disorders (St. Clair et al., 1990). In addition, studies in an American family revealed a rare frameshift mutation in *DISC-1* that co-segregated with schizophrenia and schizo-affective disorder (Sachs et al., 2005). However, it should be noted that Sullivan (2013) has analyzed the genetic data on *DISC-1* and concluded that the case has not yet been made for a statistically significant association between *DISC-1* and schizophrenia. Especially lacking is replication of findings in multiple independent samples. However, in some ways the train has left the station given the name originally attached to the gene, so I will review a selection of some of the many studies of *DISC-1* in laboratory mice.

Trangenic approach. Pletnikov et al. (2008) were the first to develop a mouse model that involved inducible expression of a mutant human *DISC-1* gene, with regulation by calcium/calmodulin-dependent protein kinase II (CAMKII), which was limited to the olfactory bulbs, cerebral cortex, hippocampus, and striatum. Expression of *hDISC-1* was first detected on GD15 in the forebrain, but the mutant protein was not detected in brainstem or cerebellum or in non-neuronal cell types. In a subsequent study (Abazyan et al., 2010), *hDISC-1* expression was first detected on GD 9. No gross neurodevelopmental or physical abnormalities were observed, but there was modest enlargement of the lateral ventricles and reductions in neurite outgrowth in primary cultures of embryonic cortical neurons. Transgenic male but not female mice displayed increased levels of locomotor activity over a 24-hour period compared to sex-matched littermate controls. Transgenic male mice also displayed reductions in social interaction and increased levels of aggression. Transgenic female but not male mice did display deficits in tests of spatial memory. These results pointed to the potential of mutant *hDISC-1* transgenic mice as a valuable animal model for studying the pathophysiology of schizophrenia.

In a subsequent report from this same group (Ayhan et al., 2011), the expression of the *hDISC-1* gene in transgenic mice was limited to the prenatal period, the postnatal period, or both. Expression of the mutant *hDISC-1* gene was specified by addition of doxycycline to the laboratory chow (200 mg/kg), with 5–7 days required for inhibiting expression or an equal amount of time required for removal of inhibition following a return to normal laboratory chow. A variety of neurobiological and behavioral measures were quantified in the course of this study. The results suggested that *DISC-1* expression during specific stages of development resulted in neurobehavioral phenotypes that were consistent with schizophrenia. Further, the results pointed to disruptions in prenatal and early postnatal development as critical components of the etiology of schizophrenia, and possibly other serious mental disorders.

Gene x environment design. Abazyan et al. (2010) incorporated the *hDISC-1* transgenic mouse model into a gene x environment experimental design, with maternal immune activation via poly(I:C) administration on GD 9 (5.0 mg/kg, i.p.) as the environmental component. Administration of the drug was by the intraperitoneal route rather than the intravenous route to minimize the possibility that poly(I:C) would exert a maximal effect, thereby masking the interaction of the *hDISC-1* mutation with prenatal maternal infection. The combination of the *hDISC-1* mutation and prenatal exposure to poly(I:C) resulted in increased anxiety-like and depression-like behaviors, diminished levels of social behavior, decreased reactivity of the HPA axis to acute restraint stress, reduced serotonin neurotransmission in the hippocampus, and decreased density of dendritic spines on hippocampal granule cells. These effects required *hDISC-1* expression throughout prenatal and postnatal life. This mouse model provided a valuable system for discoveries relating to the molecular pathways that lead to behavioral abnormalities consistent with a schizophrenia-like phenotype.

Lipina et al. (2013) also examined interactions between prenatal maternal immune activation on GD 9 using poly(I:C) (2.5 or 5.0 mg/kg, i.v.) interacting with a polymorphism (L100P$^{(+/-)}$) in *DISC-1*. DISC-1 mutants treated with poly(I:C) had a greater maternal immune response and alterations in behaviors of adult offspring compared to similarly treated wild-type (WT) mice. Behavioral alterations included disruptions in PPI, LI, and social behavior as well as spatial object recognition. DISC-1 fetuses had dramatically higher brain levels of IL-6 at 6 hours after administration of poly(I:C) to their mothers compared to the responses of WT fetuses. Remarkably, co-administration of poly(I:C) with an anti-IL-6 antibody on GD 9 normalized the behaviors of DISC-1 mutant mice when tested in adulthood. These results clearly demonstrated a gene x environment interaction in the development of a schizophrenia-like phenotype in adult mice. IL-6 appears to play a crucial role in this model of maternal immune activation in DISC-1 mutant mice (Lipina et al., 2013).

The effects of chronic social defeat stress on behaviors of male mice carrying two different point mutations in *DISC-1* were reported by Haque et al. (2012). The point mutations in *DISC-1* included L100P$^{(+/-)}$ and Q31L$^{(+/-)}$, and wild-type mice were employed as controls. Exposure to chronic social defeat stress reduced locomotor activity and rearing in L100P$^{(+/-)}$ mice but not in Q31L$^{(+/-)}$ mice or wild-type mice. Mice of the three groups that were exposed to chronic social defeat stress had similar increases in immobility time in the forced swim test and similar reductions in preference for sucrose in a two-bottle choice test. Exposure to chronic social defeat stress suppressed % time spent in the open arms of an EPM in wild-type and L100P$^{(+/-)}$ mice but not in Q31L$^{(+/-)}$ mice. In addition, this measure was much lower in the two heterozygous groups compared to wild-type mice. With respect to PPI and LI, chronic social defeat stress did not affect either of these measures. In addition, the magnitude of PPI was greatly reduced in L100P$^{(+/-)}$ mice compared to Q31L$^{(+/-)}$ and wild-type mice. LI was clearly established in wild-type mice, but not in either of the DISC-1 mutant strains. Finally, chronic social defeat stress resulted in reductions in social approach and preference for a novel social stimulus in wild-type and L100P$^{(+/-)}$ mice. In contrast, Q31L$^{(+/-)}$ mice did not display sociability in either the social approach or the novel social stimulus task. These findings provide clear evidence of gene x environment interactions across several behaviors measured in adult mice with two different *DISC-1* mutations.

Timing is everything. Underscoring the importance of DISC-1 during early postnatal development, Li et al. (2007) demonstrated that reversible disruption of the C-terminal portion of DISC-1 in laboratory mice on PND 7 but not in adulthood resulted in a complex of behavioral and neurobiological changes that resembled a schizophrenia-like phenotype. These changes included decreases in spatial working memory, shorter latency to remain immobile in the forced swim test, increased social withdrawal, reduced dendritic branching in the dentate gyrus, and reduced hippocampal synaptic transmission. The transient disruption of DISC-1 on PND 7 matched the temporal aspects of the study by Lipska et al. (2002), which employed TTX injections into the ventral hippocampus on PND 7 to block voltage-gated sodium channels.

Kellendonk et al. (2009) provided an overview of studies that employed seven different genetically modified DISC-1 mouse models. Taken together, these models demonstrated significant and consistent disruptions in schizophrenia-like endophenotypes, including sensorimotor gating, spatial working memory, and patterns of social interaction. In addition, these mouse models revealed morphological alterations in the brain that resembled parallel measures in patients with schizophrenia.

Neuregulin-1 (NRG-1)

NRG-1 is a neurotrophic factor that signals by stimulating ErbB4 receptor tyrosine kinases. This protein plays a key role in neural development, neuronal migration, and synapse formation and plasticity. In addition, evidence has accumulated in support of a role for polymorphisms in the *NRG-1* gene in the pathogenesis of schizophrenia (Mei & Xiong, 2008; Stefansson et al., 2002).

In an early study, Karl et al. (2007) sought to characterize the behavioral phenotype of heterozygous NRG-1 transmembrane domain mutant mice, with wild-type (WT) mice serving as controls. Heterozygous mice were characterized by increased locomotor and exploratory activity as well as enhanced anxiety-like behavior. Importantly, these behavioral parameters were sensitive to alterations in the environment. At a general level, these findings were consistent with gene x environment interactions and the neurodevelopmental theory of schizophrenia.

Gene x environment design. O'Leary et al. (2014) studied the effects of NRG-1 in combination with administration of poly(I:C) (5.0 mg/kg, i.p.) on GD 9 using heterozygous NRG-1 transmembrane domain mutant mice. In addition, cross-fostering was employed to control for any changes in maternal behaviors associated with prenatal exposure to the viral mimic. The combination of prenatal immune challenge and disruption in NRG-1 signaling resulted in deficits in PPI, social behavior, and cognition. In addition, the results supported previous findings that control offspring cared for by immune-challenged mothers had significant alterations in behavior in adolescence and adulthood, especially with regard to PPI. This was a surprising finding, as the cross-fostered offspring did not experience the disruptive effects of maternal immune activation during gestation.

In a direct test of gene x environment interactions in an animal model of schizophrenia, Desbonnet et al. (2012) investigated the effects in male laboratory mice of NRG-1 combined with exposure to chronic social defeat stress during adolescence (PNDs 35–45). Mice heterozygous for NRG-1 were maintained on a C57BL/6 background and were compared to wild-type mice (WT), with behavioral and immune measures obtained in adulthood (PNDs 50–85). The results revealed that NRG-1 heterozygotes exhibited phenotypic traits that were consistent with a schizophrenia-like phenotype, including enhanced activity in an open field, disruptions in sensorimotor gating, decreased preference for a novel conspecific, and increased levels of agonistic behavior. With the addition of chronic social defeat stress during adolescence, NRG-1 mice had elevated basal levels of cytokines in the spleen and altered patterns of cytokine responses of spleen cells *in vitro* following stimulation with concanavalin A. In addition, the interaction of susceptible genotype with adolescent stress resulted in brain region–specific alterations in expression of IL-1β, TNF-α, and BDNF. These results underscored the importance of gene x environment interactions in the emergence of a schizophrenia-like phenotype in mice (Desbonnet et al., 2012).

A comparable experimental paradigm was followed by Clarke et al. (2017), with wild-type and NRG-1 heterozygous mice exposed to restraint stress from PNDs 35-57. Controls were not exposed to stressful stimulation. NRG-1 heterozygous mice had increased anandamide (ANA) concentrations in the amygdala and decreased 2-arachidonoylglycerol (2-AG) concentrations in the hypothalamus. ANA and 2-AG are endocannabinoid signaling molecules. In addition, NRG-1 heterozygous mice displayed increased 2-AG concentrations in the hippocampus and impaired spatial learning performance in the Morris water maze. Chronic stress during adolescence increased ANA concentrations in the amygdala to a similar extent in wild-type and NRG-1 heterozygous mice.

Taken together, the results from these experiments highlight the complex results obtained when combining a schizophrenia risk gene, *NRG-1*, with exposure to adolescent stress.

Parental effects. A final study explored the issue of parent of origin effects when employing heterozygous NRG-1 mutant mice in experiments involving measures of schizophrenia-related behaviors (Shang et al., 2017). Heterozygous offspring were generated by crossing wild-type fathers with mutant mothers and mutant fathers with wild-type mothers. Offspring from the two crosses were tested in a battery of behavioral measures. Compared to wild-type littermates, heterozygous males from mutant fathers but not mothers displayed disruptions in fear-related memory and had increased levels of social interaction. These results clearly demonstrated that parental origin of a mutation can impact the behaviors of offspring, and served as a cautionary note to investigators that employ heterozygous mutant mice in experiments.

Nuclear Receptor Related 1 Protein (Nurr-1)

Nurr-1 is a transcription factor and orphan member of the steroid/thyroid nuclear receptor superfamily. Originally characterized by Law et al. (1992), it is expressed primarily in midbrain DA neurons, and is essential for the development of the DA phenotype (Smits et al., 2003). Because of the many lines of evidence linking abnormalities in central DA systems with the pathophysiology of schizophrenia (Grace, 2016), *Nurr-1* has attracted attention as a candidate schizophrenia risk gene.

In an elegant series of experiments, Meyer's research group (Vuillermot et al., 2012) explored the effects of maternal immune activation with poly(I:C) (2.0 mg/kg, i.v.) on GD 19 on neurobiological and behavioral parameters of wild-type and Nurr-1 heterozygous mice tested in adulthood. A low dose of poly(I:C) was employed to enhance the possibility of detecting an additive effect of maternal immune activation and the genetic manipulation. A standard dose of poly(I:C) might have produced a ceiling effect on the various behavioral and neurobiological measures. Previous data from this laboratory demonstrated a 30%–50% reduction in expression of Nurr-1 protein in the midbrain area of heterozygous mice compared to their wild-type littermate controls.

This two-hit experimental design produced additive effects on measures of total activity in an open field test, as well as activity in the center of the open field; magnitude of disruption in PPI; impairments in attentional shifting as assessed by measures of LI; a reduction in D2 receptor immunoreactivity in the core and shell subregions of the nucleus accumbens; and a significant decrease in tyrosine hydroxylase immuno-staining and a significant increase in catechol-O-methyl transferase immuno-staining in the mPFC. These results have important implications for understanding the pathophysiology of neurocognitive disruptions in schizophrenia and their association with disruptions in specific DAergic pathways. A critical feature of these results was the additive effects of the Nurr-1 deficiency with maternal immune activation, supporting the widely held view that schizophrenia results from a susceptible genotype interacting with an environmental stressor to produce cognitive and neurobiological alterations in adulthood.

In a different approach to generating an immune challenge, Eells et al. (2015) examined interactions between a schizophrenia risk gene (Nurr-1 heterozygous mice) and an immune-related environmental stressor (6-week period of infection with *Toxoplasma gondii* in adult mice). *T. gondii* is an obligate intracellular parasite that reproduces sexually in a cat host, and then sheds oocysts into the environment through cat feces that are picked up by a range of warm-blooded vertebrate hosts, including humans. Global infections rates in humans are estimated conservatively at 30% and are associated with an increased risk for development of schizophrenia (Torrey et al., 2012). The findings from this experiment revealed that the combination of heterozygous mice and *T. gondii* infection resulted in a potentiative interaction, with greater open field activity compared to wild-type mice with or without infections and heterozygous mice without infections. In addition, results were suggestive of a gene x environment effect on disruption of PPI in heterozygous mice. One complication in interpreting the results of this study was the highly variable antibody titers to *T. gondii* in wild-type and Nurr-1 heterozygous mice.

Reelin

Reelin is a glycoprotein of the extracellular matrix that subserves critical functions in neuronal migration and positioning as well as brain lamination during development. Reelin is also co-expressed with GAD67 in GABAergic neurons of the cerebral cortex and hippocampus and in glutaminergic neurons of the cerebellum. There is also evidence that reelin regulates synaptic plasticity in adulthood (Folsom & Fatemi, 2013). Many post-mortem studies of brain tissue samples have implicated abnormal reelin signaling in a variety of neuropsychiatric disorders, including schizophrenia, autism, major depressive disorder, Alzheimer's disease, and bipolar disorder (Impagnatiello et al., 1998; Lewis et al., 2005).

One approach to gaining greater insight into the role of reelin in the pathophysiology of schizophrenia has been to study heterozygous mice that are haplo-insufficient for reelin (+/*rl*) and compare them to wild-type mice (+/+). Haplo-insufficient mice are referred to as "reeler mice", which may be a source of confusion. An early report from Costa's laboratory (Costa et al., 2002) suggested that heterozygous reeler mice were worthy of consideration as a model to aid in the development of new antipsychotic drugs. These mice were characterized by behavioral, neurochemical, and neuroanatomical alterations that aligned well with those observed in schizophrenic patients. However, others did not replicate the findings from Costa's laboratory regarding the behavioral phenotype of reeler mice. In fact, when subjected to an extensive battery of behavioral tests, heterozygous reeler mice were reported to differ from wild-type mice only in very subtle ways (Podhorna & Didriksen, 2004).

Several investigators have incorporated heterozygous reeler mice into studies that employed a two-hit experimental paradigm. For example, Howell and Pillai

(2014) examined the effects of prenatal hypoxia on GD 17 (9% O_2 for 2 hours) on wild-type and heterozygous reeler mice. All testing was conducted at 3 months of age. Prenatal hypoxia resulted in anxiety-like behaviors and measures of PPI that were similar in wild-type and heterozygous reeler mice. There was no evidence that hypoxia and reelin deficiency interacted to yield additive effects on any of the behavioral or neurobiological measures assessed in this study.

A different approach was taken by Schroeder et al. (2015), who examined the effects of elevated levels of CORT from 6 to 9 weeks of age on cognitive and social behaviors in male and female WT mice and mice heterozygous for the reelin gene. Exposure to elevated levels of CORT in adolescence was associated with a significant decrement in short-term spatial memory in male and female heterozygous mice, but not in WT mice. In addition, CORT treatment resulted in an increase in reelin expression in the PFC of heterozygous females but not heterozygous males. Finally, there were PPI deficits in CORT-treated WT males, but not in WT females or in heterozygous mice. These findings provide further support for the view that schizophrenia-like phenotypic characteristics may result from gene x environment interactions, with adolescence being an especially vulnerable period.

Teixeira et al. (2011) compared wild-type mice with heterozygous reeler mice and with mice that over-expressed reelin on a variety of behavioral tests that were relevant to schizophrenia. Their results were consistent with earlier reports that wild-type and heterozygous reeler mice did not differ consistently across the various behavioral tests. However, in mice that over-expressed reelin, there was a reduction in time spent floating in the forced swim test following chronic administration of CORT, diminished behavioral sensitization to cocaine, and reductions in PPI deficits following administration of an NMDA antagonist. Reelin supplementation through bilateral injections into the lateral ventricles also normalized subtle deficits in behavioral and neurobiological parameters in adult male and female heterozygous reeler mice when tested 5 days post-injection (Rogers, Zhao, et al., 2013).

Giovanoli et al. (2014) employed an experimental approach similar to the one described in the preceding (Giovanoli et al., 2013) to examine cellular abnormalities in hippocampal GABA neurons. There were guided by strong evidence to suggest that the glutamatergic system is down-regulated in schizophrenia (Konradi and Heckers, 2003). Briefly, pregnant mice received a very low dose (1.0 mg/kg, i.v.) of poly(I:C), or vehicle, on GD 9. Offspring born to poly(I:C) or vehicle-injected control mothers were weaned on PND 21, and then exposed to an assortment of stressors from PNDs 30 to 40. Testing of adult mice occurred from PNDs 70 to 100. Mice that were exposed to maternal immune activation combined with adolescent stress exhibited a significant reduction in PV-expressing GABAergic interneurons in the ventral dentate gyrus. Neither treatment alone yielded such an effect. In addition, the number of reelin-positive cells was reduced in the dorsal CA1–CA3 regions of the hippocampus of immune-challenged mice that were exposed to adolescent stress.

Serine Racemase

It takes two to tango. N-methyl-D-aspartate receptors (NMDARs) are quite unusual in that they require co-agonists to open the cation channel and permit Ca^{++} to flow into the neuron. For this to occur, D-serine or glycine must bind to the GluN1 subunit of the NMDAR at the same time that glutamate binds to the GluN2 subunit (Johnson & Ascher, 1987; Keckner & Dingledine, 1988). Serine racemase (SR) is an enzyme that catalyzes the conversion of L-serine to D-serine in discrete areas of the brain. D-serine appears to be stored in type II astrocytes and is released upon stimulation by NMDAR agonists (Wolosker et al., 1999). Following the influx of Ca^{++}, cAMP-response-element-binding protein (CREB) increases expression of several genes, including BDNF, microRNA-132, and activity-regulated cytoskeleton-associated protein (Arc) (Balu & Coyle, 2018).

D-serine and schizophrenia. Convergent lines of evidence have implicated NMDAR hypofunction in cortical areas with the cognitive deficits and negative symptoms characteristic of schizophrenia (Coyle & Balu, 2018). To pursue the connections between NMDARs and schizophrenia in an animal model, SR knockout mice ($SR^{(-/-)}$) were generated with the expectation that elimination of SR would greatly reduce but not totally eliminate NMDAR activity because of the continued availability of glycine. Compared to controls, $SR^{(-/-)}$ mice had greater than 90% decreases in levels of D-serine in cortex and hippocampus, reduced volume and altered neuronal morphology of the hippocampus, and diminished long-term potentiation in neurons in the dentate gyrus. $SR^{(-/-)}$ mice also exhibited significant reductions in CREB binding to the promoter regions of the genes coding for BDNF, microRNA-132, and Arc (Balu & Coyle, 2018). Consistent with these findings were reduced levels of miR-132 and BDNF mRNAs, as well as the high-affinity receptor for BDNF, phosphorylated tropomyosin receptor kinase B (pTrkB). Chronic treatment of $SR^{(-/-)}$ mice with D-serine (300 mg/kg on day 1 followed by 150 mg/kg on days 2–20 s.c.) normalized hippocampal electrophysiological measures, BDNF-related signaling pathways, and measures of hippocampal-dependent trace memory tasks (Balu et al., 2013).

Labrie et al. (2009) took a different approach to develop an animal model of SR deficiency. They employed N-nitroso-N-ethylurea (ENU) mutagenesis to generate a point mutation in exon 9 of the SR gene. Mice homozygous for this point mutation displayed an absence of SR activity in several brain areas as measured by generation of D-serine. SR mutant mice did not differ overtly from controls in body weight gain, reflexes, vision, maintenance of the fur, balance, coordination, and levels of activity in an open field arena. A forced swim test and an EPM test revealed no evidence of depression-like or anxiety-like behaviors, respectively. However, several phenotypic characteristics did reflect behaviors associated with schizophrenia. These included deficits in social behaviors, PPI, spatial object discrimination, and spatial learning and memory in the Morris water maze. Transcriptome-wide screening of RNA levels in the hippocampus and frontal cortex of control and SR mutant mice using more than 25,000 unique transcripts were also undertaken. Of 171 transcripts in the brain that were altered in SR mutant mice, 130 occurred in the hippocampus, and these alterations tended to be higher in magnitude compared to values for the frontal cortex (32 transcripts changed) and cerebellum (33 transcripts changed). Several of the differentially expressed genes were associated with neural development, myelination, and cognition and have previously been implicated in schizophrenia. Treatment with D-serine (600 mg/kg, s.c.) prior to testing normalized measures of social behavior, PPI, spatial object recognition, and spatial memory. In contrast, D-serine restored some but not all transcript levels in the hippocampus to control values (Labrie et al., 2009).

These two animal models of SR deficiencies represent promising approaches to study schizophrenia. In particular, SR-deficient mice will prove valuable in screening drugs that target the glycine modulatory site of the NMDAR as a novel approach to drug discovery. The effectiveness of D-serine in restoring the molecular, structural, and behavioral changes in SR-deficient animals to control levels is an encouraging start (Labrie et al., 2012).

Summary

In their seminal review article on animal models of schizophrenia, Lipska and Weinberger (2000) foreshadowed many of the research advances in this area for the next two decades. As they pointed out, attempting to capture the most prominent features of schizophrenia (e.g., hallucinations, disordered thought processes, and delusions) in an animal model is a fool's errand. But all is not lost! The development of animal models of schizophrenia that target a particular aspect of the developmental trajectory, capture the essential features of a two-hit gene x environment model, reflect neuropathological features unmasked in postmortem brain studies of schizophrenic patients, or serve as aids in screening new therapeutic agents continue to play an essential role in the multiprong basic research approaches to this complex mental disorder (Kellendonk et al., 2009; O'Donnell, 2011; Powell & Miyakawa, 2006; Wong & Josselyn, 2016). In addition, it is critical that animal models seek to address the full range of symptoms of schizophrenia, including positive, negative and cognitive symptoms (Jones et al., 2011) (Figure 8.2).

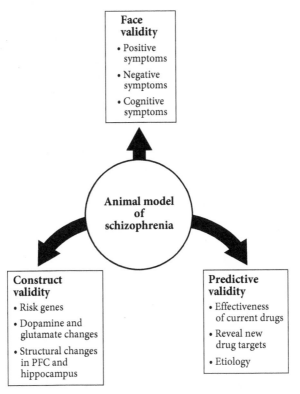

Figure 8.2. Approach to evaluating an animal model of schizophrenia based upon measures of face validity, construct validity, and predictive validity.

The foregoing discussion of experiments with animal models of schizophrenia underscores the value of gene x environment and environment x environment experimental paradigms. The various animal models discussed in this chapter fall into six distinct categories:

1. Maternal immune activation models, including prenatal administration of poly(I:C) or LPS to pregnant mice or rats, have been a popular approach. These models are based upon an extensive epidemiological literature suggesting that exposure of pregnant women to infections increases the risk of schizophrenia in their offspring.

2. Exposure of pregnant mice and rats to stressful stimulation has also been employed to stimulate the development of schizophrenia-like phenotypic characteristics in adult offspring.

3. Disruptions in mother-pup interactions in laboratory strains of mice and rats have been effective in producing schizophrenia-like changes in

the offspring when assessed in adulthood. These manipulations, usually in the form of separating mothers from their litters, occur at a neurodevelopmental stage that matches with the third trimester of human pregnancy.

4. Exposure to stressors during adolescence, including social isolation, has also been employed to model the development of schizophrenia in humans. Adolescence represents an especially sensitive period just prior to the first onset of symptoms in schizophrenic patients.

5. Stimulated by the neurodevelopmental model of schizophrenia, disruptions of neural development in laboratory mice and rats have been incorporated into basic research studies of schizophrenia. MAM, a potent mitogen, has been employed to disrupt normal patterns of brain development when administered on E17 to pregnant rats. In addition, electrolytic and drug-induced lesions of the ventral hippocampus on PND 7 have been utilized to alter neural development in rat pups.

6. Genetic approaches to the study of animal models of schizophrenia have included experiments with selectively bred strains of laboratory mice and rats, as well as models that focus upon a specific risk gene identified through GWAS. Specific risk genes discussed in the preceding included *DISC-1, NRG-1, Nurr-1*, and *reelin*.

What is clear from the highlights of these exciting studies of animal models is that the paths to onset of schizophrenia are almost certainly many and varied. In addition, animal models differ in the schizophrenia-like phenotypic alterations that have been observed in adults. This high degree of variability matches well with clinical observations of schizophrenic patients, and may be indicative of the possibility that schizophrenia is not a single disorder, but rather a complex of disorders that share symptom clusters. Going forward, investigators will depend increasingly on identification across animal models of electrophysiological, anatomical, and/or behavioral endophenotypes of schizophrenia that will inform studies of schizophrenic patients (Arnsten, 2011; Lisman et al., 2008; Rosen et al., 2015). This broad-based approach will hopefully result in the identification of new targets for drug development and novel insights for interventions that could actually prevent the symptoms of schizophrenia from occurring or may lessen their severity.

9

Stress and Autism Spectrum Disorder

Imagine taking your 2-year-old child to the pediatrician for a well-baby visit. As soon as the physician comes into the examining room, you express concern because your lovely little boy's language skills are not progressing in the same way that those of your older two children did. After a careful examination, the physician turns your world upside down when she says that your son is probably autistic. She orders a detailed evaluation by a specialist in the same practice. As you walk out of the office, you feel numb and alone in the world. This is often the starting point for becoming a parent of an autistic child.

As Gene Bensinger (Autism Speaks, 2013), a parent-advocate for Autism Speaks, Inc., describes it, families must confront a host of challenges that impact the autistic child, his or her parents, and other siblings. These include difficult-to-manage and unpredictable "meltdowns" at home or in public places, tensions that inevitably arise between exhausted parents or parents and siblings, and feelings of guilt about the lack of time available for other children in the family. The challenges for many parents continue over the years, but some parents make a contribution to public education and advocacy efforts, as Mr. and Mrs. Bensinger have done.

Clinical Aspects of Autism Spectrum Disorder

Autism spectrum disorder (ASD) is a severe and heterogeneous neurodevelopmental disorder that has its onset in infancy. The genetic heterogeneity of the disorder is reflected in the plethora of genetic risk loci (more than 100 risk genes have been identified) and copy number variations contributing to the disorder, and the variable phenotypic expression of these risk loci across individuals (Persico & Napolioni, 2013). Sanders et al. (2015) identified 71 risk loci that formed a single network of protein-protein interactions involved in chromatin regulation and synaptic function. To illustrate the genetic heterogeneity of ASD, Yuen et al. (2015) conducted whole genome sequence analyses of 85 quartet families (e.g., parents and 2 ASD siblings). In 70% of the sibling pairs, the underlying ASD-relevant genetic alterations were different between siblings, and the phenotypic expression was more variable compared to sibling pairs with similar genetic alterations.

The defining triad of symptoms for ASD includes deficits in reciprocal social interaction and verbal social communication, as well as high levels of repetitive and ritualistic behaviors. Males have a prevalence for ASD that is approximately 4 times that of females, and this sex difference may be even greater in milder forms of the disorder. The diagnostic boundaries that delineate ASD are blurred, with ASD sitting at one extreme of a spectrum of impairments relating to social interactions, verbal behavior, repetitive activities, and cognitive function. Included in this assortment of developmental disorders with ASD are Rett syndrome, Asperger's syndrome, and pervasive developmental disorder not otherwise specified (American Psychiatric Association, 2013). In a large birth cohort study in California, concordance rates for ASD ranged from 0.50–0.77 in monozygotic twins and the estimate of heritability of ASD was 38%, while the estimate of shared environmental effects was 58%. The authors suggested that future research efforts should be devoted to examining gene x environment effects on the development of ASD, particularly aspects of the prenatal environment, given the early onset of symptoms of ASD (Hallmayer et al., 2011). In contrast, studies of a British birth cohort that employed a different diagnostic strategy revealed higher heritability estimates of 56%–95%, but lower estimates for shared environmental effects compared to the previous study (Colvert et al., 2015).

The population prevalence of ASD and related disorders in the United States was 2.24%, with substantial increases in prevalence over the past two decades (Zablotsky, 2015). This significant increase in prevalence is due in large measure to improved dissemination of knowledge about ASD to parents and health-care providers and broad acceptance of diagnostic instruments among pediatricians and child psychologists who provide care and support for children with ASD and their families.

A consistent finding in post-mortem studies of brains from ASD patients has been a variety of histopathological changes in the cerebellum. These changes include a loss of Purkinje cells and granule cells, but a preservation of the numbers of stellate and basket cells. Neuroimaging studies of ASD patients have noted reduced volume of the cerebellar cortex and abnormalities in white matter connectivity, as well as disruptions in cerebellar activation under resting-state conditions and across a range of motor, executive function, and attention-related tasks. Taken together, the various disruptions in cerebellar function appear to play a critical role in the symptoms of ASD (Becker & Stoodley, 2013). Pathophysiological changes in the cerebellum have been studied in various animal models of ASD, as will be described in the sections that follow.

Gene x Environment Interactions in ASD

Although there is compelling evidence that ASD is influenced to a considerable degree by genetic factors, it has become evident that the complex and variable presentation of this disorder likely involves a combination of genetic, environmental, and epigenetic factors. In particular, several researchers have argued for a greater focus on the interaction between risk genes and environmental factors during prenatal or early postnatal life to facilitate a greater understanding of the etiology of ASD (Chaste & Leboyer, 2012; Iwata et al., 2010; Jones et al., 2010; London & Etzel, 2000; Tordjman et al., 2014).

It is beyond the scope of this chapter to review the many exciting genetic studies of ASD that have employed a wide range of methodologies (Bourgeron, 2015). These studies have identified many new risk alleles, some of which are involved in regulation of synaptic plasticity (Sanders et al., 2014) and immune system dynamics during development (Estes & McAllister, 2015). Some of these risk alleles will be featured in the following discussions of specific experiments with animal models.

Epigenetic dysregulation may also play an important role in the etiology of ASD. As discussed in Chapter 7, epigenetic changes include functional modifications in the genome that influence gene expression but do not alter the underlying base sequence of DNA. These modifications require enzymes that catalyze the methylation of DNA as well as the methylation or acetylation of histone proteins that are part of the chromatin complex. There is evidence that a subset of risk genes associated with ASD are involved in chromatin regulation (Sanders et al., 2014). Epigenetic changes may be driven by prenatal stressors and contribute to the complex phenotypic expression of ASD (Tordjman et al., 2014).

Large-scale epidemiological studies have identified an association between several pre- and perinatal risk factors and ASD. These include maternal gestational diabetes, maternal bleeding during pregnancy, maternal medications, maternal immune activation, and complications associated with birth, including hypoxia (Chaste & Leboyer, 2012). In several large population-based studies in Sweden, England, and Denmark, no evidence was found to support a role for stressful life events during pregnancy on risk of ASD in the offspring (Li et al., 2009; Rai et al., 2012). In contrast, Beversdorf et al. (2005) employed a retrospective approach and reported a higher incidence of prenatal stressors during weeks 21–32 of gestation (peak at 25–28 weeks) in mothers who later delivered children who were diagnosed with autism.

Some of these experiments have attempted to resolve the dramatically greater prevalence of ASD in males compared to females. Schaafsma and Pfaff (2014) have proposed that sex differences in ASD may be understood by adopting a three-hit model that includes one or several genetic vulnerabilities (*Hit 1*) interacting with prenatal exposure to a stressor (*Hit 2*) followed by the prenatal surge in testosterone (*Hit 3*). These findings have inspired a number of preclinical studies that will be discussed in greater detail in the sections that follow (Figure 9.1).

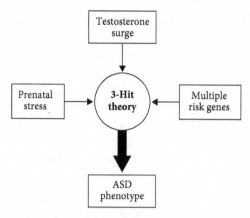

Figure 9.1. An overview of a model originally proposed by Schaafsma and Pfaff (2014) involving a three-hit theory of ASD with greater vulnerability of males compared to females. Androgenic hormones could interact with stressors during the prenatal period to impact genetically vulnerable male fetuses to a greater extent than female fetuses.

Animal Models of ASD

As part of a broad-based strategy of preclinical research on ASD, many laboratories have focused attention on the development of animal models that express some or all of the core triad of symptoms of ASD—deficits in reciprocal social interaction and language skills and repetitive behaviors. Self-grooming has been frequently employed as a measure of a repetitive behavior in laboratory mice and rats, and there is an extensive literature relating to the neurobiological control of this frequently displayed behavior (Kalueff et al., 2016). In addition to these core symptoms, several secondary symptoms that vary in prevalence and severity have been associated with ASD, including increased reactivity to sensory stimuli, reductions in prepulse inhibition (PPI), hyperactivity, increased anxiety, and occurrence of epileptic seizures. An ideal animal model of ASD would express 2–3 of the core symptoms as well as a subset of the secondary symptoms. Critical to the success of studies with animal models is the establishment of sensitive and specific behavioral measures that capture essential features of the core symptoms of autism in children (Ornoy et al., 2019; Silverman et al., 2010).

To a large extent, efforts to characterize animal models of ASD have included studies with genetically defined strains of laboratory mice, in part because methods for genetic manipulations have been developed and refined in this species. These models have been employed extensively to examine the molecular mechanisms underlying environmental risk factors, such as maternal infections and risk genes, and their contributions to the ASD phenotype (Crawley, 2012; Moy & Nadler, 2008; Patterson, 2011). However, a cautionary note has been issued regarding the care that must be exercised in interpreting behavioral and molecular findings in studies with mouse models of ASD (Hyman, 2014).

Strain Comparisons of Autistic-Like Behaviors

Inbred strains of mice. Several research groups have phenotyped inbred strains of mice in a search for valid animal models of ASD. Moy et al. (2004) compared male and female mice of five inbred strains for levels of sociality and preference for a novel conspecific. The strains included C57BL/6, DBA/2J, FVB/NJ, A/J, and B6129PF/J hybrids. With the exception of the A/J strain, juvenile and adult male and female mice of the four other strains displayed a preference for a novel conspecific compared to an empty chamber (i.e., tendency to initiate social contact), and a novel conspecific versus a familiar one (i.e., preference for social novelty). In contrast, A/J mice displayed social deficits in that they preferred an empty chamber to spending time in close proximity to a conspecific (Moy et al., 2004). Similar findings were reported by Bolivar et al. (2007) with FVB/NJ mice that displayed high levels of social behavior, while mice of the A/J and BTBR T⁺tf/J (BTBR) strains exhibited low levels of social behavior.

Mice of the Balb/c inbred strain have also been advanced as a possible animal model of ASD. Balb/c mice exhibited profound deficits in social behaviors across a variety of testing environments and stages of development. Balb/c mice also displayed high levels of anxiety-like and aggressive behaviors, impairments in the development of the corpus callosum, and low levels of brain serotonin (Brodkin, 2007; Jacome et al., 2011).

Moy et al. (2007, 2008) expanded upon their earlier study by comparing a total of 17 inbred strains of mice on a set of tasks to assess social behaviors, preference for social novelty, and reversal learning in memory tasks (a measure of resistance to change). Of the strains that were tested, BTBR and C58/J mice emerged as unusual in that they displayed low levels of social behavior, stereotypy, and resistance to change when tested repeatedly in the Morris water maze or a T-maze.

Selectively bred rat strains. In a highly creative approach to modeling autistic-like behaviors in laboratory animals, Burgsdorf et al. (2013) developed lines of Long-Evans rats that were selectively bred based upon frequency of play-related 50 kHz vocalizations (ultrasonic vocalizations; USVs) in a 2-minute play bout on PND 28. Two lines were developed: one line emitted low rates of vocalizations (Low) while the other emitted high rates of vocalizations (High). A randomly bred line from the same breeding stock was maintained as a control for the High and Low lines. Brother-sister mating was avoided for each of the three groups of rats. By the 25 generation of selective breeding, High animals emitted almost 400 USVs/2 minutes, Low animals emitted approximately 75 USVs per 2 minutes, and controls emitted approximately 175 USVs per 2 minutes.

The Low animals were evaluated as an animal model of ASD based upon their diminished rates of USVs when tested in early adolescence, with the control line serving as the point of reference. Low animals exhibited many of the classic signs of ASD, including reduced social contact with conspecifics, lower rates of play-induced USVs, and an increase in rate of non-frequency modulated USVs. In addition, there was a statistically significant overlap between the previously identified human autism-associated genes and genes differentially expressed in Low rats (Moskal et al., 2011). One of the genes that was differentially expressed in Low rats, the NMDA receptor family, was identified as a significant hub, and possibly a target for future drug development. Indeed, treatment of Low rats with an NMDA partial agonist rescued the deficits in pro-social USVs and reduced non-frequency modulated USVs compared to controls (Burgdorf et al., 2013).

The BTBR model. The BTBR inbred mouse strain was originally bred for experiments relating to insulin resistance, diabetic nephropathy, and phenylke-tonuria. The strain was originally developed in the 1950s, and was eventually acquired by the Jackson Laboratories in 1994. It is now employed in research related to dermatology, developmental biology, and neuroscience. Research in dermatology has focused on skin and hair texture defects (e.g., Nadeem et al., 2018); research in developmental biology has examined the impact of a lack of a corpus callosum and a greatly reduced hippocampal commissure (e.g., Wahlsten et al., 2003); and research in neuroscience has revolved around use of the BTBR strain as an animal model of autism (for reviews, see Meyza & Blanchard, 2017; Meyza et al., 2013).

The C57BL/6J inbred strain (BL6) has emerged as a frequently employed control strain for the BTBR strain because it is highly social, as judged by a battery of tests typically employed in basic research on autism, and displays lower levels of anxiety-like behaviors. To test for possible postnatal maternal effects on the development of autistic-like behaviors, litters of BTBR and C57BL/6 mice were fostered to mothers of the same strain (in-fostered) or the opposite strain (cross-fostered). Controls litters of both strains remained with their biological mothers. The findings of this study provided clear-cut evidence that the strain differences in juvenile social interactions, adult levels of sociality, and frequency of self-grooming were not altered by the maternal environment in either the BTBR or the C57BL/6 strains. The results strongly favored a view that these stable strain differences in behaviors related to ASD were genetically determined (Yang et al., 2007).

Behavioral measures. BTBR mice exhibited profound disruptions in initiation of social interactions, as well as avoidance of reciprocal frontal orientation in pairings with a conspecific (either a BTBR or a C57BL/6 mouse). Avoidance of reciprocal frontal orientations may be comparable to gaze aversion in children with ASD. BTBR mice also engaged in crawl-under behaviors when paired with a conspecific, perhaps reflecting the extremely aversive and anxiety-provoking nature of being in close social proximity to another mouse (Defensor et al., 2011).

BTBR mice also exhibited enhanced levels of self-grooming when tested in a variety of experimental settings. Relative to C57BL/6 controls, BTBR mice also exhibited a more rigid pattern of self-grooming and more frequent stereotypical bar-biting behavior, additional characteristics that add value in an animal model of ASD. When presented with four novel objects, BTBR mice displayed greater preference for specific objects and had more consistent patterns for sequential investigation of these same objects compared to C57BL/6 mice (Pearson et al., 2011).

McTighe et al. (2013) expanded the base of comparison of BTBR and C57BL/6 mice by employing a five-choice serial reaction time task, with an automated touch screen testing apparatus that is similar to tests given to clinical populations. They reported that BTBR mice had increased levels of impulsivity (i.e., an inability to withhold responding), decreased motivation, and decreased accuracy in detecting brief stimuli compared to C57BL/6 mice. Scattoni et al. (2013) reported that BTBR mice exhibited a lack of behavioral flexibility based upon responses in a fear conditioning task. These strain differences further enhance the validity of the BTBR strain as a model of ASD.

Intraspecific modes of communication have also been investigated in BTBR mice. Unusual patterns of ultrasonic vocalizations have been noted in infant BTBR mice, as well as adult BTBR mice, compared to age-matched C57BL/6 controls. In adult BTBR mice, the lower levels of vocalizations, together with reductions in social investigation, occurred in male-male, male-female, and female-female dyads. In addition, male BTBR mice displayed reduced scent-marking behavior and ultrasonic vocalizations in a social setting. Taken together, these studies are consistent with deficits in two modes of communication in BTBRs, another of the triad of primary deficits observed in ASD (Scattoni et al., 2008, 2011, 2013; Wöhr et al., 2011).

Responses to stress. Given the high levels of repetitive self-grooming observed in BTBR mice but not in C57BL/6 mice, Silverman et al. (2010) tested the hypothesis that these elevated levels of self-grooming might reflect a hyper-responsiveness to stressful stimuli in BTBR mice. With respect to the HPA axis, basal plasma levels of CORT were significantly elevated in BTBR mice compared to C57BL/6 controls, a difference also reported by Frye and Llaneza (2010). In addition, levels of CRF peptide and expression of CRF mRNA in the PVN were similar between mice of the two strains. Levels of GR mRNA were significantly elevated in the CA1 region of the hippocampus of BTBR mice compared to

C57BL/6 controls. Finally, levels of oxytocin were elevated in the PVN of BTBR mice compared to C57BL/6 controls. Unfortunately, this study did not include measures of circulating CORT during and after exposure to an acute stressor.

Levels of stress-induced hyperthermia were similar between mice of the two strains. BTBR and C57BL/6 mice had similar profiles when tested for stress-induced hyperthermia, behavior in an elevated plus-maze (EPM) and a light-dark box, and acoustic startle response and PPI. BTBR mice differed from C57BL/6 controls in having less immobility in the forced swim test and the tail suspension test, and a longer latency to react during hot plate testing, but the two strains did not differ in tail flick latencies, a measure of pain threshold (Silverman et al., 2010).

Benno et al. (2009) took a different approach to address the responsiveness of BTBR mice to stressful stimulation. They reported that BTBR mice had higher basal levels of plasma CORT compared to C57BL/6 controls, and BTBRs had higher plasma levels of CORT immediately following a 5-minute test on an EPM, and 15 and 45 minutes after a 90-second tail suspension test plus testing on the elevated plus-maze. BTBR and C57BL/6 mice did not differ in time spent on the open arms of the EPM. However, if mice were exposed to the brief stress of tail suspension for 90 seconds immediately prior to plus-maze testing, BTBR mice spent significantly less time in the open arms of the EPM compared to similarly treated C57BL/6 mice. These findings clearly indicated that the HPA axis of BTBR mice was hyper-responsive to acute stressors. In addition, behavioral responses of BTBR mice displayed greater sensitivity to prior exposure to a brief stressor compared to C57BL/6 controls. Gould et al. (2014) also reported higher plasma CORT responses to novelty and social interactions in adolescent and adult male BTBR mice compared to age-matched C57BL/6 and 129S1/SvlmJ male mice.

Taken together, these studies of HPA axis hyper-responsiveness in BTBR mice were consistent with findings in children with autism. For example, two studies have reported higher salivary cortisol levels in autistic children during play or following a blood stick (Corbett et al., 2010; Spratt et al., 2012). These findings suggest that BTBR mice match well with autistic children in displaying greater reactivity of the HPA axis to social and non-social stressors.

The Valproic Acid (VPA) Model of ASD

Use of VPA during pregnancy. VPA has been employed for many decades as an anti-epileptic medication, as well as a mood stabilizer in patients with bipolar disorder. It is also a potent teratogenic agent. Management of epilepsy in pregnant women is a challenge to physicians, who attempt to strike a balance between the risk of maternal seizures to the developing fetus and mother and the risk of anti-epileptic drugs to the developing fetus. In the case of VPA, studies have revealed that its use by pregnant women increases the risk of birth defects, developmental delays, reductions in cognitive function, and prevalence of autism (Meador et al., 2008; Shallcross et al., 2011). Indeed, use of VPA by women during the first trimester of pregnancy resulted in a 7-fold increase in the prevalence of ASD and related cognitive impairments in their children (Bromley et al., 2008).

VPA animal model of autism. If exposure to VPA during the first trimester of pregnancy increases the prevalence of ASD in children, then it follows that *in utero* exposure of laboratory animals to VPA could provide a valid animal model of ASD. The timing of administration and dose of VPA during gestation are critical variables, and an early study by Rodier et al. (1996) involved administration of VPA in a single dose (350 mg/kg, i.p.) to pregnant rats on either GDs 11.5, 12.0, or 12.5. In laboratory rats, the neural tube closes on GD 11, and it appeared in this study that VPA was an effective antimitotic agent that eliminated cells that formed during the time of drug exposure. This experiment focused on reductions in cell counts in the cranial nerve motor nuclei of laboratory rats compared to an autopsy case of a 21-year-old autistic female who died from sepsis. No behavioral data were collected from the laboratory rats exposed to VPA *in utero* (Rodier et al., 1996). Experiments described in the following indicate that a single dose of VPA administered around GD 12 in the range of 400–600 mg/kg resulted in an autistic-like phenotype in 70%–80% of offspring of female rats and mice. A single dose of VPA (600 mg/kg) to pregnant rats on GD 8 or later resulted in maximal levels of VPA in plasma within 1 hour and a half-life in plasma of 2.3 ± 0.7 hours, with most of the drug cleared from the circulation within 24 hours (Binkerd et al., 1988).

In a more recent study, Kim et al. (2011) compared the effects of a single dose of VPA (400 mg/kg, s.c.) administered to pregnant laboratory rats between GDs 7 and 15 on autism-like behaviors. Their findings revealed that a single dose of VPA on GD 12 in laboratory rats resulted in the most dramatic behavioral alterations compared to vehicle-injected controls, including reduced sociality and decreased preference for a novel conspecific.

In a similar study using CD-1 laboratory mice, Kataoka et al. (2013) reported that optimal parameters for a VPA mouse model of autism involved a single dose of VPA (500 mg/kg, i.p.) administered on GD 12.5. Mice exposed to VPA in utero displayed deficits in social interactions and memory function as well as increased anxiety-like behavior when tested between 4 and 8 weeks of age. In addition, VPA-exposed mice exhibited decreased numbers of neocortical neurons as a result of increased apoptosis and decreased neurogenesis. Finally, VPA administered on GD 12.5 transiently inhibited the activity of histone deacetylase (HDAC), with a concomitant increase in acetylation of histones H3 and H4 in fetal mouse brain for up to 6 hours after drug administration. This transient increase in histone acetylation, postnatal behavioral changes, and cortical anatomical changes observed in mice exposed in utero to VPA did not occur if valpromide, an analogue of VPA, was administered on GD 12.5. These authors suggested that transient hyper-acetylation of H3 and H4 was a critical molecular event in the VPA mouse model of ASD (Kataoka et al., 2013).

In an excellent review article, Roullet et al. (2013) summarized an extensive body of research on the three core behavioral symptoms of ASD that have been observed in VPA-treated mice and rats. These changes, which have been observed in male and female animals, included the following:

1. *Impairments in social behaviors*: a reduction in adolescent play behaviors, increased latency to engage in social interactions, and reduced interest in familiar or novel conspecifics.
2. *Repetitive or stereotyped behavioral patterns*: increased frequency of and time spent in repetitive behaviors, increased frequency of self-grooming, increased burying of marbles, and more frequent repeat entries into the same arm of a Y-maze.
3. *Sensory and communication impairments*: impairment in olfactory-guided nest-seeking behavior and disruptions in ultrasonic communication in neonates and adults.

Related behavioral alterations that have been noted in VPA-treated animals and that match well with findings from autistic children include increased anxiety-like behaviors, increased depression-like behaviors, and diminished cognitive function (Roullet et al., 2013).

To probe further the underlying causes of social deficits observed in VPA-treated laboratory rats, Markram et al. (2008) observed enhanced levels of anxiety-like and repetitive behaviors, reduced sensitivity to painful stimuli, impaired sensorimotor gating, and stronger and more persistent responses to fear conditioning than controls. The enhanced, overgeneralized, and extinction-resistant conditioned fear memories observed in VPA-treated rats were reflected in greater hyper-reactive and hyperplastic changes in the lateral complex of the amygdala. Based upon their findings in the VPA rat model of autism, these investigators suggested that autistic children may experience their immediate environments as highly stressful, aversive, and fearful due to dysregulation of amygdalar and cortical microcircuits. This "Intense World Theory" predicts that patients with ASD contend with their highly aversive environments beginning very early in life by withdrawing into a restricted but highly predictable internal world that minimizes surprises. Aggressive management of the early environment of autistic infants could involve filtering out extremes in the intensity of sensory and emotional experiences as well as progressive systematic desensitization to sensory experiences over time. The goals of these and other facets of a treatment protocol based upon the Intense World Theory were to prevent abnormal patterns of brain development based upon elimination to the greatest extent possible of abrupt or surprising sensory, social, or emotional experiences. After age 6 and when critical brain circuits have been established, autistic children could gradually gain broader exposure to the world around them and increase their capacity to deal with an ever-changing and at times anxiety-provoking world (Markram & Markram, 2010).

Reversing the effects of VPA. There are few therapeutic interventions that are effective in treating autistic children (DeFelippis & Wagner, 2016; Palermo & Curatolo, 2004). Thus, the VPA animal model of autism provides an ideal opportunity to explore treatments that might reverse the behavioral and neurobiological changes observed in rats and mice treated in utero with VPA. In one such study, Schneider et al. (2006) explored the effects of environmental enrichment from PNDs 7–21 and, following weaning, from PNDs 22–35. The earlier enriched environment consisted of extensive handling and exposure to a wide variety of multisensory experiences. The later time involved housing animals in groups of 12 in a large chamber that contained a range of toys and other objects that were changed every other day. After weaning, controls were housed in groups of 5 in standard laboratory cages. Testing occurred during adolescence (days 30–50 of age) or in adulthood (days 90–120 of age).

Environmental enrichment reversed most of the behavioral alterations produced by in utero exposure to VPA. These favorable changes included normal pain thresholds in the tail flick test, stronger PPI, reductions in locomotor and stereotypic behaviors, increased exploratory behaviors, decreased anxiety-like behaviors, and increases in social behaviors. These investigators were encouraged by the effects of environmental enrichment on VPA-exposed rats, and suggested that their findings may have important implications for the treatment of autistic children (Schneider et al., 2006).

In a further test of their Intense World Theory, Professor Kamila Markram and her coworkers (Favre et al., 2015) compared the effects of standard housing or predictable versus unpredictable enriched environments on the phenotype of VPA-treated laboratory rats (GD 11.5, 500 mg/kg, i.p.). After weaning, offspring of vehicle-injected or VPA-treated mothers were housed from PNDs 23–123 in one of the three housing conditions (standard, predictable-enriched, and unpredictable-enriched). The unpredictable enriched environment differed from the predictable enriched environment by having twice-weekly changes in the objects available in the enclosure, as well as cycling among four different sensory packages available to the animals. Only in the predictably enriched environment did the same technician also conduct all animal husbandry procedures throughout the experiment.

The results of this experiment clearly indicated that a predictable, but not an unpredictable, enriched environment could reverse many of the disruptive effects of in utero exposure to VPA. Specifically, a predictable enriched environment prevented the development of a hyper-emotional phenotype, but an unpredictable enriched environment did not. The hyper-emotional phenotype included elevations in fear, anxiety, social withdrawal, and sensory alterations. Further, individual variability in autism-like behaviors correlated with neurochemical profiles (e.g., protein levels of GABA receptor subunits, levels of GR protein, post-stress levels of plasma CORT) and predicted the response of VPA-exposed rats to the predictable enriched environment (Favre et al., 2015).

The results of these two environmental enrichment studies are difficult to reconcile. Schneider et al. (2006) started their enrichment condition at an earlier age and terminated it sooner than Favre et al. (2015). Favre et al. (2015) argued that their results pointed to a critical role for predictability in the effects of environmental enrichment in VPA-exposed rats. But one could argue that a standard laboratory cage environment could be made very predictable and would include fewer sensory and social stimuli than the enriched environment. Returning to the Intense World Theory of Markram and her colleagues, it was suggested that increased sensory stimulation would be deleterious to the developmental trajectory of an autistic infant. Yet, that is exactly what they did in placing VPA-exposed rats in an enriched environment. This is obviously an important issue to consider in the design and interpretation of future experiments.

Mehta et al. (2011) tested the effects of a metabotropic glutamate receptor antagonist (mGluR5) on autistic-like behaviors in VPA-exposed C57BL/6 mice (600 mg.kg, s.c. on GD 13). The mGluR5 antagonist, 2-methyl-6-phenylethylpyrididine (MPEP, 20 mg/kg, i.p.) or an equal volume of saline was administered 10 minutes prior to testing. MPEP significantly reduced repetitive behaviors (e.g., marble burying and self-grooming) but had no effect on anxiety-like behaviors during testing in an open field arena.

Kim et al. (2014) investigated the role of cholinergic signaling in the brain by treating VPA-exposed mice and rats with the acetylcholinesterase (AChE) inhibitor, donepezil (0.3 mg/kr, i.p., each day beginning on PND 14). Exposure to VPA in utero resulted in an up-regulation of AChE in the PFC of mice and rats. Acetylation of histone H3 in the AChE promoter region was increased in VPA-exposed animals. Repeated daily injections of donepezil improved sociality and reduced repetitive behaviors and hyperactivity in VPA-exposed animals. These findings point to AChE as a possible therapeutic target for the treatment of ASD.

Maternal Immune Activation

Compelling evidence has been marshaled in support of a connection between maternal immune activation during pregnancy and increased risk of ASD in off-spring (Harvey & Boksa, 2012; Hornig et al., 2018; Lydholm et al., 2019; Meltzer & Van de Water, 2017; Patterson, 2011). In addition, autistic individuals appear to have a persistently elevated inflammatory profile beginning prenatally and extending well into adulthood that involves areas of the brain as well as the periphery. The connection between maternal immune system dysfunction and symptoms of ASD in her offspring appears to be mediated by the effects of maternally produced proinflammatory cytokines on the placenta and directly on the developing fetus (Bronson & Bale, 2014; Estes & McAllister, 2015; Goines & Ashwood, 2013; Goines & Van de Water, 2010). In addition, some mothers produce anti-brain autoantibodies during pregnancy that are specific for fetal brain proteins. The combination of maternally produced cytokines and autoantibodies negatively impacts neural development in the fetus, and sets in motion a pattern of neurobehavioral development that culminates in the ASD phenotype in genetically susceptible individuals (Estes & McAllister, 2015; Meltzer & Van de Walter, 2017). A recurring theme in experiments with animal models and studies with humans is that gene x environment interactions are critical to the pathophysiology of ASD.

In this section, I will discuss several preclinical approaches to the study of immune activation during pregnancy that result in the development of an ASD-like phenotype in the offspring. An important issue to resolve at the end of this section is the shared versus distinct features that have been identified in animal models of ASD and schizophrenia.

Maternal infections. Viral and bacterial infections during pregnancy are associated with an increased risk of autism in the offspring. In support of this assertion, Atladóttir et al. (2010) studied a birth cohort of the more than 1.6 million children born in Denmark between January 1, 1980, and December 31, 2005. In this birth cohort, 10,133 children were diagnosed with autism. Diagnoses of maternal infection with and without hospitalization during pregnancy were determined for all mothers from nationwide health system registers. The results indicated a lack of association between a viral or bacterial infection over the entire course of pregnancy and risk of autism in the children. In contrast, admission to the hospital as a result of a maternal viral infection during the first trimester of pregnancy (adjusted hazard ratio = 2.98) or a maternal bacterial infection during the second trimester of pregnancy (adjusted hazard ratio = 1.42) was significantly associated with a later diagnosis of ASD in her child.

Several studies in animal models have explored the relationship between maternal infections during pregnancy and the development of ASD-like behaviors in the offspring. For example, Shi et al. (2003) infected pregnant Balb/c and C57BL/6 females with human influenza virus by intranasal infusion on GD 9.5, resulting in a transient period of illness that persisted for several days. Behaviors of adult offspring of control and infected mothers were assessed to determine the impact of in utero exposure to the human influenza virus on neurobehavioral development. Infected animals were significantly less active in the center squares of an open field arena and reared less frequently than control mice. In addition, infected mice had longer latencies to explore a novel object and made fewer approaches to the novel object compared to controls. The same was true for social contact; infected mice had significantly longer latencies to initiate contact with a social stranger. Infected mice also exhibited deficits in sensorimotor gating, as reflected in diminished PPI of the acoustic startle response. The authors reported that mice born to prenatally infected mothers did not appear to display any evidence of viral entry into brain tissue based on negative results from a variety of assays. However, other investigators have detected viral RNA and nucleoprotein in fetal brain tissue and have demonstrated that viral RNA persisted in the brains of offspring to PND 90 using a mouse model (Aronsson et al., 2002).

Fatemi et al. (2005) infected pregnant Balb/c females intra-nasally on GD 9 with human influenza virus. On the day of birth, brains of offspring from control and infected mothers were processed for microarray studies of 20,000 known mouse gene transcripts. The effects of influenza virus infection on gene transcription were highly targeted; 21 genes were up-regulated and 18 genes were down-regulated. The up-regulated genes included examples that influence neurotransmission, post-translational modification, gene expression, and signal transduction. The down-regulated genes included examples that influence gene expression, signal transduction, and axonal stability. Alterations in the expression of these genes could lead to long-lasting changes in brain structure and function and contribute to the pathophysiology of ASD and related disorders.

Poly(I:C). As noted in Chapter 8, poly(I:C) is a synthetic, double-stranded RNA molecule that stimulates a proinflammatory antiviral response when injected into laboratory animals. Malkova et al. (2012) determined if offspring exposed to maternal immune activation during gestation reflected the three defining behavioral characteristics of ASD. They subjected pregnant C57BL/6J mice to injections of poly(I:C) (5.0 mg/kg, i.p.) on GDs 10.5, 12.5, and 14.5. Pregnant female controls received injections of saline at the same times during gestation. Frequency of ultrasonic vocalizations was reduced beginning on PND8 in poly(I:C)-exposed pups. Beginning on PND10, the structure of the ultrasonic vocalizations was altered in poly(I:C)-exposed pups, and these differences persisted into adulthood. In adulthood, poly(I:C)-exposed males emitted significantly fewer ultrasonic vocalizations during encounters with male or female conspecifics, and displayed reduced scent marking in the presence of female urine. Treated animals also exhibited significant reductions in social behaviors and increases in repetitive and stereotyped behaviors. Thus, the maternal immune activation model captured the three essential behavioral characteristics of ASD.

Building upon these findings, Hsiao et al. (2012) administered poly(I:C) (20 mg/kg, i.p.) to pregnant C57BL/6N mice on GD 12.5. Following birth and weaning of the litters from control and poly(I:C) exposed mothers, adult offspring were tested in a battery of behavioral tests and were assessed for peripheral immune functioning. Maternal immune activation by poly(I:C) resulted in adult offspring that exhibited a distinct behavioral profile of deficits in PPI of the acoustic startle response, increased stereotyped behavior, decreased social preference for a novel conspecific, and increased anxiety-like behaviors in an open field test. The poly(I:C)-exposed offspring also displayed a peripheral cellular immune profile that was consistent with a proinflammatory phenotype. Interestingly, irradiation of poly(I:C)-exposed offspring and transplantation of bone marrow from control offspring reversed in part their behavioral phenotype.

Schwartzer et al. (2013) adopted a gene x environment experimental design and compared the effects of poly(I:C) on pregnant females of two inbred strains, C57BL/6J and BTBR. Poly(I:C) (20 mg/kg, i.p.) was administered on GD 12.5. Strain x treatment interactions were reported for sociality, ultrasonic vocalizations, and stereotyped and repetitive behaviors such that the effects were more dramatic in BTBR mice compared to C57BL/6J mice. The exception was in measures of social approach, where control BTBR mice had such low scores that maternal immune activation could not exert further effects. In addition, poly(I:C)-exposed BTBR but not C57BL/6J mice displayed persistent alterations in splenic responses to stimulation, as reflected in greater release of the proinflammatory cytokines IL-6, IL-10, IL-17, and TNFα.

A BIG challenge. Considerable recent attention has been directed at the brain-immune-gut (BIG) axis and its impact on brain development and behavior (Cryan & O'Mahoney, 2011; Mulle et al., 2013; Sharon et al., 2016). Three studies from the laboratories of Gloria B. Choi at MIT and Jun R. Huh, now at Harvard Medical School, unraveled the connections between maternal immune activation by administration of poly(I:C), gut bacteria, and dysfunctional brain circuits involved in behavioral abnormalities in offspring. In their initial study (Choi et al., 2016), pregnant mice were injected with poly(I:C) on E12.5 and compared to control dams that were injected with saline on E12.5. Three hours after administration of poly(I:C), pregnant dams displayed significant increases in serum levels of IL-6, TNF-α, interferon-β, and IL-1β. Two days later, there was a significant increase in serum levels of IL-17a that was dependent upon the earlier increase in IL-6. In a comprehensive series of experiments, these researchers provided convincing evidence that poly(I:C)-induced abnormalities in fetal cortical development and behavior were dependent upon T helper 17 (T_H17) cells and their production of IL-17a. Behavioral measures included ultrasonic vocalizations on PNDs 7–9, social behavior at 8 weeks of age, and repetitive behavior at 9 weeks of age. The enhanced expression of IL-17a mRNA on E14.5 was evident in mononuclear cells from the placenta and decidua of poly(I:C)-treated dams. In addition, there was a significant increase in the expression of IL-17a receptor subunit A (IL-17Ra) mRNA, but not subunit C (IL-17Rc) mRNA, on E14.5 in fetal brains of mothers treated with poly(I:C). Pretreatment of pregnant mothers with an antibody to IL-17a prevented the abnormalities in cortical development and later ASD-like behavioral abnormalities (Choi et al., 2016).

In a follow-up report, Kim et al. (2017) demonstrated a critical role for maternal intestinal bacteria in the T_H17 immune cell response to treatment of pregnant mothers with poly(I:C) on E12.5. These effects were not observed in nonpregnant female mice treated with poly(I:C). Pretreatment of pregnant dams with the broad-spectrum antibiotic vancomycin blocked the effects of poly(I:C) treatment on abnormal cortical development and ASD-like behaviors in offspring. Segmented filamentous bacteria in the intestinal tracts of pregnant dams appeared to be responsible for the induction of T_H17 cells. When pregnant mice lacking these intestinal bacteria were treated with poly(I:C) on E12.5, their offspring did not have abnormalities in cortical development and behavior. If segmented filamentous bacteria were introduced into these same mice that normally lacked them, then the offspring of poly(I:C)-treated females did display abnormalities in cortical development and behavior.

In a final report, Yim et al. (2017) focused their attention on the cortical control of ASD-like behavioral changes in offspring of dams treated on E12.5 with poly(I:C). The previously identified cortical abnormalities were localized to the dysgranular zone of the primary somatosensory cortex (S1DZ). Using optogenetic techniques to control neuronal activity in S1DZ neurons, the authors demonstrated that activating these neurons in mice that were not exposed to poly(I:C) in utero resulted in the appearance of ASD-like patterns of behavior. In addition, if S1DZ neurons were inhibited in offspring of poly(I:C)-treated dams, these mice no longer exhibited an ASD-like pattern of behavior. They further demonstrated that atypical social behaviors were regulated by S1DZ neurons that projected to the temporal association area of cortex, whereas repetitive behaviors were controlled by S1DZ neurons that projected to striatum.

Taken together, this remarkable series of reports has connected viral infections during pregnancy, immune responses mediated in part by intestinal bacteria, and abnormal development of cortical areas and behaviors in offspring. These findings have obvious implications for the development of ASD in children of mothers who were exposed to viral infections during the first or second trimesters of pregnancy. These exciting results provide a range of testable hypotheses to pursue to advance our understanding of the mechanisms at work in the development of ASD in children.

Lipopolysaccharide (LPS). As noted in Chapter 8, LPS mimics the effects of infection by gram-negative bacteria when injected into pregnant laboratory animals, and represents another experimental approach to induce maternal immune activation. In a series of experiments by Kirsten et al. (2010, 2012), pregnant Wistar rats were injected with LPS (100 μg.kg, i.p.) or saline on GD 9.5, and the offspring were studied in infancy and in adulthood. Ultrasonic vocalizations in response to maternal separation on PND 11 were reduced significantly in LPS-exposed rats compared to saline-injected controls. In addition, LPS-exposed males but not females displayed deficits in social behaviors and in learning and memory. These results are consistent with maternal immune activation by LPS as animal model of ASD.

Human antibodies. Given the heterogeneity of ASD, some have speculated that maternal autoantibodies may affect brain development in utero in a subset of children with ASD. To test this hypothesis, Zimmerman et al. (2007) tested reactivity of GD 18, PND 8, and adult rat brain proteins to serum samples collected from 11 mothers of an ASD child and compared them to serum samples from 10 control mothers. Antibodies in sera from mothers with an ASD child recognized different fetal, but not postnatal or adult rat brain proteins, compared to mothers of normal children. In contrast, serum samples from the two groups of mothers did not differ in their reactivity to myelin basic protein or glial acidic fibrillary protein. It is possible that these antibodies to prenatally expressed rat brain antigens may cross the blood-placental barrier and disrupt fetal brain development. These findings should be considered tentative given the very small sample sizes that were reported.

Singer et al. (2009), in a follow-up to the previous study, isolated and purified antibodies from pooled serum samples from 63 mothers with autistic children (ASD sample, 279 mg/dl) and from 63 mothers of unaffected children (control sample, 245 mg/dl). Pregnant mice received daily injections (i.p.) of 0.5 ml of purified IgG from either ASD or control samples from GDs 13–18. Offspring of mothers treated with the ASD sample displayed enhanced anxiety-like behaviors, greater magnitude of the acoustic startle response, and reductions in social behaviors when tested in adulthood. The authors also reported evidence of cytokine and glial activation in fetal brains of mothers injected with the ASD sample.

To obtain greater experimental control, Martin et al. (2008) tested three groups of rhesus monkeys: (i) those exposed prenatally to IgG antibodies collected from mothers with multiple children diagnosed with ASD; (ii) those exposed prenatally to IgG antibodies collected from mothers of multiple normal children; and (iii) those untreated prenatally. Following birth, monkeys were observed beginning at 1 month of age and continuing in various test situations until 1 year of age. Rhesus monkeys exposed to IgG antibodies in utero from mothers of children with ASD displayed increased stereotypical behaviors across multiple testing episodes and had significant increases in activity. Monkeys exposed in utero to IgG antibodies purified from mothers of typically developing children and untreated control monkeys did not display stereotyped behaviors or hyperactivity. These and other findings suggest the possibility that trans-placental transfer of autoantibodies from mother to developing fetus may be an etiologic factor in some cases of ASD. The possibility of therapeutic interventions, especially in women who have delivered a child later diagnosed with autism, will depend on gaining clearer insight into processes related to the generation of autoantibodies and their targets in fetal brain (Fox-Edmiston & Van de Water, 2015).

ASD or Schizophrenia?

How does one make sense of the obvious overlaps as well as the distinctions between the etiologies of ASD and schizophrenia? This same question applies to the overlaps and distinctions between animals models of these two psychiatric disorders (Garay et al., 2013). The similarities between ASD and schizophrenia complicated the evolution of psychiatric diagnostic criteria. Although Kanner's original description of infantile autism was published in 1943 (Kanner, 1943), many psychiatrists placed children that would now be diagnosed with ASD into a category labeled "childhood psychoses" as late as the 1970s (e.g., Kolvin, 1971). Infantile autism was first included as a diagnostic category in *DSM-III*, which was published in 1980.

Meyer et al. (2011) have developed an elegant model that explains the similarities and differences between autism and schizophrenia. According to their model (refer to Figure 9.2), maternal infection during critical stages of pregnancy results in acute fetal inflammation. The consequences of acute fetal neuroinflammation during the course of early neural development may promote in genetically susceptible fetuses the appearance of psychopathological and neuropathological phenotypes that are common to schizophrenia and autism.

There are two potential pathways following acute fetal inflammation; the maternal and/or fetal system may progress into a state of persistent inflammation, or it may rein in the ongoing inflammatory process. The pathway that is followed is shaped in part by an interaction with individual risk genes for schizophrenia or autism. The occurrence of persistent inflammation in utero may be explained by a failure in negative feedback control of inflammatory processes, and may eventually result in chronic inflammation that persists following birth

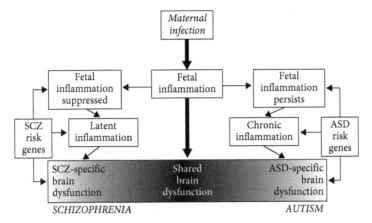

Figure 9.2. A model demonstrating how maternal immune activation following an infection during pregnancy could result in both common and disorder-specific symptoms of schizophrenia (SCZ) and autism spectrum disorders (ASD) in offspring. This model presents a dynamic interaction both prenatally and postnatally between disease-specific risk genes and immune system responses.

This model is based upon the extensive experiments of Dr. Urs Meyer and colleagues, as referenced in the text.

and into adulthood. If anti-inflammatory and immunosuppressive responses are mounted by the maternal and/or fetal systems, they may be sufficient to diminish the acute fetal inflammatory responses. However, the fetal immune system may now be primed for future latent disruptions in the immune system that extend well beyond birth. These future latent disruptions may be unmasked in adolescence or adulthood by exposure to stressors or other immune challenges (e.g., Giovanoli et al., 2013).

Persistent inflammation appears to be more relevant for the pathogenesis of autism, and thus may contribute to phenotypic abnormalities specifically seen in autism. However, latent immune abnormalities may be an important aspect of the pathogenesis of schizophrenia-specific brain abnormalities. The genetic background further contributes to the emergence of unique brain dysfunctions independently of, or interacting with, the inflammatory pathways (Meyer, 2014; Meyer et al., 2011). More than 100 risk genes have been identified thus far for the two disorders, some of which are shared; thus, the potential is established for significant heterogeneity in presentation of children with ASD and young adults with schizophrenia.

When comparing the results of maternal immune activation experiments in the preceding chapter on schizophrenia, and the current chapter on ASD, it is obvious that the animal models that have been employed are not specific for one disorder versus the other. If experiments are motivated by an interest in the etiology of schizophrenia, then the behavioral and neurobiological endpoints employed in the study reflect that bias. If, on the other hand, experiments are designed with ASD in mind, then there is a greater focus on behavioral and neurobiological endpoints that reflect what is known about ASD. As noted in Figure 9.1, the pathway from maternal immune activation in utero to a specific disorder in later life depends upon the genetic and environmental contexts in which the infection occurs, and this same level of interaction occurs following birth. Increasingly, these complexities should be reflected in the design of experiments that employ maternal immune activation as an animal model of ASD or schizophrenia (Careaga et al., 2017; Harvey & Boksa, 2012; Meyer, 2014).

Neonatal Infections

As an example of an alternative approach to viral infections, Lancaster et al. (2007) advanced an animal model of ASD based upon intracranial injection of neonatal Lewis rats with Borna disease virus (BDV) within 1 day of birth. When tested in adulthood, BDV-infected rats spent less time interacting socially with a conspecific and more time following the conspecific. Associated with these behavioral changes in BDV-infected rats were degeneration of the dentate gyrus of the hippocampus and a gradual loss of Purkinje cells in the cerebellum. Given that this model involves neonatal infection with a virus that destroys specific neuronal populations in areas of the brain, this may explain why it has not been widely adopted by other researchers.

Genetic Alterations

Risk genes. Significant advances have been made in the identification of risk genes for ASD. The general consensus is that ASD, like schizophrenia, involves hundreds of functionally diverse risk genes, each with very low penetrance. Several lines of evidence now support the concept of molecular convergence that originally emerged from studies of post-mortem gene expression and protein-network analyses in ASD compared with typically developing brain samples. These findings suggested that ASD risk genes were involved in specific neural pathways and cell types. These included synaptic function, chromatin modification, receptor signaling, and protein synthesis. In post-mortem brain samples from individuals with ASD, coordinated down-regulation of synaptic function genes and up-regulation of microglial and neural immune genes have been noted, pointing to the possibility of global dysregulation of cortical patterning and synaptic homoeostasis. Glial up-regulation may not necessarily be related to inflammatory processes per se, and instead may be reflective of disruptions in synaptic pruning (De Rubeis & Buxbaum, 2015; Geschwind & State, 2015; Roeder & State, 2015; Sanders et al., 2014; Voineagu et al., 2011; Yuen et al., 2015).

As a starting point, many investigators have manipulated individual risk genes in laboratory animals, usually mice, and have examined the impact of a given manipulation on behavioral and neurobiological measures (Banerjee et al., 2014). In this section, I will discuss a sampling of the many studies that have utilized this experimental design. The rationale behind experiments that manipulate single genes is that ASD is a neurodevelopmental disorder, and manipulations of genes that are critical for neurodevelopmental processes may illuminate some of the mechanisms that shape features of the ASD-like phenotype.

Greco et al. (2013) studied autism-like phenotypes in synapsin KO mice. Synapsins (Syn I, II, and III) are a family of synaptic vesicle-associated phosphoproteins that are critically involved in synapse development and plasticity and neurotransmission. KO mice lacking Syn I and/or II were characterized by epileptic seizures and mild cognitive impairments. Individual KO mice were generated for each of the Syn genes and were subjected to a battery of behavioral tests prior to the emergence of epileptic seizures beginning at 2–3 months of age. The results indicated that deletion of Syn I or Syn III disrupted social behaviors and repetitive behaviors, whereas deletion of Syn II produced significant changes in social and cognitive behaviors, altered exploration in a novel environment, and increased self-grooming. These changes were consistent with an involvement of synapsins in the behavioral alterations observed in ASD.

Synaptic growth-associated protein 43 (GAP43). GAP43 is a risk gene for ASD that plays a vital role in development and migration of neurons, neurotransmission, and synaptic plasticity. Zaccaria et al. (2010) studied GAP43 heterozygous $(GAP^{(+/-)})$ mice to determine if the behaviors of these mice were consistent with a pattern of ASD-like behaviors. They reported that GAP43-deficient mice exhibited reduced behavioral flexibility, were sensitive to stressful stimulation, and had reduced levels of social behaviors, confirming an ASD-like phenotype.

Engrailed-2 (En2). En2 is a homeobox transcription factor that plays an important role in nervous system development and differentiation, including the size and anatomical organization of the cerebellum and amygdala, and connections of monoaminergic neurons (Kuemerle et al., 2007). Several laboratories have reported that En2 is an ASD risk gene, and a study by Brielmaier et al. (2012) utilized a comprehensive array of behavioral tests to assess the patterns of social, communicative, stereotyped, and cognitive behaviors of WT, En2 heterozygous mice, and En2 null mutant mice. Their findings revealed that En2 null mutants displayed deficits in social behaviors, fear conditioning, performance in the Morris water maze, increased immobility in the forced swim test, reduced PPI, and mild impairments in grip strength and coordination. *En2* null mutants did not differ from WT controls in USVs in a social setting; stereotyped behaviors; or in general measures of health, exploratory behaviors, anxiety-like behaviors, and responses to painful stimuli. Thus, *En2* null mutants displayed two important behavioral measures relevant to ASD—deficits in social behaviors and in cognitive function.

Tsc1. Mutations in either *Tsc1* or *Tsc2* can result in tuberous sclerosis complex (TSC), a genetic disorder characterized by numerous benign tumors in many parts of the body, including the brain, as well as high rates of comorbid ASD. *Tsc1* and *Tsc2* produce protein products that dimerize and negatively regulate mammalian target of rapamycin (mTOR) signaling. Tsai et al. (2012) generated an animal model of ASD using heterozygous or homozygous loss of *Tsc1* in cerebellar Purkinje cells that resulted in anatomical and behavioral changes consistent with an ASD-like phenotype. These alterations included reduced numbers of Purkinje cells in the cerebellum and increased size of the soma and increased spine density in surviving Purkinje cells of homozygous mutant mice. In addition, *Tsc1* mutant mice did not display a preference for a novel test mouse compared to a familiar one, exhibited impairments in discrimination of social olfactory cues, encountered difficulties in a reversal learning and a motor learning paradigm, and had increased pup vocalizations from PNDs 5–12. Disturbances in cerebellar morphology and behaviors were prevented in *Tsc1* mutant mice by treatment with the mTOR inhibitor, rapamycin, beginning on PND 7.

In follow-up experiments, Stoodley et al. (2017) focused their attention on Right Crus I (RCrusI) as a critical mediator of ASD-related pathologies in the *Tsc1* mouse model and in children with ASD. Using a chemogenetic approach, these investigators inhibited Purkinje cell activity in RCrusI in wild-type mice and produced impairments in social behavior and reduced responsiveness to social olfactory stimuli as well as repetitive grooming episodes and behavioral inflexibility during water Y-maze testing. These behavioral effects of Purkinje cell inhibition were not observed if chemogenetic inhibition occurred in the Left Crus I. To explore further the connection between RCrusI activity and ASD-related behavioral changes, RCrusI Purkinje cell activity was increased chemogenetically in *Tsc1* mutant mice, which resulted in restoration of social behaviors but not repetitive grooming behaviors and behavioral inflexibility in water Y-maze testing. Further experiments are needed to explore additional cerebellar circuits that influence repetitive grooming and behavioral inflexibility. But this experimental approach holds promise in developing cerebellar-specific treatment strategies for ASD patients.

PTEN. Lugo et al. (2014) examined the behavioral and molecular consequences in mice with neuron subset-specific deletion of the negative repressor phosphatase and tensin homolog, PTEN. Compared to WT mice, PTEN

KO mice exhibited deficits in social behaviors, decreases in marble-burying behavior, reduced anxiety-like behavior in the EPM, and increased activity in an open field arena. PTEN KO mice were similar to WT mice in frequency of USVs emitted on PNDs 10 and 12. In an earlier study, Kwon et al. (2006) reported that PTEN KO mice had macrocephaly, enhanced patterns of axonal and dendritic growth, deficits in social behavior, impaired cognitive function, reduced anxiety-like behavior in the EPM, but enhanced anxiety-like behaviors in an open field arena and a light-dark box, and exaggerated responses to sensory stimuli. Thus, PTEN KO mice may serve as a suitable animal model for ASD.

NLGN4. Loss of function mutations in any of several genes have been associated with some forms of monogenic heritable ASD. In an approach using an animal model, laboratory mice with a loss-of-function mutation in the murine *NLGN4* ortholog, *Nlgn4*, which codes for the synaptic cell adhesion protein, Neuroligin-4, exhibited deficits in reciprocal social interactions with familiar and novel conspecifics, a reduced latency to emit USVs and reduced frequency of USVs when male KO mice were paired with a female in estrus, and increased repetitive behaviors. In contrast, sensory function, locomotor and exploratory behaviors, anxiety-like behavior, and learning and memory were not disrupted in KO mice. In addition, KO mice had significant reductions in total brain volume, volume of the brainstem, and volume of the cerebellum. These investigators suggested that a gene network that includes *Nlgn4* regulates the maturation and function of synapses in the brain, and may influence some of the core symptoms of ASD (El-Kordi et al., 2013; Jamain et al., 2008). A different profile of changes was noted in *Nlgn2* KO mice, which included developmental delays and reduced pup USVs in response to maternal separation. In contrast, *Nlgn2* KO mice did not differ from WT controls in levels of social behaviors, repetitive behaviors, or PPI (Wöhr et al., 2013).

SERT. The 5-HT transporter (SERT) gene (*SLC6A4*) has been associated with whole blood 5-HT levels and ASD susceptibility. Several gain-of-function SERT coding variants in children with ASD have been identified. Blakeley and his coworkers (Veenstra-Vanderweele et al., 2016) reported that transgenic mice expressing the most common of these variants, *SERT Ala56*, exhibited elevated p38 MAPK-dependent transporter phosphorylation, enhanced serotonin (5-HT) clearance rates, and hyperserotonemia. These effects were accompanied by altered basal firing rates of raphe 5-HT neurons, as well as $5HT_{1A}$ and $5HT_{2A}$ receptor hypersensitivity. In addition, *SERT Ala56* mice exhibited alterations in social function, communication, and repetitive behaviors. These data suggest that altered 5-HT signaling may increase risk for ASD-like traits and may contribute to the etiology of ASD.

DAT. The dopamine transporter (DAT) is a presynaptic membrane protein that regulates the availability of DA in the synapse by rapidly clearing it following release. DiCarlo et al. (2019) took a reverse translational approach by developing a knockin mouse model using a DAT mutation previously identified in ASD and attention deficit hyperactivity disorder (ADHD) patients. This mutation involves a threonine → methionine substitution at site 356 (DAT T356M). DAT T356M$^{(+/+)}$ mutant mice differed from wild-type controls in having reduced DAT transporter activity, increased DA content in the synapse, and reduced DA synthesis in the striatum. These alterations in DA neuronal activity were associated with increased repetitive rearing, increased locomotion, and disturbances in social behaviors. These behavioral changes capture some of the key features of ASD as well as ADHD and suggest that striatal DAT dysfunction may be associated with these developmental disorders in children.

Oxytocin. Mice with a null mutation of the oxytocin gene (OXT KO) display several interesting cognitive and behavioral alterations that may have special relevance to ASD (Winslow & Insel, 2002). Contrary to studies in rats, mice do not appear to require OXT for normal sexual or maternal behaviors; however, OXT is required for the milk ejection reflex during lactation. OXT KO pups do develop normally up to weaning if they are raised by a lactating WT foster mother. Studies of OXT KO pups revealed that they emit fewer USVs following maternal separation. OXT KO adults were more aggressive than WT mice, but they were unable to recognize familiar conspecifics after repeated social encounters. It should be noted that OXT KO mice exhibited normal olfactory and non-social memory functions. Central administration of OXT into the amygdala restored social recognition in OXT KO mice.

In a complementary approach, Sala et al. (2011) reported that OXT receptor-null mutant mice (OXTR$^{(-/-)}$) displayed deficits in social behavior and memory for a conspecific, reductions in behavioral flexibility, increased levels of aggression, and increased susceptibility to epileptic seizures. These ASD-like behavioral characteristics of OXTR$^{(-/-)}$ mice were reversed by acute i.c.v. administration of OXT or AVP, both of which act on vasopressin 1a receptors. The behavioral phenotypes of OXT and OXTR KO mice provided a novel approach to the study of ASD, and pointed to potential new targets for drug development (Sala et al., 2011).

Teng et al. (2013) extended the early findings with OXT by comparing two inbred mouse strains, BALB/cByJ and C58/J, which exhibited phenotypes relevant to core ASD symptoms. Mice from both strains received acute or sub-chronic injections (4 times every other day) of OXT (i.p.). Acute OXT did not increase sociability in BALB/cByJ mice, but did result in decreased motor stereotypy in C58/J mice without affecting open field behavior. The sub-chronic OXT regimen resulted in significant prosocial effects in both BALB/cByJ and C58/J mice, more rapidly in the former than the latter. Thus, peripheral administration of OXT attenuated social deficits and repetitive behaviors in these two inbred mouse models of ASD. These findings related to actions of OXT are especially relevant for the disruptions in social behavior and the repetitive behaviors observed in ASD patients (Carter, 2007; Lukas & Neumann, 2013; Modi & Young, 2012).

Contactin-associated protein-like 2 (CNTNAP2). CNTNAP2 is a neuronal trans-membrane protein member of the neurexin superfamily that plays a role in neuron-glia interactions and clustering of K^+ channels in myelinated axons. $Cntnap2^{(-/-)}$ KO mice display key features of ASD, including communication deficits, repetitive movements, disturbances in social behavior, epileptic seizures, and hyperactivity, and have been advanced as an animal model of ASD (Peñagarikano et al., 2011). Selimbeyoglu et al. (2017) employed $Cntnap2^{(-/-)}$ KO mice to explore the contributions of disturbances in the balance between excitation and inhibition (E:I balance) in neurons of the mPFC to the ASD-like phenotype. They utilized optogenetic techniques to increase the excitability of inhibitory parvalbumin-positive (PV) neurons or to decrease the excitability of excitatory pyramidal neurons in the mPFC in freely behaving mice during behavioral testing. As expected, KO mice differed from WT mice in having dramatic decreases in social interaction and higher levels of locomotor activity during tests of social interaction. Increasing the excitability of PV neurons or decreasing the excitability of mPFC pyramidal neurons had the same dramatic effects. Each of these interventions reversed the deficits in social behaviors and hyperactivity that characterized KO mice. Additional experiments with WT mice revealed that PV neuronal activity increased to a greater extent during novel social interactions compared to interactions with a novel object. Similar patterns of PV neuronal activity during social versus novel object interactions were not observed in KO mice. In addition, PV neuronal activity was greater in KO mice during interactions with a novel mouse compared to a familiar mouse. WT mice did not display this differential pattern of activation. These exciting results suggest that real-time modulation of E:I balance in the mPFC may reverse deficits in social behaviors and locomotor activity in a mouse model of ASD. The translational potential of these findings for treatment of children with ASD is very high (Selimbeyoglu et al., 2017).

Kim et al. (2019) also employed $Cntnap2^{(-/-)}$ KO mice to investigate the role of abnormal AMPA receptor function on ASD-like social behaviors. Their methods for manipulating receptor function were much less precise and their findings were not concordant with the report of Selimbeyoglu et al. (2017). However, the results of Kim et al. (2019) were generally consistent with the E/I imbalance hypothesis.

SHANK2. SHANK is a family of postsynaptic scaffolding proteins that regulate the development and function of excitatory synapses and may impact the expression of ASD-like symptoms (Sala et al., 2015). One member of this family of proteins, SHANK2, has been implicated in ASD and schizophrenia. Chung et al. (2019) utilized $Shank2^{(-/-)}$ KO mice and WT controls to explore the effects of NMDA receptor function on the development of ASD-like deficits in behaviors. Prior to weaning (PND 14), *Shank2*$^{(-/-)}$ mice displayed hyperfunction of NMDA receptors in Schaffer collateral-CA1 pyramidal synapses and in pyramidal neuron synapses in the mPFC that changed to hypofunction beginning soon after weaning (PND 24). Chronic treatment (PNDs 7–21) with the NMDA receptor antagonist, memantine (20 mg/kg, p.o., twice daily), prevented NMDA receptor hyperfunction early in life and blocked later expression of ASD-like social behaviors in adolescence and early adulthood. However, memantine did not affect other ASD-like behaviors, including reduced USVs, enhanced repetitive behaviors, and enhanced levels of locomotor activity. Memantine had no effects on social behaviors of WT mice.

Chromosomal modifications. Hemizygosity of a segment of human chromosome 22q11.2, which encompasses more than 30 genes, has been associated with ASD in children. *Tbx1* is a risk gene for ASD that is contained within the segment of DNA that is deleted from the long arm of chromosome 22. Hiramoto et al. (2011) generated mice that were heterozygous for *Tbx1*$^{(+/-)}$ and compared them to WT control mice with regard to expression of the mRNA and presence of the protein for Tbx1 in brain areas and behaviors in a variety of tests. The results revealed that Tbx1 mRNA and protein were expressed throughout the brains of adult C57BL/6J mice, with levels especially high in areas that exhibit neurogenesis in adulthood (e.g., olfactory bulbs and dentate gyrus). *Tbx1* heterozygous mice displayed significant impairments in social behaviors, neonatal ultrasonic vocalizations, and working memory as reflected in a spontaneous alternation task. These investigators suggested that the behavioral changes observed in *Tbx1* heterozygotes were consistent with patterns observed in ASD and in schizophrenia.

On the basis of conserved human/mouse chromosomal linkage, Nakatani et al. (2009) modeled duplication of human chromosome 15q11–13, a mutation observed in some cases of ASD, by generating mice with a 6.3 Mb duplication of the conserved linkage group on mouse chromosome 7. Mice with a maternally or paternally inherited chromosomal segment duplication on a C57BL/6 genetic background bred normally and were fertile. Compared to WT mice, mice with a paternal duplication exhibited deficits in social behavior, behavioral inflexibility in a reversal task in the Morris water maze, increased USVs following maternal separation on PNDs 7 and 14, and heightened levels of anxiety-like behaviors. One possible mechanism to explain these behavioral changes may involve the 5-HT$_{2C}$ receptor.

Using a mouse model of a copy number variation on chromosome 16p11.2 previously observed in ASD patients, Walsh et al. (2018) explored the impact on neuronal activity in 5-HT dorsal raphe neurons projecting to the nucleus accumbens. Genetic deletion of the syntenic region of the chromosome from 5-HT neurons produced deficits in social behavior and decreases in dorsal raphe 5-HT neuronal activity. The deficits in social behaviors in the mutant mouse model were reversed by optogenetic enhancement of 5-HT neuronal activity in the dorsal raphe that signaled through 5-HT$_{1B}$ receptors in the nucleus accumbens. In addition, optogenetic inhibition of firing by dorsal raphe neurons reduced social interactions. Taken together, these results make the case for a critical role for 5-HT signaling in the nucleus accumbens in modulation of social behaviors.

Summary. Manipulations of risk genes and chromosomal deletions and duplications in laboratory animals have revealed important connections between genetic alterations and behavioral and neurobiological changes relevant to ASD. However, few experiments in this area of research have adopted a gene x environment experimental design such that the genetically manipulated laboratory mice or rats are exposed to stressful stimuli, followed by behavioral and neurobiological assessments related to ASD. This has been a profitable strategy in animal models of other mental disorders, and could be helpful in explicating the variety of mechanisms underlying the development of ASD.

The Stress of Birth

GABA serves as the principal inhibitory neurotransmitter of the mature nervous system, and a system of GABAergic interneurons influences the generation of behaviorally relevant central neural oscillations. In contrast, GABA's effects are the opposite polarity during prenatal development, when it functions as an excitatory neurotransmitter. The key to this change from excitatory to inhibitory action is determined by a shift in intracellular chloride concentrations ($[Cl^-]_i$) that is regulated by two membrane proteins, NKCC1 and KCC2, which serve as chloride importers and exporters, respectively. Progressive alterations in the balance of these two chloride transporter molecules during neural development lead ultimately to a switch from an excitatory to an inhibitory action of GABA. The polarity change in GABA neurons at birth is driven in part by the neurohormone, oxytocin (OXT). OXT also exerts a range of neuroprotective effects on the newborn, including an analgesic effect and buffering against anoxia (Ben-Ari, 2015).

The polarity shift in GABAergic neurons at birth from excitatory to inhibitory may be disrupted in children with ASD as well as in animal models of ASD (Lee et al., 2017). Some of the many genetic modifications that have been reported for ASD are associated with excitatory/inhibitory imbalances in interneurons and their associated circuits. To test these hypotheses, Tyzio et al. (2014) employed two very different animal models of ASD—rats exposed prenatally to VPA and KO mice lacking the *fmr1* gene (FRX KO), which serves as an animal model of the fragile X syndrome. In control rats and WT mice, the driving force of GABA$_A$ receptors was elevated in fetal hippocampal neurons on GDs 20–21, decreased dramatically on the day of birth, rebounded to higher levels on PND 2, and then decreased progressively to reach low adult levels by PND 30. Acute application of an antagonist to the NKCC1 chloride importer, bumetanide (10 μM), or oxytocin (1 μM) decreased $[Cl^-]_i$ and the driving force of GABA on PND 0 in VPA rats and FRX KO mice. In addition, the chloride exporter, KCC2, was down-regulated in hippocampal neurons of juvenile VPA rats and FRX KO mice. In hippocampal neurons from control rats and WT mice on PNDs 0 and 15, the GABA$_A$ agonist, isoguvacine (10 mM), had no effect or inhibited spike frequency. In striking contrast, administration of isoguvacine stimulated spike frequency in hippocampal neurons from PND 0 and PND 15 VPA rats and FRX KO mice.

Two critical experiments extended the findings described in the preceding and firmly established the vital role played by the disruption in the polarity shift in GABA neurons to an ASD-like phenotype (Figure 9.3). In the first experiment,

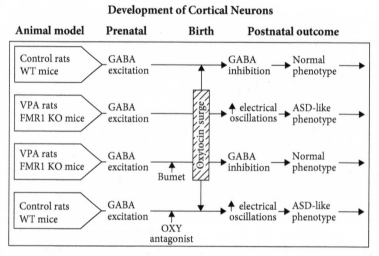

Figure 9.3. Three experimental approaches reveal the critical role played by the surge in oxytocin (OXY) during the transition from prenatal to postnatal life. During prenatal life, GABA signaling exerts excitatory effects on cortical neurons. There is a switch from excitatory to inhibitory GABA signaling that is mediated by the OXY surge around the time of birth, as revealed by studies with normally developing rats and wild-type (WT) mice. The transition from excitatory to inhibitory cortical GABA signaling did not occur in two animal models of autism spectrum disorder (ASD): *Fragile X Mental Retardation* 1 (FMR1) knockout (KO) mice (ASD) and rats exposed prenatally to valproic acid (VPA). Disruptions in the development of GABA signaling could be blocked in VPA rats and FMR1 mice by oral administration of bumetanide (Bumet) to pregnant dams. In addition, the normal transition from excitatory to inhibitory cortical GABA signaling could be blocked in WT mice and control rats by administration of an OXY antagonist prior to the surge in the hormone beginning just prior to birth. Refer to the text for details.

pretreatment of near-term pregnant female VPA rats and FRX KO mice with bumetanide restored electrophysiological properties of hippocampal GABA neurons and normalized ultrasonic vocalizations of PND 4 VPA rat pups and PND 8 FRX KO mouse pups following separation from their mothers. In the second experiment, administration on the day before birth of a selective OXT receptor antagonist to pregnant female rats and WT mice resulted in offspring with electrophysiological properties and behavioral changes that matched with the ASD-like phenotype of VPA rats and FRX KO mice, respectively.

In a third experimental approach, Corradini et al (2018) administered poly(I:C) to pregnant mice on GD 9, and demonstrated a delay in the polarity shift of GABAergic neurons in their offspring from excitatory to inhibitory. This delay in the GABA switch was confirmed by direct neuronal recordings in vitro and quantification of elevated intracellular levels of Cl⁻ in PND 20 offspring. Offspring of poly(I:C)-treated dams could be rescued from delays in the GABA switch by pretreatment of their dams with magnesium sulfate just prior to dosing with poly(I:C), a pretreatment which prevented the increases in cytokine levels in poly(I:C)-treated developing fetuses.

This remarkable set of findings in a drug-induced model of ASD using rats, a genetic model of ASD in mice, and a maternal immune activation model using mice points to the transition from prenatal life to postnatal life as a critical period for the expression of the ASD-like phenotype. Several possible targets for drug intervention in pregnant mothers around the time of birth or in infants and young children emerged from these experiments (Ben-Ari, 2015, 2017; Tyzio et al., 2014; Zimmerman & Connors, 2014). Indeed, treatment of young autistic children with bumetanide has yielded encouraging results, although there are concerns about the poor penetration of the blood-brain barrier by the drug and its associated side effects on fluid and electrolyte balance (e.g., Lemonnier et al., 2017). For those pregnant women exposed to infections near the end of the first trimester when fetal cortical development is underway, magnesium sulfate may prevent the untoward effects of immune activation on fetal development (Corradini et al., 2018).

Summary

Many investigators have taken up the significant challenge of developing animal models of ASD that capture to varying degrees the core triad of symptoms. Comparisons of multiple inbred mouse strains have identified several promising models, including the Balb/c and the BTBR strains of mice. In addition, Long-Evans rats have been selectively bred for high and low rates of ultrasonic vocalizations as a means of modeling disruptions in communication associated with ASD. A significant effort has also been devoted to examining the effects of prenatal insults, including maternal immune activation, on offspring development. Studies of individual ASD risk genes have also been a valuable component of this broad-based effort to learn more about the underlying mechanisms of ASD. A recent promising line of research has involved studies of the polarity shift in GABAergic neurons during the transition from prenatal to postnatal life in three very different animal models of ASD. These exciting findings point the way to treating ASD in utero by reversing this defect in GABA neurons.

Work on several of these animal models has followed a reverse translational strategy, where the generation of the animal model has benefited from knowledge gained in the treatment of children with ASD or through results gleaned from clinical research projects or population-based epidemiological studies. A major benefit of several of these experimental approaches with animal models has been the ability to alter the prenatal environment in a highly controlled way and then follow the affected offspring well into adulthood. This level of experimental precision is simply not possible in prospective studies of human infants and children. More importantly, results from experiments like these open the way for improvements in the treatment of children with ASD.

10

Stress and Bipolar Disorder

De Moore and Westmore (2016), in the prologue to their excellent biography of the Australian psychiatrist John Cade, provide a vivid description of the plight of bipolar patients before Cade's accidental discovery of lithium as a first-line treatment. It was early 1948 in Sydney, and "Edward" walked along Bondi Beach and hatched the grand idea of selling the beach grain by grain. Surely this would make him one of the richest people in the world. Edward was in the full throws of a manic episode that had been going on for weeks, a state he had experienced frequently over almost 20 years of suffering from bipolar disorder. He was no stranger to insane asylums, where the mentally ill were then relegated for their own protection.

As Edward walked along the beach to contemplate the great riches that awaited him, he sensed that the excitement of the manic high of the previous weeks was starting to fade, and he felt "the black chill of depression seep into his body." This rapid cycling from the highest high to the lowest low is one of the classic symptoms of bipolar disorder. As the depressed state overwhelmed him, Edward went across town to the Sydney Harbour Bridge and contemplated suicide (De Moore & Westmore, 2016).

Clinical Aspects of Bipolar Disorder

Bipolar disorder is a severe mental disorder that affects approximately 1%–2% of the population worldwide. Individuals with bipolar I disorder exhibit at least one episode of mania, while those with bipolar II disorder display at least one hypomanic episode and one depressive episode (Figure 10.1). Hypomania is less intense than mania, but both conditions involve some level of sleep reductions, higher than normal energy levels, restlessness, increased self-esteem, having many new ideas and plans, decreased inhibitions, and increased risk-taking. The age of onset for this debilitating disorder is approximately 20 years of age, with similar rates of occurrence of bipolar I disorder in males and females, but a higher prevalence of bipolar II disorder in females. There is a high rate of suicide attempts associated with bipolar disorder, and affected individuals may experience significant levels of disability over the life span (Belmaker, 2004; Phillips & Kupfer, 2013; Vieta et al., 2018).

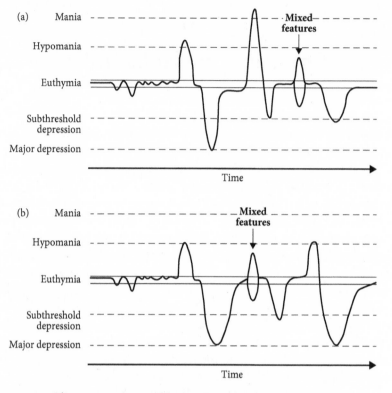

Figure 10.1. There are two main subtypes of bipolar disorder. A: Bipolar I disorder is characterized by at least one episode of mania. B: Bipolar II disorder is characterized by at least one hypomanic and one depressive episode. Note that mixed features can occur in both disorders.

Adapted from Vieta et al. (2018) and used with permission of the publisher.

The heritability of bipolar disorder is extremely high, with estimates up to 85%, and the genetic architecture is quite complex, with many risk genes thought to be involved, each contributing a small effect. There is also considerable evidence to support a powerful role for environmental factors interacting with these risk genes at different stages of development as described in Chapter 2, including prenatal maternal infections, traumatic experiences in childhood, drug use and abuse, and stressful life experiences. Patients with bipolar disorder often express comorbidities for other psychiatric disorders, including attention deficit hyperactivity disorder, anxiety disorders, and substance use disorders (Vieta et al., 2018).

Lithium was the first drug approved by the US Food and Drug Administration for the treatment of acute mania. Valproic acid, an anti-epilepsy medication, has also been employed for the treatment of acute mania, in addition to several other drugs. Cognitive-behavioral therapy and electroconvulsive therapy have also been utilized in the treatment of mania. Bipolar patients spend much more time in depressive episodes than in manic episodes, but there are limited options for the treatment of bipolar depression. A major concern in the treatment of bipolar depression is susceptibility to mood switching and the onset of hypomania or mania, as well as an increase in cycling from mania to depression or vice versa. Long-term management of bipolar disorder typically involves administration of a mood stabilizer such as lithium or lamotrigine, often in combination with an antipsychotic or an antidepressant drug (Geddes & Miklowitz, 2013).

Stressful life events appear to play a critical role in the onset and recurrence of bipolar disorder over the life course. Kapczinski et al. (2008) have suggested that bipolar patients who experience frequent switching between mood states are more susceptible to the adverse effects of environmental stressors on brain signaling pathways. This increased level of susceptibility to stressors may place bipolar patients at greater risk of subsequent swings in mood and increased likelihood of comorbid drug use. Brain-derived neurotrophic factor (BDNF), which plays a role in regulating multiple signaling pathways involved in survival and growth of neurons and synaptic plasticity, may play a pivotal role in connecting environmental stressors to early onset of symptoms and/or rapid cycling in bipolar patients (Post, 2007).

Several years before the announcement of the RDoC framework, Hasler et al. (2006) proposed a series of endophenotypes of bipolar disorder based upon a broad survey of the relevant literature. Possible cognitive endophenotypes included attention deficits, deficits in verbal learning and memory, and deficits in executive functions following depletion of tryptophan. Endophenotypes related to changes in brain structure included reduced volume of the anterior cingulate cortex and white matter abnormalities, including reductions in myelin content, based on neuroimaging studies. Instability of circadian rhythms in bipolar patients may represent another physiological endophenotype, especially as it relates to sleep disturbances and sensitivity to seasonal changes in day length. Disturbances in brain motivation and reward pathways were also advanced as an endophenotype. Finally, patterns of bipolar symptom provocation following sleep deprivation or administration of psychostimulant drugs or cholinergic agonists or antagonists may also serve as a basis for the delineation of response-based endophenotypes. This research strategy also matches well with experiments that employ a range of animal models, where each model system may capture one or several features of bipolar disorder.

An Evolutionary View of Bipolar Disorder

It is not unreasonable to ask why bipolar disorder, which has a very high heritability, has been maintained at a stable rate in most ethnic groups when it appears to be so deleterious. You may recall that a similar question was raised regarding schizophrenia in Chapter 8. And we can't simply blame everything on our distant Neanderthal cousins, or can we?

Modern humans (*Homo sapiens*) originated in Africa in close proximity to the equator. This place of origin provided an environment with a relatively un-changing photoperiod of approximately equal amounts of daylight and darkness each day throughout each year. As early humans began to migrate north into Europe and Asia, two major moderating influences were encountered that are relevant to our discussion of bipolar disorder. First, the migration north took early humans into an environment characterized by seasonal rhythms in light-dark cycles over the course of each year. Second, there was some interbreeding of *H. sapiens* of African origin with their more northern Neanderthal cousins (*H. neanderthalensis*).

At the time early humans ventured north, Neanderthals had been living in Europe and Asia for tens of thousands of years, sufficient time for optimization of physiological and behavioral adjustments to seasonal variations in the light-dark cycle. These adjustments would have included reductions in energy levels, loco-motion, and social interactions, as well as increased sleep during short days (e.g., fall and winter), and increases in energy levels, affect, and goal-directed activities associated with foraging for food and sexual partners during long days (e.g., spring and summer). Extremes in these seasonally driven changes in behavioral pheno-type among Neanderthals could have been the source of risk genes for modern-day bipolar disorder, and would have been passed along to offspring through infre-quent matings with *H. sapiens* partners (Sherman, 2012; Young & Dulcis, 2015).

A critical piece of evidence in support of these hypotheses comes from comparisons of the genome sequencing of Neanderthal DNA and DNA samples from present-day Europeans, Asians, and sub-Saharan Africans. These genomic data support the view that interbreeding of modern humans with Neanderthals did occur on a very limited basis, such that present day non-African humans de-rived approximately 1%–4% of their DNA from Neanderthals. In addition, these genomic comparisons revealed that Neanderthals shared more derived alleles with non-Africans compared to Africans (Green et al., 2010). Another piece of this ev-olutionary puzzle is reflected in the finding that present-day Africans are less likely than non-Africans to receive a diagnosis of bipolar disorder. Thus, even a trace of Neanderthal-derived DNA appears to increase the risk for bipolar disorder.

Animal Models of Bipolar Disorder

Two features of bipolar disorder that are especially relevant for those interested in modeling this disorder in laboratory animals include the process of switching from a manic or hypomanic episode to depression (or vice versa), and the possible disruption of circadian systems in bipolar individuals, including alterations in sleep-wake patterns and seasonal variations in susceptibility to the onset of mania or bipolar depression. There is also the challenge of dealing with significant inter-individual variability among bipolar disorder patients in the switching process and in the extent of involvement of circadian systems and occurrence of seasonal variability. What is clear at this time is that the underlying neural and molecular mechanisms that regulate the switch process are incompletely understood in bipolar patients, and there is an urgent need for animal models that permit a detailed exploration of these underlying mechanisms (Salvadore et al., 2010; Vieta et al., 2018).

In the sections that follow, the primary focus will be on manic-like behavioral phenotypes in various animal models and the mechanisms involved in switching from mania to depression (or vice versa). Some aspects of depression will be captured in particular animal models of bipolar disorder where there is a mixed state of depression-like and mania-like behaviors or when an animal model does include a switch from mania-like to depression-like behaviors. A detailed discussion of animal models of depression will be presented in Chapters 12 and 13.

The Holy Grail

Developing animal models of bipolar disorder is not for the faint of heart. This challenge is magnified when one confronts the unique aspect of bipolar disorder that sets it apart from all other psychiatric diagnoses—the switch process from one extreme mood state to another extreme mood state of opposite polarity. As will be discussed in the following, not all developers of animal models have attempted to capture aspects of the switching process, preferring instead to focus on modeling mania-like behaviors or depression-like behaviors. However, there are now animal models that have provided compelling evidence of switching between mood states of opposite polarity, and these models open the way for a careful dissection of the molecular mechanisms involved in regulating this process. A more complete understanding of the mechanisms involved in the switch process could reveal new targets for drug development that would represent a major step forward in the management of bipolar disorder patients.

A Focus on Dopamine

The CAs, DA and NE, have been at the center of efforts to describe the pathophysiology of mood disorders since the 1960s (Schildkraut, 1965), and that focus has continued to the present (e.g., Ashok et al., 2017). With respect to bipolar disorder, DA and, to a lesser extent, NE have been proposed to contribute to mania, while cholinergic activity is thought to underlie depression (van Enkhuizen et al., 2015). A major component that is missing from this formulation is the mechanism that directs the switching process from one mood state to another of opposite polarity.

DAergic signaling pathways have been a special focus of preclinical research in laboratories interested in developing drugs to treat bipolar disorder and depression. In this section, we will begin with a look at acute and chronic amphetamine models of mania-like behavior, and then move to more targeted strategies for disruption of DA signaling, including pharmacological and genetic manipulations of the DA transporter (DAT).

Speed it up. Early efforts to model bipolar mania were focused on producing laboratory animals that reliably displayed mania-like behaviors. Given that a key symptom of mania in humans is excessive locomotion, some laboratories produced mania-like behavior in laboratory animals by peripheral administration of amphetamine. The use of amphetamine was also consistent with the hypothesis that bipolar mania involved a disruption of DAergic signaling in brain. In one early experiment, Davies et al. (1974) administered a combination of d-amphetamine and chlordiazepoxide to laboratory mice and observed a significant increase in head dips in a hole board test and activity in a Y-maze. The hyperactivity following administration of the drug mixture tended to occur only in a novel environment. The behavioral effects of the drug combination were blocked by pretreatment with lithium, a mood stabilizer, or α-methyl-p-tyrosine, an inhibitor of tyrosine hydroxylase, the rate-limiting step in the synthesis of CAs. The effects of lithium on the activity of mice was most evident when animals were hyperactive based upon a combination of drug administration, prior test experience, and test environment.

Cappeliez and Moore (1990) extended these findings by subjecting laboratory rats to chronic daily doses of lithium for 21 days. From days 7–16, rats also received daily injections of d-amphetamine (3.0 mg/kg) or saline, and from days 17–21, d-amphetamine was withheld. Administration of d-amphetamine resulted in significant increases in locomotor activity that were not blocked by co-administration of lithium. Locomotor activity returned to control levels after the cessation of d-amphetamine and was unaffected by lithium. The authors concluded that amphetamine and lithium act on different neurotransmitter systems to affect locomotor activity.

In an indirect approach, Rezin et al. (2014) studied the effects of acute versus chronic i.p. administration of fenproporex, a commonly used anorectic agent, which is rapidly converted into amphetamine in vivo. Fenproporex stimulated an increase in locomotor activity in laboratory rats that was prevented or reversed by administration of the mood stabilizers lithium or valproate. These investigators presented their results in the context of a new animal model for mania-like behavior.

Pathak et al. (2015) followed a sensitization protocol by administration of d-amphetamine (1.8 mg/kg, s.c.) to CD-1 mice each day for 5 consecutive days, while controls received vehicle injections. From days 6–31 of withdrawal from d-amphetamine, both groups of mice were evaluated on a battery of behavioral tests. Locomotor activity levels were similar in mice of the two groups. However, relative to vehicle-injected controls, mice that received d-amphetamine on days 1–5 exhibited long-lasting locomotor hyperactivity following either acute re-straint stress for 30 minutes (day 17 of withdrawal) or administration of a low chal-lenge dose of d-amphetamine (1.0 mg/kg, s.c.) (days 4–31 of withdrawal). In both instances, the locomotor hyperactivity was greatly attenuated by treatment with the mood-stabilizers lithium or quetiapine. Amphetamine-treated mice also dis-played significant reductions in sucrose preference from days 7–17 of withdrawal. Amphetamine-treated mice were less adept at nest building, an ongoing ethologic-ally relevant activity of mice. When these experiments were repeated in C57BL/6J mice, the effects of amphetamine sensitization were blunted relative to CD-1 mice.

These authors provided a detailed justification for the value of the amphet-amine sensitization protocol as a model for bipolar disorder. Under basal conditions, amphetamine-sensitized mice displayed a depression-like pheno-type based upon a reduced preference for a sucrose solution and the decrease in the normal daily maintenance activity of nest building. When presented with a challenge dose of amphetamine or when exposed to acute restraint stress, the sensitized mice displayed more of a mania-like phenotype, with increased lo-comotor activity levels. In addition, these findings varied across two different inbred strains of mice, underscoring the importance of genotype in the sensiti-zation model. Finally, these results are consistent with a critical role for DA sig-naling in the sensitization model and in bipolar disorder.

Don't be so sensitive. Dr. Seymour Antelman and his colleagues at the University of Pittsburgh School of Medicine worked for more than two decades on a most unusual phenomenon. They reported that a single exposure to any of a variety of drugs or non-drug stressors led to physiological and behavioral effects that grew over time on a scale of weeks to months. They termed this phenom-enon *time-dependent sensitization* (TDS) (Antelman et al., 2000).

TDS demonstrates that exposure to a stressor (including some drugs) can have a delayed impact when an animal is exposed to another stressor or drug at some point in the future. Some of these delayed effects of stressors do not result in sensitization of the response, but rather a decrease in the later physiological or behavioral response. Thus, *time-dependent modulation* might have been a more appropriate term than TDS.

A critical aspect of TDS is the interchangeability of drugs and stressors in producing a sensitized (or decremented) response. In a landmark paper, Antelman et al. (1980) demonstrated that daily exposure of laboratory rats to the mild stress of tail pinch sensitized them to the behavioral effects of a later dose of amphetamine. Similarly, a single dose of amphetamine led to an amplification of tail pinch–induced behaviors up to 30 days after the single drug injection. That tail pinch and amphetamine shared the ability to enhance later responses suggested that these two treatments shared a common set of neural and endocrine effects. In addition, the findings opened the way for a view of drugs as a special category of stressors (Antelman et al., 1992, 2000).

Of special relevance to modeling bipolar disorder was their observation that repeated exposure of laboratory animals to drugs or stressors resulted in an oscillation or cycling of their effects on several neurochemical and physiological systems (Antelman & Caggiula, 1996; Antelman et al., 1995, 1998; Caggiula et al., 1996). Antelman and his colleagues proposed that these oscillations resulted from over-stimulation of a system, especially one that was already highly sensitized. Briefly, the model stated that sensitization, which results from repeated exposure to drugs (e.g., amphetamine or cocaine, drugs that impact brain DA neurons) or environmental stressors, increases as long as the relevant physiological or neural systems are within their normal functional range. However, if the extremes of those functional ranges are approached or if the prior stress history or genotype of the animal places these systems near that functional limit, then countervailing homeostatic processes are activated and an oscillatory pattern of responsiveness to subsequent exposures ensues, such that cycling follows prior sensitization (Antelman & Caggiula, 1996). Although this model emphasizes the condition in which extreme sensitization leads to oscillations, it does not require that all oscillatory processes must be preceded by sensitization. Rather, it leaves open the possibility that other factors, including risk genes or prior history with stressors, may also promote the development of oscillatory patterns in neural systems and behavior, including those relevant to bipolar disorder.

This body of research on TDS and oscillatory processes could enrich the design and interpretation of amphetamine sensitization models of mania-like behavior. In addition, the model proposed by Antelman et al. (1998), which included supporting data and reversibility of in vitro neurochemical effects and in vivo behavioral effects by lithium, still holds considerable potential for expanding the validity of other animal models of bipolar disorder.

Down but not out. Using a variety of approaches to manipulate DAergic signaling, the laboratories of Professors Mark A. Geyer and Jared W. Young of the Department of Psychiatry at the University of California, San Diego, have been at the forefront of efforts to translate these strategies into valid mouse models of bipolar mania. I will highlight their work and the works of others in the following sections.

What's DAT? The DAT protein has been a molecular target of interest for a number of psychiatric disorders, including schizophrenia, attention deficit hyperactivity disorder, and bipolar disorder (Logan & McClung, 2016; Salatino-Oliveira et al., 2018; Sharma et al., 2016). Although early efforts to generate DAT$^{(-/-)}$ KO mice were successful (Gainetdinov et al., 1999), these animals exhibited many extreme physiological alterations, including impaired growth rates due to pituitary hypoplasia, that made them less than ideal as animal models for psychiatric disorders. An alternative approach to disrupt DAT function was to produce a knockdown (DAT-KD) model, where DAT expression in brain was reduced by approximately 90% compared to WT controls (Zhuang et al., 2001). DAT-KD mice did not differ from WT controls in growth rates, mortality rates, lactation, or gross anatomy of the pituitary.

Experiments with striatal slices maintained in vitro in a recording chamber revealed that DA release following electrical stimulation was cleared at a much slower rate in DAT-KD mice compared to WT controls. However, the amount of DA released by DAT-KD striatal slices was approximately 25% of WT levels, probably because of inefficient recycling of released DA back into presynaptic vesicles. Tissue content of DA was reduced by 55%, and extracellular levels of DA in the striatum were 70% higher in DAT-KD mice compared to WT controls.

Several behavioral changes were noted in DAT-KD mice. They had normal levels of activity in their home cages, but displayed hyperactivity and increased rearing in a 3-hour test in an open field arena. In addition, DAT-KD mice habituated more slowly to a prolonged open field test. DAT-KD mice also exhibited greater levels of activity when a novel object was placed in the center of the open field arena. Finally, both the indirect DA receptor agonist amphetamine and the direct-acting DA agonists apomorphine and quinpirole inhibited locomotor activity in DAT-KD mice (Zhuang et al., 2001).

In a subsequent report, behavioral differences relevant to bipolar disorder were further explored in DAT-KD and WT mice (Ralph-Williams et al., 2003). DAT-KD mice were hyperactive and displayed greater perseverative motor patterns in an open field arena compared to WT controls. Somewhat surprisingly, measures of PPI and habituation of the acoustic startle response were similar in mice of the two strains. In contrast, DAT KO mice exhibited significant deficits in PPI relative to WT controls (Powell et al., 2008). Startle magnitude was greater in DAT-KD mice in one experiment but was similar to WT mice in a replication. Acute administration of the mood stabilizer valproate (100 mg/kg, i.p.) significantly reduced the hyperactivity and perseverative locomotor behavior of DAT-KD mice but had no effect on behaviors of WT controls.

Additional studies have expanded the range of behavioral alterations observed in DAT-KD mice. In a modification of the Iowa Gambling Task that was tailored to laboratory mice, DAT-KD mice were characterized by increased risk-taking behavior relative to WT controls, a finding that was similar to the riskier choices made by manic patients in the same task. In addition, DAT-KD mice displayed a behavioral profile in the Behavioral Pattern Monitor that matched well with a similar set of measures in bipolar patients (Kwiatkowski et al., 2019; van Enkhuizen et al., 2014; Young et al., 2011). DAT-KD mice also exhibited increased levels of motivation and reward-seeking, as well as enhanced reversal learning (Milienne-Petiot et al., 2017).

Seasonal changes. One clinical observation that opens a window onto an aspect of the process of switching from mania to depression (or vice versa) in bipolar patients relates to seasonal effects on mood states. Manic states are more likely to occur in the spring and early summer with increasing day length, while depressive episodes are more likely to occur in fall and winter as day length shortens (Wang & Chen, 2013). In addition, bipolar patients have reduced expression of DAT, and this alteration in DAergic signaling may render these patients more susceptible to seasonal changes in photoperiod.

Based upon these clinical findings, Young et al. (2018) examined seasonal extremes of light-dark cycles on behavioral and neural measures of WT mice and DAT$^{(+/-)}$ heterozygous (DAT-HZ) mice that expressed ~50% of WT levels of DAT protein. Prior to training and behavioral testing, all mice were maintained for at least 2 weeks on one of the following three photoperiods: long-active (LA, 5:19 light-dark cycle), short-active (SA, 19:5 light-dark cycle), or control (NA, 12:12 light-dark cycle). The time of lights-on for the three chambers was adjusted such that they shared a 5-hour period of darkness each day when behavioral testing occurred.

WT and DAT-HZ mice housed in an SA photoperiod exhibited increased immobility in the forced swim test, with the depression-relevant effect being much greater in DAT-HZ mice. In an elevated plus-maze (EPM), WT and DAT-HZ mice housed in an LA photoperiod displayed more frequent open-arm entries, and the mania-relevant effect was much greater in DAT-HZ mice. In addition, DAT-HZ mice but not WT mice displayed acceleration of collection of rewards under LA conditions. Relative to an NA photoperiod, DAT-HZ mice in LA conditions were more sensitive to rewards, while in SA conditions they were more sensitive to punishment and loss in a probabilistic learning task and a progressive ratio breakpoint response task.

Photoperiod also affected the balance between tyrosine hydroxylase (TH)-positive and somatostatin-positive neurons in the hypothalamic PVN. Compared to the NA photoperiod, WT and DAT-HZ mice had similar magnitude reductions in TH-positive cells but similar magnitude increases in somatostatin-positive cells when mice were housed in an SA photoperiod. The opposite was true for the LA photoperiod, with increases in TH-positive cells and decreases in somatostatin-positive cells. DAT mRNA levels increased substantially in WT mice under an LA photoperiod. In contrast, DAT mRNA levels were unaffected by photoperiod in DAT-HZ mice (refer to Table 10.1).

This series of experiments represents a major advance in modeling bipolar disorder in laboratory animals. These findings revealed that variations in photoperiod can drive changes in neurotransmitter phenotype in the PVN as well as several behavioral endpoints that have great relevance to bipolar disorder. However, one can certainly find things to criticize regarding the design of the

Table 10.1 Summary of Main Photoperiod-Induced Changes in Behavior and Neurochemistry of Wild-Type (WT) Control Mice and Mice Heterozygous (HZ) for the Dopamine Transporter (DAT$^{(+/-)}$)

Behavioral Domains	Dependent Measures	WT Control		DAT HZ	
Photoperiod		SA	LA	SA	LA
Depression-relevant	Forced swim test immobility	↑	0	↑↑	0
Mania-relevant	EPM open arm entries	0	↑	0	↑↑
Reward learning	PLT accuracy	0	0	↓↓	0
Punishment sensitivity	PLT time-out perseveration	0	0	↑↑	0
	PLT target lose shift	0	0	↑↑	0
Reward sensitivity	Reward collection latency	0	0	0	↓↓
Neurochemical Measures					
TH-positive cells in the PVN		↓↓	↑↑	↓↓	↑↑
STN-positive cells in the PVN		↑↑	↓↓	↑↑	↓↓
Relative DAT mRNA levels	DAT-WT (NA = 1.0)	0.5	5.5		
in the HYP (estimated)	DAT-HZ (NA = 2.0)			2.5	2.4

Results are summarized from the report by Young et al. (2018).

Abbreviations: SA: short-active photoperiod with 19:5 light-dark cycle; LA: long-active photoperiod with 5-19 light:dark cycle; EPM: elevated plus-maze; PLT: probabilistic learning task; TH: tyrosine hydroxylase; PVN: paraventricular nucleus of the hypothalamus; STN: somatostatin; HYP: hypothalamus; NA: normal photoperiod with 12:12 light-dark cycle.

study. Mice were only maintained for 2 weeks in a given photoperiod, and longer periods of acclimation may have exerted more dramatic effects on the DAT-HZ mice. In addition, future experiments may address the issue of dynamically changing day length (increasing or decreasing in the spring and fall, respectively, in the Northern Hemisphere) that is often mentioned by bipolar patients as a challenge to regulation of mood. Finally, although the authors of this article associated the 5:19 light-dark LA photoperiods to increased summertime activity, in fact, this is a photoperiod characteristic of winter seasons and not summer seasons. The reverse is true for the 19:5 light-dark SA photoperiod, which is characteristic of summer seasons and not winter seasons. Finally, would neurotransmitter phenotype and behavioral measures have changed in the expected directions if mice maintained in an LA photoperiod were switched to an SA photoperiod, and vice versa? Such an additional experiment would have made the findings regarding seasonality-specific mood regulation even more compelling. At the very least, the interpretation of these findings should be reassessed given these and other criticisms (Rosenthal & McCarty, 2019).

Summary. The experimental approaches taken to manipulate brain DAergic signaling described in the preceding—acute versus chronic administration of amphetamine, time-dependent sensitization to the effects of amphetamine, and knockdown of DAT—all point to a critical role for DA in the regulation of bipolar mania. Given the additional indications that DA signaling may be a component of the switching process from mania to depression during seasonal changes, these models hold great promise for novel approaches to targeted drug therapies.

The Sodium Hypothesis

Singh (1970) was one of the first to suggest that a fundamental disturbance in regulation of sodium metabolism across neuronal membranes was an underlying feature of affective disorders, including bipolar disorder. The defect in sodium metabolism in bipolar disorder was later attributed by El-Mallakh (1983) to the sodium, potassium-activated adenosine triphosphatase (Na,K-ATPase) pump, and he argued that this membrane defect could explain the manic as well as the depressive episodes that characterize bipolar disorder. Additional studies documented that patients who were in a manic phase or a bipolar depressive phase exhibited increases in intracellular levels of Na^+ and Ca^{++} and decreases in Na,K-ATPase activity as measured in erythrocytes (Pedroso et al., 2018).

The ouabain model. Ouabain is a plant-derived toxin that was once used to coat the tips of poisoned arrows. It is a cardiac glycoside, a potent inhibitor of the Na,K-ATPase pump, and is lethal in high doses. Because ouabain is highly lipophobic, the drug must be administered directly into brain to induce mania-like behaviors (Herman et al., 2007). El-Mallakh et al. (1995) first reported on their attempts to develop an animal model of mania by acute administration of ouabain into the lateral cerebral ventricle of laboratory rats. The highest sublethal dose of ouabain (5 μl of a 1.0 mM solution) resulted in significant increases in locomotor activity that persisted for up to 30 minutes. Yu et al. (2010) expanded upon this experimental paradigm and reported that i.c.v. administration of higher doses of ouabain (0.5 and 1.0 mM) to laboratory rats resulted in significant increases in locomotor activity that persisted for up to 8 hours.

Ouabain-induced hyperactivity in laboratory rats was blocked by chronic pretreatment with lithium or valproate. In addition, both mood stabilizers prevented in large part ouabain-induced increases in oxidative stress levels and activation of apoptotic signaling pathways in neurons and glial cells (Valvassori et al., 2015). This same research group expanded their focus by examining alterations in brain glycogen synthase kinase-3β (GSK-3β) in the ouabain model of mania. GSK-3β is of special significance to the etiology of bipolar disorder because lithium acts as a selective inhibitor of GSK-3β as well as other enzymes. In addition, the effects of lithium, valproate, and an inhibitor of GSK-3β (AR-A014418) on hyperactivity were examined. Ank and other enzymes catalyze the phosphorylation of GSK-3β, which reduces its activity. Administration of lithium or valproate blocked the increased open field activity, rearing, sniffing, and grooming episodes associated with i.c.v. administration of ouabain. In addition, both of these mood stabilizers reversed the significant ouabain-induced decreases in phosphorylation of GSK-3β in the frontal cortex and hippocampus. Lastly, AR-A014418 blocked the increased levels of locomotor activity and rearing in the open field in ouabain-treated rats. These investigators suggested that the manic-like effects of ouabain are mediated in part by the GSK-3β signaling pathway and that lithium and valproate reverse the effects of ouabain by increasing phosphorylation of GSK-3β (Valvassori et al., 2017).

To expand beyond simple measures of locomotor activity following administration of ouabain, Amodeo et al. (2017) investigated changes in learning and memory and cognitive flexibility in the ouabain model of mania, as these behaviors are also characteristic of bipolar disorder. Compared to control rats that received i.c.v. injections of artificial CSF, rats that received ouabain (5 μl of a 1.0 mM solution, i.c.v.) had comparable scores for spontaneous alternation in a Y-maze, although ouabain-treated rats had significantly more arm entries, reflecting increased locomotion. However, i.c.v. administration of ouabain resulted in impairments in reversal learning in a spatial discrimination task that were attributable to an inability to maintain a new choice pattern and decreased sensitivity to negative feedback during the initial phases of reversal learning. These findings expand upon the behavioral changes that occurred following i.c.v.

administration of ouabain to laboratory rats and enhance the value of this model in the study of bipolar mania.

The ouabain model of mania comports well with changes in the Na,K-ATPase pump as reported in bipolar patients. In addition, mania-like behaviors are normalized by treatment of animals with lithium or valproate. To date, laboratory rats have been the preferred species as i.c.v. injections are more easily accomplished in this species than in laboratory mice. Unfortunately, a complete behavioral phenotype of the ouabain model has not yet been completed.

The Myshkin mouse. There is an interesting story behind the generation of Myshkin mice in the laboratory of Professor John C. Roder (1950–2018) at the University of Toronto. Clapcote et al. (2009) employed in vivo mutagenesis with N-nitroso-N-ethylurea to generate a mutant mouse referred to as Myshkin (Myk), which was characterized in heterozygotes (Myk$^{(-/+)}$) by neuronal hyperexcitability and epileptic seizures, but in homozygotes (Myk$^{(-/-)}$) death occurred soon after birth. Myshkin was selected as the name for the mutant mouse strain for two reasons: Myshkin was a character who suffered from epilepsy in Dostoevsky's novel The Idiot. In addition, "Mysh" is derived from the Russian word for mouse. The Myshkin allele contained a point mutation in the Na$^+$,K$^+$-ATPase α3-isoform that inactivated this enzyme and was totally responsible for the neuronal hyper-excitability and epileptic seizures observed in these mice. The epilepsy and neuronal hyper-excitability in Myk mice could be prevented by delivery of additional copies of the wild-type Na,K-ATPase α3-isoform and its promoter by transgenesis using a bacterial artificial chromosome.

Serendipitously, Myk mice were observed to display a manic-like behavioral phenotype that could be reversed by treatment with lithium or valproate or by transgenic expression of a functional Na,K-ATPase α3-isoform. Compared to wild-type controls, the pattern of manic-like behaviors included: increased exploration of a novel object, increased frequency of nose pokes in a hole board test, increased activity in an open field test with a chaotic pattern of ambulation and lack of habituation to repeated testing, increased sensitivity to a low dose of amphetamine (0.5 mg/kg) in an open field test, decreased REM and non-REM sleep during the light phase of a 24-hour photoperiod, an extended endogenous circadian period of 25 hours in constant darkness, reduced anxiety-like behaviors in the EPM and light-dark box, increased consumption of and preference for a sucrose solution, increased activity in a forced swim test, and deficits in PPI and habituation of the acoustic startle response (Kirshenbaum et al., 2011).

Myk mice also displayed increased Ca^{++} signaling in cultured cortical neurons and phospho-activation of extracellular signal-regulated kinase (ERK) and protein kinase B (Akt) in the hippocampus. Acute administration of an inhibitor of ERK (SL327) that had no effect of locomotor activity in wild-type mice reduced total activity of Myk mice in the open field, reduced anxiety-like behavior in the EPM, and reduced head pokes in a hole board test. Finally, chronic administration of rostafuroxin, a compound that displaces endogenous ouabain from Na,K-ATPase, also reversed some of the manic-like behaviors of Myk mice. These results point to the Na,K-ATPase α3 isoform, its physiological regulators, and downstream signal transduction pathways as critical links in the control of mania-like behaviors and as possible targets for novel therapeutics (Kirshenbaum et al., 2011).

In a follow-up experiment, Kirshenbaum et al. (2012) examined the effects of agrin in Myk mice. Agrin is a proteoglycan that appears to act as a regulator of synapses and an inhibitor of Na,K-ATPase α3 activity. Myk$^{(+/-)}$ mice were crossed with agrin heterozygous knock-out mice (Agrn$^{(-/+)}$) to produce mice that had a null allele that affected all isoforms of agrin (Myk/+/Agrn). Myk/+/Agrn mice did not display the pattern of mania-like behaviors that were characteristic of Myk mice. In Myk mice, suppression of agrin increased brain Na,K-ATPase activity by 11% ± 4%, but had no effect on Na,K-ATPase activity in wild-type mice.

Two novel treatments were explored for their effects on mania-like behaviors in Myk mice. Melatonin and aerobic exercise have shown promising effects as potential mood stabilizers in studies with bipolar disorder patients. In Myk mice and wild-type controls, melatonin (~2 mg/kg/day) was included in the drinking water for 21 days prior to behavioral testing. Other groups of Myk and wild-type mice had access to a running wheel in their home cages for 42 days prior to behavioral testing. Both treatments reduced mania-like behaviors in Myk mice, but had no effect of behaviors of wild-type mice (Kirshenbaum et al., 2014).

The Myk mouse shows considerable promise as an animal model of mania. The extensive phenotyping of these mice provided convincing evidence for a consistent pattern of behavioral changes that matched well with the behavioral profile of bipolar disorder patients during a manic episode. Several molecular targets relating to the neuron-specific Na,K-ATPase-α3 isoform have been identified and may hold promise in the development of new therapies for the treatment of manic episodes.

Mouse Models of Mania

Black Swiss mice. All outbred Black Swiss mice are not created equal. Black Swiss mice obtained from Taconic Biosciences displayed increased preference for saccharin solutions, reduced immobility in the forced swim test, and elevated levels of locomotor activity compared to mice obtained from Charles River. In addition, lithium reduced the elevated locomotor activity of Taconic mice but not Charles River mice (Juetten & Einat, 2012). All studies that are discussed in the following that employed Black Swiss mice had Taconic as the supplier.

In comparisons of several strains of mice, Black Swiss mice have stood out because they exhibit mania-like behaviors, including increased levels of reward-seeking, risk-taking, and aggression. In addition, Black Swiss mice were also more sensitive to the effects of amphetamine. In a comparison of four strains of mice (Black Swiss, C57BL/6, CBA/J, and A/J), Flaisher-Grinberg and Einat (2010) reported that Black Swiss mice were the most aggressive strain in a resident-intruder test, had dramatically lower times spent immobile in a forced swim test, exhibited a strong preference for a saccharin solution, spent more time in the light portion of a light-dark box, were more active, and had greater levels of activity following acute administration of amphetamine (1.0 mg/kg, i.p.). Further experiments with Black Swiss mice revealed that lithium and valproate significantly reduced some mania-like behaviors (e.g., saccharin preference and amphetamine-induced hyperactivity) but not others (spontaneous activity, resident-intruder aggression, behavior in a light-dark box). In contrast, the antidepressant, imipramine, was without effect on any of the normally occurring mania-like behaviors in mice of this strain.

Sánchez-Blázquez et al. (2018) examined the role of sigma receptors type 1 (σ1Rs) in the Black Swiss model of mania. The σ1R is a chaperone that resides at the interface between the endoplasmic reticulum (ER) and mitochondria and plays a role in Ca^{++} signaling and modulation of various ion channels, neurotransmitter receptors, and kinases (Kourrich et al., 2012). Evidence suggests that σ1Rs modulate NMDA receptors, which are involved in the increased locomotor activity of animal models of mania. Acute administration of amphetamine (2.0 mg/kg, i.p.) resulted in a significant increase in locomotor activity in Black Swiss mice that was blocked by i.c.v. injection of a GSK-3β inhibitor or each of three different σ1R antagonists. Preference of Black Swiss mice for a sucrose solution was blocked by an i.p. injection of valproate or an i.c.v. injection of any one of several σ1R antagonists. In the forced swim test, Black Swiss mice typically have very low immobility times. These low immobility times were increased substantially when mice received an i.p. injection of valproate or an i.c.v. injection of either a GSK-3β inhibitor or a σ1R antagonist. Importantly, these mood stabilizers did not have significant effects of the behavior of Black Swiss mice from Charles River, which served as a control group in these studies.

In a related study, Garzón-Niño et al. (2017) reported that total levels of GSK-3β levels in frontal cortex were similar between Black Swiss mice from Taconic and Charles River, whereas Akt-mediated inhibitory phosphorylation of GSK-3β at serine 9 was decreased in Black Swiss mice from Taconic. Given that activating phosphorylation of GSK-3β at tyrosine 216 predominated over inhibitory phosphorylation at serine 9 for Black Swiss mice from Taconic, it is likely that functional GSK-3β activity was higher than in Black Swiss controls from Charles River.

The Madison (MSN) strain. MSN inbred mice were derived from outbred hsd:ICR mice for an experiment on exercise physiology in the 1990s. At the time of this initial experiment, the mice were estimated to be >90% inbred (Scotti et al., 2011). In this initial characterization, MSN male mice displayed a manic-like phenotype compared to control mice, with home cage locomotor hyperactivity during the light and dark phases of the light-dark cycle, decreased immobility in the forced swim test, reduced daytime sleeping, and increased frequency of mounting a receptive female. Chronic administration of olanzapine (1.0 mg/kg/day), a first-line treatment for acute mania, and lithium (0.2%–0.4% in food), a mood stabilizer, significantly decreased home cage levels of locomotor activity. This initial study provided promising results and supported further experiments on the utility of the MSN strain as a mouse model for mania-like behavior.

In a follow-up experiment from the same laboratory, Saul et al. (2012) replicated the finding of home cage hyperactivity in another generation of MSN mice relative to ICR control mice. They then performed a gene expression microarray experiment by comparing samples of the hippocampus from MSN and ICR mice. Their results revealed dysregulation of multiple transcripts with human orthologs that have been previously linked with bipolar disorder and other psychiatric disorders. These genes included *Epor, Smarca4, Cmklr1, Cat, Tac1, Npsr1, Fhit*, and *P2rx7*. The results for seven of the genes from the microarray experiment were confirmed with reverse transcriptase-quantitative polymerase chain reaction (RT-qPCR). For each gene, the magnitude of dysregulation and the direction of change matched well with the microarray data. Using a functional network analysis, these investigators reported alterations in a gene system involved in chromatin packaging, a finding that matches well with recent data from patients with bipolar disorder. Their findings were consistent with MSN mice serving as a polygenic model for the manic pole of bipolar disorder, and capturing some of the genetic complexity of this disorder.

To characterize further the locomotor hyperactivity of MSN mice, Saul et al. (2013) reported that home cage locomotor activity was significantly higher in female compared to male MSN mice. Further, this sex difference in activity was not a result of activity changes over the course of the estrus cycle. Locomotor hyperactivity was evident in MSN mice as early as PND 28. Continuous monitoring of home cage activity levels for 1 month revealed that MSN mice were consistently hyperactive relative to ISR control mice. In addition, there was no evidence of a cycling from hyperactivity to normal or low activity levels over the course of the recording period. MSN mice tended to wake up earlier and go to sleep earlier than ICR controls. When housed in an 18:6 light:dark photoperiod, MSN mice exhibited increases in locomotor hyperactivity relative to 12:12 and 6:18 light-dark photoperiods. Control ICR mice had stable levels of activity across all three light-dark photoperiods, and their activity levels were significantly lower in each of the photoperiods compared to MSN mice. These results suggest that MSN mice are sensitive to seasonal changes in photoperiod, which is a characteristic shared in common with many bipolar patients.

To explore further the genetic underpinnings of mania-like behavior in MSC mice, Saul et al. (2018) examined differences in naturally occurring candidate genetic variants using whole exome re-sequencing on a small sample of animals. These results were confirmed in a larger population with genotyping. Re-sequencing identified 447 structural variants that were mostly fixed in MSN mice compared to control mice. They distilled their results down to 11 nonsynonymous variants in MSN mice that appeared to alter protein function. The allelic frequencies for 6 of these variants were associated with locomotor hyperactivity in the MSN strain. The variants included *Npas2, Cp, Polr3c, Smarca4, Trpv1*, and *Slc5a7* genes, and many of the proteins coded by these genes are in pathways implicated in human bipolar disorders. When combined, variants in *Smarca4* and *Polr3c* accounted for more than 40% of the variance in locomotor behavior in the Hsd:ICR founder strain. These results support the construct validity of the MSN strain as a model for bipolar disorder, and implicate altered nucleosome structure and transcriptional regulation as important molecular pathways underpinning mania-like behavior in this genetic model of mania-like behavior.

A possibility for the future suggested by these investigators would involve using CRISPR technology to generate transgenic mice bearing each of these gene variants, by creating a knockin of each variant identified in the MSN strain to an unrelated mouse strain such as the C57BL/6J. Such an experimental approach would allow for behavioral characterization of each variant as well as measurement of protein function using assays specific to each gene. The looming challenge would be to put all of the variants together in a single transgenic strain as the whole (behavioral phenotype) may be greater than the sum of the six individual variants.

In summary, the MSN strain shows considerable promise as an animal model for the manic component of bipolar disorder. Unfortunately, this strain is only available at the University of Wisconsin, Madison, and other laboratories have not yet replicated and extended the findings reported from Professor Stephen Gammie's laboratory.

Tick-Tock

On the *Clock*. Given the well-described circadian and seasonal disruptions that are characteristic of bipolar disorder, several laboratories have explored the role of genes involved in circadian time-keeping on mania-like behavior (McClung,

2013). The *Clock* gene (circadian locomotor output cycles kaput) has been critical to this effort. It was originally identified as a single locus, semi-dominant autosomal mutation by treating C57BL/6J male mice with N-ethyl-N-nitrosourea, then mating them with untreated C57BL/6J females, and screening their offspring for disruptions in circadian rhythms (Vitaterna et al., 1994). The *Clock* gene was later cloned, and the mutation was identified as a deletion of exon 19, which prevents transcriptional activation by the CLOCK protein (King et al., 1997).

The basic molecular oscillator within the hypothalamic suprachiasmatic nuclei (SCN) is composed of interconnected negative feedback loops that consist of transcription factors regulating their own expression over a period of approximately 24 hours. CLOCK protein binds to brain and muscle ARNT-like protein 1 (BMAL1). The resulting heterodimer then regulates the expression of the *period* (*Per*) and *cryptochrome* (*Cry*) genes, which bind together as proteins, enter the nucleus, and inhibit further transcription of CLOCK and BMAL1. Further regulation is provided by a feedback loop involving D-box binding protein, as well as post-translational mechanisms. These molecular oscillators are further entrained by light via the retinohypothalamic tract (Chen et al., 2018).

Roybal et al. (2007) reported that *Clock* mutant mice exhibited a behavioral and neurobiological phenotype that was consistent with the key features of bipolar mania in humans. Compared to wild-type controls, *Clock* mutant mice displayed less anxiety-like behavior in an EPM, during an open field test, or when confronted with a cracker in a novel or a stressful test environment. *Clock* mutant mice also displayed higher levels of locomotor activity as well as reductions in all stages of sleep. In the forced swim test, *Clock* mutant mice spent significantly less time immobile. When tested in a learned helplessness paradigm, *Clock* mutant mice made fewer escape failures than wild-type mice. *Clock* mutant mice also exhibited an increased preference for a sucrose solution and were more sensitive to the rewarding effects of self-stimulation of the medial forebrain bundle. In addition, mutant mice were also more sensitive to the rewarding effects of cocaine. Taken together, these striking features of the phenotype of *Clock* mutant mice matched well with the characteristics of the manic state in bipolar disorder patients.

Most of the behavioral changes observed in *Clock* mutant mice were reversed by chronic administration of a low dose of lithium (600 mg/liter in drinking water for 10 days), a commonly employed mood stabilizer in bipolar disorder patients. In addition, these investigators employed a viral vector to deliver a functional *Clock* gene to the ventral tegmental area (VTA) of mutant mice. The VTA is a brain region rich in DAergic neurons that is known to play a critical role in brain reward mechanisms, including those associated with drugs of abuse. Placement of a functional *Clock* gene into the VTA of mutant mice reduced their locomotor hyperactivity to near-normal levels and altered their behavior on an EPM to match well with behaviors of wild-type mice. These important findings support the use of *Clock* mutant mice as an animal model of mania-like behavior and suggest a critical role for the *Clock* gene as a regulator of behavior through its effects on DAergic neurons in the VTA (Roybal et al., 2007).

In a follow-up experiment from this same laboratory, Mukherjee et al. (2010) employed RNA interference to effect a knockdown (KD) of *Clock* that was limited to the VTA. *Clock* KD mice exhibited increased locomotor activity over a 2-hour period after placement in a novel environment, reduced home cage locomotor activity over a 24-hour period, a decrease in the circadian period of approximately 15 minutes, and reduced anxiety-like behaviors across three different behavioral tasks. These behavioral changes were consistent with a mania-like phenotype. In contrast, *Clock* KD mice also displayed behaviors consistent with a depression-like phenotype, including increased immobility in the forced swim test and increased latency to escape and a greater number of escape errors in a learned helplessness task. *Clock* KD mice also exhibited increased firing rates of DAergic neurons in the VTA that expressed the inhibitor gene. This mixture of depression-like and mania-like behaviors resembled the mixed features in bipolar patients, as illustrated in Figure 10.1.

To assess *Clock*-related behavioral alterations in mice using tasks that have translational relevance to patients with bipolar disorder, Van Enkhuizen et al. (2013) employed measures of exploratory behavior in a behavior pattern monitor and sensory motor gating of the acoustic startle response, both of which have been studied in patients with bipolar disorder (Henry et al., 2010; Young et al., 2007). In addition, they assessed preference for a 1.0% saccharin solution and monitored circadian rhythms in running wheel activity. Their results indicated that *Clock* mutant mice displayed hyperactivity and increased specific exploration of the test chamber, and reduced sensorimotor gating of the acoustic startle response. In addition, *Clock* mutant mice exhibited a greater preference for a 1.0% saccharin solution and a greater sensitivity to alterations in photoperiod compared to wild-type controls.

Kristensen et al. (2018) conducted a systematic review of 22 published studies (of a total of 910 publications that were screened) relating to the behavior of *Clock* mutant mice. As presented in the preceding, their results consistently demonstrated a behavioral phenotype of *Clock* mutant mice that included hyperactivity, decreased anxiety-like behaviors, decreased depression-like behaviors, and increased preference for rewarding stimuli (e.g., sucrose, saccharin, cocaine, and intracranial self-stimulation). In addition, *Clock* mutant mice exhibited changes in activity patterns within a 24-hour period (a more manic-like phenotype during the day, followed by closer to normal levels of activity at night). Chronic administration of lithium, a drug with well-established mood-stabilizing effects in patients with bipolar disorder, reversed a majority of the mania-like traits of *Clock* mutant mice. These investigators concluded that this putative model of mania-like behavior had significant face validity as an animal model for mania. However, the predictive validity of this model is limited by the dependence on experiments with lithium. An important issue to address in future studies is the inclusion of other mood-stabilizing drugs, including valproate, lamotrigine, and carbamazepine to strengthen the predictive validity of this animal model of mania-like behavior.

Into D-box. A major challenge to researchers involved in developing animal models of bipolar disorder has been the rapid cycling of patients from mania to depression, as was described for Edward at the beginning of this chapter. One of the first animal models to capture a stress-induced switch from a depressive-like state to a manic-like state was presented by Le-Niculescu et al. (2008), using mice with a homozygous deletion of the clock gene, D-box binding protein (DBP). DBP mice were originally derived on a 129/ola genetic background at the University of Geneva, but were re-derived on a C57BL/6 background at the University of California, San Diego. This mixed genetic background made it less likely that any experimental results were unique to a particular mouse strain that served as the background and were not more broadly generalizable.

Male and female $DBP^{+/-}$ mice were bred to produced mixed litters of $DBP^{(+/+)}$, $DBP^{(+/-)}$, and $DBP^{(-/-)}$ pups. All experiments involved studies with $DBP^{+/+}$ (WT) and $DBP^{(-/-)}$ (KO) mice. Compared to WT mice, DBP KO mice had reduced levels of locomotor activity but comparable levels of stereotyped behavior under basal conditions. Following a challenge dose of methamphetamine (10.0 mg/kg, i.p.), WT mice had levels of locomotor activity and stereotyped behavior that were similar to values for saline-injected controls. In contrast, methamphetamine-treated DBP KO mice had increases in locomotor activity and decreases in stereotyped behavior compared to saline-injected KO mice. When exposed to a 4-week chronic stress paradigm (isolation housing plus acute stressors in week 3), WT mice displayed a reduction in locomotor activity, whereas DBP KO mice had an increase in locomotor activity (interaction term: P <0.02). Sleep deprivation of DBP KO mice for 1 day increased locomotor activity relative to DBP KO mice on a standard light-dark cycle, and this mania-like effect was abolished by pretreatment of mice with valproate.

The next major phase of these experiments was to perform microarray studies of gene expression in samples of PFC, amygdala, and blood of WT and DBP KO mice under basal conditions and following chronic stress. A selected sample of the genes from unstressed and stressed DBP KO mice that scored highest based upon a convergent functional genomics approach (Niculescu et al., 2000) is included in Table 10.2. The genes listed in Table 10.2 have been reported to influence risk of addiction and drug abuse, abnormal levels of emotion, and altered

Table 10.2 Selected Bipolar Disorder Risk Genes from Unstressed DBP KO Mice Maintained under Basal Conditions and DBP KO Mice Exposed to Chronic Stress

Gene Symbol and Description	Brain region (↑ or ↓)	Mouse Genetics	BP Human Genetics	BP Post-mortem Brain	BP Human Blood	CFG Score
Unstressed DBP KO mice						
Cnp: cyclic nucleotide phospodiesterase I	PFC: ↓	XXX				5
Drd2: dopamine receptor 2	AMY: ↓	XXX		XXX	XXX	4.5
Scg2: secretogranin II	AMY: ↓	XXX				4
Nos1: nitric oxide synthase 1	AMY: ↓	XXX	XXX	XXX		4
Camk2a: calcium/ calmodulin- dependent protein kinase IIα	AMY: ↑	XXX	XXX	XXX		4
Stressed DBP KO mice						
Snca: synuclein α	AMY: ↓	XXX	XXX			5.5
Drd2: dopamine receptor 2	PFC: ↓	XXX		XXX		4.5
Hspa1a: heat shock protein 1A	PFC: ↓	XXX	XXX			4.5
Sfpg: splicing factor proline/glutathione rich	AMY: ↑	XXX		XXX		4.5
Fos: FBJ osteosarcoma oncogene	AMY: ↑	XXX				4

Note: Risk genes were selected from a more extensive list of risk genes based upon their elevated CFG scores. Each gene was evaluated based upon its change relative to controls in the PFC or AMY, previous reports on behavioral or physiological effects in mice and humans, and previous reports on changes in the gene based upon human post-mortem brain or blood studies. CFG scores were computed as reported in Le-Niculescu et al. (2008).

Abbreviations: BP: bipolar disorder; CFG Score: Convergent Functional Genomics Score; DBP: D-box binding protein; KO: knockout; PFC: prefrontal cortex; AMY: amygdala.

sleep and circadian rhythms in studies of laboratory mice. Also of interest are those nine genes that exhibited significant changes in brain and blood samples. Data from selected genes in blood samples provide a valuable starting point for characterizing potential biomarkers for identifying patients with bipolar disorder and tracking their responses to drugs (Le-Niculescu et al., 2008).

Although the DBP KO mouse model of bipolar disorder represents a major step forward, there are serious limitations with the underlying methodology. First, the behavioral phenotyping was quite limited, and the behavioral differences between WT and DBP KO mice were not as clear-cut as one would have hoped. In addition, the stress protocol left much to be desired as the focus was on social isolation with a minor overlay of acute stressors, as opposed to a better characterized model of stressful stimulation (e.g., chronic social defeat stress or restraint stress). Still, the suggestion of a switch between a depression-like state and a mania-like state was intriguing and is well worth follow-up experiments.

DA in the driver's seat. Sidor et al. (2015) made the surprising observation that *ClockΔ19* mice exhibited rapid "mood" cycling, with a mania-like pattern of behavior during the daytime followed by a more normal behavior pattern at night. For example, compared to WT controls, *ClockΔ19* mice displayed more entries into and more time spent in the center of an open field arena, more entries into and more time spent in the light portion of a light-dark box, increased struggling time during a forced swim test, and increased preference for a sucrose solution. These differences between WT mice and *ClockΔ19* mice were normalized during the dark portion of the 12:12 light-dark cycle.

The next question addressed by these investigators centered on how VTA DA neuronal activity changed over the course of the 12:12 light-dark cycle in WT controls and *ClockΔ19* mice. Firing rates of VTA DA neurons were elevated significantly during daylight hours in *ClockΔ19* mice, and there was an absence of a diurnal rhythm in DA neuronal activity in *ClockΔ19* mice. Tyrosine hydroxylase, the rate-limiting enzyme in CA biosynthesis, was elevated during the daylight hours in *ClockΔ19* mice compared to WT controls. Elevations in tyrosine hydroxylase resulted in significant increases in DA synthesis in the nucleus accumbens during daylight hours in *ClockΔ19* mice. Using an optogenetic stimulation protocol to selectively increase VTA DA neuronal activity resulted in a mania-like behavioral phenotype in WT mice, whereas dampening of the elevations in tyrosine hydroxylase activity during the daylight hours reversed the mania-like behaviors. Evidence was presented that CLOCK protein acted as a negative regulator of tyrosine hydroxylase activity. These findings provide a link between disruptions in circadian genes and regulation of mania-like behaviors, leading to rapid cycling from mania-like behavior during daylight hours to WT patterns of behavior at night (Sidor et al., 2015).

Knock Out or Knock In

Give me a HINT. Mice with a deletion of the gene for histidine triad nucleotide-binding protein 1 (HINT1$^{(-/-)}$) display a stress-induced switch that different from the DBP model described earlier; that is, a switch from a manic-like state to a depressive-like state occurs. The HINT1 protein, which includes 126 amino acids, is widely expressed in the brain, where it binds to membrane-bound σ1Rs to coordinate activities of G protein-coupled receptors and NMDA receptors. In HINT1$^{(-/-)}$ mice, protein kinase C (PKC) activity increased, cross-regulation between G protein-coupled receptors and NMDA receptors was diminished, and responsiveness of NMDA receptors to direct activation increased. Earlier GWAS findings suggested a connection between the *HINT1* gene and risk of bipolar disorder.

In a comprehensive series of experiments from the Instituto Cajal in Madrid (Garzón-Niño et al., 2017; Sánchez-Blázquez et al., 2018), HINT1$^{(-/-)}$ mice were compared to wild-type (WT) littermate controls across a range of behavioral tasks and pharmacological challenges. The results of these experiments revealed that HINT1$^{(-/-)}$ mice exhibited a mania-like pattern of behavior. For example, HINT1$^{(-/-)}$ mice had higher levels of activity and spent more time in the center of an open field test arena, displayed higher levels of aggression in a resident-intruder test, had an increased preference for a sucrose solution, were immobile for less time during the forced swim and tail suspension tests, and had greater increases in locomotor activity following administration of apomorphine (5.0 mg/kg, i.p.). In addition, HINT1$^{(-/-)}$ mice had higher levels of PKA and PKC activities in brain synaptosomal membrane preparations from frontal cortex compared to WT controls. HINT1$^{(-/-)}$ mice also had increased serine-41 phosphorylation of the PKC substrate neuromodulin (GAP43). Treatment with valproate (200 mg/kg, i.p.) resulted in increased immobility times of HINT1$^{(-/-)}$ mice to levels of WT mice during the forced swim test but had no effect on immobility times of WT controls.

HINT1$^{(-/-)}$ mice had greater increases in locomotor activity than WT controls when challenged with a dose of amphetamine (2.0 mg/kg, i.p.). Pretreatment of HINT1$^{(-/-)}$ mice with an i.c.v. injection of an inhibitor of GSK-3β (TDZD8) or PKC (Gö7874) reduced significantly the locomotor hyperactivity following amphetamine administration, but these enzyme inhibitors had little to no effect on locomotor activity of WT controls.

Manic-like behavior is typically associated with high levels of GSK-3β activity but mania-like behavior decreases significantly after inhibition of GSK-3β. Although total levels of GSK-3β in frontal cortex were similar between HINT1$^{(-/-)}$ mice and WT controls, Akt-mediated inhibition of phosphorylation of GSK-3β at serine 9 was decreased in HINT1$^{(-/-)}$ mice. Given that activating phosphorylation of GSK-3β at tyrosine 216 predominated over inhibitory phosphorylation at serine 9 for HINT1$^{(-/-)}$ mice, it is likely that functional GSK-3β activity was higher than in WT controls.

Administration of antidepressants had no effect on the time spent immobile in the forced swim test for HINT1$^{(-/-)}$ mice, but decreased immobility times in

WT mice to levels seen in HINT1$^{(-/-)}$ mice. The NMDA receptor antagonist, MK801, decreased immobility times in WT mice in the forced swim test, and reduced further the immobility times of HINT1$^{(-/-)}$ mice. Inhibitors of PKC, PKA, and GSK-3β as well as valproate and lamotrigine increased immobility times of HINT1$^{(-/-)}$ mice in the forced swim test to levels seen in WT mice. These same compounds were without effect in WT mice.

The stress of being exposed acutely to the forced swim test had a dramatic impact on HINT1$^{(-/-)}$ mice that persisted for more than 10 days. Between 1–10 days following an initial forced swim test, HINT1$^{(-/-)}$ mice exhibited increases in immobility times that were significantly greater than levels of immobility in first-time stressed HINT1$^{(-/-)}$ mice. In contrast, WT mice were unaffected by the forced swim test. Administration of antidepressants restored the immobility times of previously stressed HINT1$^{(-/-)}$ mice to levels observed in first-time stressed HINT1$^{(-/-)}$ mice. In contrast, a σ1R antagonist was without effect on immobility times of HINT1$^{(-/-)}$ mice during a second exposure to the forced swim test. This important finding is consistent with a stress-promoted switch from mania-like behavior to a depressive phenotype. In addition, pretreatment of HINT1$^{(-/-)}$ mice with MK801 prior to the forced swim test blocked the development of a depressive-like phenotype in the days that followed.

What we don't know at this point is how much the mania-like behavioral phenotype of HINT1$^{(-/-)}$ mice is affected by acute stress. The only behavioral measure reported in the preceding study was time spent immobile in a subsequent forced swim test. It is critical to know if other behaviors (e.g., locomotor activity, aggression, preference for sweet solutions, response to stimulants, etc.) are altered in a similar way. In addition, if acute stress precipitates the change from mania-like to depression-like patterns of behavior, what would be the effect of exposure to chronic intermittent stress?

These and other findings led Garzón-Niño et al. (2017) to suggest a radically different view of the relationship between mania and depression in HINT1$^{(-/-)}$ mice and bipolar patients. They reasoned that depression and mania may coexist as opposing forces instead of cycling from one state to the other over time. The consequence of these two oppositional forces vying for predominance would result in alterations in mood swings that are typical of this mental disorder. Importantly, stressful life events appear to tip the balance away from manic-like behavior and in favor of a depression-like state in genetically susceptible animals and possibly humans. The HINT1 KO mouse is an unusual animal model of bipolar disorder that may be especially valuable in identifying new drug targets to prevent the manic and depressive mood swings that are characteristic of the disorder.

Where the action is. *Ankyrin 3* (*ANK3*), the gene that codes for a large scaffold protein (Ankyrin-G), has been identified as a shared risk gene with a modest effect size for both bipolar disorder and schizophrenia, based upon several GWAS. The most studied function associated with this gene involves the formation and maintenance of the axon initial segment, which includes a high density of voltage-gated Na^+ and K^+ channels. This unmyelinated region at the origin of the axon hillock is where axon potentials originate (Kole & Stewart, 2012). Reports from two laboratories using different methodologies indicated that disruption of ANK3 resulted in mania-like behavioral patterns that switched to depression-like behaviors following exposure of animals to chronic stress. (Note: homozygous ANK3$^{(-/-)}$ KO mice cannot be studied as an animal model of mania-like behavior due to early-onset ataxia that affects overall locomotor activity.)

Leussis et al. (2013) utilized C57BL/6J mice for RNA interference studies targeting the dentate gyrus (45%–62% reduction in transcription of ANK3 in the axon initial segment) and to generate ANK3$^{(+/-)}$ heterozygotes and ANK3$^{(+/+)}$ WT controls by breeding males and females that were heterozygous for the ANK3 gene. Reduced transcription of ANK3 in the dentate gyrus as a result of RNA interference led to a behavioral profile characterized by a significant reduction in anxiety-like behaviors (or perhaps an increase in impulsive or risk-taking behaviors) in the EPM, light-dark box, and anxiety-suppressed feeding task and increased locomotor activity during the light phase of the light-dark cycle. These differences between ANK3 knockdown mice and controls were reversed by treatment with lithium (85 mg/kg, i.p. for 14$^+$ days).

Experiments with WT and ANK3$^{(+/-)}$ mice yielded results that were consistent with the ANK3 knockdown experiments described earlier. ANK3$^{(+/-)}$ mice displayed 39% and 41% decreases in ANK3 expression in the dentate gyrus and cortex, respectively, compared to WT controls. ANK3$^{(+/-)}$ mice displayed reductions in anxiety-like behaviors in the EPM, light-dark box, and novelty-suppressed feeding task. In addition, these mice had an increased preference for a 1% sucrose solution in a two-bottle choice test. It should be noted that ANK3 knockdown mice and ANK3$^{(+/-)}$ heterozygous mice did not differ from their respective controls in a range of other behavioral tasks, including open field activity, acoustic startle, prepulse inhibition, and contextual and cued fear conditioning.

These investigators chose isolation housing for 6 weeks as the chronic stressor. Isolation housing had no discernible effect on the behaviors of WT mice. In contrast, isolation-housed ANK3$^{(+/-)}$ heterozygous mice differed from group-housed controls in the following measures: increased anxiety-like behavior in the EPM, light-dark box, and novelty-suppressed feeding task; reduced preference for a sucrose solution; and increased immobility in the forced swim test. In addition, isolation-housed and group-housed ANK3$^{(+/-)}$ heterozygous mice had increased plasma CORT levels under resting conditions and following acute restraint stress compared to WT mice. These results suggest that housing in isolation stimulated a switch from a mania-like behavioral phenotype to a depression-like phenotype in $ANK3^{(+/-)}$ heterozygous mice but not in WT mice, providing strong evidence of a gene x environment interaction in mice with a reduction in Ank3 expression in brain. However, the behavioral changes in these two ANK3 disruption models were reminiscent of some but not all aspects of mania-like and depression-like phenotypes.

In a second study, Zhu et al. (2017) utilized a protocol for targeted homozygous conditional deletion of ANK3 (ANK3 cKO) from pyramidal neurons in the forebrain (cortex, hippocampus, and striatum) of mice. When tested in adulthood, ANK3 expression was lost from more than 60% of cortical neurons in ANK3 cKO mice. There was also evidence of disinhibition of cortical neurons due to loss of inhibitory GABAergic cartridge synapses. Further support for disinhibition of cortical neurons was revealed by increased expression of c-fos, a marker of neuronal activity. ANK3 cKO mice displayed a behavioral phenotype consistent with aspects of bipolar mania (persistent locomotor hyperactivity, reduced anxiety-like behavior, reduced immobility in the forced swim and tail suspension tests, but no effect on PPI), and these behavioral changes were reversed by chronic treatment with lithium or valproate.

Next, these investigators exposed control and ANK3 cKO mice to chronic social defeat stress for 14 days. This chronic stress protocol has been employed as a way to induce depression-like behavior in laboratory mice. When ANK3 cKO mice were exposed to chronic social defeat stress, they displayed significant changes in behavior that were of greater magnitude than similarly stressed control mice and that were consistent with a depression-like phenotype. Remarkably, within 7 days after the end of chronic social defeat stress, ANK3 cKO mice reverted to high levels of locomotor activity consistent with a switch back to a mania-like phenotype. Re-exposure to chronic social defeat stress again resulted in a depression-like phenotype in ANK3 cKO mice but not in controls (Zhu et al., 2017).

This model represents a substantial step forward in the development of an animal model of bipolar disorder. Indeed, it provides a gold standard for how investigators should approach the study of identified risk genes associated with human psychiatric disorders. Although the switching process from mania → depression → mania in this study was dependent on the onset and then withdrawal of chronic social defeat stress, such a pattern is not inconsistent with findings from bipolar patients. There are many strengths to this series of experiments, including the targeted depletion of forebrain ANK3, the anatomical characterization of the extent of ANK3 depletion and its consequences for disinhibition of neuronal activity, use of a broad array of tasks for behavioral phenotyping, selection of a chronic stress paradigm that is well characterized and relevant for inducing depression-like behaviors, and following animals through two cyclic changes from mania-like to depression-like to mania-like behaviors.

Too much of a good thing. GSK-3β plays a critical role in several signaling pathways coupled to neuronal receptors, and these signaling pathways in turn inhibit GSK-3β activity by phosphorylation at serine 9, an effect catalyzed by PKC, PKA, and Akt-1. Prickaerts et al. (2006) explored the impact of overexpressing GSK-3β on behavioral measures and molecular regulatory pathways in transgenic mice. Compared to WT controls, transgenic mice exhibited an increase in locomotor activity in a 1-hour open field test; significant reductions in food intake; an enhanced acoustic startle response, but with a decrease in habituation; and reduced immobility in a forced swim test. There were no differences between groups in baseline and stress-induced activation of the HPA axis. The increased expression of GSK-3β in the striatum resulted in a compensatory decrease in the endogenous GSK-3β signaling pathway via up-regulation of Akt-1 expression. The behavioral changes in mice overexpressing GSK-3β resembled in part a mania-like phenotype. However, this model is not as well-documented or as clear-cut as others in modeling bipolar mania.

Kozikowski et al. (2007) explored the effectiveness of various inhibitors of GSK-3β that penetrate the blood-brain barrier on an amphetamine + chlordiazepoxide mouse model of mania. A more targeted approach in the design of GSK-3β inhibitors may improve the effectiveness of these newer drugs over standard mood stabilizers such as lithium and valproate, as well as reduce their undesirable side effects.

Close the gates. The L-type voltage-gated calcium channel family includes four distinct isoforms, referred to as $Ca_v1.1$, $Ca_v1.2$, $Ca_v1.3$, and $Ca_v1.4$. CACNA1C codes for the pore-forming α-1C subunit of the $Ca_v1.2$ isoform. In the mouse brain, $Ca_v1.2$ accounts for ~85% of the L-type channels, while $Ca_v1.3$ accounts for most of the remainder (Zamponi et al., 2015). Single nucleotide polymorphisms in CACNA1C have been associated with bipolar disorder in a meta-analysis of GWAS data for bipolar disorder and major depressive disorder, and this finding was the most robust of the meta-analysis and exceeded genome-wide significance levels (Liu et al., 2011).

Based upon the findings from a GWAS of bipolar disorder, Dao et al. (2010) investigated the role of CACNA1C on a battery of behavioral tests in male and female $Cacna1c^{(+/-)}$ heterozygous mice, and compared the results to $Cacna1c^{(+/+)}$ WT littermate controls. $Cacna1c^{(+/-)}$ heterozygous mice displayed several behavioral changes, some of which were sex-specific. These included reduced exploratory behavior in the hole board test, a decreased locomotor response to repeated daily injections of d-amphetamine, and decreased immobility in the forced swim and tail suspension tests. Female, but not male, heterozygous mice displayed decreased risk-taking behavior and/or increased anxiety in the EPM, light-dark box, and an open field area; greater attenuation of d-amphetamine-induced lo-comotor behavior; decreased escape failures in the learned helplessness task; and decreased amplitude of the acoustic startle response. These investigators suggested that $Cacna1c^{(+/-)}$ heterozygous mice had a mood-stabilized phenotype that was modified by sex for some but not all behaviors. These intriguing findings should be explored further given the strong association between polymorphisms in *CACNA1C* and risk of bipolar disorder (Dao et al., 2010).

BDNF. Patients diagnosed with bipolar disorder display volumetric reductions in specific brain areas that are associated with atrophy or loss of neurons. These morphological changes in various brain areas may reflect reductions in neuro-trophic signaling pathways. In addition, circulating levels of BDNF are reduced during manic or depressive episodes as well as with the progression of bipolar illness (Shaltiel et al., 2007).

Stress-responsive gene transcription may play an important role in trans-ducing the interaction between risk genes and life stressors with the onset and progression of bipolar disorder and the cycling from one mood state to an-other mood state of opposite polarity (Liu et al., 2008). In particular, BDNF has been the focus of numerous preclinical and clinical studies on the molec-ular mechanisms that contribute to bipolar disorder, especially the depressive component. BDNF stimulates neuronal connectivity and plasticity as well as neurogenesis in adult animals through activation of its tyrosine receptor kinase (TrkB). A rich literature has emerged regarding stress-induced decreases in the expression of BDNF mRNA in limbic brain regions. In addition, administration of antidepressants blocked the deleterious effects of stress on BDNF signaling in brain (Duman & Monteggia, 2006; Lindholm & Castrén, 2014). Finally, mood stabilizers such as lithium and valproate have been shown to stimulate increased levels of BDNF in the hippocampus in a rat model of amphetamine-induced mania (Frey et al., 2006).

A number of laboratories have studied knockdown or knockin mouse models of BDNF or TrkB, but the results to date have been conflicting. An alternative strategy has been to move downstream of BDNF signaling to evaluate the role of a member of the immediate early gene family, early growth response gene 3 (*Egr3*), which is decreased significantly in postmortem samples of prefrontal cortex from bipolar patients. $Egr3^{(-/-)}$ KO mice displayed greater behavioral and HPA axis reactivity to handling, elevated locomotor activity when placed in an open field arena, lack of habituation to social cues and to acoustic stimuli, and deficits in spontaneous alternation behavior. They also displayed increased levels of aggression and other behaviors that were suggestive of greater impulsivity compared to WT controls (Gallitano-Mendel et al., 2007, 2008). In another ex-periment, the stress of sleep deprivation for 6 hours was accompanied by a 2-fold increase in *Htr2a* mRNA levels, and this effect was dependent upon *Erg3* (Maple et al., 2015). Finally, Francis et al. (2017) reported that EGR3 was increased in D1 receptor-containing medium spiny neurons in nucleus accumbens in mice susceptible to the deleterious effects of chronic social defeat stress. Targeted reduction of *Egr3* activity in these same neurons reversed their depressive-like behaviors, blocked dendritic atrophy, and altered their *in vivo* activity.

These and other findings led Pfaffenseller et al. (2018) to propose that disruptions in *Bdnf* and *Egr3* signaling are critically involved in the onset and progression of bipolar disorder. Lower BDNF levels reported in patients with bipolar disorder would result in reductions in EGR3 levels as BDNF is a key regulator of *Egr3* transcription. EGR3 may also indirectly induce BDNF expression via regulation of NMDA receptors. In addition, reductions in *Egr3* expression would further reduce BDNF levels. Based on these findings, they proposed a feedback loop that reinforces this dysfunctional pathway, and that would increase vulnerability to life stressors, and could result in alterations in several behavioral, cognitive, and biological processes that contribute to the neuroprogression characteristic of bipolar disorder (Figure 10.2). Ultimately, individuals at risk for bipolar disorder would display increasing vulnerability to the deleterious effects of stressors and to disturbances in regulation of mood, and reduced responsiveness to mood-stabilizing drugs. The net result of these alterations would be a feed-forward cycle of illness progression.

Conclusions

In spite of the significant challenges to investigators of capturing the essential features of bipolar disorder in animal models, there are many promising leads, including some that have emerged from clinically based studies, as was described earlier (see also Beyer & Freund, 2017; Malkesman et al., 2009). It is important to keep in mind that no single animal model will perfectly reproduce the symptoms of bipolar disorder, and the same is true for any other psychiatric disorder. But each animal model that is successful in capturing an endophenotype of relevance to bipolar disorder provides valuable information that must then be combined with findings from other models. In addition, when behavioral findings from several animal models are consistent for a given behavioral endophenotype, there is the added possibility that these models will provide a convergence on a common mechanism to explain the disrupted patterns of behavior.

A major hurdle that has now been cleared is the development of an animal model that exhibits the essential features of switching from mania-like behavior to depression-like behavior (or vice versa). The switching process is often dependent upon exposure of laboratory animals to stressful stimuli, which also matches well with the clinical literature (refer to Chapter 2). Unfortunately, some

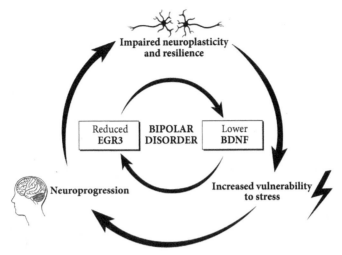

Figure 10.2. Proposed link between BDNF and EGR3 and their potential role in bipolar disorder (BD). Lower BDNF levels observed in BD patients may influence the reduced EGR3 levels seen in BD since BDNF regulates EGR3. EGR3 may also indirectly induce BDNF expression via regulation of NMDAR. Thus, reduced EGR3 expression, as has seen in BD patients, could contribute to lower BDNF levels associated with this illness. Based upon these findings, a feedback loop reinforcing this dysfunctional pathway is proposed that could impair neuroplasticity and resilience. This process could ultimately lead to increased vulnerability to stress, and could result in alterations in several biological factors that contribute to BD, such as abnormal structural brain changes and the associated cognitive and functional decline (a process called neuroprogression). The neural circuits additionally disrupted in this process could contribute to impaired neuroplasticity and resilience, increasing vulnerability to stress and mood episodes and reducing responsiveness to pharmacotherapy, thus perpetuating a vicious cycle of illness progression.
Adapted from Pfaffenseller et al. (2018) and used with permission of the first author.

of the stressor paradigms have not been carefully designed, and there is much room for improvement in this area.

A host of challenges remains. Some promising animal models have been developed and evaluated in only one laboratory, and this is a major limitation that must be addressed going forward. Only when findings with a given model can be replicated and extended by experiments in multiple laboratories can the true value of the animal model be assessed. In some animal models of mania-like behavior, investigators have utilized the EPM as a means of assessing risk-taking behavior. This is a slippery slope when a task that has been widely used to assess anxiety-like behaviors is suddenly reinterpreted to provide measures of increased risk-taking behavior. There are tasks that can be employed to quantify risk-taking behavior in laboratory animals (e.g., van Enkhuizen et al., 2014), and others should be developed. This is a key symptom of mania in bipolar patients, and it should be the subject of careful experimentation in several of the available animal models.

Several clinical observations have as yet not been examined carefully in animal models to begin the process of identifying underlying mechanisms. For example, some bipolar patients experience a progressive refractoriness to mood-stabilizing drugs, while others are not helped significantly by treatment with currently available drugs. Another issue concerns the onset and management of psychiatric and medical comorbidities in bipolar patients. These are some of the many research opportunities that remain to be explored in detail in animal models of bipolar disorder.

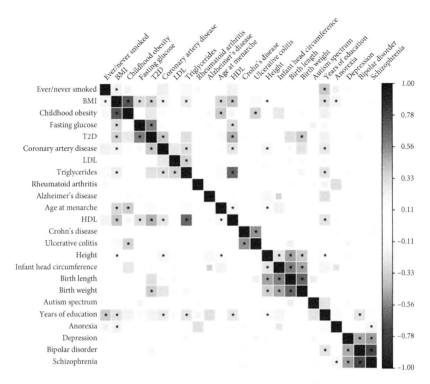

Color Plate 2.1. Genetic correlations among 24 traits analyzed by genome-wide association. Blue: positive genetic correlation; red: negative genetic correlation. Larger squares correspond to more significant *P* values. Genetic correlations that are different from zero at a false discovery rate (FDR) of 1% are shown as full-sized squares. Genetic correlations that are significantly different from zero after Bonferroni correction for the 300 tests in this analysis are marked with an asterisk. Results that did not pass multiple-testing correction are shown as smaller squares, to avoid obscuring positive controls, where the estimates point in the expected direction but do not achieve statistical significance owing to small sample sizes. The correction for multiple testing is conservative as the tests are not independent. To keep this figure to a reasonable size, representatives of several clusters of highly correlated traits were presented. Additional details and supplemental materials are available in the original publication.

Reproduced from Bulik-Sullivan et al. (2015) and used with permission of the publisher.

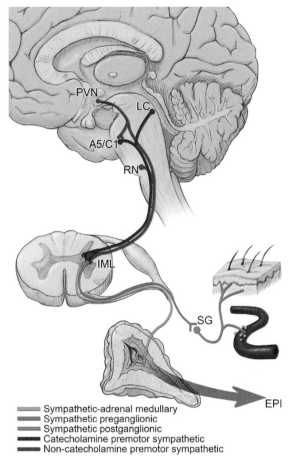

Sympathetic-adrenal medullary
Sympathetic preganglionic
Sympathetic postganglionic
Catecholamine premotor sympathetic
Non-catecholamine premotor sympathetic

Color Plate 4.1. Neural pathways regulating the sympathetic-adrenal medullary system response to stress. Depicted in this illustration are sympathetic postganglionic projections to skin and a section of a blood vessel, where norepinephrine is released from nerve terminals (blue dots), and sympathetic preganglionic projections to the adrenal medulla, where epinephrine (EPI) is released into the circulation from chromaffin cells.

Abbreviations: PVN: paraventricular nucleus of the hypothalamus; LC: locus coeruleus; A5/C1: A5 noradrenergic and C1 adrenergic neuronal cell groups; RN: raphe nuclei; IML: intermediolateral column of the spinal cord; SG; sympathetic ganglion; EPI: epinephrine.

Adapted from McCarty (2016) and used with permission.

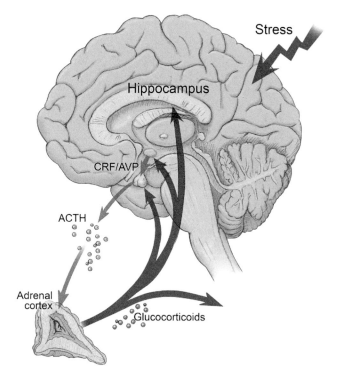

Color Plate 4.2. Influence of stress on the HPA axis, illustrating negative feedback effects of circulating glucocorticoids at the level of the anterior pituitary, the paraventricular nucleus of the hypothalamus (PVN), and higher brain centers (e.g., hippocampus).

Abbreviations: CRF: corticotropin releasing factor; AVP: arginine vasopressin; ACTH: adrenocorticotropic hormone.

Adapted from McCarty (2016) and used with permission.

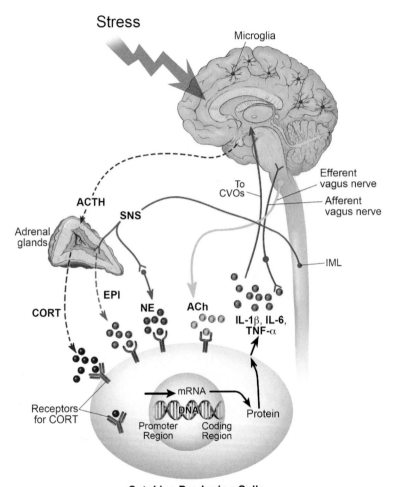

Cytokine Producing Cells

Color Plate 4.3. Stress stimulates the release of cytokines in the periphery. Cytokine-producing cells have receptors for glucocorticoids (CORT, blue dots), NE (red dots), EPI (orange dots), and acetylcholine (ACh, yellow dots). There are outer membrane receptors for CORT, NE, EPI, and Ach, as well as cytoplasmic receptors for CORT. The proinflammatory cytokines IL-1β, IL-6, and TNF-α (green dots) can provide feedback to brain areas by binding to receptors on afferent vagal nerve fibers or by entry into the brain at the circumventricular organs that lack a fully formed blood-brain barrier. One consequence of cytokine signaling to the brain is the activation of brain microglia.

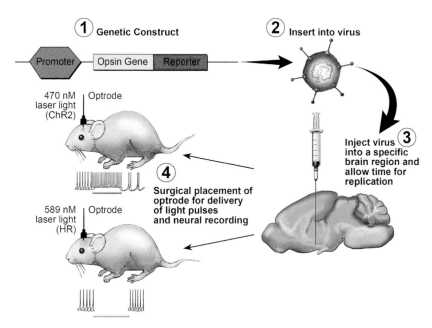

Color Plate 5.1. Optogenetic control of neuronal activity in freely behaving laboratory mice. 1. Pairing of a bacterial opsin gene with a promoter sequence that conveys neuronal specificity together with a reporter that identifies those neurons that express the opsin gene. 2. Insertion of the construct into a virus, typically an adreno-associated virus. 3. Stereotaxically guided injection of the virus into a brain area of interest, with several weeks allowed for uptake and replication of the DNA construct. 4. Surgical placement of an optrode that permits delivery of controlled fiber optic light pulses in proximity to the brain area under study as well as direct recordings of neuronal activity. Two simple examples are presented: use of channelrhodopsin-2 (ChR2) paired with blue light at 470 nM to stimulate neuronal activity, and use of halorhodopsin (HR) paired with yellow light at 589 nM to inhibit neuronal activity. Additional details are provided in the text.

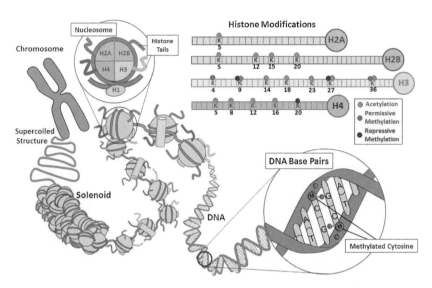

Color Plate 7.1. The dynamic (epi)genome: DNA methylation, histone post-translational modifications, and chromatin structural organization. Within the nucleus of eukaryotic cells, chromosomes are composed of DNA coiled around an octamer of histone proteins to form nucleosomes, the basic repeating unit of chromatin. Histone H1 proteins stabilize the coupling, wrapping, and stacking of nucleosomes into a 30 nm solenoid and higher order supercoiled chromatin fiber. The histone octamers are composed of four pairs of histone proteins (H2A, H2B, H3, and H4), which have globular domains and N-terminal tails that protrude from the nucleosome (H2A also has a C-terminal tail). Each histone tail can undergo numerous post-translational modifications. The most common forms of mammalian acetylation and methylation modifications of lysine (K) residues are shown. Additionally, mammalian DNA can be chemically modified by methylation and hydoxymethylation (M) of the 5' position of the cytosine base of 5'-cytosine-phosphodiester-guanine (CpG) dinucleotides. Chromatin structure directs the activity (expression) of genes: genes within tightly packed nucleosomes are silenced, whereas genes within relatively spaced nucleosomes are actively transcribed (expressed). The process of remodeling chromatin into domains of different transcriptional potentials is regulated by reciprocal changes of DNA methylation and histone modification in response to extrinsic cues and/or changes in intrinsic properties of cells.

Adapted from Weaver et al. (2017) and used with permission of Dr. Weaver.

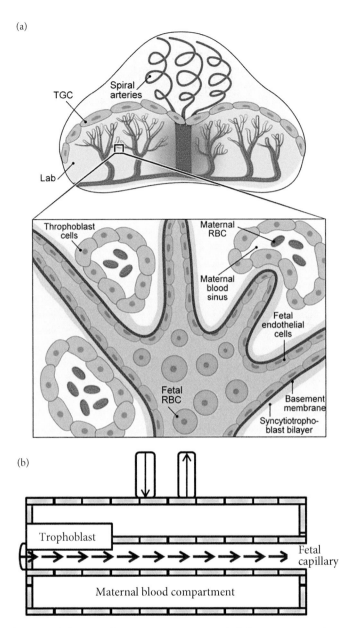

Color Plate 7.2. Schematic diagrams summarizing (A) the structure and main components of a mouse placenta and (B) the movement of fluids in each of these main compartments as visualized by diffusion MRI. Inset in A details the fetal–maternal–trophoblastic interactions in the labyrinth (Lab) area: fetal cells are surrounded by endothelial cells and membranes; fetal capillaries are surrounded by maternal blood sinuses, which conduct red blood cells (RBC) and are lined by trophoblast cells. Fluid exchanges between the fetal capillaries and the maternal blood pools are mediated by the trophoblasts, including the trophoblast giant cells (TGC).

Reproduced from Solomon et al. (2014) and used with permission of the senior author, Dr. M. Neeman.

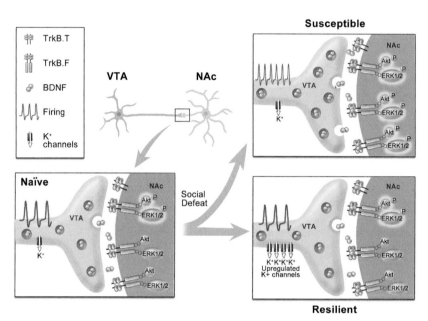

Color Plate 15.1. In susceptible mice, CSDS increases the firing rate of VTA DA neurons, which subsequently gives rise to heightened BDNF signaling within the nucleus accumbens (NAc). Resilient mice display a resistance to this adverse cascade of events by up-regulating various K$^+$ channels in presynaptic VTA neurons.

Adapted from Krishnan et al. (2007) and used with permission of the publisher.

11

Stress and Anxiety Disorders

In 1947, W. H. Auden published a book-length poem in six parts, *The Age of Anxiety*, which won the Pulitzer Prize for Poetry the following year (Auden, 1947). The poem centers on four strangers who meet in a bar in New York City during World War II and engage in active discussions over the course of the evening, ending at dawn the following day. The poem captured the sense of loneliness, lack of purpose, and anxiety in a time of global conflict, rise of technology, and displacement of peoples. The title is much more widely remembered than the poem itself, and it seems to capture the feelings of many people decades removed from the original publication date. Indeed, many would argue we now live in a perpetual age of anxiety.

Overview of Anxiety Disorders

Clinical Overview of Anxiety

Survey data support the suggestion that we currently live in an age of anxiety. Anxiety disorders comprise specific phobias, social phobias, agoraphobia, childhood and adult-onset separation anxiety, panic disorder, and generalized anxiety disorder. As a group, the anxiety disorders are chronic and disabling and occur in people in countries around the globe. The combination of these diagnoses represents the highest lifetime prevalence of any mental disorder, ranging as high as 29% for the United States and Western Europe. Heritability estimates for anxiety disorders are modest, and range from 30% to 40% (Hettema et al., 2001). A meta-analysis of seven independent GWAS of various anxiety disorders that included data from more than 18,000 individuals revealed several genetic markers of the disorders, including a gene involved in calcium-dependent neuronal signaling. However, this GWAS was still significantly under-powered, and dramatic increases in sample sizes will be required to detect what are expected to be multiple risk genes of anxiety disorders, each with low effect (Otowa et al., 2016).

The various anxiety disorders exact a high cost emotionally and economically on individuals, families, and communities throughout the world (Craske et al., 2017; Kessler et al., 2009). Based upon global data for 2010, anxiety disorders were the sixth leading cause of disability, with 65% of the disability-adjusted life years occurring in females and the highest burden of disability in males and females between 15 and 34 years of age (Baxter et al., 2014).

For some of the anxiety disorders, the age of onset is in childhood, while others first occur in late adolescence or early adulthood. The symptoms tend to wax and wane throughout the life span, quite often in combination with other anxiety disorders or other mental and substance use disorders or chronic medical conditions. Individuals who are diagnosed with an anxiety disorder tend to have lower educational attainment, unstable social relationships, and reduced earning potential. To make matters worse, there is often a significant delay from the onset of symptoms to the time when treatment is first received.

With the publication of *DSM-5* (American Psychiatric Association, 2013), the chapter on anxiety disorders reflected several important changes from the previous edition. Obsessive-compulsive disorder was moved to a new chapter, as was post-traumatic stress disorder. Separation anxiety disorder and selective mutism are now classified as anxiety disorders. In addition, the chapter on anxiety now takes a developmental approach. Finally, the chapter on anxiety disorders is placed between chapters on depressive disorders and obsessive-compulsive disorders to emphasize the similarities shared across these diagnoses (Kupfer, 2015; Stein et al., 2014).

Translating Anxiety

In forging a connection between stressful stimulation and symptoms of anxiety in animal models, a useful starting point might be to establish a definition of anxiety that is roughly translatable from humans to laboratory animals and back again. All humans worry to varying degrees about uncertainties associated with future events, but all humans do not have an anxiety disorder. According to Barlow's highly influential monograph (Barlow, 2002), anxiety is a diffuse mood state that focuses on the potential for negative events to occur at some point in the future, and includes recurring symptoms of worry, hyper-arousal, avoidance behaviors, and muscular tension. However, individuals with generalized anxiety disorder do not exhibit activation of the sympathetic-adrenal medullary system. In contrast, fear is an immediate alarm reaction (e.g., fight-or-flight response) to imminent danger, be it real or perceived. Fear symptoms comprise thoughts of immediate danger, escape behaviors, and sympathetic nervous system activation. In detailed analyses of clinical symptoms, the accumulated data tend to sort into two separate buckets—one is related to fear and/or panic, while the other involves worry and apprehension. The criteria for anxiety disorders contained in *DSM-5* are also associated with recurring thoughts and worries about the debilitating symptoms, which lead to long-term distress and impairment of normal activities (Craske et al., 2009; Craske et al., 2017; Stein et al., 2014).

Stress Effects on Anxiety

As with many other mental disorders, current etiologic models of anxiety disorders focus on the interaction between internal risk factors that confer vulnerability (e.g., diatheses) and external stressors in the onset and maintenance of these disorders (Chorpita & Barlow, 1998; Mineka & Oehlberg, 2007). Internal risk factors include genetic predispositions, specific personality traits, and various early experiences. External stressors include a range of stressful life events, including trauma-related events. Later in this chapter, we will have a detailed look at animal models that capture this gene x environment or environment x environment dynamic.

Another consideration is the role of physiological responses to stressors in patients with specific anxiety disorders compared to healthy controls. In one such study, Grillon et al. (1994) examined fear-potentiated startle responses in patients diagnosed with a panic disorder compared to healthy controls. Startle responses were significantly greater in patients less than 40 years of age compared to controls of a similar age range. This difference in startle amplitude was observed during fear-potentiated startle and during a safe period when no shocks were delivered. The investigators suggested that these differences between younger panic disorder patients and controls were due to a higher level of anxiety related to the experimental context. In addition, Blechert et al. (2007) reported that panic disorder patients had lower levels of P_{CO2} and higher levels of cardiovascular sympathetic activation compared to controls.

An Uncertain World

In developing their uncertainty and anticipation model of anxiety (UAMA), Grupe and Nitschke (2013) integrated findings from a variety of perspectives and advanced five processes to explain why uncertainty about future threats becomes so disruptive in the lives of patients with anxiety. These disruptions, all revolving around the common theme of uncertainty, included the following: (i) inflated estimates of the likelihood and costs of a potential threat; (ii) increased attention to potential threats; (iii) deficits in safety learning regarding potential threats; (iv) behavioral and cognitive avoidance and associated worry about potential threats; and (v) elevated reactivity to the uncertainty surrounding a potential threat.

These five disruptions in behavioral responses to uncertainty were associated with perturbations of neural circuits that normally function in adaptive responses to threat assessment. These circuits, which were informed by translational studies in animal models and revealed by fMRI studies in humans, included the dorsomedial and dorsolateral PFC, the orbitofrontal cortex, rostral cingulate cortex, anterior mid-cingulate cortex, parietal cortex, anterior insula, striatum, amygdala, hypothalamus, pons, periaqueductal gray, and the BNST (Grupe & Nitschke, 2013). These anxiety-relevant circuits will be discussed in greater detail in the sections to follow that describe research with animal models of anxiety.

Another approach to examining the diasthesis-stress model in the etiology of anxiety disorders is through the perspective of classical conditioning paradigms of fear and anxiety learning (Bouton et al., 2001; Mineka & Oehlberg, 2007). The results of several studies highlight small but significant differences in the rate of fear acquisition and extinction between individuals with a diagnosis of clinical anxiety compared to healthy controls, or in comparisons of individuals who are high versus low in trait anxiety. In addition, the speed and the strength of the acquisition and extinction of fear learning are moderately heritable. Evidence has been presented in support of the view that conditioning of fear and conditioning of anxiety involve two different types of learning processes, which may explain in part the distinctive features of the various anxiety disorders.

Animal Models of Anxiety Disorders

Refining Animal Models

In February 1999, the National Institute of Mental Health invited a distinguished group of basic and clinical researchers to evaluate existing animal models of anxiety disorders, to compare findings using animal models with what was known at the time about symptom profiles of patients with anxiety disorders, to enhance existing animal models of anxiety disorders, and to consider opportunities for the development of new animal models. A summary of this workshop was published and provides an interesting look back at identified challenges with animal models and how well these shortcomings have been addressed (Shekhar et al., 2001). One such challenge related to the fact that many preclinical studies have employed generic animal models of anxiety, even though there are clear distinctions among the various *DSM-5* descriptions of anxiety disorders. Another concern related to the fact that many animal models of anxiety involved exposing "normal" animals acutely to an anxiety-provoking test environment, such as an elevated plus-maze (EPM). This approach ignores the widely held view that anxiety disorders reflect an underlying vulnerability that may be unmasked by exposure to an environmental trigger. Also of importance was the need to employ a battery of tests to assess levels of anxiety in animal models, as there was no single "gold standard" test for anxiety, especially in experiments with genetically modified animals. Very few experiments with animal models of anxiety have included female subjects, in spite of the fact that females are more susceptible to developing anxiety disorders than males (Maeng & Milad, 2015). Given the comorbidity of anxiety disorders with other mental disorders and medical conditions, the workshop participants also encouraged studies of gene x environment and environment x environment interactions on the expression of anxiety as well as other disorder-specific phenotypes (e.g., depression). Finally, taking advantage of novel anxiety-like behavioral phenotypes in breeds of dogs was encouraged as an out-of-the-box approach to anxiety research (Overall, 2000).

Much of the research on animal models of anxiety has been motivated by a search for more effective medications to treat anxiety disorders in patients (Bourin, 2015; Rodgers, 1997; Treit et al., 2010). Several of these experimental approaches have actually modeled state anxiety; that is, animals were exposed acutely to a test environment designed to provoke anxiety, such as an EPM or T-maze or a black-white test chamber. This approach represents a test of acute levels of anxiety, not a model of anxiety! Unfortunately, as noted earlier, these tests of state anxiety do not accurately capture the essential features of trait anxiety in patients, or in animals either for that matter (Belzung & Griebel, 2001; Cryan & Sweeney, 2011; Kalueff et al., 2007; Lister, 1990; Steimer, 2011). A further complication occurs in validating genetic animal models of trait anxiety, in that these same acute tests are used to assess levels of trait anxiety. Therefore, one must be mindful that genetic models may have excessive levels of state anxiety rather than elevated levels of trait anxiety, and this concern should be reflected in the control groups included in any experiment (Allsop et al., 2014).

Tests of Anxiety in Laboratory Animals

A range of tests of anxiety has been developed over the past several decades, with most being employed in experiments with laboratory strains of rats and mice. Most of these tests have been used to screen new compounds or test the effectiveness of existing anxiolytic drugs. Tests of anxiety-like behaviors have been organized into five major groupings (see also Table 11.1):

- *Exploration-based*: behavioral measures of freely moving animals in various test environments, including measures of social behavior in pairings with a conspecific.

Table 11.1 Laboratory Paradigms for Measuring Anxiety and Fear in Laboratory Strains of Mice and Rats

Test	Description	Assumptions	References
Exploration-based			
Elevated plus-maze (EPM)	Animals are allowed free exploration of an elevated plus-shaped maze that includes two open arms and two closed arms.	Open arms are more anxiety-provoking than closed arms.	Carobrez & Bertoglio (2005) Hogg (1996) Lister (1987) Pellow et al. (1985) Wall & Messier (2001)
Light-dark box	Apparatus with two compartments, one brightly lit and the other dimly lit or dark, and connected by an opening at floor level	Light compartment more anxiety-provoking than dark compartment. Measures include freezing behavior.	Bourin & Hascoët (2003) Costall et al. (1989) Crawley (1981) Crawley & Goodwin (1980)
Open field arena	Animals are allowed free access to a large arena that may be square or circular.	Time spent and activity in central part of arena reflect lower levels of anxiety.	Prut & Belzung (2003) Walsh & Cummins (1976)
Hole board test	Animals placed on a board with holes equally spaced along its length.	Measures of head dips into the holes, with higher numbers reflecting less anxiety.	Crawley (1985) Nolan & Parkes (1973)
Social interaction test	Test animals are placed with a novel conspecific and behaviors are monitored.	Decreased levels of social interaction reflect higher levels of anxiety.	File (1980) File & Seth (2003)
Stress-related			
Defense burying test	Test animals are placed into a novel cage containing bedding material and either several marbles or a shock probe.	Burying of the marbles or the shock probe is taken as measure of anxiety.	De Boer & Koolhaas (2003) Njung'e & Handley (1981) Treit et al. (1981)

Table 11.1 Continued

Test	Description	Assumptions	References
Four-plate test	Animal freely explores a cage with a floor made up of four metal plates. Crossing from one plate to the next results in a shock.	Shock is avoided by remaining immobile. High levels of immobility reflect increased anxiety.	Bourin et al. (2005) Hascoët et al. (2000)
Physiological			
Stress-induced hyperthermia	Mice are housed in isolation overnight and then rectal temperature is measured two times within 10–15 min.	Increased rectal temperature from the first to second measurement is an indication of anxiety.	Van Der Heydena et al (1997) Olivier et al. (2003)
Autonomic activation	Remote monitoring of heart rate, blood pressure, etc., in response to stressors	Elevated autonomic responses are associated with fear.	Van Bogaert et al. (2006)
Conflict-based			
Geller-Seifter task	Food-deprived animals are trained to press a lever to receive food. Later, lever pressing is paired with shock.	A conflict between approach to secure food and fear of shock. Less approach reflects increased anxiety.	Geller & Seifter (1960) Heilig et al. (1992) Pollard & Howard (1979)
Vogel task	Water-deprived animals are given access to water, then drinking is paired with electric shocks.	Lack of punished drinking behavior is taken to reflect increased anxiety.	Moreira et al. (2006) Vogel et al. (1971)
Novelty-suppressed feeding	Food-deprived animals are placed in a strange environment where food is available.	Less food consumed is associated with increased anxiety.	Dulawa & Hen (2005) Shephard & Broadhurst (1982)
Novelty-induced hypophagia	Animals are trained to consume a desirable food (e.g., sweetened milk) and then placed with the food in a novel environment.	Hesitation to consume the desirable food is a measure of anxiety and anhedonia.	Dulawa & Hen (2005) Chen et al. (2006)

(Continued)

Table 11.1 Continued

Test	Description	Assumptions	References
Conditioned Responses			
Pavlovian fear conditioning	Animals are trained to associate a conditioned stimulus (CS) with an electric shock (unconditioned stimulus, UCS). The animal learns to respond (i.e., freezing) to the CS alone.	Freezing behavior in response to the CS without the UCS is a measure of fear.	Maren (2001) Schafe et al. (2001)
Fear-potentiated startle	Conditioned fear is measured as an increase in the acoustic startle reflex in the presence of a cue previously paired with shock.	An increase in the magnitude of the startle response reflects an increase in fear/anxiety.	Davis (2006) Davis et al. (1993)

- *Stress-related*: animals are exposed to acute stressors and behaviors are monitored.
- *Conflict-based*: animals are exposed to aversive stimulation or punishment in the form of electric shock. This creates a conflict between the need for food/water or the tendency to explore and fear of the electric shock.
- *Physiological*: autonomic responses to stressors, including blood pressure, heart rate, and body temperature are measured.
- *Cognitive*: animals are trained to associate a specific stimulus or a behavioral response with an aversive stimulus.

Genetically Selected Strains of Anxious Rats and Mice

The HAB rat and mouse models of trait anxiety developed at the Max Planck Institute of Psychiatry in Munich are without doubt the most intensively studied animal models of anxiety disorders. Behavioral phenotyping of these lines of rats and mice have also revealed that the high anxiety-like lines also displayed a passive coping style during stressful stimulation, suggestive of a connection to depressive-like behaviors. Dr. Ranier Landgraf and his Institute colleagues, together with collaborators from other universities, have taken a multidisciplinary translational approach to characterize these two model systems, with an ultimate goal of improving the diagnosis and treatment of anxiety disorders in humans.

HAB/LAB lines of rats. Landgraf and Wigger (2002, 2003) provided a detailed summary of the procedures that were followed to establish two lines of Wistar rats, one with high levels of trait anxiety (rHAB) and another with low levels of trait anxiety (rLAB), beginning in the 1990s. The selection criterion for establishment of these two lines was based upon behaviors in the EPM, with rHAB rats spending significantly less time and having fewer entries into the open arms compared to rLAB rats. rHAB and rLAB rats have also been tested in laboratories in France and Austria, and the anxiety-like behavioral differences between strains were consistent across all three locations (Salomé et al., 2002).

State or trait? One obvious question relates to the description of rHAB rats as an animal model of trait anxiety. A novel approach to distinguishing between trait anxiety and state anxiety involved selecting the highest (HA) and lowest scoring (LA) Wistar rats based upon time spent on the open arms of an EPM. These rats had been purchased from the same supplier that provided the original breeders for the rHAB and rLAB lines. The HA and LA rats had scores for time spent on the open arms that matched well with scores for rats of the rHAB and rLAB lines, respectively. However, HA and LA rats did not differ in their patterns of coping behavior during a forced swim test. Although HA rats displayed greater activation of the HPA axis following acute stress compared to LA rats, this difference was not driven by elevated expression of AVP in the PVN. Thus, some but not all facets of the anxiety-like phenotype of rHAB rats were evident in HA rats, and these distinctions appeared to provide a reasonable basis for associating trait anxiety with rHAB rats and state anxiety with HA rats (Landgraf & Wigger, 2003).

One could argue that this process was a classic example of circular reasoning. Specifically, if behavior in the EPM is a valid measure of state anxiety, and if Wistar rats can be selected for extremes of behavior in the EPM, then the resulting strains would serve as a valid animal model of trait anxiety. Let's keep this concern in mind as we consider some of the findings in experiments with the rHAB and rLAB lines.

Rats of the rHAB and rLAB lines have also been compared in additional tests that are relevant for an anxiety-like phenotype. These include the open field test, the modified hole board test, behavior in a black-white box, social interaction tests, exposure to social defeat, and neonatal ultrasonic vocalizations. In all comparisons, behaviors of rHAB and rLAB rats differed in the expected direction. rHAB rats also exhibited a more passive coping strategy and a greater HPA responsiveness to an acute stressor, as reflected in higher levels of circulating ACTH and CORT. The greater reactivity of the HPA axis appeared to be driven by increased synthesis of vasopressin (AVP) in the PVN and increased release of AVP into the pituitary portal blood supply. Interestingly, intra-PVN administration of an AVP V1 receptor antagonist by inverse microdialysis resulted in decreases in anxiety-related behaviors in rHAB rats (Wigger et al., 2004). Further studies detected a polymorphism in the AVP promoter of rHAB rats that resulted in elevated transcription of the AVP gene in the PVN (Murgatroyd et al., 2004).

When subjected to fear-sensitized acoustic startle tests, the results were somewhat surprising; rLAB rats displayed higher baseline and fear-sensitized acoustic startle responses compared to rHAB rats. The two lines of rats did not differ in amount of time spent freezing during the inter-stimulus interval with or without delivery of footshocks. When tested in an EPM, rats of the two lines displayed consistent differences in anxiety-like behaviors, with rHAB rats having fewer entries into and less time spent on the open arms. These data suggest that the EPM and the fear-sensitized acoustic startle test tap into different qualities of fear and anxiety (Yilmazer-Hanke et al., 2004).

rHAB and rLAB rats also differed in their patterns of Fos expression following the mild stress of placement in an open field arena or on the open arm of an EPM. rHAB rats had higher numbers of Fos-positive cells in the PVN, the lateral and anterior hypothalamic areas, and the medial preoptic area. In contrast, rLAB rats had higher numbers of Fos-positive cells in the cingulate cortex (Salomé et al., 2004).

Stress and anxiety. In a related study that employed social defeat as a stressor, rHAB rats spent more time freezing and emitted more ultrasonic vocalizations (USVs), while rLAB rats spent more time rearing and grooming, reflecting passive and active coping styles, respectively. Surprisingly, rLAB rats had higher circulating levels of ACTH and CORT compared to rHAB rats in response to the stress of social defeat. Finally, rHAB rats exhibited greater numbers of Fos-positive cells in the medial preoptic area, periventricular hypothalamic area, central nucleus of the amygdala, and medial portions of the amygdala. In contrast, rLAB rats had greater numbers of Fos-positive cells in the dorsomedial PAG, paraventricular nucleus of the thalamus, cingulate cortex, primary and secondary motor cortex, and the ventrolateral septal nucleus (Frank et al., 2006).

Using LPS (30 µg/kg, i.p.) as an immune challenge, Salomé and coworkers (2008) measured plasma levels of ACTH, CORT, and IL-6 under basal conditions and at 2 and 4 hours after administration of LPS in rHAB and rLAB rats. Under basal conditions, plasma levels of ACTH and CORT were similar in rats of the two strains. In contrast, basal plasma levels of IL-6 were significantly lower in rHAB rats. Plasma CORT was significantly higher in rHAB rats at 2 hours post-LPS, but this difference between lines was not observed at 4 hours post-LPS. Although plasma levels of IL-6 increased to a similar extent in rats of the two lines, the ratio of 2-hour values versus basal values was significantly greater in rHAB rats.

rHAB and rLAB rats also differed in regulation of heart rate (HR) under basal conditions and following stressful stimulation. Surgically placed radiotelemetry transmitters allowed recordings of the electrocardiogram (ECG), body temperature, and locomotor activity in freely behaving rats of the two lines. Under resting conditions, HR was similar between rats of the two lines, although cardiac vagal tone was significantly reduced in rHAB rats. rHAB rats had approximately twice the number of episodes of ventricular arrhythmias following administration of the β-adrenergic agonist, isoproterenol, compared to rLAB rats. HR responses to a 15-minute period of restraint stress were lower in rHAB compared to rLAB rats, and these differences between lines were maintained up to 30 minutes following restraint stress. Body temperatures over the course of a 24-hour period were significantly elevated in rHAB rats, suggesting increased sympathetic tone. The disturbances in cardiac regulation in rHAB rats in this study compared favorably with reported disturbances in cardiovascular regulation in patients with anxiety disorders (Carnevali et al., 2014).

The effects of the postnatal maternal environment on the development of anxiety-related behaviors in rats of the rHAB and rLAB lines were also explored. Cross-fostering litters from soon after birth until weaning between mothers of the two lines had no significant impact on anxiety-related behaviors in control or foster-reared offspring (Wigger et al., 2001).

Prenatal stress and anxiety. Gene x environment interactions may play a role in the development of an anxiety-like phenotype in animal models of trait anxiety. Several experiments have examined the effects of prenatal stress on rats of the rHAB and rLAB strains. In the first experiment, between days 4 and 10 of pregnancy, individual female rats of the two lines were placed into the home cage of a lactating female rat for 45 minutes each day (maternal defeat stress), and were also exposed to restraint stress for 1 hour each day. From days 11 to 18 of pregnancy, female rats were exposed to maternal defeat stress for 60 minutes each day. Control females of each line were left undisturbed in their home cages except for bedding changes. Prenatal stress reduced behavioral indices of anxiety-like behaviors (e.g., EPM and hole board tests) in adult male rHAB rats, but increased them in adult male rLAB rats. In addition, prenatal stress reduced mRNA levels of CRF in the PVN of adult rHAB males, but increased mRNA levels of AVP in the PVN of adult rLAB males. Plasma CORT responses to brief exposure to an elevated platform were reduced in prenatally stressed adult rHAB females compared to rHAB controls. Plasma CORT responses to acute stress did not differ between prenatally stressed and control adult LAB females. The strain differences in response to prenatal stress could not be explained by differences in CORT levels in pregnant females of the two lines or in their behaviors directed toward their litters (Bosch et al., 2006).

In a second experiment, Lucassen et al. (2009) exposed pregnant rHAB and rLAB females each day from days 5–20 of pregnancy to a combination of maternal defeat stress (15 minutes) followed by restraint stress (45 minutes). Control females of the two lines were left undisturbed in their home cages. At 43 days of age, control rHAB males had significantly lower rates of hippocampal neurogenesis compared to control rLAB males. rHAB males exposed to prenatal stress displayed further reductions in rates of hippocampal neurogenesis, but prenatally stressed rLAB males were unaffected. A possible mechanism to explain these strain differences in response to prenatal stress could be a failure of pregnant rHAB females but not rLAB females to increase activity of placental 11β-hydroxysteroid dehydrogenase type 2 (11β-HSD2) in response to prenatal stress. Placental 11β-HSD2 inactivates maternal CORT, thereby protecting the fetal brain from high levels of the adrenal steroid, which was especially critical given the daily increases in HPA activity of pregnant females following exposure to stress (Seckl & Holmes, 2007). The results of these two experiments highlight the very different patterns of responses to prenatal stress in rHAB and rLAB pregnant females and their offspring.

Postnatal stressors and anxiety. The recurring stress of daily bouts of separation of litters from their mothers provides another approach for studying gene x environment effects in rHAB and rLAB rats. From PNDs 2–15, rHAB and rLAB litters were separated from their mothers and maintained in a separate room at 32°C for 3 hours. Control litters of the two lines were left undisturbed with their mothers from birth until weaning. Compared to rLAB mothers, rHAB mothers spent more time with their litters from birth until PND5, although rates of licking and grooming were similar between mothers of the two strains prior to separation of the litters, and increased to a similar extent during the 1-hour period following reunion of mothers and their litters. When tested in adulthood, postnatally stressed rHAB rats exhibited reductions in anxiety-like behaviors compared to controls, whereas postnatally stressed rLAB rats exhibited increases in anxiety-like behaviors. In addition, postnatally stressed rHAB rats displayed reductions in HPA axis responses to acute stress compared to rHAB controls. In contrast, the stress of repeated maternal separation did not affect HPA axis responsivity in rLAB rats (Neumann et al., 2005).

The rHAB and rLAB lines also differed in their responses to an enriched environment (EE) versus chronic mild stress exposure (CMS) beginning prior to weaning and extending to PND 42. A critical aspect of this study was an examination of the involvement of the gene that codes for the CRF_1 receptor (*Crfr1*) in the amygdala on the expression of an anxiety-like phenotype. When exposed to an enriched environment, rHAB rats exhibited reductions in CORT responses to acute stress and reduced expression of *Crfr1* in the basolateral amygdala. In contrast, exposure of rLAB rats to CMS resulted in elevations in CORT responses to acute stress and enhanced expression of *Crfr1* in the basolateral amygdala. The bidirectional changes in *Crfr1* expression were associated with changes in the methylation status of its promoter, and provided evidence that *Crfr1* serves as a plasticity gene in the amygdala to regulate the expression of the anxiety pheno-type (Slotnikov et al., 2014).

HAB/LAB lines of mice. A parallel selective breeding effort was undertaken to establish lines of mice derived from the Swiss CD-1 outbred strain that displayed high levels of anxiety-like behavior (mHAB) or low levels of anxiety-like behavior (mLAB) based upon EPM tests, and these differences were also reflected across an array of other behavioral tests (Krömer et al., 2005). Consistent with findings from rHAB rats, mHAB mice have higher levels of expression of AVP in the PVN compared to mLAB mice (Landgraf et al., 2007).

HPA activity and anxiety. In a series of experiments relating to the HPA axis, Slotnikov et al. (2014a,b) compared responses in mice of the mHAB and mLAB lines to normal CD1 (mNAB) mice. These lines were at approximately the 50th generation of selective breeding. The percentage of time spent on the open arms of an EPM was as follows: mHAB (<15%), mNAB (35%–45%), and mLAB (>60%). Time spent floating in the forced swim test was greatest for mHAB, lowest in the mLAB, and intermediate in the mNAB. Swim-stress induced increases in plasma CORT were significantly reduced in mHAB compared to mice of the other two lines. Finally, mHABs displayed significant blunting of plasma CORT levels following administration of dexamethasone (DEX), and had diminished plasma CORT responses to exogenous administration of CRF.

In further studies of HPA regulation, these investigators reported that gluco-corticoid receptor (GR) levels were significantly higher in the pituitary, PVN, and hippocampus of mHAB mice compared to mLAB and mNAB mice. CRF expression was significantly higher in the PVN of mHAB mice compared to mice of the two other lines. Expression of the CRF_1 receptor (*Crfr1*) gene was significantly higher in the PFC but significantly reduced in the pituitary of mHAB mice compared to mice of the other two lines.

Chronic administration of CORT through the drinking water for 6 weeks resulted in reductions in anxiety-like and passive coping behaviors in mHAB mice. In contrast, chronic administration of CORT resulted in increased anxiety-like behavior in mNAB mice. In mHAB and mNAB mice, chronic ad-ministration of CORT led to significant reductions in levels of GR expression but not *Crfr1* expression. Based upon the results of this series of experiments, Slotnikov et al. (2014b) proposed that HAB mice resembled patients who present with pathological levels of anxiety together with symptoms of depression.

Risk genes and anxiety. Landgraf et al. (2007) reported that expression of glyoxylase-I, an enzyme in the glyoxal pathway, was 5-fold higher in samples of hypothalamus, amygdala, and motor cortex of mLAB compared to mHAB mice.

In addition, levels of expression of glyoxylase-I in 17 unidentified blood samples could be used to accurately identify mHAB and mLAB animals. Finally, similar differences in expression of glyoxylase-I in blood samples were observed in less anxious BALB/c mice (higher levels of glyoxylase-I) compared to more anxious C57BL/6 mice (lower levels of glyoxylase-I). Levels of glyoxylase-I may be a marker of trait anxiety in mice, or it may be an important risk gene for the onset of anxiety-like behaviors. Additional experiments will be required to address these possibilities.

In another line of inquiry, experiments focused on TMEM132D, a single pass transmembrane protein thought to serve as a cell surface marker for oligodendrocyte differentiation. *Tmem132d* has been advanced as a risk gene for anxiety disorders in humans based upon GWAS and post-mortem studies. In addition, *Tmem132d* mRNA is more highly expressed in the anterior cingulate cortex but not in other brain areas of mHAB mice compared to mLAB mice. Lastly, experiments with an F2 population derived from crossing mHAB and mLAB mice revealed that a single nucleotide polymorphism (SNP) associated with *Tmem132d* co-segregated with anxiety-related behaviors in an EPM test in males and females (Erhardt et al., 2011).

Naik et al. (2018) extended these findings by employing an adeno-associated viral vector to over-express *Tmem132d* in the anterior cingulate cortex of C57BL/6 mice. Compared to controls, mice that over-expressed *Tmem132d* by 1.7-fold spent significantly less time in the open arms of an EPM and spent less time in the illuminated portion of a light-dark box, confirming that an anxiety-like phenotype was associated with enhanced expression of *Tmem132d*.

F1 offspring. Chekmareva et al. (2014) utilized an interesting approach to examine molecular regulation of anxiety-like behavior. They generated F1 hybrids by crossing mHAB and mLAB lines of mice, and then exposed them to a standard laboratory environment (controls), an enriched environment (EE), or chronic mild stress treatment (CMS). The latter two treatments were initiated on PND 15 and continued until PND 42. When tested in an EPM, EE mice spent significantly more time in the open arms compared to mice of the other two groups. In addition, CMS mice had fewer and EE mice had more entries into the open arms compared to controls. Finally, CMS mice had significantly longer latencies to enter the open arms compared to mice of the other two groups. Similar behavioral results were obtained for testing of mice in a light-dark box, with EE mice showing less anxiety-like behaviors and CMS mice displaying elevated levels of anxiety-like behaviors.

Studies were also conducted on two anxiety-related genes in the basolateral amygdala, high mobility group nucleosome binding domain 3 (*Hmgn3*) and *Crfr1*, in mice of the three treatment groups. Results indicated that total expression of *Hmgn3* was reduced by EE and increased by CMS. Total expression of *Crfr1* did not change in response to either of the environmental manipulations (Chekmareva et al., 2014).

Maternal effects on anxiety. Cross-fostering experiments have also been reported using high and low anxiety lines of CD1 mice. Compared to mLAB mice, mHAB mice had increased levels of maternal care, higher levels of expression of AVP in the PVN, and elevations in anxiety-like behaviors. These behavioral and neuroendocrine differences between lines were not altered significantly by cross-fostering of litters from soon after birth until weaning (Kessler et al., 2011).

Will the real Fawn-Hooded rat please stand up? The Fawn-Hooded rat strain (FH) has been employed as an animal model of anxiety, but there are many complications associated with this strain. The foundation breeding stock for FH rats included a mixture of German Brown, Lashley albino, and Long-Evans rats, and was maintained as an outbred line. These outbred rats were provided to the University of Northern Iowa (FH/Har) and the New York State Department of Health (FH/wjd), where they were inbred over many generations. Another group of rats was dispatched to Erasmus University, where two inbred strains were developed, FH rats with high blood pressure (FHH) and FH rats with low blood pressure (FHL). There are at least three primary strains/lines of FH rats currently in use, and there are clear differences in their behavioral phenotypes, including differences in anxiety-like behaviors and alcohol preferences. In addition, FH rats have been reported to have a number of somatic abnormalities, including a bleeding disorder, proteinuria, high blood pressure, and renal pathology.

One major problem with FH rats is the lack of a simultaneously selected control strain. Some published studies have employed Wistar rats as a control, while others have included Long-Evans rats or Sprague-Dawley rats. Another problem relates to significant behavioral differences between two currently employed inbred strains of FH rats, the FH/Har strain, now maintained at the National Cancer Institute, and the FH/wjd strain, now maintained at the University of North Carolina. In a comparative study, rats of the FH/wjd strain exhibited less struggling in the forced swim test, spent more time in the open arms of an EPM, and voluntarily drank more saccharin and alcohol compared to rats of the FH/Har strain (Overstreet & Rezvani, 1996).

High and low anxiety lines of Sprague-Dawley rats. Stead et al. (2006) selected outbred Sprague-Dawley rats for high (HR) and low (LR) behavioral responses to placement in a novel environment. After only eight generations of selective breeding but without brother-sister mating, there was a 2-fold difference in locomotor behavior in a novel environment between HRs and LRs. A battery of behavioral tests (EPM, light-dark box, open field arena) further revealed that LRs had greater levels of anxiety-like behaviors than HRs.

Maternal effects on anxiety. A cross-fostering experiment examined the impact of the postnatal maternal environment on the development of the anxiety-like phenotype in HRs and LRs tested in adulthood. Cross-fostering had no effect on the behavior of HRs and LRs in an open field arena. In contrast, HR males reared by LR or HR foster mothers spent less time in the open arms of the EPM compared to control HR males. Testing in the light-dark box revealed that LR males reared by HR or LR foster mothers had reduced latencies to enter the light compartment of a light-dark box compared to control LRs. Thus, cross-fostering per se had an effect on the two measures of anxiety, and the results suggested that the behaviors of the foster mothers may have been altered when the strange litters were introduced.

HR and LR mothers also differed in their patterns of maternal behavior, and these differences between lines have in large measure been attributed to geno-typic differences and not early rearing experiences. Compared to LR mothers, HR mothers displayed less engagement with their pups during the dark phase of the light-dark cycle. However, during the light phase of the light-dark cycle, HR mothers were in contact with their litters and engaged in passive nursing to a greater extent than LR mothers. During the dark phase of the light-dark cycle, LR mothers spent more time licking and grooming their pups and engaged in arched-back nursing bouts more frequently than HR mothers (Clinton, 2015; Clinton et al., 2007; 2010).

Brain circuits and anxiety. Significant connections exist between neural circuits that regulate HPA responses to stress and anxiety-like behaviors in Sprague-Dawley rats classified as HR and LR based upon an initial test in a novel environment. HRs were in the top 1/3 of all animals tested for locomotor ac-tivity while LRs were in the lowest 1/3 of all animals tested for locomotor ac-tivity (Kabbaj et al., 2000). When HR rats were placed into a light-dark box for 5 minutes, they displayed marked differences in exploration and had signif-icantly greater increases in plasma levels of CORT compared to LR rats. HRs also exhibited higher levels of CRF mRNA in the PVN but lower levels in the central nucleus of the amygdala. In the hippocampus, HRs had lower levels of GR mRNA but comparable levels of MR mRNA compared to LRs. Intra-hippocampal injections of RU38486 (100 or 200 ng), a GR antagonist, eliminated the strain differences in behaviors in the light-dark box such that LRs behaved more like HRs. These results forged a connection between stress circuits in the brain and anxiety-like behaviors, and raised the possibility that hippocampal GRs may contribute in part to the strain differences in anxiety-like responses to novel environments (Kabbaj et al., 2000).

Genes and anxiety. Building upon these initial studies, Cohen et al. (2015) examined developmental patterns of gene expression in the hippocampus and amygdala and anxiety-like behaviors of LR pups reared by their biolog-ical mothers or by LR or HR foster mothers. LRs reared by HR foster mothers exhibited a developmental shift in gene expression in the amygdala but not the hippocampus, as well as reductions in anxiety-like behaviors and enhanced patterns of social interactions in adulthood. These findings, when combined with earlier studies from this laboratory, point to critical differences in the hippocampus and the amygdala of LRs that may explain their elevated levels of anxiety-like behaviors.

Further experiments focused on the role of hippocampal gene expression on adult levels of anxiety-like behaviors in HR and LR rats. Initial experiments demonstrated that hippocampal expression of fibroblast growth factor-2 (FGF2) was elevated in low-anxiety HRs compared to high-anxiety LRs. In addition, environmental enrichment for 3 weeks increased expression of hippocampal FGF2 and reduced anxiety-like behaviors to a greater extent in LRs compared to HRs. Chronic daily administration of FGF2 via i.p. injections for 3 weeks also reduced anxiety-like behaviors and enhanced survival of adult-born neurons and glial cells in the hippocampus (Perez et al., 2009).

The role of FGF2 during development was assessed in HR and LR rats. On the day after birth, HR and LR pups were injected with FGF2 or vehicle (s.c.). In adulthood, LRs that received neonatal FGF2 exhibited decreased anxiety-like behaviors, had increased numbers of neurons in the dentate gyrus, and altered expression of 226 gene transcripts in the dentate gyrus. Of these, two were selected for further study. Levels of expression of neurotrophin tyrosine kinase receptor 3 (*ntrk3*) and glucose-1-phosphate thymidylyltransferase (*bc1212*) were elevated significantly in the dentate gyrus of FGF2-injected LRs compared to vehicle-injected LRs. Both genes promote the survival of post-mitotic neurons, and *ntrk3* has been shown to exert anti-anxiety effects (Turner et al., 2011; Turner et al., 2012).

Taken together, these exciting findings and related research point to FGF2 as a modulator of stress responsiveness and anxiety-like behaviors. FGF2 exerts a profound effect on the developing hippocampus of animals with an anxiety-prone genotype, and it can also alter behaviors and gene expression in these adult animals when administered peripherally. Related research by Salmaso et al. (2016) on FGF2 knockout (KO) mice suggested that GR was necessary for the anxiety-reducing effects of FGF2. This body of research expands the array of potential new molecular targets for the treatment of anxiety disorders (Turner et al., 2016).

Maternal Environment and Development of Anxiety-Like Behaviors

Prenatal Stress

Prenatal restraint stress (PS, 45 minutes × 3 times per day from GDs 14 to 21) was employed by Barros et al. (2006) to induce anxiety in offspring. Control pregnant females remained undisturbed in their home cages. Soon after birth, litters of control and PS mothers were assigned to 1 of 3 groups: (i) controls: reared by the biological mother; (ii) in-fostered: reared by a foster mother of the same treatment group; or (ii) cross-fostered: reared by a foster mother of the opposite group. Weaning occurred on PND 21 and male offspring were studied beginning at 90 days of age. Offspring of control mothers spent significantly more time in the open arms of an EPM and had a greater number of open-arm entries compared to offspring of prenatally stressed mothers. In addition, benzodiazepine (BDZ) binding sites were reduced significantly in the CA1, CA3, and dentate gyrus areas of the hippocampus as well as the central nucleus of the amygdala.

When offspring of control mothers were reared by PS foster mothers, they had a significant decrease in open-arm entries compared to in-fostered controls. Open-arm entries did not differ between offspring of PS mothers reared by control foster mothers versus in-fostered controls. BDZ binding sites did not correspond well to the behavioral changes in the EPM for in-fostered and cross-fostered PS and control offspring (Barros et al., 2006).

Strain Differences in Response to a Novel Environment

Chronic social instability (twice weekly reconstitution of social groups of 4 CD-1 mice per cage for 2 months beginning at 27 days of age) is an experimental manipulation that produced a phenotype characterized by anxiety-like behaviors and decreases in social interactions with conspecifics. These behavioral alterations were also transmitted across generations. To examine the role of the postnatal maternal environment on the development of anxiety-like behaviors, Saavedra-Rodríguez and Feig (2013) reciprocally cross-fostered litters soon after birth between mothers that were previously exposed to social stress or mothers that were housed in stable social groups. The results of this experiment revealed that the maternal environment did not influence the transmission of anxiety-like behaviors in the F1 generation. Specifically, offspring of socially stressed mothers that were reared by control foster mothers still exhibited an anxiety-like phenotype based upon their behaviors in an EPM, an open field test, and a social interaction test. Similarly, offspring of control females reared by socially stressed mothers did not exhibit anxiety-like behaviors when tested in adulthood.

LG-ABN in Long-Evans Rats

A novel approach to linking the early maternal environment with the development of anxiety in offspring is by taking advantage of naturally occurring differences in maternal behaviors of female Long-Evans hooded rats (Caldji et al., 1998; Liu et al., 1997). Among these differences are frequency of licking and grooming of pups and arched-back nursing episodes by mothers (LG-ABN). Two groups of lactating females were designated as high LG-ABN (above the mean for the group) or low LG-ABN (below the mean for the group) based upon observations during the first 10 days following birth of the litters. Male offspring from the two groups of mothers were tested in adulthood on several behavioral tasks, blood samples were collected during and after exposure to stress, and brains were analyzed for changes in areas related to fear and anxiety.

Offspring of high LG-ABN mothers had lower plasma levels of ACTH and CORT in response to restraint stress. In addition, levels of CRF mRNA were significantly reduced in the PVN of high LG-ABN offspring. GR mRNA levels were significantly higher in the hippocampus of high LG-ABN offspring. The hippocampus is an important brain area involved in negative feedback regulation of the HPA axis. Adult offspring of high LG-ABN mothers also exhibited less fearfulness in an open field arena (i.e., increased activity) and had reduced latencies to begin eating in a strange environment compared to offspring of low LG-ABN mothers. In studies of the fear circuits of the brain, BDZ receptor density was greater in several nuclei of the amygdala and in the locus coeruleus of high LG-ABN offspring. Also, α_2-adrenergic receptor density was higher and CRF receptor density was lower in the locus coeruleus of adult offspring of high LG-ABN mothers. These results are consistent with an anxiogenic effect of CRF projections from the amygdala to the locus coeruleus, as well as an anxiolytic effect of BDZs in the amygdala. Taken together, the results of these two studies provide convincing evidence that naturally occurring differences in maternal care over the first 10 days of postnatal life program later stress and anxiety responses in adult offspring by alterations in brain systems that regulate the HPA axis and fear responses. Further, these programmed changes endure well into adulthood (Caldji et al., 1998; Liu et al., 1997).

In an extension of these studies, van Hasselt et al. (2012a) focused on individual litters and recorded differences between littermates in levels of licking and grooming (LG) received from their mothers. Surprisingly, maternal LG scores for pups in a single litter varied over a wide range. LG scores correlated positively with levels of GR mRNA in the adult hippocampus (van Hasselt et al., 2012b), less anxiety-like behavior, and improved cognitive function (van Hasselt et al., 2012c). In males but not females, LG scores also correlated positively with total apical dendrite branch length and dendritic complexity (van Hasselt et al., 2011).

C57BL/6 and Balb/c Mice

In an elegant experiment with C57BL/6 and Balb/c inbred mice, Francis et al. (2003) employed embryo transfer and/or cross-fostering of C57BL/6 mice to either Balb/c or C57BL/6 foster mothers to generate four experimental groups based upon prenatal environment → postnatal environment: (i) C57BL/6 → C57BL/6; (ii) C57BL/6 → Balb/c; (iii) Balb/c → Balb/c; and (iv) Balb/c → C57BL/6. Strain differences in behaviors in the open field, EPM, and Morris water maze were established with adult male C57BL/6 and Balb/c mice. C57BL/6 mice from the following three experimental groups were similar to control C57BL/6 mice in their behavioral profiles: C57BL/6 → C57BL/6; C57BL/6 → Balb/c; and Balb/c → C57BL/6. In contrast, C57BL/6 mice that developed in a Balb/c uterine environment *and* were nursed by a Balb/c foster mother from birth to weaning (Balb/c → Balb/c) displayed a behavioral profile that matched with Balb/c controls. Unfortunately, Balb/c mice were not exposed to the various prenatal/postnatal environmental conditions to determine if they would respond in a manner similar to C57BL/6 prenatal + postnatal environments. The authors suggested that the prenatal environment may in some manner prime the developing fetus to respond to specific elements of postnatal maternal care, resulting in a characteristic behavioral phenotype (Francis et al., 2003).

In a subsequent study using the C57BL/6 and Balb/c strains, Priebe et al. (2005) found that C57BL/6 mothers engaged in significantly more LG-ABN, while Balb/c mothers spent significantly more time away from the nest. Open field and EPM tests revealed that C57BL/6 mice exhibited less anxiety-like behaviors compared to Balb/c mice (e.g., more active in the center squares of the open field arena and higher ratio of entries into the open arms of the EPM). Balb/c mice had higher plasma levels of CORT immediately following a 30-minute restraint stress bout compared to C57BL/6 mice. Basal plasma levels of CORT and levels at 30 and 60 minutes post-restraint were similar between mice of the two strains.

To explore the role of the maternal environment in programming these strain differences in behavior and CORT responses to acute stress, litters of C57BL/6 and Balb/c mice were in-fostered to a mother of the same strain or cross-fostered to a mother of the opposite strain within 1 day following birth. Mice were weaned at 21 days of age and males were studied in adulthood. Observations of maternal behavior revealed that foster-rearing of litters of the same or opposite strain did not alter the significant strain differences in maternal behaviors as determined in the first part of the experiment. In an open field test, C57BL/6 mice reared by Balb/c foster mothers spent significantly less time in the center squares compared to C57BL/6 mice reared by C57BL/6 foster mothers. In the EPM, Balb/c mice reared by a C57BL/6 foster mother had a greater ratio of open-arm entries to total arm entries compared to Balb/c mice reared by Balb/c foster mothers. Basal levels of plasma CORT were higher in cross-fostered C57BL/6 mice compared to in-fostered C57BL/6 mice. Restraint-stress induced levels of plasma CORT were not affected by cross-fostering in either strain. These results clearly point to a gene x maternal environment interaction in affecting strain differences in anxiety-like behaviors and stress responses in these two inbred strains of mice (Priebe et al., 2005).

LPS and Anxiety

Building upon earlier studies in their laboratory, Walker et al. (2012) employed neonatal injections of lipopolysaccharide (LPS) to male and female Wistar rats on PNDs 3 and 5 to induce anxiety-like behaviors when the animals were tested in adulthood. LPS-treated males and females were then bred with untreated mates, and their offspring were evaluated for anxiety-like behaviors in adulthood. The adult offspring of LPS-treated females displayed anxiety-like behaviors and had enhanced plasma CORT responses to acute restraint stress. Adult offspring of LPS-treated males also displayed anxiety-related behaviors, but did not have elevated plasma CORT responses to acute restraint stress. Observations of maternal behaviors revealed that LPS-treated mothers had lower scores for LG-ABN but higher scores for blanket nursing of pups. In addition, LPS-treated females had higher scores for non-pup-directed behaviors.

To assess how differences in maternal behaviors affected the development of anxiety in adulthood, litters of LPS-treated females were reciprocally cross-fostered with saline-treated females soon after birth. Offspring of LPS-treated females that were reared by saline-treated foster mothers had reductions in plasma levels of CORT following acute restraint stress and reductions in anxiety-like behaviors. The opposite was true of offspring of saline-treated females reared by LPS-treated females; the phenotype of these animals matched with the anxiety profile of LPS-treated animals.

The offspring of LPS-treated males also displayed an anxiety-like phenotype, but this was not explained by patterns of maternal behavior. The authors suggested that neonatal LPS treatment may have altered the methylation status of male gametes, thus providing a means for trans-generational transmission of an anxiety-like phenotype (Walker et al., 2012).

Risk Genes for Anxiety

5-HT$_{1A}$ Receptors

One approach to the study of anxiety disorders using animal models has involved experiments with 5-HT$_{1A}$ receptor KO mice (Akimova et al., 2009). 5-HT$_{1A}$ receptors are expressed in two distinct neuronal populations in the brain: autoreceptors on serotonin-containing neurons of the raphe nuclei, and postsynaptic receptors on non-serotonin-containing neurons of the hippo-campus, septum, and cerebral cortex. Activation of both receptor populations results in membrane hyperpolarization and decreased neuronal excitability.

An early study by Ramboz et al. (1998) examined the anxiety-like behaviors of KO mice[(-/-)] and heterozygotes[(+/-)] compared to WT controls[(+/+)]. They re-ported that KO mice displayed lower levels of exploratory activity and increased aversion to open spaces (i.e., open field and open arms of EPM) while having decreased immobility in a forced swim test. In most cases, heterozygotes were in-termediate in behavioral measures between WT and KO mice. The investigators argued for a link between 5-HT_{1A} receptors and the development of an anxiety-like phenotype.

Building upon these initial results, this same laboratory employed a more targeted approach anatomically to eliminating 5HT_{1A} receptors and examining the effects on anxiety-like behaviors (Gross et al., 2002). Using a tissue-specific, conditional rescue strategy, these researchers were able to generate transgenic mice that had near-normal patterns of 5-HT_{1A} receptor binding in the hippo-campus and cerebral cortex, but lacked expression of 5-HT_{1A} receptors in the raphe nuclei. The transgenic mice expressing 5-HT_{1A} in the cerebral cortex and hippocampus were indistinguishable from WT control mice, but differed signifi-cantly from 5-HT_{1A} KO mice in displaying less anxiety-like behaviors in an EPM, open field arena, and a novelty-suppressed feeding task.

Also addressed was how the 5-HT_{1A} receptor exerts its anti-anxiety effect over the course of postnatal development. If forebrain 5-HT_{1A} receptors were not expressed during embryonic development and extended through weaning at PND 21, then anxiety-like behaviors were similar to 5-HT_{1A} KO mice. In con-trast, if forebrain 5-HT_{1A} receptor expression occurred during embryonic devel-opment and continued through weaning on PND 21, then anxiety-like behaviors were similar to WT mice. Additional experiments pointed to the period between PNDs 5 and 21 as the time when expression of forebrain 5-HT_{1A} receptors were related to the development of forebrain circuits essential for the appearance of WT levels of anxiety-like behaviors in adult mice (Gross et al., 2002).

Gleason et al. (2010, 2011), in a remarkable series of experiments, combined embryo transfers and postnatal cross-fostering between wild-type (WT) and 5-HT_{1A} KO mothers to evaluate prenatal and postnatal maternal contributions to anxiety-like behaviors (e.g., EPM, open field test, forced swim test). Cross-fostering WT litters to 5-HT_{1A} KO foster mothers resulted in a partial anxiety-like phenotype. However, cross-fostering 5-HT_{1A} KO litters to WT foster mothers did not affect development of the anxiety-like phenotype. Surprisingly, WT embryos implanted in 5-HT_{1A} KO females and then cross-fostered to WT foster mothers exhibited a pronounced anxiety-like phenotype. These results were consistent with a dual-risk model of 5-HT$_{1A}$ receptor defects, involving genetic and non-genetic modes of transmission. The abnormalities in behavior associated with nongenetic transmission may have been linked with developmental delays in the dentate gyrus due to effects of the 5-HT$_{1A}$ KO uterine environment alone.

5-HT Transporter (5-HTTP)

Anxiety-like behaviors, including EPM, open field behavior, novelty-suppressed feeding, and latency to emerge from the home cage, were studied in male and female 5-HTTP KO laboratory rats and compared to behaviors of male and female WT rats (Olivier et al., 2008). Compared to WT rats, 5-HTTP KO rats spent significantly less time in the central portion of an open field arena, spent significantly less time in the open arms of an EPM, exhibited a significantly longer latency to begin eating in the novelty-suppressed feeding task, and had dramatically higher levels of 5-HT in the hippocampus as measured by microdialysis. The majority of these effects were consistent across male and female 5-HTTP KO rats. Similar anxiety-like behavioral profiles have been reported for male and female 5-HTTP KO mice compared to their WT controls (Holmes et al., 2003).

Manipulations of CRF Signaling

Selective CRF deletion. CRF signaling in the brain has been implicated in the regulation of stress responses and in anxiety-like phenotypes in various animal models (Bakshi & Kalin, 2000). Zhang et al. (2017) took a creative approach to selectively deplete CRF from the PVN and determine the effects on neuroendocrine regulation and anxiety-like behaviors. They created *Sim1Crf* KO mice on a C57BL/6 background by taking advantage of the fact that expression of the transcription factor, *Sim1*, is required for normal development of the supraoptic nucleus and the PVN (Duplan et al., 2009). In the PVN, *Crf* expression was almost completely eliminated in *Sim1Crf* KO mice but was largely unaffected in other brain areas, including the amygdala, cerebral cortex, and hippocampus. This highly targeted genetic manipulation, combined with delivery of CORT in the drinking water of pregnant females carrying the KO fetuses, normalized fetal lung development and allowed a focused examination of the role of PVN *Crf* expression on neuroendocrine regulation and behavioral responses to acute stress in adult animals.

Sim1Crf KO male mice displayed atrophy of the adrenal glands as well as dramatic decreases in basal and restraint stress-induced increases in CORT and basal levels of ACTH. In addition, these same mice displayed significant reductions in anxiety-like behaviors when tested in an open field arena, an EPM, a hole-board apparatus, a light-dark box, and a novel object recognition test relative to controls (WT, heterozygous *Sim1Crf* WT, or homozygous *Crf*flox male mice, depending on the experiment). In addition, CORT supplementation did not alter the anxiolytic behavioral pattern of *Sim1Crf* KO mice. These findings confirm a causal link between the stress-responsive CRF system in the PVN and the regulation of anxiety-like behaviors (Zhang et al., 2017).

CRF$_1$ receptor (CRFR1) and CRFR2 double-mutant mice. Bale et al. (2002) successfully generated double-mutant mice for *Crfr1* and *Crfr2* by crossing null mutant *Crfr2* female mice with null mutant *Crfr1* male mice. The resulting F1 offspring, which were heterozygous for both genes, were crossed to yield offspring that included control mice, *Crfr1* mutant mice, *Crfr2* mutant mice, and double-mutant mice. If the mother was homozygous or heterozygous for the *Crfr2* mutation, her male but not female pups, regardless of genotype, displayed significantly higher levels of anxiety-like behavior during testing on an EPM. In contrast to these effects, *Crfr1* mothers did not affect the anxiety-like behaviors of their pups. Finally, the genotype of the father did not affect anxiety-like behaviors of the offspring.

CRF and the locus coeruleus. NE neurons of the locus coeruleus (LC-NE) are highly sensitive to stressful stimulation and play an essential role in the development of anxiety-like behaviors. McCall et al. (2015) employed a variety of techniques to demonstrate that tonic activity of LC-NE neurons is necessary and sufficient for the development of restraint stress-induced anxiety-like behaviors. Chemogenetic inhibition of LC-NE neurons blocked the development of anxiety-like behaviors following restraint stress, whereas optogenetically controlled increases in tonic LC-NE neuronal activity in the absence of stress still enhanced anxiety-like behaviors. CRF neurons that project from the central nucleus of the amygdala to the LC drive tonic LC neuronal activity by signaling through CRFR1, which increases anxiety-like behaviors.

Urocortin-1 and -2 signaling. The urocortins 1–3 are members of the family of neuropeptides that includes CRF. All three urocortins are endogenous ligands for CRFR2, and they appear to have a role in regulation of the HPA axis and serotonergic activity in the dorsal raphe nucleus. Urocortin-1 and -2 double-deficient (dKO) mice were generated to study the involvement of these peptides in adaptation to stress. Compared to WT controls, dKO male and female mice spent significantly more time in the open arms of an EPM and spent more time in the central portion of an open field arena. In addition, dKO mice displayed lower levels of anxiety-like behaviors immediately following exposure to restraint stress for 30 minutes compared to WT controls. dKO mice also displayed elevated CORT responses following acute restraint stress and had higher levels of CRF expression in the PVN. Finally, dKO mice had elevated levels of 5-HT and its metabolite, 5-HIAA, in areas of the brain receiving projections from the dorsal raphe nucleus, including the basolateral nucleus of the amygdala, lateral entorhinal cortex, and the CA1 area of the hippocampus. These results point to a relationship between CRFR2 signaling and an anxiolytic phenotype (Neufeld-Cohen et al., 2010).

In an earlier series of experiments with CRFR2 KO mice, Bale et al. (2000) reported that mice lacking CRFR2 receptors had enhanced HPA responsivity to acute restraint stress and greater levels of anxiety-like behaviors based upon testing in an EPM and an open field arena. The discrepancy between the findings of Neufeld et al. (2010) versus those of Bale et al. (2000) may be explained by higher expression of CRF mRNA in the central nucleus of the amygdala of CRFR2 KO mice relative to dKO mice (Neufeld-Cohen et al., 2010).

Neuropeptide Y (NPY)

NPY is a 36-amino acid peptide that is widely distributed in the central nervous system and plays a key role in emotionality and adaptation to stressful stimulation (Sabban et al., 2016). A range of studies provides a compelling connection between adaptive responses to stress and anxiolytic effects of NPY acting at Y1 and Y5 receptors. For example, central administration of NPY exerts anti-anxiety effects when animals were tested in several different paradigms, including an EPM, a light-dark box, fear-potentiated startle, a social interaction test, the Vogel test, and the Geller-Seifter test. These anti-anxiety effects of NPY appeared to be mediated in large part by binding of NPY to Y1 receptors. In addition, central administration of the nonpeptide selective Y1 antagonists, BIBP3226 and BIBO3304, increased anxiety-like behaviors, and also blocked the anxiolytic effects of exogenously administered NPY (for a review, see Heilig, 2004).

Another facet of NPY signaling in the brain is the presence of presynaptic Y2 receptors, which regulate the release of endogenous NPY. Redrobe et al. (2003) assessed the effects in Y2 receptor KO mice of testing in an EPM and an open field arena. Compared to WT mice, Y2 KO mice spend significantly more time in the open arms of an EPM and the central portion of the open field arena. To increase the anatomical precision of the Y2 receptor-mediated effects on anxiety-like behavior, Tasan et al. (2010) ablated the Y2 gene in the basolateral and central nuclei of the amygdala, and this manipulation was associated with a reduction in levels of anxiety-like behaviors. In contrast, ablation of Y2 receptors in the medial amygdala or the BNST was without effect. Taken together, these two reports indicate that NPY acts at presynaptic Y2 receptors to inhibit release of NPY and/or GABA from interneurons and/or projection neurons of the basolateral and central nuclei of the amygdala.

To assess the role of NPY Y1 receptors in the limbic forebrain, conditional Y1 KO mice were generated such that inactivation of the *Npy1r* gene was in full effect after weaning and was limited to excitatory neurons. Compared to appropriate groups of control mice, Y1 KO male mice reared by FVB/J foster mothers exhibited greater body weight gain beginning on PND 6 and increased anxiety-like behaviors during testing in an EPM and an open field arena. In addition, FVB/J-reared Y1 KO mice had higher basal levels of plasma CORT and elevated expression of CRF and NPY in the PVN.

These striking neural and behavioral differences between Y1 KO mice and controls were not apparent when litters were reared by C57BL/6J foster mothers. FVB/J foster mothers engaged more frequently in arched-back nursing postures compared to C57BL/6J foster mothers, and these differences in maternal behaviors are known to influence regulation of the HPA axis response to stress as well as behavioral characteristics in the offspring (Meaney & Szyf, 2005b). These results pointed to limbic Y1 receptors as targets of maternal care-induced programming of offspring stress and anxiety responses (Bertocchi et al., 2011).

A more recent study from this same research group included a refinement of their experimental approach by adopting a strategy of conditional inactivation of Y1 receptors in Y5 receptor-expressing neurons. These more targeted Y1 KO mice displayed increased anxiety-like behaviors but no changes in regulation of the HPA axis or in growth rates. Importantly, these alterations were independent of the strain of foster mother, as mice reared by C57BL/6J or FVB/J foster mothers displayed similar phenotypes. Finally, a key conclusion of this series of experiments was that GABAergic interneurons in the basolateral amygdala that co-express Y1 and Y5 receptors appeared to play a critical role in regulation of anxiety (Longo et al., 2014).

Neuropeptide S

Dealing with an orphan receptor is like having a lock but not knowing which of many keys to use. The superfamily of G protein-coupled receptors includes more than 800 seven-transmembrane domain receptors, and the endogenous ligands have as yet not been identified for more than 100. These receptors are referred to as *orphan receptors* until the endogenous ligand is identified (Tang et al., 2012).

Discovery of NPS. Xu et al. (2004) described a series of experiments on an orphan receptor and its newly discovered endogenous peptide ligand, neuropeptide S (NPS). NPS, a 20-amino acid peptide, and the mRNA for its receptor (NPSR1) were found in the brain as well as peripheral tissues. In the brain, expression of NPS mRNA was localized to a cluster of cell bodies that was interposed between Barrington's nucleus (primarily CRF-expressing neurons) and noradrenergic cell bodies of the locus coeruleus (LC). A more detailed neuro-anatomical study (Xu et al., 2007) revealed that the majority of NPS-positive neurons in the LC area were glutamatergic, whereas the NPS-positive neurons in the vicinity of the lateral parabrachial nucleus co-expressed CRF. NPSR1 mRNA was highly expressed in several brain areas involved in anxiety and stress responses, including the amygdala, PVN, raphe nuclei, posterior paraventricular nucleus of the thalamus, ventral tegmental area, and hippocampus.

Central effects of NPS. Intracerebroventricular (i.c.v.) administration of NPS in C57BL/6 mice at a dose of 0.01, 0.1, or 1.0 nmol resulted in increased wake-fulness, enhanced locomotor activity, and decreased anxiety-like behaviors. With regard to its anxiolytic properties, i.c.v. administration of NPS increased time spent in the open arms of an EPM, increased center zone entries and total activity in the outer zones of an open field arena, increased time spent in the light portion of a light-dark box, and decreased burying of marbles. Each of these behavioral changes was consistent with an anxiolytic effect of NPS (Xu et al., 2004).

Experiments by Smith et al. (2006) revealed that administration of NPS into the third ventricle or directly into the PVN resulted in significant increases in plasma levels of ACTH and CORT. Using in vitro studies of hypothalamic explants, these investigators demonstrated that administration of NPS selec-tively stimulated the co-release of CRF and AVP from PVN neurons. In contrast, NPS failed to stimulate release of ACTH from fragments of anterior pituitary, indicating lack of a direct effect of NPS on the anterior pituitary gland.

These results have been replicated and extended by a number of other labo-ratories. Npsr1 KO mice provided further evidence of anxiolytic effects of cen-tral NPS circuits (Duangdao et al., 2009; Ruzza et al., 2012). In addition, NPS was quite effective in reducing anxiety-like behaviors when administered i.c.v. or intra-nasally in laboratory rats (Lukas & Neumann, 2012) and in reducing fear-potentiated startle in mice when injected directly into the amygdala (Fendt et al., 2010).

NPS circuitry also appears to play a role in neural and neuroimmune adaptations to acute stressors. For example, brainstem NPS neurons were acti-vated in response to acute immobilization stress-induced local release of CRF (Jüngling et al., 2012). In comparing the responses of WT and Npsr1 KO mice to acute immobilization stress, Donner et al. (2010) noted that plasma CORT responses to 1 hour of immobilization stress did not differ between WT and Npsr1 KO mice. Compared to Npsr1 KO mice, WT mice exhibited greater stress-induced expression of NPSR1 in the cerebral cortex and neurotrophin-3 in the cerebral cortex and striatum. In contrast, stress-induced expression of IL-1β was greater in the cerebral cortex and hypothalamus of Npsr1 KO mice compared to WT controls.

NPS and anxious mice and rats. The high-anxiety lines of mice and rats that were described in the preceding provided an interesting platform for evaluating the effects of NPS circuits on anxiety-like behaviors. In an extensive series of experiments, Slattery et al. (2015) reported that basal *Npsr1* expression was reduced significantly in the PVN of rHABs versus rLABs and in the basolateral amygdala of mHABs versus mLABs. Basal *Nps* expression was elevated in the LC of rHABs relative to rLABs, but there were no differences in this measure between mice of the two lines. Further studies indicated that a single nucleotide polymorphism (SNP) in the exonal region increased NPSR1 signal transduction following administration of the NPS ligand in the HAB lines of rats and mice. This alteration counteracted the effects of SNPs in the promoter region of *Npsr1* that caused transcriptional inhibition. A critical set of experiments revealed that i.c.v. administration of NPS reduced significantly levels of anxiety-like behaviors in the HAB lines of mice and rats, as well as impaired cued-fear extinction in rHABs and enhanced fear expression in mHABs relative to their respective LAB control lines.

Clinical studies of NPS. Not surprisingly, notice was taken of the discovery of NPS by psychiatrists involved in clinical research on anxiety disorders. Building on early studies that identified *Npsr1* as a risk gene for asthma (Laitinen et al., 2004), Donner et al. (2010) were among the first to report an association between asthma and anxiety in studies of two population-based cohorts. In addition, SNPs within the genes coding for *Nps* and *Npsr1* associated significantly with diagnoses of panic disorder in two adult samples and with parent-reported levels of anxiety/depression in a birth cohort of Swedish children.

Rapid progress has been made in studying the impact of SNPs associated with *Npsr1* on anxiety symptoms in humans. For example, the locus for *Npsr1* has been mapped to a chromosomal region that has consistently been associated with panic disorder (Logue et al., 2003). The frequently encountered Asn[107]Ile variant of *Npsr1*, stemming from an A → T single nucleotide polymorphism, resulted in a dramatic 10-fold greater efficacy of NPS signaling in vitro, as reported by Reinscheid et al (2005). Raczka et al. (2010) exposed healthy volunteers, some of whom were carriers of the *Npsr1* variant, to a classical fear conditioning paradigm. Carriers of the *Npsr1* variant (AT and TT) rated their fear reactions to conditioned stimuli (painful electric shocks) as more intense than non-carriers (AA) in spite of the fact that their skin conductance responses were similar. In addition, carriers of the *Npsr1* variant displayed more pronounced activation of the rostral portion of the dorsomedial PFC following exposure to electric shocks. This cortical area has been linked to appraisal of threatening stimuli. These findings were interpreted as evidence of a causal link between the Asn[107]Ile polymorphism and panic disorder (Raczka et al., 2010).

In a related study, investigators combined several German clinical populations totaling 766 patients with panic disorder and other comorbidities, including agoraphobia and depression, and an equal number of controls. In this combined sample, there was a significant association of the T risk allele for *Npsr1* with female but not male patients with panic disorder. In a subset of these patients, the anxiety sensitivity score was significantly higher in female but not male patients with the T risk allele versus those without the T risk allele. During a behavioral avoidance task, carriers of the T risk allele had elevated heart rates throughout the test procedure and higher symptom reports during confinement in a closed chamber. Finally, carriers of the T risk allele exhibited diminished activation in the dorsolateral prefrontal, lateral orbitofrontal, and anterior cingulate cortex in response to presentation of fearful faces versus no faces as the control. Activation of the amygdala was similar in patients with an AA genotype versus carriers of the T risk allele (Domschke et al., 2011).

In a further study of the *Npsr1* risk allele, Laas et al. (2014) reported that females but not males with the least active AA genotype combined with prior exposure to stressful life events had a higher incidence of affective and anxiety disorders and more self-reported suicidal behaviors compared to individuals with the AT or TT genotypes. These findings, while consistent with studies in animal models, are clearly at odds with the prior two reports on panic disorder using clinical samples. However, Laas et al. (2014) did not focus on panic disorder, and were more concerned with a broad spectrum of affective and anxiety disorders, and patients with a diagnosis of panic disorder represented a very small percentage of the total study sample. An explanation advanced by Domschke et al. (2010) to explain these conflicting findings was that panic disorder in humans is associated with an increased level of arousal, which in animal models results from increased NPS activity. Increased arousal associated with the more active T allele was also consistent with the report described earlier of NPS stimulating the HPA axis and leading to increased arousal in rats (Smith et al., 2006).

NPTX2

Nptx2 encodes one of a family of neuronal activity-regulated pentraxins (also known as NARPs), a group of synaptic proteins that are related to C-reactive protein. NPTX2 plays important roles in the formation of excitatory synapses and the clustering of AMPA-type glutamate receptors. In addition, it is rapidly regulated by neuronal activity and may be involved in neuronal plasticity (Tsui et al., 1996). Chang et al. (2018) explored a possible role for NPTX2 in the regulation of anxiety-like behaviors in genetically modified and control laboratory mice. They reported that conditional knockout of *Nptx2* expression in the hippocampus but not the amygdala was followed by an increase in anxiety-like behaviors, decreased rates of cellular proliferation and the number of new neurons in the dentate gyrus, a greater HPA axis response to acute stress, and increased expression of GR target genes following acute stress. In contrast, over-expression of *Nptx2* in the hippocampus reversed anxiety-like behaviors and alterations in GR-related gene expression. NPTX2 presents yet another potential therapeutic target for treatment of anxiety disorders.

Immune Mechanisms of Anxiety

It's a Two-Way Street

Stressors stimulate peripheral immune activation as well as anxiety-like behaviors in laboratory mice and rats. Several experiments have examined the interactions between stressful stimulation, immune system activation, stress-responsive brain circuits, and the development of anxiety-like behaviors. In their comprehensive review, Wohleb et al. (2015) described the immune → brain and the brain → immune pathways that are activated during chronic exposure to psychological stressors, including chronic social defeat stress. This two-way communication between the brain and the immune system also results in a range of behavioral alterations, among them an increase in anxiety-like behaviors. Following activation of stress-responsive brain circuits, there is an increase in sympathetic-adrenal medullary outflow and HPA axis activity. Elevations in circulating levels of NE, EPI, and CORT signal immune cells in lymphoid tissues, including bone marrow, lymph nodes, and spleen. Under conditions of chronic intermittent stress (e.g., chronic social defeat stress or chronic unpredictable stress), NE signaling in bone marrow results in enhanced production and release of monocytes and granulocytes and a gradual accumulation of these immune cells in the circulation. These monocytes have a phenotype characterized by being less mature and more prone to inflammatory effects as they traffic throughout the body. There is also enhanced proinflammatory transcriptional activity and a corresponding decrease in sensitivity to CORT (Wohleb et al., 2015).

Macrophages and microglia. An important consequence of the stress-induced activation of bone marrow–derived monocytes is their recruitment to inflamed tissues, including the central nervous system. Chronic exposure to stress results in a significant increase in macrophages in close proximity to blood vessels and brain parenchyma, where they are effective at antigen presentation and elicitation of inflammatory responses from brain microglia. Another important response to repeated stress exposure is the infiltration of macrophages into stress-responsive brain areas, which contributes to increases in anxiety-like behaviors. These infiltrating macrophages/monocytes respond to local environmental cues and resemble microglia in their morphology and in the protein markers they express. Cells of the neurovascular unit produce cytokines, chemokines, and cell adhesion molecules that promote the continued infiltration of macrophages into the brain. The associated increase in inflammatory signaling within key brain areas results in the development of recurring bouts of anxiety-like behaviors. There is also evidence that spleen-to-brain monocyte trafficking contributes to stress-sensitization and recurring anxiety (Wohleb et al., 2015) (Figure 11.1).

Cytokines alert the brain. Three experiments from the laboratories of John Sheridan and Jonathan Godbout expand on the involvement of stress-induced increases in immune system to brain signaling and the onset of anxiety-like behaviors. Using chronic social defeat stress in mice as a model, McKim et al. (2018) demonstrated that brain endothelial IL-1β signaling provides a key pathway through which chronic social defeat drives increasing levels of

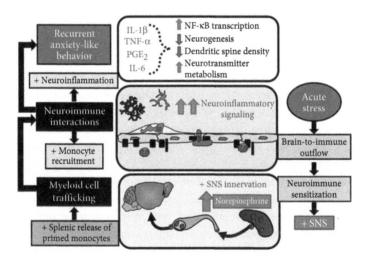

Figure 11.1. Stress-induced neuroimmune sensitization and spleen-to-brain macrophage trafficking after acute stress leads to recurrent anxiety-like behavior. Repeated stress exposure leads to neuroimmune sensitization and redistribution of immature monocyte progenitors in the spleen. Following acute stress, sympathetic nervous system (SNS) activation leads to rapid release of monocytes that traffic to the brain and enhance neuroinflammatory signaling initiated by primed microglia. In these conditions, elevated neuroinflammatory mediators (IL-1β, TNF-α, IL-6, prostaglandins) likely provoke recurrent anxiety-like behavior by reinforcing neurobiological alterations caused by prior stress exposure.

Reproduced from Wohleb et al. (2015) and used with permission of the corresponding author, Dr. Godbout.

anxiety-like behaviors through activation of brain threat appraisal areas, including the prelimbic cortex, central nucleus of the amygdala, and the CA3 region of hippocampus. Further experiments revealed that brain microglia were essential in the process of monocyte recruitment to the brain and for the expression of anxiety-like behaviors.

As a follow-up to these experiments, Niraula et al. (2019) described a critical role for IL-6 signaling in shaping the inflammatory profile of bone marrow–derived monocytes released following chronic social defeat stress that are so critical to the development of anxiety-like behaviors. Behavioral changes and the proinflammatory profile of monocytes recruited to the brain during chronic exposure to social defeat stress were prevented in IL-6 KO mice or in WT mice treated with an antibody to IL-6.

In a third study, Weber et al. (2019) highlighted the long-lasting sensitization of microglia and neurons for up to 24 days following exposure to chronic social defeat stress. Sensitization rendered previously stressed individuals more susceptible to exposure to a stressor at a later time point. For example, 24 days following chronic social defeat stress, mice exposed to an acute episode of defeat displayed monocyte accumulation in the brain and increased anxiety-like behaviors. In addition, administration of LPS to these stress-sensitized mice resulted in microglial activation and the onset of sickness behavior. Further experiments included elimination and repopulation of microglia in mice immediately following exposure to chronic social defeat stress. Repopulation of microglia occurred within 21 days following chronic stress, and exposure to acute social defeat still resulted in monocyte accumulation in the brain and anxiety-like behaviors. However, in mice that experienced microglial elimination and repopulation, the immune response to LPS was attenuated.

Taken together, these three sets of experiments revealed the complex nature of stress sensitization of brain microglia and immune-to-brain communication. Microglia and neurons remain sensitized for at least 24 days and peripheral immune tissues, including bone marrow and spleen, continued to provide activated monocytes that were actively recruited to the brain. Finally, these results underscore the fact that microglia are not required for the occurrence of sensitization but are essential for the expression of stress-induced sensitization (Weber et al., 2019).

Insights from Anxious Monkeys

In a remarkable example of translational psychiatry at its best, Dr. Ned Kalin and his colleagues at the University of Wisconsin at Madison established a nonhuman primate model of childhood anxious temperament to study neural contributions to the development of anxiety-like phenotypes in adulthood (Fox & Kalin, 2014). Their model was based upon observations of children who display behavioral inhibition (BI) or an anxious temperament (AT) at an early age. Up to 50% of children with extreme levels of BI will go on to develop social anxiety disorder (Fox & Kalin, 2014).

Modeling Anxiety in Infant Monkeys

If infant rhesus monkeys (~6–12 months of age) are separated from their mothers and, after a brief period alone, are exposed to a strange human who remains motionless, they display one of two distinct behavioral responses. If a human intruder stares directly at an infant monkey, the infant responds with coo and barking vocalizations. In contrast, if a human intruder does not make direct eye contact with the infant, the infant engages in freezing behavior and often does not emit vocalizations. The freezing behavior is considered highly adaptive given that it is a successful strategy for avoiding detection by predators under naturalistic conditions (Kalin & Shelton, 1989).

Using the no-eye-contact (NEC) paradigm, Kalin et al. have developed a protocol to assess AT in infant monkeys using three distinct measures: extent of freezing behavior, reduction in coo vocalizations, and elevations in circulating levels of CORT. Their studies of laboratory-reared infants and infants in free-ranging social groups on the island of Cayo Santiago established strong connections between children and rhesus infants with extreme AT. Importantly, some rhesus infants with high levels of AT do go on to develop normal social relationships later in life, similar to children with high AT. However, other monkeys with unusually high AT display extreme levels of fearfulness and functional impairments in social behaviors into adulthood, and tend to avoid contact with peers. In monkeys as in humans, the high AT phenotype appears to be ~20%–40% heritable, based in part on a study of 238 young rhesus monkeys from a multigenerational single-family pedigree of 1,500 individuals (Oler et al., 2010).

Brain Circuits and Anxiety

Using ^{18}F-fluoro-deoxyglucose positron emission tomography (FDG-PET), Kalin and his coworkers have identified the neural structures that are critical for the expression of the AT phenotype, including the central nucleus of the amygdala, BNST, hippocampus, anterior temporal pole, and PAG. Increased metabolism in these critical brain areas occurred during stressful situations (NEC paradigm) or when the animals were resting in their home cages. Importantly, these patterns of elevated brain metabolism were stable over repeated measurements and strongly correlated with individual AT scores, consistent with the trait-like nature of AT in young rhesus monkeys (Fox et al., 2012).

In a sample of more than 200 juvenile monkeys, AT was shown to be a variable mixture of the three primary components (e.g., freezing, vocalizations, and CORT levels). CORT levels were weakly correlated with freezing and reductions in vocalizations, while the latter two variables were highly correlated. A critical next step was to examine the degree to which variability in the three principal components of AT in young monkeys was related to specific patterns of brain circuit activation as measured by FDG-PET. The results pointed to a core set of brain areas that were shared among individual monkeys with extremes of AT, and a set of selective brain areas that were associated with specific expressions of the AT phenotype. The core brain areas included the lateral portion of the central nucleus of the amygdala and the anterior hippocampus. The selective brain areas included the lateral anterior hippocampus (CORT response), primary motor cortex (freezing behavior), and ventrolateral PFC (reductions in coo vocalizations), which are essential elements in contributing to the individual expressions of AT.

These results suggested that early interventions in children with AT may be particularly effective in preventing, or at the very least diminishing, the likelihood of later development of an anxiety disorder in adulthood (Shackman et al., 2013). Further experiments with a much larger sample of monkeys from an extended multigenerational pedigree revealed that differences in brain metabolism in the orbital frontal cortex–anterior insular cortex, the extended amygdala, and the PAG formed the critical link between genotype and risk of developing AT and depression (Fox et al., 2015).

In a detailed follow-up study that focused on freezing as a stable measure of BI, 23 rhesus monkeys (mean age = 2.2 years) were selected for further study based upon initial testing of a larger group of 109 rhesus monkeys in three conditions: alone in the home cage, in the NEC paradigm with a human intruder, and presence of a live snake in a transparent enclosed box that had a preferred food item placed on the top of the box. The 23 animals were selected from the extremes of the distribution of freezing behavior scores that were stable across testing. High BI animals averaged 61% time spent freezing, while low BI animals averaged 3% time spent freezing.

Approximately 18 months after initial phenotyping, FDG-PET imaging was performed after each monkey was tested in the alone condition and the NEC condition. The findings revealed increased metabolic activity in the BNST, a key area of the extended amygdala that is involved in defensive responses to diffuse and temporally remote threatening stimuli (Shackman et al., 2017).

Gene Expression and Anxiety

Molecular signatures associated with AT have also been investigated in juvenile rhesus monkeys. In an initial series of experiments, Fox et al. (2012) conducted a transcriptome-wide study of gene expression within the central nucleus of the amygdala 4–5 days following the final exposure of subjects to the NEC paradigm, maximizing the possibility that observed transcriptional changes would reflect trait-like properties rather than residual responses to a threatening test environment. There were 139 transcripts from the central nucleus of the amygdala that predicted AT, reflecting a diverse array of biological processes. In this initial engagement with the data, these investigators focused their attention on neurotrophic tyrosine kinase receptor 3 (*ntrk3*) and insulin receptor substrate 2 (*irs2*), which play a role in cell survival and synaptic plasticity. *Ntrkr3* expression was negatively correlated with AT, but positively correlated with metabolic activity within the central nucleus of the amygdala. In contrast, *ntrk3* expression in motor cortex was unrelated to AT or metabolic rate in the central nucleus of the amygdala. In addition, differentially methylated neural plasticity genes in the central nucleus of the amygdala also predicted AT (Alisch et al., 2014). Based upon these findings, these investigators argued for a neurodevelopmental pathway to the development of AT in rhesus monkeys (Fox et al., 2012).

Polymorphisms in the gene *crfr1* can affect responses to stressful stimuli and risk of anxiety and depression, especially in individuals with a history of exposure to childhood trauma (Binder & Nemeroff, 2010). Using a sample of young rhesus monkeys, Rogers, Raveendran, et al. (2013) identified three SNPs affecting exon 6 of *crfr1* that impacted AT as well as metabolic activity in the anterior hippocampus, amygdala, and selected areas of cerebral cortex. Variations in *crfr1* may interact with childhood trauma or other stressful experiences to influence the development of anxiety and depression. In a related study, overexpression of *crf* in the dorsal amygdala of young monkeys was associated with increases in AT as well as metabolic changes in components of the neural circuitry underlying anxiety (Kalin et al., 2016).

Using similar strategies, Kalin's group (Roseboom et al., 2014) reported a negative correlation between levels of expression of NPY receptor 1 (Y1) and Y5 in the central nucleus of the amygdala and AT. In addition, alterations in expression of Y1 and Y5 were linked to alterations in metabolic activity in components of the anxiety circuitry of the brain, including the dorsolateral PFC and cingulate cortex. These results were consistent with NPY serving a role in promoting resilience (see Chapter 14), and the authors suggested that NPY signaling could be a therapeutic target to prevent the development of anxiety disorders.

In summary, the studies of the NEC model in young rhesus monkeys have provided important insights from the perspective of a nonhuman primate translational model of extreme behavioral inhibition, anxious temperament, and shyness in young children. This phenotypic pattern leads approximately 50% of the time to the onset of social anxiety disorder in the late teenage years. Using a multidisciplinary approach, Kalin and his coworkers have revealed neural circuits and molecular pathways that play a critical role in the development of the AT phenotype. These studies provided an encouraging advance in identifying molecular targets for the treatment of anxiety disorders in children and adults (Fox & Kalin, 2014).

Summary

Experiments with animal models of anxiety are impressive for their breadth as well as their depth. Much of this research hinges on the validity of behavioral paradigms for assessing anxiety in laboratory strains of mice and rats (refer to Table 11.1). Several inbred strains of mice and rats have been developed by selective breeding for many generations, and these models have been utilized in gene x environment studies of anxiety-like behaviors. A particular focus of several laboratories has been on the role of the maternal environment in the development of anxiety-like behaviors.

Another facet of this research area has involved studies of risk genes for anxiety-like behaviors in laboratory mice. Among the risk genes that have been studies are those involved in signaling pathways associated with 5-HT, CRF, NPY, and NPS. In the case of NPS, initial findings in laboratory animals progressed very quickly, and led to clinical studies of genetic variants in receptors for NPS and the potential use of NPS delivered intra-nasally in patients. An added strength of this area of research is the remarkable series of experiments from Kalin's laboratory on the development of anxious temperament in rhesus monkeys. It is rare to have the benefit of a wealth of experimental findings in a nonhuman primate model, as is the case for anxiety research.

Taken together, the animal models described in this chapter have provided important insights into the neural circuitry involved in the regulation of anxiety-like behaviors. These experiments have also identified a wealth of potential new targets for drug development, and now the difficult work begins in evaluating the effectiveness of some of these new treatments.

12

Stress and Depression

Part 1

Much more effort has been devoted to developing animal models of depression over the years compared to any other mental disorder. One could argue that it is much easier to imagine that laboratory animals naturally exhibit symptoms of depression (e.g., reduced social interaction, reduced food intake, reduced interest in pleasurable activities) over the life span compared to symptoms of other mental disorders, such as those associated with schizophrenia or bipolar disorder or autism spectrum disorder. This enhanced effort by basic scientists to model depression in the laboratory also matches well with data on the devastating worldwide impact of depression on disability. In this first of two chapters on depression, I will provide a brief overview of clinical aspects of depression, followed by a consideration of the challenges associated with developing animal models of this disorder. The remainder of the chapter will be taken up with summaries of research findings from genetically selected animal models of depression, as well as animal models based upon exposure to chronic stressors.

Clinical Overview of Major Depressive Disorder (MDD)

Kay Redfield Jamison, a distinguished clinical psychologist in the Department of Psychiatry at The Johns Hopkins Hospital and an award-winning author, is most often associated with her intimate portrait of bipolar disorder, a disorder which she developed while in graduate school. However, her description of the symptoms of depression captures the struggles of so many individuals who suffer from MDD (Jamison, 1996, pp. 217–218).

> Others imply that they know what it is like to be depressed because they have gone through a divorce, lost a job, or broken up with someone. But these experiences carry with them feelings. Depression, instead, is flat, hollow, and unendurable. It is also tiresome. People cannot abide being around you when you are depressed. They might think that they ought to, and they might even try, but you know and they know that you are tedious beyond belief: you are irritable and paranoid and humorless and lifeless and critical and demanding

and no reassurance is ever enough. You're frightened, and you're frightening, and you're "not at all like yourself but will be soon," but you know you won't.

Hippocrates (460–377 BCE) thought that melancholia was caused by an abundance of one of the four humors, black bile. The treatment of choice at that time consisted of purging and removal of blood to reduce the negative impact of black bile. Today, MDD is viewed as a debilitating psychiatric disorder characterized by one or more bouts of depression lasting for at least 2 weeks and resulting in a depressed mood state, lack of interest in pleasurable activities, reduced energy levels, sleep disturbances, decreases in ability to concentrate, feelings of worthlessness, and recurrent thoughts of death and possibly suicidal ideation. Some or all of these symptoms cause great distress and result in impairments in normal functioning at home, at school, and in the workplace.

Howard et al. (2019) combined data from three large-scale GWAS of depression to increase statistical power in their efforts to identify risk gene variants for MDD. They reported 102 independent gene variants, 269 genes, and 15 gene sets associated with depression, including genes and gene pathways involved in synaptic structure and neurotransmission. Supporting evidence of the importance of prefrontal brain regions in depression was provided by an enrichment analysis. In an independent replication sample of more than 1.5 million people, 87 of the original 102 associated gene variants were significant for an effect of MDD following correction for multiple comparisons. Surprisingly, none of the risk variants was associated with serotonin neurons or their postsynaptic receptors.

MDD is moderately heritable (~40%), and there is also evidence that epigenetic alterations play an important role in the pathophysiology of the disorder. Females are about twice as likely to be diagnosed with MDD as males. The lifetime prevalence of MDD is approximately 16%, and it occurs across racial and demographic groups. The median age of onset of a first depressive episode is approximately 25 years, and the peak risk period extends into the 40s. A strong case has been made that life stressors play a critical role in the onset and recurrence of symptoms (refer to Chapter 2), and alterations in the regulation of the HPA axis have been a focus of research over the years (Otte et al., 2016).

MDD is a significant contributor to the global burden of disease based upon estimates of years of life lost to disability (DALYs), and this effect is magnified given that MDD is also associated with higher risks of developing other chronic medical conditions, including Type II diabetes, cardiovascular disease, and obesity. Patients with MDD are also 20 times more likely to die from suicide than individuals in the general population.

Based upon the symptom checklist in *DSM-5*, there are 681 combinations of symptoms that satisfy the *DSM* criteria for a diagnosis of MDD. This observation alone underscores the heterogeneity of this disorder and its associated subtypes (psychotic, melancholic, seasonal, atypical, postpartum, etc.). Add to this the fact that some depressive symptoms are also characteristic of other psychiatric disorders, including anxiety disorders, schizophrenia, and bipolar disorder.

In spite of the worldwide negative impact of MDD on human health, the current outlook for treatment options for MDD is anything but encouraging (Wong & Licinio, 2001). Up to 50% of patients diagnosed with MDD do not respond favorably to currently available psychological and pharmacological interventions. In addition, the approach taken by psychiatrists to develop treatment plans for many patients remains one of trial and error. Even though more than 40 years have passed since the introduction of the first antidepressants, we still do not have reliable biomarkers to guide drug selection and many patients develop resistance to medications over time (Akil et al., 2018).

Is Depression an Adaptive Trait?

Given the very high incidence of MDD in the population, it strikes me as logical to ask why a mental disorder that has such a life-altering impact on individuals and their loved ones could persist in the population. Shouldn't there be strong selection pressure against the genetic contributions to the behavioral traits associated with MDD? (Recall that a similar question was posed in Chapters 8 and 10 in relation to the relatively high incidence of schizophrenia and bipolar disorder, respectively, in the population.) While it is true that depression is only modestly heritable (~40%), there is substantial evidence that other factors also contribute to the etiology of this disorder, including environmental stressors acting upon a susceptible genotype, as well as epigenetic changes in DNA or histone proteins. Could the sum total of these biological and environmental contributions to MDD be viewed through an evolutionary lens such that the resulting behavioral characteristics might confer an adaptive advantage under certain circumstances?

In dealing with the possible adaptive advantages of depression, most evolutionary analyses begin by separating out depressive mood states from MDD. However, there is not a bright line between the transition from a low mood state to MDD, and this difficulty further complicates such an approach (Hagen, 2011; Nesse, 2000). In tackling this subject matter, we are also delving deeply into the realm of "thought experiments," as many of these hypotheses regarding adaptive advantages of depressed mood cannot be tested directly, only bolstered by indirect evidence. Given the prevalence of risk genes for depression (Wray et al., 2018), it would appear that these genes confer net benefits within the population. Such benefits could result from two different processes. In the first, the depression phenotype could have conveyed adaptive advantages in spite of its obvious costs to the depressed individual. Second, risk genes for depression may have conferred adaptive advantages through pleiotropic effects on other advantageous traits that outweighed the disadvantages of depression.

Theories of Depression

Socially based theories. Several theories relating to the adaptive advantages of MDD have been advanced and often revolve around the costs and benefits of social interactions (Hagen, 2011). The *social competition hypothesis* emphasizes submission and posits that an individual will display submissive behaviors toward higher ranking individuals, and in so doing will adopt a sense of powerlessness, thereby inhibiting further aggression originating from those of higher rank. The *social risk hypothesis* argues that those individuals who are not adept at forming and maintaining social relationships are less likely to engage in social risk-taking. Such individuals perceive themselves as having low social value, are very sensitive to social threats, and expect to experience failure in their social interactions. The *psychic pain hypothesis* suggests that sadness and generally low affect are adaptive responses to conditions of social adversity. The *situation-symptom congruence hypothesis* advances a more finely tuned system of affective responses to a variety of challenges. For example, sadness and crying often occur following the loss of a loved one, whereas pessimism and fatigue are typical responses following failure to achieve a major goal or exposure to severe life stressors or hardships.

Watson and Andrews (2002) have proposed the *social navigation hypothesis* to account for the adaptive significance of depression. In their elegant description and analysis, they presented two complementary functions of depression that address difficulties in social relations. The first function, involving rumination, relates to the cognitive changes associated with depression that permit a greater attention to analyzing complex social problems and developing strategies to resolve them. The second function, involving social motivation, capitalizes on the loss of pleasurable activities and the fatigue and relative inactivity of the depressed individual to motivate social partners to become more engaged and to extend assistance.

The positive side of rumination. Somewhat later, Andrews and Thomson (2009) advanced the *analytical rumination hypothesis*, which expands greatly the rumination function from the social navigation hypothesis described in the preceding. The analytical rumination hypothesis views some of the symptoms associated with MDD as an adaptive response to deal with complex problems, often associated with social relationships. The loss of interest in most daily activities affords the depressed individual the luxury of focused and largely uninterrupted attention to develop strategies to solve the complex problem. There is an element of rumination, but the rumination is focused and devoted to finding a solution to a particular problem, while other activities, including pleasurable ones, are forsaken.

Focus on the immune system. Miller and Raison (2016) also offered an evolutionary perspective as part of their discussions of stress, the immune system, and depression. Consider the following observations on physiological responses to a laboratory stressor, the Trier Social Stress Test (Allen et al., 2014). An individual is brought into a laboratory and asked to deliver a speech to a highly critical panel of three experts. Not surprisingly, as this person prepares and then delivers the speech, a classic fight-or-flight response is mounted, with increases in blood pressure and heart rate and secretion of EPI and CORT into the circulation. But something surprising also occurs—exposure to this laboratory stressor activates white blood cells and leads to increases in proinflammatory cytokines, including IL-1β, IL-6, and TNFα. Why would immune activation occur in the absence of a pathogen or an injury? Presumably, the only thing at stake in experiencing this laboratory stressor is a threat to one's ego. And of critical importance to the theme of this chapter, why would individuals at high risk of developing depression have a greater proinflammatory response to laboratory stressors compared to low-risk individuals?

In their analysis of these issues, Miller and Raison (2016) argued that modern humans have continued a genomic bias toward inflammation that may be traced back to our ancient ancestors, who evolved in a pathogen-rich environment and were constantly confronting risks of severe wounding and associated infections from predators or human competitors. When dealing with an infection, early humans developed a constellation of "sickness behaviors" that enhanced survival through strategic alterations in behavior. These behavioral changes included conservation of energy through social avoidance and anhedonia, and hypervigilance to reduce the chance of a subsequent confrontation and further risk of infection. These sickness behaviors bear a striking resemblance to modern-day symptoms of depression (Figure 12.1).

In the end, it all comes down to reproductive success, and contributing genes to subsequent generations. Slavich and Irwin (2014) have advanced the *social signal transduction theory of depression* to support the notion that evolution favored those individuals who marshaled preemptive proinflammatory responses to stressors, even if the response was occasionally a false alarm. Unfortunately, modern humans live for the most part under sanitary conditions, and the very proinflammatory processes that served early humans so well have now turned into a decided liability (Figure 12.1).

Summary. These and other theories of the adaptive aspects of MDD will not halt the search for new and more effective antidepressants, nor should they. However, these theories do inform efforts by therapists working with patients

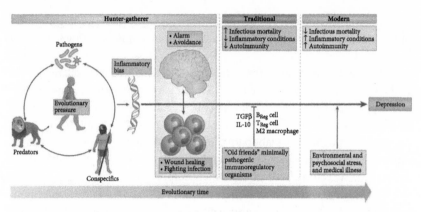

Figure 12.1. Early evolutionary pressures derived from human interactions with pathogens, predators and human conspecifics (such as rivals) resulted in an inflammatory bias that included an integrated suite of immunological and behavioral responses that conserved energy for fighting infection and healing wounds, while maintaining vigilance against attack. This inflammatory bias is believed to have been held in check during much of human evolution by exposure to minimally pathogenic, tolerogenic organisms in traditional (that is, rural) environments that engendered immunological responses characterized by the induction of regulatory T (TReg) cells, regulatory B (BReg) cells, and immunoregulatory M2 macrophages, as well as the production of the anti-inflammatory cytokines interleukin-10 (IL-10) and transforming growth factor-β (TGFβ). In modern times, sanitized urban environments of more developed societies are rife with psychological challenges but generally lacking in the types of infectious challenges that were primary sources of morbidity and mortality across most of human evolution. In the absence of traditional immunological checks and balances, the psychological challenges of the modern world instigate ancestral immunological and behavioral repertoires that represent a decided liability, such as high rates of various inflammation-related disorders, including depression. Adapted from Miller & Raison (2016) and used with permission of the publisher.

with MDD to look more broadly at the potential benefits of some symptoms of MDD. Consider the following quote from Watson and Andrews (2002, p. 11):

> The social navigation hypothesis implies that anti-depressant medications risk handicapping the client's ability to navigate and control their social environment; this could, in the long run, hinder the depressive from making key improvements in quality of life. If the social navigation hypothesis is correct, then a therapeutic prime directive to reduce suffering per se may be an irresponsible approach. Even when a therapist can implement a helpful talking therapy, it may be best to let depression work its miserable yet potentially

adaptive magic on the social network under protective supervision. The social navigation hypothesis suggests that drugs should not be given unless the causative social problems are also being addressed, and that drugs not be allowed to emasculate the ruminative and motivational functions of a potentially adaptive depression.

Animal Models of Major Depressive Disorder

Nature of the Challenge

In late 2000, 10 distinguished workgroups of scientists and clinicians were convened by the US National Institute of Mental Health as part of a broad-based strategic planning process to identify gaps in knowledge relating to mood disorders research and ways to address them. The workgroup on preclinical models issued a detailed report, which included four areas of highest priority. The first of these highest priorities was the development of better animal models of mood disorders with the hope that these models would lead to the development of a new generation of antidepressants (Nestler et al., 2002). Some of the recommendations of this workgroup foreshadowed advances in the field since the time of its publication. In particular, risk genes identified in humans through GWAS have been studied in mouse models. Genetically selected animal models have assumed a more important role in basic research on MDD, and emphasis has been placed on disruptions in mood-regulating circuits. Finally, ethologically relevant animal models for MDD have been employed with greater frequency, and chronic mild stress models of MDD have been standardized to a greater degree than before the time of this workgroup report. Unfortunately, translational research on animal models has still not tackled the important issue of why there are sex differences in the frequency of MDD in humans. Most studies using animal models have continued to focus solely on males, and this issue must be addressed for the field to move forward. These and other areas of research will be described in detail in the following.

Taking Up the Challenge

MDD presents a clear and compelling challenge to basic and clinical researchers given its very high prevalence in the global population and the level of debilitation associated with this mental disorder. Animal models of depression occupy an important niche within this comprehensive effort to enhance the diagnosis, treatment, and prevention of MDD across the life span (Han & Nestler, 2017;

Ménard et al., 2016). However, developing valid animal models of MDD remains a significant challenge for several important reasons. First, the relatively low heritability of MDD precludes a focused effort on studies of risk genes in animal models. There is certainly an important role for environmental stressors in the etiology of MDD, but how does one begin to model these stressful experiences in animals. A related issue concerns the stages during development when these stressors exert their maximal impact on a susceptible genotype. Another challenge to basic researchers is the inherent variability in the disorder in humans, such that no single animal model of MDD, regardless of its sophistication, will ever capture the many facets of the disorder in patients. As is true for virtually all psychiatric disorders, there are no valid biomarkers of MDD that can inform efforts to develop valid animal models. Finally, many current animal models are evaluated in part by their responses to currently available antidepressant medications. Such an approach is fraught with problems. Most of the medications employed to treat MDD were developed more than 50 years ago, largely by serendipitous observations. These medications for the most part target monoamine neurotransmitter signaling pathways, especially NE and 5-HT, and their effects in patients are inconsistent at best. In addition, a significant percentage of patients with MDD are classified as treatment-resistant. Based upon these concerns, one could argue that using currently available medications as a means to validate a given animal model are inappropriate and could well negate a model system that could reveal promising new targets for drug discovery (Akil et al., 2018; Belzung, 2014; Berton et al., 2012; Matthews et al., 2005).

The success rate for identifying new targets for the treatment of MDD using animal models has been a major disappointment. What explains this major source of disappointment? In her excellent review, Belzung (2014) argued that results from animal models have failed to identify new treatments that are effective in clinical trials. In other instances, clinical trials have not been optimized to detect the beneficial effects of some new drugs that interact with novel molecular targets identified through the use of animal models.

Several suggestions for improving the current state of affairs have been advanced. Animal models should be developed that mimic defined subpopulations of patients with MDD (including females) or specific endophenotypes of MDD. Clinical findings from patients with MDD using imaging techniques, potential blood biomarkers, or newly identified risk genes could be the basis for the development of new animal models. In addition, species differences in pharmacogenetic parameters that affect drug metabolism and brain levels of a new drug must be a critical part of experimental designs for clinical trials. In addition, careful patient stratification may reveal highly effective new drugs that work well in one subpopulation but not another. A final recommendation was for a greater dialogue between basic researchers who work with animal models and clinicians who work with patients and conduct clinical trials (Belzung, 2014; Willner & Belzung, 2015).

Sink or Swim (or Float)

Porsolt et al. (1977, 1978) initially reported on a new animal model for the study of depression that appeared particularly useful in identifying new antidepressant medications. In the second of these two publications, the animal model was referred to as a behavioral screening test for antidepressants. Briefly, laboratory rats were placed into a cylindrical chamber filled with 25°C water from which they could not escape for 15 minutes. The next day, the rats were again placed into the water for a 5-minute period and the total time spent immobile was measured. Time spent immobile in the second exposure usually comprised 75% of the test period. A variety of antidepressant drugs significantly reduced the time spent immobile, as did electroconvulsive shock and REM sleep deprivation. More recently, latency to immobility has been employed as another measure of behavioral despair in the forced swim test (Castagné et al., 2009). These investigators argued that this very simple and highly reproducible protocol for inducing behavioral despair in rats could be a valuable screening procedure for new antidepressants, including those with novel mechanisms of action. Kara et al. (2018) presented a systematic review and meta-analysis of the effects of antidepressants on the forced swim test and concluded that the forced swim test is useful in screening antidepressant effects of various compounds. However, it is not possible to compare the results of different compounds on the forced swim test across experiments, which represents a major limitation.

But let's be clear, the forced swim test **is not** an animal model for MDD. However, over time, the forced swim test has become the most frequently employed assessment of depression-like behavior in a range of genetically selected and environmentally induced animal models, as well as in animals with manipulations of specific risk genes for depression. According to Google Scholar, the two initial publications by Porsolt et al. (1977, 1978) have been cited more than 7,000 times! This very high number of citations reflects the broad impact this test has had on the continued development of animal models of depression. In this chapter and the one to follow, I will describe many studies that have employed the forced swim test as an assessment of depression-like behavior in a given animal model. I have avoided studies that employed the forced swim test to model depression. Please keep that distinction in mind for these two chapters.

In their insightful analysis, Molendijk and de Kloet (2015) argued that the forced swim test reflects an adaptive switch from active (struggling) to passive (floating) coping that is shaped by prior experience. Exposure of laboratory animals to swim stress for 15 minutes on day 1 results in memory formation for that experience. On day 2, when immobility is measured to reflect depression-like behavior, it would be more appropriate to interpret time spent immobile as a measure of memory for the experience on day 1. Molendijk and de Kloet (2015) and others (e.g., Prince & Anisman, 1984) over the years have argued that immobility is in fact an adaptive coping response to an inescapable stressor. It may be that antidepressants disrupt memory storage for the forced swim on day 1, resulting in reductions in time spent immobile on day 2. Consistent with this suggestion is the finding that administration of a protein synthesis inhibitor following swim stress on day 1 resulted in disruption of memory storage processes, and animals spent less time immobile on day 2 compared to vehicle-injected controls (De Pablo et al., 1989). An alternative, as suggested by Anyan and Amir (2018), is that the forced swim test is capturing aspects of depression as well as anxiety, with active escape behaviors reflecting levels of anxiety in laboratory animals.

What will be evident in the remainder of this chapter is that many investigators have either ignored these valid concerns about the forced swim test, felt they were unjustified, or were somehow unaware of them. The net result is that many genetic and environmental animal models of depression have been built upon the shifting sands of a questionable laboratory test. In the sections that follow, these concerns should be kept in mind in interpreting the results of experiments on various animal models.

Genetically Selected Animal Models

Flinders Sensitive Line. This genetic model of depression evolved quite by accident. Professor David Overstreet, then at Flinders University in Australia, set out to establish a line of laboratory rats that would be resistant to the anticholinesterase agent, diisopropyl fluorophosphate (DFP). What he ended up with instead was a line of rats that became progressively more sensitive to the effects of DFP (Flinders Sensitive Line, FSL) and a line that was similar to outbred Sprague-Dawley rats in its resistance to DFP (Flinders Resistant Line, FRL). The enhanced cholinergic sensitivity of FSL rats, which was associated with an increased expression of muscarinic receptors, was the phenotypic characteristic that led Overstreet to focus on the use of FSL rats as a model of human depression (Overstreet & Wegener, 2013). For a comprehensive review of basic and clinical studies linking increased central cholinergic signaling to depressed mood states, refer to the article by Dulawa and Janowsky (2019).

Experiments with rats of the FSL strain have revealed several characteristics that match well with findings from patients with MDD. These include reduced bar pressing for food or water rewards, reduced appetite and lower body weights, reductions in social behavior, elevated levels of REM sleep and latency to enter a REM sleep bout, alterations in immune function, and increased levels of anxiety-like behaviors.

Several facets of the FSL model are particularly interesting within the context of a genotype x environment interaction in shaping the depression-like phenotype of FSL rats. The maternal environment appears to have a significant impact on FSL pups. For example, problems arose for Overstreet and colleagues when litters of FSL pups were cross-fostered soon after birth to FRL mothers to rid the FSL pups of maternally conveyed viruses and other pathogens over the course of the selective breeding program. The unanticipated result of cross-fostering was that the depression-like phenotype, especially as reflected in the forced swim test, was lost in FSL rats that were reared by FRL foster mothers. In contrast, FRL pups reared by FSL mothers did not develop a depression-like behavioral phenotype (cited in Overstreet & Wegener, 2013). These observations during selective breeding to establish the two lines were confirmed in a later series of experiments involving cross-fostering of FSL and FRL litters (Friedman et al., 2006).

Results presented by Gómez-Galán et al. (2016) revealed that voluntary wheel running by FSL rats diminished stress-induced mechanisms of depression-like behaviors, but without altering predisposing genetic factors. Voluntary exercise in the form of wheel running has consistently improved behavioral outcomes in stress-induced animal models of depression, but the results are far less dramatic for patients with MDD (Cooney et al., 2013).

A second line of evidence relates to the effects of stressful stimulation on behaviors of FSL rats. One hour following a single bout of swim stress for 5 minutes, there was a significant suppression of saccharin consumption in FSL rats but not in FRL rats. Following a 4-week protocol of daily exposure to chronic mild stressors, FSL but not FRL rats exhibited significant decreases in saccharin consumption as well as saccharin preference. These data support the view that acute and chronic stressors had a greater anhedonic effect in FSL versus FRL rats (Pucilowski et al., 1993). Exposure to acute footshock stress also impacts the behaviors of FSL rats to a greater extent than FRL rats (see Overstreet et al., 2005). Finally, chronic exposure to escapable/inescapable swim stress enhanced nitric oxide signaling in the hippocampus of FSL rats but not FRL rats (Wegener et al., 2010).

FSL rats have also been employed as an animal model of childhood depression. Experiments in prepubertal rats (PNDs 30–40) revealed that FSL rats weighed significantly less than FRL rats, exhibited increased immobility in the forced swim test, displayed lower levels of non-play-related social behaviors, and had lower levels of HPA activity as indicated by reductions in circulating ACTH and CORT. Based upon these findings, Malkesman et al. (2006) concluded that

FSL rats could prove valuable in studying the early onset of depression in children and adolescents.

WKY rats and related models. The Wistar-Kyoto (WKY) rat was originally inbred to serve as the normotensive control for a genetic model of hypertension, the spontaneously hypertensive rat (SHR) (Okamoto & Aoki, 1963). WKYs have exaggerated sympathetic-adrenal medullary and hypothalamic-pituitary-adrenocortical responses to stressful stimulation and altered behavioral responses to open field testing (McCarty & Kirby, 1982; McCarty & Kopin, 1978; Owens et al., 1991). Paré (1989, 1994) was among the first to suggest that WKY rats might be valuable as an animal model of depression and anxiety based upon behavioral and physiological comparisons with other normotensive rats strains, including Fisher-344, Wistar, Long-Evans, and Sprague-Dawley rats. Specifically, WKYs were more susceptible to stress-induced gastric ulcers, had lower levels of activity in an open field test, were deficient in acquisition of a shuttle box escape response following inescapable shock, exhibited reduced levels of conditioned defensive burying behavior, and were immobile a greater percentage of the time in the forced swim test.

Lahmame et al. (1997) expanded upon these initial findings by comparing the behavioral responses of WKY, Sprague-Dawley, and Brown-Norway rats in the forced swim test before and following acute versus chronic administration of imipramine, an antidepressant. WKYs were clearly different from rats of the other two strains in levels of depression-like behaviors in the forced swim test, lack of response to acute administration of imipramine, and a diminished response to chronic treatment with imipramine. These investigators suggested that the WKY strain might serve as a model of treatment-resistant depression. In addition, WKYs have also been employed as an animal model of childhood depression. Experiments in prepubertal rats (PNDs 30–40) revealed that WKY rats weighed significantly less than Wistar controls, exhibited increased immobility in the forced swim test, displayed lower levels of social play and other social behaviors, and had higher levels of HPA activity as indicated by elevations in circulating ACTH and CORT. Based upon these findings, Malkesman et al. (2006) concluded that WKYs could prove valuable in studying some types of depression in children.

Additional experiments have revealed neurochemical differences between WKY rats and various control strains in basal and stressed-induced activities of DA, NE, 5-HT, and CRF systems in brain areas involved in regulation of mood states, including the PFC, hippocampus, amygdala, and nucleus accumbens (De La Garza & Mahoney, 2004; Jiao et al., 2003; Tejani-Butt et al., 1994).

Selective breeding of WKYs. Professor Eva Redei and her colleagues at Northwestern University were troubled by the high phenotypic and genotypic variability among WKY rats within their closed breeding colony as well as in

WKYs from different commercial suppliers, and these levels of variability were much higher than for other inbred rat strains. They took the novel approach of selectively breeding WKYs, using extremes of immobility in the forced swim test as the basis for selection. Brother-sister matings were avoided until after generation 5. Within several generations, they produced two lines, WKY Most Immobile (WMI) and WKY Least Immobile (WLI) that differed dramatically in behavioral responses to stress and antidepressants. Compared to WLI rats, WMI rats exhibited greater immobility in the forced swim test, decreased activity in an open field test, reduced and less variable plasma CORT responses to acute restraint stress, and greater responses to some antidepressants (e.g., desipramine) but no response to others (e.g., fluoxetine). Rats of the two lines did not differ in patterns of conditioned defensive burying behavior. This novel experimental approach afforded an opportunity to explore the underlying molecular genetic mechanisms that contributed to the differences between WMI and WLI rats (Will et al., 2003).

Using WMI rats as a model of endogenous depression, Andrus et al. (2012) confirmed the behavioral differences with WLI rats, which included higher levels of immobility in the forced swim test and lower activity levels in an open field test. In contrast, rats of the two lines did not differ in tests of anxiety-like or fear-related behaviors. Differentially expressed genes were identified in the hippocampus and amygdala of WMI and WLI rats using genome-wide microarray analyses; 638 genes in the amygdala and 463 genes in the hippocampus were differentially expressed between the WMI and WLI rats. Twenty-seven genes were differentially expressed in both brain regions and in the same direction between WMI and WLI rats. These results were confirmed for a subset of genes using RT-PCR. Genes associated with the integrin signaling pathway, cellular processes, cell communication, and signal transduction were highlighted in the WMI-WLI comparisons. Interestingly, no genes associated with NE or 5-HT neurotransmission were represented among the differentially expressed genes.

Building upon these initial findings, Pajer et al. (2012) utilized WMI and WLI rats from the 13th generation of selective breeding to identify gene expression patterns in blood and brain samples. Following this stage of the experiment, a set of differentially expressed genes between the two lines was selected such that the directional changes were similar in blood and in either hippocampus or amygdala. When combined with results from another animal model of depression, a collection of 26 potential blood transcriptomic markers were employed to distinguish human subjects with early onset MDD from controls. These blood-based biomarkers have the potential to identify patients with MDD and to support efforts to enhance the effectiveness of treatments through precision psychiatry. These blood biomarker differences between WMI and WLI rats were resistant to environmental perturbations and appeared to be trait-like biomarkers (Mehta-Raghavan et al., 2016).

Mixing it up. Heterogeneous stock (HS) rats provided another approach to examining genetic contributions to depression-like behaviors in laboratory rats. I have included the section on HS rats here because the WKY strain is one of the inbred rat strains employed to generate the HS breeders. We would anticipate that the WKY traits of increased immobility in the forced swim test and resistance to the effects of fluoxetine would carry over to the HS rats, but in a much-diluted fashion.

HS rats were originally developed by Hansen and Spuhler (1984) at the US National Institutes of Health by designing an 8-way cross of 8 different inbred strains of rats of various origins over 3 generations to achieve maximum genetic variability. These animals have been valuable in a range of experiments addressing genetic contributions to biomedical as well as behavioral disturbances (Solberg Woods, 2014).

Holl et al. (2018) measured the heritability of immobility in the forced swim test and the response to sub-acute fluoxetine treatment in 4-week-old HS rats. In addition, these researchers examined in HS rats blood levels of biomarkers that were previously found to be associated with depression-like behaviors in WHI rats and patients with MDD. Their findings revealed that many of the HS rats were unresponsive to treatment with fluoxetine. In addition, three genes that were differentially expressed in blood in previous research with an animal model and with patients with MDD were also differentially expressed in HS rats with high versus low immobility scores. These encouraging results suggested the translational power of identifying blood-borne biomarkers in animal models and then carefully assessing their diagnostic relevance in clinical populations.

A feeling of helplessness. Henn and Vollmayr (2005) summarized their efforts with outbred Sprague-Dawley rats to develop a line that was highly susceptible to the learned helplessness paradigm (cLH line), and a comparison line that was relatively resistant to learned helplessness (cNLH strain). Their selective breeding program avoided brother-sister matings and included frequent backcrosses to Sprague-Dawley breeding stock to minimize inbreeding and to reduce the possibility of co-selection of genes unrelated to learned helpless behavior. Differences between lines were evident after 5 generations, and after many generations of selective breeding, cLH rats displayed a "helpless" phenotype without prior exposure to inescapable shock. Given the lack of exposure to inescapable shock, the developers renamed the cLH line the negative cognitive state (NC) line and the cNLH line the positive cognitive state (PC) line beginning in 2016. For this section, however, I will follow the initial designations for these lines (i.e., cLH and cNLH) to minimize confusion with published results.

The behavioral phenotype of cLH rats is as follows: higher immobility scores in a forced swim test, more escape failures in an escape-avoidance task, reductions in persistence in a bar-pressing task, reduced response to treatment with antidepressants or electroconvulsive shock, and anhedonia. In contrast, cLH rats were more active than cNLH rats in an open field test and were similar to cNLH rats in acquisition of operant responding for a sucrose reward and spatial memory in the Morris water maze (Vollmayr & Gass, 2013). In addition, exposure to acute footshock stress triggered anhedonic-like behavior in cLH rats and a reduction in the pleasure-attenuated startle response, suggesting a deficit in perception of a palatable reward (sweetened condensed milk) (Enkel et al., 2010). The cLH line has been advanced by its developers as an animal model of treatment-resistant depression.

Focus on the lateral habenula. A continuing focus of research with the cLH and cNLH lines has been on the role of neural circuits and signaling pathways in the expression of the depression-like phenotype. In particular, the lateral habenula has been the subject of several experiments with cLH and cNLH rats. The lateral habenula reciprocally interacts with DA neurons in the ventral tegmental area (VTA) and 5-HT neurons in the median and dorsal raphe nuclei and is involved in behavioral responses to stressful stimuli, including inhibition of motor activity. Lateral habenula neurons appear to be hyperactive in patients with MDD, and have been a target for development of novel therapies (Hikosaka, 2010).

To explore this relationship further, Li et al. (2011) injected a retrograde tracer into the VTA of cLH and cNLH rats 2–3 days before preparation of brain slices for in vitro recording. They demonstrated that excitatory synapses onto lateral habenula neurons that projected to the DA-rich VTA were potentiated relative to cNLH controls, and identified these VTA-projecting lateral habenula neurons as glutamatergic. This synaptic potentiation was associated with depression-like behaviors and resulted from an enhanced probability of presynaptic neurotransmitter release. If presynaptic neurotransmitter content was reduced by repeated electrical stimulation of lateral habenular afferents, there was a significant decrease in synaptic drive onto VTA-projecting lateral habenula neurons that was promptly reversed with cessation of electrical stimulation. Moving to intact animals exposed to a learned helplessness protocol, deep brain stimulation but not sham stimulation of the lateral habenula greatly decreased immobility in the forced swim test. As an additional control, if the stimulating electrode was placed in the thalamus, there was no effect of stimulation on immobility in the forced swim test. The stimulation parameters in this experiment with laboratory rats were similar to two reports where deep brain stimulation of the lateral habenula resulted in marked improvement of two patients with treatment-resistant depression. In both cases, the improvements in outcome were temporarily reversed when the pacemaker malfunctioned or was replaced due to an infection (Kiening & Sartorius, 2013; Sartorius et al., 2010).

The findings by Li et al. (2011) were extended in several ways. For example, Winter et al. (2011) employed bilateral microinjections of muscimol (0.5 ng), a GABA agonist, into the lateral habenulae of cLH rats to reduce neuronal activation. One week after administration of muscimol, cLH rats exhibited significant decreases in percentage of errors in a learned helplessness test that were no longer apparent 2 weeks post–drug administration. These findings were consistent with the earlier report by Li et al. (2011) and demonstrated that tonic suppression of lateral habenula neuronal activity was required for improvement of depression-like behaviors in cLH rats.

Functional connectivity. To probe circuit-level differences between anesthetized cLH and cNLH rats, a 9.4 T scanner was employed to measure regional cerebral blood volume and resting-state functional connectivity in rats of the two lines (Gass et al., 2014). cLH rats exhibited significant reductions in regional cerebral blood volume in the lateral habenula, dentate gyrus, and subiculum. In contrast, cLH rats had significant increases in regional cerebral blood volume in the BNST. Functional connectivity was enhanced in cLH rats with respect to serotonergic projections from the dorsal raphe nucleus to the forebrain, within the hippocampal-PFC network, and between the BNST and the lateral frontal cortical areas. These authors noted the discrepancy between increased activity in VTA-projecting lateral habenula neurons of cLH rats and decreased regional cerebral blood volume measures in the lateral habenula. However, the VTA-projecting neurons make up a small percentage of all neurons in the lateral habenula, and the spatial resolution of the blood volume measures were not sufficient to capture differences within the lateral habenula. In a related experiment, cLH and cNLH rats were subjected to resting-state fMRI time series analyses before and after exposure to stressful stimulation. Acute exposure to stress affected the anterior cingulate cortex and prelimbic cortex to a greater extent in cLH compared to cNLH rats, possibly creating a bias in attention to negative information, as is often observed in patients with MDD (Gass et al., 2014; Gass et al., 2016).

Glutamate. Accumulating evidence suggests that alterations in glutamatergic neurotransmission and reduced astroglial uptake of glutamate may be involved in the etiology of MDD (Zink et al., 2010). Expanding upon these reports, Seese et al. (2013) employed 3-D reconstructions of layer I of the infralimbic cortex, an area associated with mood disorders, to quantify excitatory synapses by fluorescence deconvolution tomography in cLH, cNLH, and outbred Sprague-Dawley rats. Their results revealed that the density of synapse-sized clusters of PSD95 (a marker of postsynaptic density) was reduced in layer I sample fields of infralimbic cortex of cLH rats. Similarly, the numerical density of synapse-sized clusters of the AMPA receptor subunit, GluA1, was also reduced in cLH rats. In contrast, these investigators did not find any differences in the incidence or immunofluorescence intensity of GABAergic (i.e., $GABA_A R^+$) contacts between cLH and cNLH rats.

Building on earlier work in humans (Raichle et al., 2001) and in rats (Lu et al., 2012), von Hohenberg et al. (2018) examined default-mode network connectivity using fMRI with a 9.4 T scanner in anesthetized cLH rats under resting conditions and following optogenetic inactivation of a portion of the neurons in the lateral habenula. Broadly speaking, the default mode network may serve to integrate multimodal sensory and affective information to alter behavior in anticipation of changes in the environment. Von Hohenberg et al. (2018) reported a connectivity decrease in the default-mode network following optogenetic inactivation of the lateral habenula. These results are consistent with studies in patients with MDD, where hyperconnectivity of the default-mode network as assessed by fMRI has been a consistent finding (for a review, see Mulders et al., 2015). Unfortunately, comparable studies were not performed in cNLH rats.

Enrichment. Environmental factors may alter the trajectory of depression-like behaviors in cLH rats. One study examined the effects of environmental enrichment on a range of depression-like behaviors in cLH and cNLH rats. Rats of both lines were housed in pairs in standard cages or enriched environment cages for 5 weeks beginning at 14 or 28 weeks of age. Environmental enrichment significantly reduced the depression-like phenotype in 14-week-old but not 28-week-old cLH rats during testing in a learned helplessness paradigm. In a test of anhedonia, cNLH rats consumed more sweetened condensed milk than cLH rats, and this difference between lines was not altered by environmental enrichment. Older cLH rats appeared to be more resistant to the benefits of environmental enrichment than younger cLH rats, and these benefits were evident in some but not all aspects of the depression-like phenotype (Richter et al., 2013).

Reactivity, stress, and depression. As described in Chapter 11, Stead et al. (2006) selected outbred Sprague-Dawley rats for high (HR) and low (LR) locomotor responses to placement in a novel environment. After only 8 generations of selective breeding but without brother-sister mating, there was a 2-fold difference in locomotor behavior in a novel environment between HRs and LRs. To examine interactions between responses to novelty and exposure to stress, Stedenfeld et al. (2011) employed HR and LR male rats from the 20th generation of selective breeding and exposed them to 4 weeks of chronic mild stress (CMS). Sucrose preference was measured weekly, and anxiety was measured using the novelty-suppressed feeding test. LRs exposed to CMS displayed a lack of preference for a sucrose solution sooner than HRs and the magnitude of change was greater in CMS-exposed LRs. In addition, novelty-suppressed feeding was increased significantly in CMS-exposed LRs, but was unaffected in CMS-exposed

HRs. These investigators concluded that emotional reactivity, as reflected in rats selected for differences in locomotor responses to a novel environment, affected susceptibility to stressful stimulation and the onset of depression-related behavioral changes. These behavioral findings underscore the importance of a gene x environment interaction model in the etiology of depression.

Summary. Genetically selected animal models have a proper place in the broad-based effort to describe the neural mechanisms controlling the onset of depression-like behaviors. Flinders Sensitive rats and WKY rats were originally developed with other purposes in mind (cholinergic sensitivity and normotensive control for the SHR strain, respectively). Over time, both of these strains were recognized as potential animal models of depression. Selective breeding strategies were employed to develop the cLH and HR strains based upon their responses to a learned helplessness paradigm and novelty, respectively. Although these animal models are not currently at the forefront of research on neural and molecular mechanisms of depression, they have contributed in important ways to advancing our understanding of genetic risk and susceptibility to depression.

Chronic Stress Animal Models

In Chapter 2, I summarized research studies in humans that clearly pointed to an association between stressful life events and the onset, severity, and recurrence of MDD. Early life stressors may also interact with a susceptible genotype to increase the risk of MDD later in life. This strong connection between stress and depression has led to the development of a range of animal models that examine behavioral and neurobiological consequences of exposure to chronic intermittent stress. In the subsections that follow, I will provide an overview of some of the animal models of depression that involve chronic intermittent exposure of laboratory animals to stressful stimuli. One challenge in developing these models is the tendency of laboratory animals to habituate behaviorally and physiologically to repeated exposure to a homotypic stressor (McCarty, 2016). As we will see in the following, there are ways to overcome this homeostatic process in the variety of stressors that is employed.

Chronic social defeat stress (CSDS). CSDS is an ethologically valid animal model for studying depression-like behaviors as well as resilience to chronic stress, as will be discussed in Chapter 15. This paradigm produces a state of chronic emotional stress in a large percentage of adult male laboratory mice and rats with minimal risk of injury and with no indication that the behavioral and physiological responses to repeated exposures habituate over time. There are two major drawbacks with CSDS: it is not as helpful in modeling depression-like behaviors in female mice and rats, and it is typically started when experimental animals are adults. Exclusive use of adult animals precludes an ability to study the developmental trajectory of a depression-like phenotype (Hollis & Kabbaj, 2014). Takahashi et al. (2017) developed a procedure for exposing adult female mice to repeated brief bouts of aggression by a resident male. In addition, Newman et al. (2019) used brief daily exposure of C57BL/6J females to a resident Swiss-Webster female and her castrated male consort as a model of social defeat stress in female mice. These substantial modifications of the standard CSDS protocol will be a welcome addition for those investigators who wish to include female mice in their experiments.

One exception to the dependence upon adult animals for experiments involving CSDS was the report by Iñiguez et al. (2014). These investigators explored the effects of CSDS for 10 consecutive days in C57BL/6 mice during PNDs 35–44. One day after the tenth exposure to social defeat, mice displayed a pattern of depression- and anxiety-like changes relative to handled controls. These changes included increased social avoidance, increased immobility in the forced swim test, decreased preference for a sucrose solution, and reduced time spent in the open arms of an EPM. This paradigm could be useful in studies of the role of stress in the onset of depression-like behaviors in adolescent mice exposed to CSDS.

Embracing variability. Focusing on models of depression-like behavior, Krishnan et al. (2007) exposed inbred C57BL/6 male mice to CSDS for 10 consecutive days. The daily protocol involved placing a C57BL/6 male into the cage of a resident and highly aggressive CD-1 male for 10 minutes, during which time the resident approached and occasionally attacked the intruder. After 10 minutes, a perforated plexiglas barrier was placed into the cage to subdivide it into two equal compartments. In this way, C57BL/6 mice were physically separated from their resident male aggressors but remained in sensory contact. This process was repeated each day, with each C57BL/6 male being placed into the cage of a different CD-1 resident male for a 24-hour period. On days 11 or 39, males exposed to CSDS and controls were subjected to a battery of tests to assess levels of depression-like or resilient behaviors.

The most obvious result from the CSDS experiment was that highly inbred C57BL/6 mice exhibited surprisingly variable behavioral responses. Approximately 40%–50% of C57BL/6 mice subjected to CSDS resembled control mice in a measure of social interaction and were characterized as *resilient*. The remaining mice displayed a lack of interest in or an aversion to social interaction with a CD-1 stranger and were labeled as *susceptible* to a depression-like phenotype. Other behavioral changes in susceptible mice that distinguished them from their resilient counterparts included a reduced preference for a 1% sucrose solution in a two-bottle choice test, blunted amplitude of the circadian rhythm in body temperature, a reduction in body weight, and a greater increase in body temperature following exposure to a CD-1 male. Compared to control mice not exposed to CSDS, both susceptible and resilient mice displayed comparable reductions in time spent in the open arms of an EPM, similar increases in stress-induced polydipsia, similar immobility scores in the forced swim and tail suspension tests, comparable levels of locomotor activity in a test chamber, and similar elevations in plasma CORT levels following brief exposure to a forced swim test. Some of these differences in behavior persisted for up to 4 weeks, including increased social avoidance, increased body temperature response upon exposure to a CD-1 male, and lower morning plasma CORT levels. For resilient mice, there was a cost to adapting to the recurring stress of CSDS—a slow-developing cardiac hypertrophy that was only evident 4 weeks after CSDS and that reflected an increased sympathetic drive to the heart (Krishnan et al., 2007).

Acetylcholine sets the tone. For many years, enhanced cholinergic signaling in the brain following stressful stimulation has been thought to play a role in the etiology of MDD in humans (for a review, see Dulawa & Janowsky, 2019). To probe this relationship, Mineur et al. (2013) examined the effects of targeted manipulations of cholinergic signaling in the hippocampus of mice exposed to CSDS. Two experimental approaches were employed to block acetylcholinesterase (AChE) in the hippocampus, thereby increasing levels of acetylcholine in the synaptic space: local infusion of physostigmine or viral delivery of short hairpin (sh) inhibitory RNAs to knockdown the various isoforms of AChE. Micro-infusion of physostigmine into the hippocampus of mice increased the time spent immobile in a tail suspension test. Unfortunately, this was the only behavioral measure taken. Virally mediated knockdown of AChE in the hippocampus resulted in behavioral changes in mice consistent with increased levels of anxiety-like and depression-like behaviors based upon tests in the EPM, light-dark box, tail suspension test, and forced swim test. These behavioral effects were reversed by co-infusion of a human AChE transgene that was resistant to the effects of the virally delivered shRNAs.

To explore the effects of hippocampal acetylcholine signaling on emotional stress, mice were exposed to a modified CSDS paradigm that consisted of three episodes of social defeat in a single day. The following day, mice were tested for levels of social interaction with a novel test mouse. In control mice, exposure to a modified CSDS protocol did not affect social interaction scores compared to unstressed mice. In contrast, mice that received virally delivered shRNAs to knockdown the various isoforms of AChE displayed significant reductions in social interactions following the modified CSDS protocol. It is important to note, however, that knockdown of hippocampal AChE in unstressed mice had no effect on levels of social interaction compared to mice receiving control infusions. As noted earlier, co-infusion of a human AChE transgene that was resistant to the effects of the virally delivered shRNAs reversed the effects of AChE knockdown on social interaction scores of mice exposed to the modified CSDS protocol. Finally, chronic administration of fluoxetine (15 mg/kg x 15 days) also blocked the effects of hippocampal AChE knockdown on social interaction in the modified CSDS protocol. These results clearly indicated that maintenance of hippocampal acetylcholine within appropriate levels was important for regulation of depression-like behavioral responses to social stressors.

BDNF joins forces with DA. Dr. Eric Nestler and his colleagues have conducted a series of experiments to delineate the neural and molecular changes that account for the depression-like behavioral phenotype described in the preceding for mice exposed to CSDS (Koo et al., 2019). These experiments explored the involvement of the mesolimbic DA pathway, as well as a key regulator of DA neurons, brain-derived neurotrophic factor (BDNF). BDNF enhances DA release in the nucleus accumbens through activation of its TrkB receptors on DA nerve terminals. An initial experiment reported a 90% increase in levels of BDNF protein but not TrkB receptors or BDNF mRNA in the nucleus accumbens of susceptible mice. There was also significant activation of signaling molecules downstream of BDNF, including phosphorylated Akt, glycogen synthase kinase 3β, and extracellular signal regulated kinase (ERK 1/2). However, these patterns of activation were not accompanied by increases in levels of the three proteins. Bilateral infusions of BDNF into the nucleus accumbens of mice decreased measures of social interaction following an abbreviated CSDS paradigm. In contrast, blockade of ERK signaling in the nucleus accumbens increased measures of social interaction in otherwise depression-susceptible mice. Local virally mediated knockdown of *bdnf* in the nucleus accumbens did not alter levels of social avoidance in mice subjected to CSDS. In contrast, virally mediated knockdown of *bdnf* in the VTA prevented the social avoidance that typically accompanies CSDS. Levels of social interaction in control mice that lacked *bdnf* but that were not exposed to CSDS were similar to uninjected controls, indicating that the effects of BDNF knockdown on social behavior was dependent upon exposure to stress (Berton et al., 2006; Krishnan et al., 2007). Finally, DNA microarray studies in the nucleus accumbens of mice one day after exposure to CSDS revealed the following: up-regulation of 309 genes and down-regulation of 17 genes in the nucleus accumbens compared to nonstressed control mice. Some of these alterations in gene expression persisted for up to 4 weeks. Most of these changes in gene expression in the nucleus accumbens were blocked by local knockdown of BDNF or chronic treatment with the antidepressant fluoxetine (Berton et al., 2006).

Phasic or tonic—that is the question. To further establish a causal relationship between activity of VTA DA neurons and susceptibility to CSDS, Chaudhury et al. (2013) documented two distinct in vivo patterns of neuronal activity—low-frequency tonic firing and high-frequency phasic firing. Phasic firing of DA neurons, which has been shown to encode reward signals (Tobler et al., 2005), was increased by CSDS in susceptible mice but not in resilient mice. Using an optogenetic approach to achieve precise regulation of tyrosine hydroxylase-containing VTA neurons, it was possible to alter firing patterns of DA neurons during an abbreviated encounter with a CD-1 resident male. On day 1 of the experiment, C57BL/6 male mice were placed individually into the home cage of a resident CD-1 mouse for 2 minutes, followed by sensory but not physical contact with the aggressor for 10 minutes. During the 10 minutes of sensory contact, photo-stimulation of DA neurons occurred in a tonic pattern (0.5 Hz) or a phasic pattern (20 Hz), with both groups receiving 5 spikes per 10-second period for 10 minutes. Two measures of susceptibility to a depression-like phenotype were taken: levels of social interaction for 2.5 minutes, followed by preference for a 1% sucrose solution over a 12-hour period.

The results of this series of experiments were quite striking in that optogenetic induction of tonic stimulation of VTA DA neurons had no effect on social avoidance or sucrose preference relative to controls. In contrast, optogenetic induction of phasic stimulation of VTA DA neurons resulted in significant decreases in measures of social proximity and sucrose preference compared to controls and to mice that received tonic stimulation. This same pattern of phasic stimulation of VTA DA neurons in mice previously documented to be resilient following CSDS also caused them to display a susceptible phenotype. Phasic stimulation of VTA DA neurons had no effect on naïve mice that had not experienced the stress associated with the abbreviated social defeat paradigm. This finding underscores the importance of prior experience interacting with the pattern of VTA DA activity to influence a susceptible behavioral phenotype.

Chaudhury et al. (2013) extended their findings by focusing on the specificity of the projection pathways from VTA DA neurons. Optogenetic phasic activation of VTA DA neurons projecting to the nucleus accumbens but not to the PFC resulted in susceptibility to social defeat stress. In contrast, optogenetic inhibition of the VTA → nucleus accumbens pathway resulted in a pattern of resilience to CSDS. Finally, optogenetic inhibition of the VTA → mPFC pathway resulted in susceptibility to CSDS.

Taken together, these impressive findings emphasize the critical role played by VTA DA neurons in regulating depression-like behavioral responses to CSDS. These effects of VTA DA neurons are finely tuned with respect to firing patterns and targets of innervation. These results have particular relevance to those interested in targeted therapies for the treatment of MDD.

Delving further into the complex reward circuitry that may underlie depression-like behaviors, Bagot et al. (2015) examined the role of glutamatergic input to the nucleus accumbens following exposure of mice to CSDS. The nucleus accumbens receives glutamatergic input from three brain areas: the mPFC, the basolateral amygdala, and the ventral hippocampus. Enhanced excitatory input to the nucleus accumbens from the ventral hippocampus was associated with a depression-like phenotype in mice exposed to CSDS. In contrast, enhancing excitatory input from the mPFC or the basolateral amygdala to the nucleus accumbens in mice exposed to CSDS had the opposite effect, promoting a resilient behavioral phenotype.

Circuits and symptoms. A critical issue addressed by Knowland et al. (2017) was the way in which individual elements of the brain circuits associated with a depression-like phenotype affected specific symptoms of depression. Their experiments revolved around the ventral pallidum, a point of convergence in depression-sensitive brain circuits involved in motivation and reward. Within the ventral pallidum, parvalbumin-expressing (PV$^+$) neurons that project to the lateral habenula and the VTA were identified as distinct subpopulations. PV$^+$ neurons projecting to the lateral habenula were excitatory, whereas PV$^+$ neurons projecting to the VTA were a mixture of inhibitory inputs to GABAergic neurons and mostly excitatory inputs to DA neurons. Track-tracing studies revealed that PV$^+$ neurons that projected to the lateral habenula received substantial input from the BNST and medial shell of the nucleus accumbens. In contrast, PV$^+$ neurons that projected to the VTA received input from the lateral shell of the nucleus accumbens, subthalamic nucleus, and the central nucleus of the amygdala.

Next, Knowland et al. (2017) examined the impact of these two subpopulations of ventral pallidal neurons in mice exposed to CSDS. They characterized mice that were susceptible to the effects of CSDS as having higher immobility scores in the tail suspension test, reduced preference for a sucrose solution, and increased social withdrawal. Electrophysiological studies of brain slices following CSDS revealed that both types of PV$^+$ neurons had more frequent spiking in susceptible mice compared to resilient mice. Reducing the activity of PV$^+$ neurons by targeted expression of Kir$_{2.1}$, a hyperpolarizing K$^+$ channel, blocked the effects of CSDS on the tail suspension test and the social withdrawal test, but had no effect of anhedonia as measured by sucrose preference. In naïve mice, optogenetic activation of PV$^+$ neurons projecting to the VTA induced social withdrawal. Targeted inhibition of PV$^+$ neurons projecting to the lateral habenula normalized behavior in the tail suspension test, but did not affect social withdrawal in CSDS-exposed mice. In contrast, targeted inhibition of PV$^+$ neurons projecting to the VTA normalized social interaction but had no effect of the tail suspension test. These results are important because they demonstrate that different elements of the complex neural circuitry that underlies reward and aversive behaviors control different depression-like behaviors. Further, stressful stimulation is a critical component in activating some of these neuronal pathways and the resulting onset of a depression-like behavioral phenotype.

You're not my type. Medium spiny neurons (MSNs) of the nucleus accumbens are critical in translating exposure to CSDS into depression-like behavioral responses. MSNs make up the majority of the nucleus accumbens and come in two types, one expressing D1 receptors and playing a role in reward, and the other expressing D2 receptors and playing a role in aversion. Using a variety of optogenetic and pharmacogenetic approaches, Francis et al. (2015) reported that the frequency of excitatory synaptic input was decreased in D1-expressing MSNs and increased in D2-expressing MSNs in mice that displayed depression-like behaviors following exposure to CSDS. If neuronal activity was increased in D1-expressing MSNs, there was a substantial reduction in depression-like behaviors following CSDS. In contrast, inhibition of neuronal activity in D1-expressing MSNs enhanced depression-like behaviors following CSDS. Modulation of activity in D2-expressing MSNs did not affect behavioral outcomes to CSDS. However, repeated activation of D2-expressing MSNs in naïve animals resulted in enhanced social avoidance following an abbreviated social defeat paradigm.

The power of prediction. As described earlier when C57BL/6 inbred mice are subjected to CSDS, they segregate into two distinct behavioral phenotypes: those that are susceptible to depression-like behaviors, and those that are resilient. A major question for some researchers has been if this susceptibility to depression can be detected prior to exposure to CSDS. If there were biomarkers of susceptibility to depression that would translate to humans, this advance would open the door to identifying individuals at high risk for the disorder and developing treatment options before the symptoms of the disorder were evident. Included in the following are two studies that have tackled this fascinating question using different methodologies.

In the first study, Muir et al. (2018) used fiber photometry Ca^{++} imaging to record Ca^{++} transients in the two types of MSNs in the nucleus accumbens in freely behaving mice prior to CSDS. Those mice that were susceptible to later CSDS displayed lower basal peak amplitudes of Ca^{++} transients but not peak frequencies in D1-expressing MSNs relative to those mice that were resilient to CSDS. These differences between groups were erased by a single exposure to social defeat. No differences between groups were detected in basal peak amplitudes or frequencies in D2-expressing MSNs. Importantly, there were no behavioral differences between groups of mice in a social interaction test that occurred prior to CSDS. One limitation of this study related to the use of fiber photometry Ca^{++} imaging. This technique provides a readout of the activity of a population of neurons, and as such, the interpretation of differences in peak amplitudes or peak frequencies of neuronal activity must wait until single-unit recordings can be employed. However, these results are a major step forward in the quest to identify a biosignature of susceptibility to a depression-like phenotype in an animal model.

In the second study, Hultman et al. (2018) tested the hypothesis that susceptibility to a depression-like phenotype following CSDS in mice could be unmasked by in vivo recordings of alterations in neuronal activity between spatially distinct brain areas over time. Recording electrode bundles targeted the following brain areas: amygdala, nucleus accumbens, VTA, PFC, and ventral hippocampus. This experimental approach was grounded in the understanding that emotional behaviors arise from the coordinated interaction of many brain circuits acting as a functional network as opposed to individual brain circuits acting in isolation. Their experiments in C57BL/6 mice revealed a spatiotemporal dynamic network that predicted the later appearance of depression-like behavioral characteristics following exposure to CSDS. Network activity originated in PFC and ventral striatum, relayed through the amygdala and VTA, and converged on the ventral hippocampus. Activity in this spatiotemporal network (Electome Factor 1) was increased during acute threat by an aggressive CD-1 mouse as well as three other manipulations that enhanced susceptibility to a depression-like phenotype. These included over-expression of a depression risk gene, *Sdk1*, in the ventral hippocampus; chronic daily administration of interferon-alpha for 5 weeks; or exposure to maternal separation for 3 hours per day from birth until PND 14. Electome Factor 1 was distinct from two other networks (Electome Factors 2 and 3) that reflected the transition to a depression-like behavioral phenotype following exposure to CSDS. Further, Electome Factor 1 was not altered following exposure of susceptible mice to two treatments that reduced depression-like behaviors: electrical stimulation of infralimbic cortex, or acute administration of the rapid-acting antidepressant ketamine. These exciting findings have significant translational potential in that a susceptibility electome was revealed that could be a target for future drug development or personalized environmental interventions in patients (Hultman et al., 2018).

Circuits, genes, and antidepressants. Bagot et al. (2017) further exploited the CSDS protocol to characterize the transcriptional profiles of susceptible and resilient C57BL/6 mice in the PFC, nucleus accumbens, amygdala, and hippocampus. Mice were identified as susceptible or resilient based upon their social interaction scores the day following 10 consecutive days of exposure to social defeat. These four brain areas are key components of the brain circuitry involved in the expression of a depression-like phenotype. Relative to controls, mice exposed to CSDS displayed the following numbers of differentially expressed genes:

- In PFC: 113 genes were up-regulated and 137 genes were down-regulated.
- In nucleus accumbens: 163 genes were up-regulated and 151 genes were down-regulated.
- In amygdala: 230 genes were up-regulated and 140 genes were down-regulated
- In hippocampus: 92 genes were up-regulated and 72 genes were down-regulated.

Susceptible mice were further divided into three groups: saline-injected controls, chronic treatment with imipramine (20 mg/kg/day for 14 days), or a single dose of ketamine (10 mg/kg). Using the social interaction test as a basis for determining a positive response to imipramine or ketamine, the results revealed that approximately equal numbers of susceptible mice were responders versus non-responders. Acute administration of ketamine resulted in more gene expression changes in the hippocampus, whereas chronic administration of imipramine led to more gene expression changes in the nucleus accumbens and amygdala. Transcriptional profiles in drug responders were most similar in the PFC. In mice that responded favorably to the drug treatments, there was a reversal of susceptibility-associated transcriptional changes and an induction of resilience-associated transcriptional changes. The results of this comprehensive study revealed that susceptible mice were heterogeneous with respect to responsiveness to drug treatment, and that each drug had shared as well as brain region–specific effects. The database of gene expression changes from this study provided a wealth of information for investigators with an interest in identifying molecular targets for more effective treatments for depression.

Summary. A bright light in basic research on depression has been the development of CSDS as a valid animal model of depression-like behaviors in male mice. Much of this work has been conducted in the laboratory of Dr. Eric J. Nestler at the Mount Sinai Medical Center in New York using C57BL/6J mice. A surprising early finding was that inbred C57BL/6J mice reacted to the stress of chronic social defeat in a highly variable manner, with some mice clearly susceptible to the effects of CSDS, while others displayed resilience to the effects of CSDS. This variability of responses quickly became an essential element in the experiments that followed given that groups of susceptible and resilient mice could be compared to understand the neural and molecular contributions to depression-like behaviors. Another important advance from the Nestler laboratory has been the use of sub-threshold CSDS to reveal a susceptible phenotype following prior exposure of mice to an experimental manipulation.

A major focus of these experiments has been the stress-sensitive reward circuitry of the brain, including the VTA and the nucleus accumbens. A particular strength of the experimental approach by the Nestler laboratory has been the use of multiple behavioral measures of a depression-like phenotype and the variety of experimental techniques employed, including direct measures of neuronal activity, optogenetic control of neuronal activity in specific populations of neurons within reward areas of the brain, and measurement of transcriptional profiles in discrete brain areas (Muir et al., 2019). In addition, several experiments focused on identifying neural markers of susceptibility to depression-like behaviors prior to exposure of mice to CSDS. This body of research has underscored powerful connections between brain reward pathways, stress, and depression that have revealed many new targets for drug development for the treatment of MDD (Slattery & Cryan, 2017).

Chronic mild stress (CMS). In contrast to the relatively consistent paradigm for CSDS that has been adopted in laboratories around the world, animal models of depression that have utilized chronic intermittent exposure of laboratory mice or rats to a variety of stressors have been hampered somewhat by variability in experimental designs, stressors employed, number of stress sessions per day, frequency of exposure to stressors, and duration of stressor protocols (Yin et al., 2016). Katz (1981) was one of the first to propose that a complex array of stressors presented in such a way as to minimize predictability of the type of stressor delivered on a given day and the time of day when the stressor would occur could be the basis for an animal model of depression. Some of the stressors employed by Katz were quite intense (e.g., cold water immersion, 48 hours of food and water deprivation, high levels of inescapable footshock) and were at odds with newer regulations governing laboratory animal welfare in several countries, including the United Kingdom.

In a recent review, Willner (2017) traced the origins of the CMS model and presented its strengths and limitations. To comply with the Animals (Scientific Procedures) Act (1986) in the United Kingdom and resulting efforts to minimize stress, Willner and his colleagues set out to develop a protocol that involved constant exposure of laboratory rats to a combination of relatively mild stressors over a period of 5–9 weeks. When combined, these mild stressors were labeled as "moderately stressful." This labor-intensive protocol included brief periods of food or water deprivation, continuous periods of lights on, cages tilted by 30°–50°, group housing, wet bedding, placement in a cold room, intermittent white noise (85 dB), strobe lights (300 flashes per minute), strange odors, and a strange object placed into the home cages. They found that rats exposed to CMS for at least 2 weeks displayed reduced intake of saccharin or sucrose solutions, and this anhedonic response persisted for up to 2 weeks after termination of CMS. Treatment with desmethylimipramine (DMI, 6.0 mg/kg/day, i.p.) for 2 weeks restored the preference for a sucrose solution without affecting the sucrose preference of unstressed control rats. They concluded that the CMS protocol represented a valid animal model of MDD (Willner et al., 1987).

CMS as a useful model. Since the early report by Willner et al. (1987), the CMS model has been employed extensively to study the neural mechanisms underlying the depression-like phenotype, and as a means of identifying new targets for drug discovery. At the end of 2015, more than 1,300 papers that employed the CMS paradigm had been published. Over time, the CMS paradigm has been modified to include chronic unpredictable mild stress (CUMS) or chronic variable stress (CVS). I view these modifications as variations on a theme, and will, for simplicity's sake, combine both of them under the umbrella of CMS for this section.

Many experiments have added to the original findings by Willner et al. (1987) on the ways in which animals exposed to CMS mimic many of the key symptoms of MDD. For example, laboratory mice and rats exposed to CMS display anhedonic responses in tests of rewarded behaviors; decreases in motivated behaviors, including sexual and aggressive behaviors; reductions in body weight gain relative to controls; disruptions in sleep patterns; reduced locomotor activity; and cognitive impairments across a range of tasks. Anxiety is often a comorbid trait in patients with MDD, and elevations in anxiety-like behaviors have also been reported in some but not all studies that have employed CMS. Finally, animals exposed to CMS responded favorably to current front-line antidepressants as well as several newer therapies, including ECT, repetitive transcranial magnetic stimulation, deep brain stimulation, and the NMDA glutamate antagonist, ketamine (Willner, 2017).

The literature on CMS, CUMS, or CVS as animal models of depression is far too extensive to review in detail in this chapter (Antoniuk et al., 2019). As an alternative, I will highlight experiments that provide a comparison with some of the findings summarized earlier that relate to the effects of CSDS on neural systems and behavior.

Targeting DA neurons. DA neurons within the mesolimbic system appear to be well-positioned to respond to a diverse array of stressful stimuli, thereby influencing the expression of depression-related behavioral responses in laboratory animals. To explore the role of DA neurons, Tye et al. (2013) selectively and reversibly inhibited VTA DA neurons optogenetically by light-induced activation of a virally delivered halorhodopsin (HR) that was inserted into tyrosine hydroxylase-positive neurons of the VTA, resulting in hyperpolarization of neuronal membranes when constantly illuminated by light at 593 nm. When compared to control mice, HR mice displayed a significant and reversible reduction in active struggling during illumination for minutes 4–6 of a 9-minute tail suspension test. Similarly, in a 90-minute, two-bottle sucrose preference test, HR mice displayed a significant and reversible reduction in sucrose preference during illumination for minutes 30–60 compared to control mice. However, control mice and HR mice did not differ in locomotor activity in an open field arena during periods of illumination.

To examine the role of VTA DA neurons in stress-induced depressive-like behaviors, mice were exposed to CMS for 8–12 weeks or were left undisturbed in their home cages. Optogenetic activation of DA neurons was achieved by activation of virally delivered channelrhodopsin-2 (ChR-2) that was inserted into tyrosine hydroxylase-positive neurons of the VTA. Phasic activation of VTA DA neurons was achieved by a physiologically relevant illumination pattern (473 nm, 8 pulses at 30 Hz, 5 millisecond pulse width, every 5 seconds) during behavioral testing. Compared to unstressed controls, CMS-exposed mice displayed significant decreases in active struggling during the tail suspension test and reduced preference for a sucrose solution in a two-bottle preference test. In contrast, CMS-exposed mice did not differ from unstressed controls in levels of activity in an open field arena. Optogenetic activation of VTA DA neurons in CMS-exposed ChR-2 mice reversed the decrease in active struggling during the tail suspension test and restored sucrose preference to levels seen in unstressed controls. These findings point to the important role played by VTA DA neurons in the neural encoding of depression-like behaviors within a circumscribed limbic circuit (Tye et al., 2013).

Vulnerability to depression. As noted earlier, it has been challenging to identify individuals who are at high risk of developing depression following exposure to stressful stimulation. To address this issue, Castro et al. (2012) subjected outbred male Sprague-Dawley rats to a battery of behavioral tests prior to exposure to CMS for 2 or 4 weeks. The behavioral tests were designed to capture the following behavioral traits: anxiety, exploration, and locomotor activity. Following exposure to CMS, rats were subjected to three behavioral tests to assess depression-like behaviors. These included a saccharin preference test, a social preference test, and a forced swim test. In addition, plasma CORT was measured following the forced swim test. Based upon their behavioral and physiological responses, rats distributed across the following four groups:

- Low anxiety–low exploration: social behavior similar to unstressed controls, CORT responses to stress higher than controls;
- Low anxiety–high exploration: social behavior decreased relative to controls, CORT levels similar to controls;
- High anxiety–low exploration: social behaviors decreased relative to controls, CORT levels similar to controls;
- High anxiety–high exploration: social behavior decreased relative to controls, CORT responses to stress higher than controls.

These findings indicated that behavioral profiles predict in part the depression-like behavioral responses of genetically heterogeneous outbred rats of the Sprague-Dawley strain following 4 weeks of CMS (Castro et al., 2012).

A behavioral antidepressant. Experiments by Rescorla (1969) demonstrated that a conditioned stimulus (CS) that is negatively correlated with delivery of an aversive unconditioned stimulus (US) can become a safety signal, with a corresponding reduction in conditioned fear. Building of these early studies of safety signals, Pollak et al. (2008) examined the impact of a safety signal on behavioral and molecular responses to CMS. Safety training consisted of one session per day for 3 consecutive days, and in each session there were 4 unpaired CS (350 Hz tone, 72 dB, 20 seconds duration) and US presentations (0.6 mA footshock for 2 seconds). In fear conditioning, the US always followed at the end of the CS. On the fourth day, mice from the safety training and fear conditioning groups were placed individually into the test chamber, and their time spent freezing was measured. Mice that received safety training exhibited significantly less freezing behavior than mice that received fear conditioning, even though mice in both groups received the same number of footshocks.

Following exposure to a CMS paradigm for 5 weeks, mice were tested for sucrose preference in a two-bottle choice test. This measure of anhedonia is often taken as a reflection of a depression-like phenotype. Compared to unstressed controls, CMS-exposed mice exhibited a significant decrease in sucrose preference. If CMS-exposed mice were previously exposed to safety training, the presence of the safety signal during the two-bottle choice test resulted in a level of preference for sucrose that matched the sucrose preference level of unstressed controls. These investigators also presented findings that were consistent with learned safety being as effective as fluoxetine in preventing the emergence of depression-like behavioral changes. Importantly, the effects of learned safety appeared to be mediated by molecular pathways that were different from those of fluoxetine. Interestingly, learned safety also promoted the survival of adult-born neurons in the dentate gyrus, which, as described in the following, may protect against stress-induced depression-like behaviors (Pollak et al., 2008).

Summary. Experiments with the CMS model have dove-tailed nicely with the CSDS model to reveal brain circuits and molecules involved in the expression of a depression-like behavioral phenotype. Rewards circuits in brain have been studied in laboratory animals exposed to CMS, and the results are generally consistent with experiments described earlier for the CSDS model. Another line of research identified behavioral markers of susceptibility prior to exposure to a CMS paradigm. Finally, use of a safety signal had an effect that was similar in magnitude to an antidepressant in animals exposed to CMS, even though the molecular pathways involved differed between the safety signal group and the fluoxetine-treated group.

Looking Ahead

In the next chapter, we will continue our discussions of animal models of stress and depression. The heterogeneity of depression will be emphasized in the next chapter, with sections on sex differences in depression, the role of adult-born neurons in depression, how epigenetic modifications of DNA and histones play a role in depression, and the importance of inflammatory responses to stress in promoting a depression-like phenotype.

13

Stress and Depression

Part 2

Phillip W. Gold, a distinguished physician-scientist who spent most of his career at the National Institute of Mental Health in Bethesda, Maryland, concluded a major review article with this overarching view of depression (Gold, 2015, p. 45):

> Depression affects ways of feeling and thinking that intrude upon the features that help define our humanity. It is a neurodegenerative disease that affects key sites of the prefrontal cortex, limbic system and multiple cortical areas. In its severe manifestations, it is like a cancer of the self that impairs our self-respect, sense of well-being and capacity to think clearly. It metastasizes from the brain to the periphery to influence the functional integrity of the HPA axis and the SNS system, and is associated with a prothrombotic state, inflammation and insulin resistance.

As Dr. Gold notes, depression is much more than a mental disorder. Because it leads to activation of the three major peripheral stress effector systems, depression also brings with it major medical problems that further reduce quality of life and add to the overall burden of disease of this disruptive illness.

In this second chapter on the topic of "Stress and Depression," I will discuss some of the risk genes associated with this disorder, followed by a brief review of studies on stress during early life as a risk factor for depression in adulthood. Next, I will present experiments that have attempted to model in laboratory animals the greater incidence of MDD in females compared to males. This chapter will conclude with three relatively new areas of investigation: the connection between birth of new neurons in the adult brain and antidepressant actions, the role of epigenetics in depression, and the impact of the immune system on depression. Exciting research advances have been made in each of these topical areas, and a host of new targets for the development of next-generation therapies has been identified.

In spite of devoting two chapters to research on animal models of depression, I was still forced to be highly selective in the experiments that are featured. The sheer volume of research on animal models of stress and depression that has been conducted over the past 5 decades could easily justify a complete volume devoted solely to this topic.

Risk Genes and Depression

GWAS have provided clear evidence that depression in humans is influenced by a large number of risk variants. In addition, MDD has a relatively low heritability of ~35%–40%. In spite of this heterogeneity in the genetics of MDD, many basic scientists and clinicians have focused remarkable levels of attention on serotonin signaling in brain, especially the 5-HT transporter. However, as a general rule, experiments focusing on individual genes have not taken center stage in this broad area of research. In spite of the reluctance to focus on individual genes, there have been several studies of individual risk genes that have provided important mechanistic insights into depression, and I will feature a selection of them in the next section.

As the Stomach Churns

Acyl-ghrelin (AG) was introduced in Chapter 4 and plays an important role in stimulating feeding and in the regulation of energy balance. The hormone is synthesized largely in specialized cells of the gastrointestinal system and interacts with growth hormone secretagogue receptor 1a (GHSR1a). Lutter et al. (2008) explored the involvement of AG in the CSDS model of depression. C57BL/6J male mice subjected to CSDS for 10 days exhibited significant increases in circulating AG that persisted for up to 4 weeks after the last defeat. To examine the role of GHSR1a in the CSDS model of depression, null mutant mice ($Ghsr^{(-/-)}$) and WT littermate controls were subjected to 10 days of CSDS. $Ghsr^{(-/-)}$ mice displayed significantly greater levels of avoidance of a social stranger than WT controls, a key behavioral measure of depressive-like symptoms in this model of stress-induced depression. These investigators also provided evidence that endogenously released AG influenced depression-like behaviors in mice. Caloric restriction for 10 days (60% of normal calories) resulted in a 4-fold increase in circulating levels of AG, lower levels of anxiety-like behaviors in an EPM, and lower levels of depression-like behavior in the forced swim test. Similar results were obtained with exogenously administered AG. The behavioral effects of endogenously released or exogenously administered AG were absent in $Ghsr^{(-/-)}$ mice. These findings revealed that AG may play an important role in regulation of mood, especially in animals (and perhaps humans) exposed to chronic stress (Lutter et al., 2008).

These results were extended by Huang et al. (2017), who exposed C57BL/6J male mice or Sprague-Dawley male rats to a chronic unpredictable mild stress (CUMS) paradigm for 8 weeks. Administration of ghrelin (5 nmol/kg/day i.p. for 2 weeks) reversed the anxiety- and depression-like behaviors that resulted from CUMS. Consistent with results from other laboratories, plasma AG levels were increased significantly following CUMS. In addition, transcription of the ghrelin gene was up-regulated in the stomach and hippocampus and transcription of the GHSR1a gene was up-regulated in the hippocampus of mice exposed to CUMS. In a final experiment, central administration of ghrelin (10 µg/rat/day, i.c.v., for 2 weeks) or growth hormone releasing peptide (10 µg/rat/day, i.c.v., for 2 weeks) also blunted the effects of CUMS for 6 weeks on depression-like behaviors (forced swim and sucrose preference tests). These findings further underscored the important of a coordinated peripheral → central signaling pathway involving AG and GHSR1a in regulation of mood states following chronic exposure to stressors (Huang et al., 2017). Finally, Gupta et al. (2019) demonstrated that blockade of ß1-adrenoceptors with atenolol during exposure to CSDS reduced the plasma AG response and enhanced the occurrence of depressive-like behaviors.

Problems with Transport

A single nucleotide polymorphism (SNP) in the neuron-specific neutral amino acid transporter gene (*SLC6A15*) was advanced by Kohli et al. (2011) as a risk gene for stress vulnerability and major depressive disorder in humans. Their results indicated that lower SLC6A15 expression, especially in the hippocampus, could increase an individual's stress susceptibility by altering neuronal integrity, hippocampal volume, and excitatory neurotransmission in this stress-responsive brain region. They extended their results to a mouse model of chronic social stress by selecting animals that were among the most susceptible and most resilient to a chronic stress paradigm. They found that stress-susceptible mice had an almost 2-fold reduction in expression of SLC6A15 in the CA1 region of the hippocampus compared to stress-resilient mice.

To understand the mechanisms by which this SNP places humans at risk for the development of major depressive disorder, Santarelli et al. (2016) examined the impact of this gene on behavioral and neurobiological measures in laboratory mice. Two approaches were taken: studies with *slc6a15* (SLC) KO mice compared to their WT littermate controls, and mice with virally mediated over-expression of *slc6a15* (SLC-OE) in the hippocampus compared to vehicle-injected controls. Mice were studied under basal conditions and following 3 weeks of CSDS.

Under basal conditions, WT and SLC-KO mice had similar behavioral phenotypes based upon an EPM, open field arena, and forced swim test. Following CSDS, SLC-KO mice displayed lower levels of anxiety- and depression-like behaviors compared to WT controls. A complementary pattern of results was reported for SLC-OE mice, which displayed increased anxiety-like behaviors under basal conditions compared to controls. These investigators suggested that GluR1 expression in the dentate gyrus appeared to be influenced by expression of *slc6a15* and may have explained the differences in responses to CSDS between SLC-KO mice and WT controls.

The Serotonin Connection

Tryptophan hydroxylase (Tph2) converts typtophan to 5-hydroxytryptophan, a key step in the biosynthesis of the neurotransmitter serotonin (5-HT). Many theories relating to the etiology of depression have focused on a possible role for a 5-HT deficiency in depressive patients. To characterize the effects of a targeted 5-HT deficiency in an animal model, Caron's laboratory at Duke University generated a knockin mouse model that involved substituting histidine for arginine at position 439 (his[439]) of Tph2 (Tph2KI). The Tph2KI mouse mimicked a genetic polymorphism detected in a small group of depressed geriatric patients from the eastern United States (Beaulieu et al., 2008). Compared to WT controls, Tph2KI mice displayed 60%–80% reductions in synthesis and tissue content of 5-HT and 95% reductions in levels of the principal 5-HT metabolite, 5-hydroxyindoleacetic acid. A battery of tests revealed that Tph2KI mice displayed elevated levels of depression-like and anxiety-like behaviors. The Tph2KI mouse model offers major advantages over the TphKO mouse model in that some residual 5-HT activity remains, a characteristic more in keeping with levels of 5-HT signaling in patients with MDD (Jacobsen et al., 2012).

Two experiments demonstrated an interactive effect of a susceptible genotype (Tph2KI) and stressful stimulation on susceptibility to depression-like behaviors. In the first experiment, exposure of Tph2KI mice to CSDS resulted in increases in social avoidance that were unresponsive to treatment with fluoxetine. This finding is important because it indicates that SSRIs require a reasonable level of biosynthetic activity of 5-HT to exert a favorable impact on depression-like behaviors in mice. Using a chemogenetic approach to selectively inhibit neuronal activity in the lateral habenula, a target of deep brain stimulation experiments in patients with MDD, these investigators reported reduced levels of social avoidance in WT mice and in Tph2KI mice following 7–10 days of CSDS. Tph2KI mice may prove valuable as an animal model for some forms of treatment-resistant depression (Sachs et al., 2015).

In a prior experiment, Sachs et al. (2014) examined sex differences in responses to CMS in WT mice and Tph2KI mice. CMS resulted in increased anxiety-like behavior in an EPM, but there was no additional effect of sex or 5-HT genotype on the behavioral measures. Following CMS, female mice displayed increased levels of immobility in the forced swim test. Female Tph2KI mice exhibited reduced preference for a sucrose solution compared to male Tph2KI mice. In addition, cell proliferation in the dentate gyrus was much greater in female compared to male Tph2KI mice. These results were consistent with a dynamic interplay between sex, susceptible genotype, and stressful stimulation in shaping alterations in emotional behaviors.

Knocking Out Transporters

Several laboratories have generated mouse knockout models of key neuronal membrane transporter molecules, including 5-HT (SERT), norepinephrine (NET), and dopamine (DAT). In the forced swim test, DAT-KO mice were exceedingly active and struggled to escape from the container and had low immobility scores. NET-KO mice also had low immobility scores, and were active in swimming and climbing. In contrast, SERT-KO mice did not differ from their WT controls in their behaviors during the forced swim test. In the tail suspension test, DAT-KO, NET-KO, and SERT-KO mice exhibited significant reductions in time spent immobile relative to their WT controls. In the sucrose preference test, DAT-KO mice displayed a significant preference for sucrose. In contrast, sucrose consumption was not affected in NE-KO and SERT-KO mice. Finally, levels of activity were significantly enhanced in DAT-KO mice, but were unaffected in NE-KO and SERT-KO mice. These investigators suggested that the DAT should be considered a target for development of new antidepressants (Perona et al., 2008).

In a study of the NE transporter, Haenisch et al. (2009) compared the behavioral and molecular responses of WT mice and NET-KO mice following exposure to chronic restraint stress or CSDS. Immobility times in the forced swim test were significantly lower in NET-KO mice compared to WT controls. WT mice exposed to either stressor exhibited increased immobility scores relative to unstressed WT controls. In contrast, NET-KO mice exposed to chronic stress had immobility scores that were similar to unstressed NET-KO mice. A similar pattern of differences between WT mice and NET-KO mice was observed for tests of sucrose preference and social avoidance. In addition, WT mice but not NET-KO mice responded favorably to an antidepressant following exposure to chronic stress. Exposure of WT and NET-KO mice to chronic stressors resulted in downregulation of BDNF in the hippocampus and cerebral cortex. These changes in

BDNF could be prevented by chronic administration of various antidepressants in WT mice but not in NET-KO mice.

Summary

Although MDD is influenced by multiple genetic variants, experiments that have focused on manipulations of individual risk genes have revealed important effects on depression-related behaviors. Manipulations of ghrelin are noteworthy in that this gastrointestinal hormone connects disruptions in mood with alterations in food intake and energy balance, all of which are key features of MDD. SLC6A15 has been identified as a possible risk gene for MDD, and it has been the subject of experiments in laboratory mice exposed to chronic stress. Not surprisingly, genetic manipulations of 5-HT synthesis or reuptake have been explored, especially within the context of gene x environment experimental designs. Unfortunately, in the long run, manipulations of single genes will not get us closer to an animal model that matches well with what is known about the etiology of MDD.

Early Life Stress

Sex Differences in Response to Early Life Stress

Goodwill et al. (2019) employed a model of early life stress (ELS) that involved disrupting patterns of maternal care by transferring C57BL/6N females and their litters on PND 4 from a solid bottom maternity cage with bedding material to a wire mesh cage with a limited amount of cotton nesting material. Mothers and their litters remained in these limited nesting conditions for 1 week, when they were returned to standard maternity cages. Control mothers and litters were left undisturbed. Male and female offspring of control and ELS females were tested during adolescence and early adulthood on several behavioral tests of depression-like behaviors. ELS females but not males exhibited depression-like behaviors on tests of sucrose preference and behavior in a forced swim test. Novelty-induced hypophagia was especially evident in adult females. Continuous monitoring of home cage behaviors yielded a similar pattern, with ELS females spending more time sleeping, less time active, and less time grooming. In contrast, ELS did not affect anxiety-like behaviors in males or females compared to controls. The behavioral changes produced in ELS females were rapidly reversed by treatment with ketamine (0.6 mg/kg, i.p.) as assessed by continuous monitoring of home cage behaviors over multiple days. These results point to a new animal model of depression that results in greater vulnerability of females than males.

Two Hits Are Better than One

In a remarkable series of experiments, Peña et al. (2017) reported that exposure of litters of C57BL/6J mice to stress for 7–10 days beginning on PND 10 but not on PND 2 increased their susceptibility to a battery of depression-like behavioral measures following CSDS in adulthood. The early life stress protocol involved maintaining mothers with their litters in cages with limited bedding material and separation of the litters from their mothers for 4 hours per day for the specified periods. Following CSDS, those mice exposed to stress from PNDs 10–20 displayed social avoidance, reduced preference for sucrose in a two-bottle choice test, increased immobility in a forced swim test, and fewer movement in the center portion of an open field arena. In addition, exposure to early life stress dramatically increased the percentage of mice that were characterized as susceptible to the effects of CSDS in adulthood compared to mice that were not stressed prior to weaning.

To explore the molecular underpinnings of exposure to early life stress, these investigators examined transcriptome-wide changes in the ventral tegmental area (VTA), a brain reward region. Although the expression of many genes was altered by stress prior to weaning and/or CSDS in adulthood, their analyses revealed that exposure to stress prior to weaning primed the VTA to be in a depression-like state based upon transcriptional activity. This pattern of transcriptional changes resulting from early life stress was long-lasting and was unmasked only after these at-risk individuals were exposed to CSDS in adulthood.

Further analyses revealed that a key upstream regulator of this depression-like state in the VTA was orthodenticle homeobox 2 (OTX2), a transcription factor involved in neural development, especially within the VTA. As a positive control, similar analyses in the nucleus accumbens, a primary target of VTA neurons, failed to detect comparable molecular changes. Approximately 70% of OTX2-positive cells in the VTA are DAergic. Interestingly, early life stress alone had no effect on *Otx2* mRNA levels in the VTA of adult animals. However, *Otx2* was transiently down-regulated on PND 21 in the VTA of mice exposed to late postnatal stress. If this transient down-regulation of *Otx2* around PND 21 was prevented by time-limited over-expression of *Otx2* using viral delivery to the VTA, the enhanced susceptibility of mice exposed to early life stress was blocked. Similarly, transient knockdown of *Otx2* in mice reared under control conditions rendered them sensitive to the effects of CSDS in adulthood. These findings revealed a highly sensitive period during postnatal development (PNDs 10–20) when the stress of maternal separation resulted in long-lasting latent vulnerability to a depression-like phenotype that was unmasked by exposure of mice to CSDS in adulthood.

These findings from a mouse model of early life stress pointed the way to a related study in children to explore the mechanisms by which exposure to stressful experiences in childhood increased risk for later development of psychiatric disorders. Early findings based upon peripheral biomarkers and brain imaging studies were consistent with a possible role for OTX2 and related genes in the onset of depression in children with a history of maltreatment (Kaufman et al., 2018).

Sex Differences in Depression

Although experiments with animal models have revealed important mechanistic insights into the pathophysiology of MDD, one issue has been all but overlooked for many decades. Women are about twice as likely as men to develop MDD, their symptoms of depression tend to be more severe than those of men, and they tend to exhibit different subsets of symptoms of depression than men (Issler & Nestler, 2018). In spite of these important clinical and diagnostic findings, very few studies with animal models of depression have even bothered to include females in the design of experiments.

In their detailed review article, Beery and Zucker (2011) reported that a sex bias in basic research favoring males over females was evident in 8 of the 10 fields of the biological sciences they analyzed, with the greatest bias in neuroscience research. They also noted that females were often underrepresented in experiments involving animal models of various diseases, including psychiatric disorders. One explanation for the bias in favor of experiments with only male animals is the concern that female mammals are inherently more variable than males because of fluctuations in ovarian hormones during the estrus cycle (Shansky, 2019). This concern about female variability has now largely been dismissed based upon empirical evidence. Another barrier that should be considered is a much simpler one—we have always done it this way, and why should we change now?

In 1993, the US National Institutes of Health (NIH) required that women be included in NIH-funded clinical research studies. It took less than two decades after this policy change for women to make up slightly more than 50% of participants in all NIH-funded clinical research projects. To catalyze a similar change in the basic biomedical sciences, the NIH developed new policies and associated training materials that sought to achieve a more balanced approach in experiments with laboratory animals, such that females and males would be included in experimental designs detailed in grant proposals (Clayton & Collins,

2014). Another important area that has often neglected the importance of gender is GWAS, where the majority of reports have neglected to include the X chromosome. Still others have neglected to include the Y chromosome. The net result of these omissions has been an underrepresentation of genes from the sex chromosomes among gene variants associated with human diseases, including MDD (Anonymous, 2017).

Are Females More Susceptible to Stress?

To address this question, Schmitz et al. (2002) exposed pregnant female rats to a single 20-minute period of restraint stress on gestational day 18. Controls were handled but not stressed. When male and female offspring of control and prenatally stressed females reached 75 days of age, the numbers of granule cells and pyramidal cells in the hippocampus were quantified using an optical fractionator. Females but not males that were exposed to stress *in utero* exhibited reductions in granule cells in the hippocampus compared to unstressed controls. These investigators suggested that the loss of granule cells in prenatally stressed females may serve as a risk factor for depression in adulthood, with a greater impact on females than males.

McCormick and Green (2013) reviewed the relevant literature regarding the impact of stressors applied during adolescence on the later development of anxiety-like and depression-like behaviors in adulthood. This period of development is a time of heightened sensitivity to stressors, which may alter the trajectory of stress-sensitive brain circuits. To explore sex differences in sensitivity to depression-like behaviors, male and female Sprague-Dawley rats were exposed to individual housing or remained group-housed from PNDs 30–35 (Leussis & Andersen, 2008). Group-housed females displayed higher levels of depression-like behaviors than grouped-housed males in both a forced swim test and a learned helplessness paradigm. Isolation housing had a greater impact on depression-like behaviors in male rats compared to female rats. Additional studies of proteins associated with brain plasticity pointed to the PFC as an especially vulnerable brain area in adolescent rats exposed to stress. These findings are especially interesting in that they revealed the emergence of sex differences in the susceptibility to depression-like behaviors in male and female rats in the period between weaning and the onset of sexual maturity in adulthood.

Adult Females and Stress

In an early experiment on stress and depression, Kennett et al. (1986) took the unusual approach of comparing the responses of adult male and female

Sprague-Dawley rats to acute versus chronic stress in the form of restraint stress for 2 hours. In males, a single bout of restraint stress resulted in reduced levels of locomotion and increased defecation during open field testing. These effects were no longer observed following 5 consecutive days of restraint stress, indicating adaptive responses (i.e., habituation) to repeated restraint stress. Accompanying this adaptation was an increased sensitivity to the 5-HT ago-nist, 5-methoxy-N,N-dimethyltryptamine (DMT). In contrast, female rats were much less affected by a single bout of restraint stress, but were significantly af-fected by repeated exposure to restraint stress over a 5-day period. After 5 days of restraint stress, female rats did not display increased sensitivity to DMT. The authors suggested that females may have different patterns of adaptation to chronic stressors compared to males, and these differences may explain in part the higher incidence of MDD in females (Kennett et al., 1986). Unfortunately, these intriguing findings did not stimulate a broad-based interest in studying sex differences in depression-like behaviors in animal models.

Female mice and chronic stress. To develop an animal model that captured the greater incidence of MDD in females versus males, Hodes et al. (2015) em-ployed a sub-chronic variable stress (SCVS) paradigm such that C57BL/6 female and male mice were exposed to stressors for only 3 or 6 days. The standard du-ration for CVS is typically 21 days. Three different stressors were employed, in-cluding footshock (100 mild footshocks over a 1-hour period), a tail suspension test for 1 hour, and restraint stress for 1 hour. Alternation of the stressors reduced the chances of habituation.

Female mice were highly susceptible to SCVS, displaying a depression-like behavioral phenotype after 6 days based upon the results of a battery of tests, and increased levels of circulating CORT. In contrast, the behaviors and plasma CORT levels of male mice exposed to SCVS were similar to unstressed controls. Samples of the nucleus accumbens, a key brain area involved in processing re-warding and emotional stimuli, were collected the day after SCVS, and transcrip-tional analyses were performed. Although male mice did not display behavioral changes following SCVS, they did display significant transcriptional alterations, with more genes up- or down-regulated following SCVS in stressed males versus control males compared to stressed females versus control females. This sex dif-ference in transcriptional responses to stress in the nucleus accumbens may ex-plain in part the greater susceptibility to a depression-like phenotype in female mice compared to male mice. In addition, only a small percentage of the genes that were regulated by stress in males overlapped with the genes regulated by stress in females.

Expression of the DNA methyltransferase, *Dnmt3a*, but not *Dnmt3b* or *Dnmt1*, was significantly elevated in the nucleus accumbens of both male and fe-male mice 1 day after exposure to SCVS. In male and female mice, overexpression

of *Dnmt3a* in the nucleus accumbens was sufficient to induce increased susceptibility to a sub-threshold form of SCVS, which included only 3 days of stressor exposure. In contrast, the selective knockout of *Dnmt3a* in the nucleus accumbens
of female mice resulted in a more male-like pattern of resilience to SCVS, as
well as a more male-like transcriptional response in the nucleus accumbens following SCVS. Knockdown of *Dnmt3a* in the nucleus accumbens of male mice
was without effect.

Taken together, these findings demonstrate that female mice are more susceptible to the effects of an abbreviated regimen of chronic variable stress, lasting
only 6 days, compared to male mice. In addition, the transcriptional responses
to SCVS in the nucleus accumbens differed dramatically between males and
females. Thus, the sex-specific behavioral responses to SCVS were mirrored
by sex-specific transcriptional responses in a key brain area related to depression. *Dnmt3a* was identified as one gene that plays a critical role in the differing
responses of male and female mice to SCVS. These exciting results suggested a
range of strategies for developing more effective antidepressant medications for
females (Hodes et al., 2015).

Females and social instability. Herzog et al. (2009) also developed a meaningful approach to stressful stimulation in studies of adult female Wistar rats.
Over a 4-week period, female rats were exposed to alternating periods of isolation or crowding with different social partners for varying lengths of time. This
social instability paradigm resulted in increased activity of the HPA axis and disruption of the hypothalamic-pituitary-gonadal axis. In addition, stressed female
rats displayed a reduced preference for sucrose and reduced food intake, but no
change in behavior during the forced swim test. This experiment developed a
useful approach for exposing adult female rats to chronic stress without evidence
of habituation over a 4-week period. It appeared that social instability was the key
variable that resulted in the neuroendocrine and behavioral changes that were
observed (Pryce & Fuchs, 2017). Unfortunately, this model has not been widely
employed by other laboratories to study the effects of stress on depression-like
behaviors in female mice and rats.

SERT-KO rats. Olivier et al. (2008) compared male and female SERT-KO
rats with their WT controls in a battery of behavioral tests designed to assess
levels of anxiety and depression. They did not observe any differences between
male and female SERT-KO rats, perhaps because of a ceiling effect of completely
eliminating the 5-HT transporter protein. Unfortunately, they did not include
SERT$^{(+/-)}$ heterozygotes in their study. SERT-KO male and female rats displayed
high levels of anxiety-like and depression-like behavioral responses.

CRF receptors. Bale and Vale (2003) reasoned that individual sensitivity to
stressful stimulation may explain why some people exposed to stressors develop
depression while others do not. They directed their attention to CRF signaling

because of its role in regulating the HPA axis and its possible role in the development of depression. They conducted experiments with (*Crfr2*) null mutant mice and WT controls and documented a lack of CRFR2 mRNA in key brain areas, with preservation of normal levels of CRFR1 mRNA levels. CRFR2 mutant male and female mice were tested in a forced swim test and exhibited increased immobility scores, decreased time spent swimming, and decreased time spent climbing compared to sex-matched WT controls. CRFR2 mutant female mice displayed more extreme levels of all three behavioral measures compared to CRFR2 mutant male mice.

In a second experiment, antalarmin (7.5 mg/kg), a non-peptide CRFR1 antagonist, was administered to WT mice and CRFR2 mutant mice 1, 24, or 72 hours prior to a forced swim test. Antalarmin was employed to determine if there was a compensatory increase in CRFR1 signaling activity in the absence of CRFR2. The results indicated that antalarmin decreased immobility times and increased swim times in CRFR2 mutant males and females. In addition, there was a significant effect of sex for time spent immobile and time spent swimming following antalarmin treatment. These findings suggested that sex differences in CRF signaling in brain during exposure to stress may explain in part the increased prevalence of MDD in females (Bale & Vale, 2002).

Sex, stress, and transcriptional signatures. In a landmark study, Labonté et al. (2017) employed post-mortem brain samples to compare the transcriptional profiles of two cohorts (*N* = 98 participants in total) that included males and females with MDD and male and female controls without MDD. Data from high throughput sequencing were used to identify gene targets and molecular pathways underlying sex differences in MDD in an unbiased manner. To identify these molecular pathways, these investigators employed advanced Weighted Gene Co-expression Network Analysis such that the expression levels of all transcripts across all samples were compared to identify subsets of genes that were co-regulated under control or depressed conditions. These classes of co-regulated genes are referred to as gene modules, and within them are hub genes that are highly connected with other genes within the module.

Labonté et al. (2017) detected a sexually dimorphic pattern in levels of differentially expressed genes in post-mortem brain samples from individuals with MDD compared to brain samples from controls. A striking result was the very low (~5%–10%) overlap in differentially expressed genes between males and females with MDD. There was also a low level of overlap between males and females with MDD in depression-specific disease modules across brain regions. Using network analysis, they identified sex-specific hub genes that were highly interconnected to various differentially expressed genes across disease modules and brain regions. For example, in brain samples from females with MDD, one of the most highly ranked modules was enriched for MAPK activity and included

18 genes, four of which were hubs, with multiple down-regulated genes. In brain samples from males with MDD, one of the most highly ranked modules included 311 genes involved with synaptic transmission, with 43 serving as hubs, and with many up-regulated transcripts, especially in the ventromedial PFC.

Armed with these powerful comparisons in transcriptional signatures between human males and females with MDD and their respective controls, Labonté et al. (2017) next embarked on a reverse translational strategy by comparing sex differences in gene expression signatures between male and female mice exposed to a chronic variable stress (CVS) paradigm. This stress protocol, when employed for 21 days, was highly effective in producing a depression-like behavioral phenotype in male as well as female mice. When these investigators compared differentially expressed genes in mice exposed to CVS, they found substantial overlap between female mice and human females with MDD and between male mice and human males with MDD. In one brain area studied in humans and in mice, the ventromedial PFC, there were 251 up- or down-regulated transcripts in common in females of the two species, and 152 up- or down-regulated transcripts in common in males of the two species.

DUSP6, a protein phosphatase that inactivates ERK signaling, is a highly interconnected hub gene in the ventromedial PFC that was decreased significantly in females with MDD. Similarly, expression of *Dusp6* was decreased in the PFC of female mice exposed to CVS. A targeted reduction in *Dusp6* expression in the PFC of female mice but not male mice increased behaviors associated with a depression-like phenotype and alterations in gene transcription that compared favorably with changes following exposure to CVS. The transcription factor, *EMX1*, a highly interconnected hub gene that regulates the development of cortical neurons, was differentially expressed in the PFC of males with MDD and male mice exposed to CVS. Targeted overexpression of *Emx1* in the PFC of male mice but not female mice resulted in some but not all facets of a depression-like phenotype. Finally, decreased expression of *Dusp6* in female mice and increased expression of *Emx1* in male mice both converged onto a common physiological output, increased activity of pyramidal neurons in the PFC. This finding points to a common mechanism activated by different pathways in males and females that could drive the overlapping behavioral changes following exposure to CVS.

This report by Labonté et al. (2017) was the breakthrough study that was so desperately needed in clinical research with depressed humans and basic research with mouse models of depression, where careful comparisons of males and females were at the heart of the experimental design. The commonalities in gene expression patterns in brain between human males and females and their mouse counterparts argued strongly for the validity of the CVS model of depression. It also opens the way for understanding the developmental trajectories of these gender-specific gene expression patterns in the mouse brain, and how they in turn influence behaviors associated with depression. Finally, these findings will be crucial in guiding the continuing quest for development of personalized treatments for MDD.

Stress and depression in female monkeys. Nonhuman primate models of MDD are relatively rare given the high costs associated with maintaining a large colony of animals, the length of time required for conduct of experiments, and concerns about the welfare of nonhuman primates in the laboratory or under captive conditions at primate centers. One exception to this general rule is the very large and successful colony of cynomolgous monkeys (*Macaca fascicularis*) maintained for several decades at the Wake Forest University School of Medicine. There are some obvious benefits to modeling MDD in a macaque species, particularly in experiments on sex differences in depression. Among the benefits of employing nonhuman primates instead of laboratory mice and rats are a 95% homology with the genetic code of humans, a larger and more highly evolved brain that can be studied with imaging methods similar to those employed in humans, a true menstrual cycle that is similar to human females, and a more complex social structure.

Naturally occurring depression. Shively and her colleagues (for a review, see Willard & Shively, 2012) have capitalized on these advantages of studying female macaques and have conducted an extensive series of experiments on cynomolgous monkeys that were wild-caught from an island breeding colony in Indonesia and shipped to the United States. Upon arrival in the laboratory, female monkeys were housed in small groups of 3–5 adults. In such a setting, female monkeys quickly establish a linear dominance hierarchy that can be assessed by frequent behavioral observations. In such a social group, the 2 top-ranked females are considered dominant and the 2–3 remaining females are considered subordinate based upon their behaviors. Compared to dominant females, subordinate females were the recipients of more aggression, they were groomed less frequently, they were constantly vigilant, and they were alone more frequently. Some subordinate females over time displayed a slumped body posture, with head below the level of the shoulders and eyes open, but with a blank stare. Such females typically lacked interest in and were unresponsive to changes in the environment. These investigators have characterized this body posture and lack of interest in ongoing events as "behavioral depression." Their initial observations revealed that behavioral depression occurred in some but not all subordinate females, but rarely occurred in dominant females. Thus, there were clear-cut individual differences in the responses of subordinate females to the ongoing stress associated with social interactions within the group (Shively et al., 1997).

Behaviorally depressed female monkeys differed from socially stressed subordinate females in a number of ways, and these differences reflected many of the cardinal symptoms of MDD in humans. Behaviorally depressed female monkeys had lower body mass, impaired ovarian function, increased coronary artery atherosclerosis, elevated heart rates at night, decreased activity levels, and spent more time in contact with conspecifics. In addition, behaviorally depressed female monkeys were relatively insensitive to glucocorticoid negative feedback of the HPA axis, but had normal responsiveness of the adrenal cortex to exogenously administered ACTH. Behaviorally depressed females also had a blunted ACTH response to exogenous CRF, suggesting a reduced responsiveness of pituitary corticotropes. These findings matched well with clinical studies of the HPA axis in depressed patients (Gold, 2015). Neurobiological correlates of depression in female monkeys also compared favorably with changes that have been observed in patients with MDD. Depressed female monkeys exhibited reductions in 5-HT_{1A} receptor binding in several brain areas and total volume of the hippocampus, both of which are consistent with findings in patients with MDD (Willard & Shively, 2012).

Behavioral depression in female cynomolgous monkeys represents an excellent animal model of MDD in humans. Importantly, the behavioral depression resulted from normal social interactions among adult female monkeys, and did not require exposure to chronic stressors. The monkey model also provided further evidence of an association between depression and cardiovascular disease, an association that has been noted in studies of rodent models and depressed patients (Grippo & Johnson, 2002; Rudisch & Nemeroff, 2003). Finally, depressed premenopausal female monkeys exhibited a mixed response to the antidepressant sertraline, an SSRI, with reductions in anxious behaviors, increases in affiliative behaviors, and a reduction in aggression. However, sertraline did not reduce depressive behaviors in these female monkeys in a dosing regimen that matched well with those utilized by MDD patients, and it exacerbated the level of atherosclerosis (Shively et al., 2017).

Replication in China. More recently, Shively teamed with a research group from Chongqing, People's Republic of China, to study female cynomolgous monkeys in semi-naturalistic enclosed social groups consisting of 2 adult males and 15–20 adult females. The total study population included 1,007 monkeys distributed across 52 enclosures. Over time, 1–2 females per social group displayed the characteristic depressive phenotype described earlier, and administration of the fast-acting antidepressant ketamine to a very small sample of depressed female monkeys was without favorable effects (Xu et al., 2015).

Taken together, these laboratory and semi-natural experiments with cynomolgous monkeys have provided extensive validation of the effectiveness of this animal model of MDD. It may also be the case that behavioral depression in these monkeys closely resembles treatment-resistant depression in humans. Thus, the failure to reverse behavioral symptoms of depression in monkeys treated with sertraline or ketamine may reflect the extent of the re-sistance to treatments currently employed for humans. However, these semi-natural populations could prove extremely valuable in testing newly developed antidepressants in a nonhuman primate model.

Summary

A gaping hole in the literature on animal models of depression involves the rela-tive lack of experiments on sex differences in the development of a depression-like phenotype. This lack of interest is surprising given the fact that women are ap-proximately twice as likely as men to develop depression. From the experiments that were summarized in the preceding, several tantalizing leads have been de-veloped. Female laboratory animals appear to be more susceptible to stressful stimuli during the prenatal period, infancy, and adolescence, and these effects carry over into adulthood. Sex differences may also occur within stress-sensitive brain circuits that result in greater susceptibility of females to depression-like behaviors. Finally, research by Labonté et al. (2017) demonstrated strikingly dif-ferent molecular genetic responses to chronic stress between male and female mice. These experiments were informed by experiments with post-mortem brain samples from human males and females. The experiments on sex differences in transcriptional signatures in laboratory mice generated a wealth of data that will inform future experiments directed at mechanisms to explain the greater suscep-tibility of females to develop depression. In addition, many of the gene networks that differed between male and female mice exposed to chronic stress will open up novel targets for development of new antidepressants. Finally, the develop-ment of a nonhuman primate model of depression in females affords an oppor-tunity to explore neural and genomic differences between subordinate females that develop symptoms of depression and those that do not.

Stress, Neurogenesis, and Depression

Death of a Dogma

A series of reports from the laboratory of Joseph Altman (e.g., Altman & Das, 1965) called into question the prevailing and deeply held dogma that neurogen-esis did not occur after puberty in the brains of higher vertebrates, including mammals. Altman and his colleagues injected ^{3}H-thymidine and observed that a substantial number of cells (including some neurons) of the dentate gyrus were labeled, indicating uptake of the molecule and incorporation into DNA during cell division. These basic findings were replicated by others, but it took more than 25 years before the dogma died a quiet death and there was general acceptance of Altman's original findings.

As Gross (2000) has recounted in rich detail, the general acceptance of neurogenesis in adulthood hinged upon new empirical findings as well as methodological advances. For example, Nottebohm's laboratory conducted a series of elegant experiments on neurogenesis in adult songbirds, and demonstrated that newly born neurons became incorporated into functional brain circuits in adult songbirds (Paton & Nottebohm, 1984). But the inevitable question arose: were findings from songbirds the exception rather than the rule for higher vertebrates? New methodologies were developed in the early 1990s for labeling dividing cells with an analogue of thymidine, 5-bromo-3'-deoxyuridine (BrdU), and newly available antibodies were employed to distinguish glial cells from neurons. BrdU staining of new nerve cells could be visualized with immunocytochemical techniques, which allowed stereological estimation of numbers of newly born neurons in specific brain areas. With these methodological advances, numerous publications appeared in the 1990s that replicated Altman's original findings for laboratory mice and rats, rhesus monkeys, and humans, and led to the general acceptance of neurogenesis in the hippocampus and olfactory bulbs and possibly other brain areas of adult animals (Gross, 2000). Quantitative studies have reported that approximately 700 new dentate granule cells are added each day to the human hippocampus.

Birth of a Theory

Jacobs, van Praag, and Gage (2000) proposed a new theory to explain the development of MDD, which was labeled the *neurogenic theory of depression.* This theory was based upon the following experimental observations. The birth of new neurons (i.e., neurogenesis) continues well into adulthood in the brains of many species, including humans, and especially in the dentate gyrus and the olfactory bulbs. Stressful stimulation was shown to suppress neurogenesis in adulthood, probably as a result of CORT release from the adrenal cortex. In contrast, elevations in brain levels of 5-HT enhanced neurogenesis in the dentate gyrus. In weaving together these findings from a number of laboratories, these authors proposed that stress-induced decreases in neurogenesis in the dentate gyrus of adult humans were an important element in the pathophysiology of MDD. They also argued that drugs that acted to increase synaptic concentrations of 5-HT produced elevations in neurogenesis in the dentate gyrus that promoted recovery from MDD. A further caveat was that the delay in the time between starting an antidepressant and receiving some therapeutic benefit corresponded to the time required for newly born neurons in the dentate gyrus to become incorporated into functional circuits within the hippocampus (Jacobs et al., 2000).

The neurogenic theory of depression continues to be a powerful stimulus for research relating to the connections between stress, neurogenesis, and depression (for reviews, see Duman, 2004; Eisch & Petrik, 2012; Schoenfeld & Cameron, 2015; Vollmayr et al., 2007). A major and continuing challenge for this area of research has been the lack of reliable methods for quantifying rates of neurogenesis in intact humans (Jessberger & Gage, 2014). In addition, a recent review by leading experts in neurogenesis addressed conflicting findings on whether neurogenesis actually occurs in the adult human hippocampus. Their very clear conclusion was that "adult-generated neurons make important functional contribution to neural plasticity and cognition across the human lifespan" (Kempermann et al., 2018, p. 25). Moreno-Jiménez et al. (2019) collected and processed post mortem brain tissue samples using highly controlled conditions and reported that robust rates of neurogenesis in neurologically healthy individuals up to the nineth decade of life. Thus, the stakes for translational studies with animal models are very high and will continue to inform research in humans, as well as drug development strategies targeting neurogenesis.

Miller and Hen (2015) proposed five criteria that should be met before the neurogenic theory of depression can be confirmed (Table 13.1). In their analysis of the five criteria, Miller and Hen noted that studies with laboratory strains of mice and rats that have been used to model features of MDD have consistently reported impairments in neurogenesis. A variety of antidepressants as well as electroconvulsive therapy (ECT) have resulted in enhanced levels of

Table 13.1 Five Criteria for Testing the Neurogenic Theory of Depression in Animal Models

---

1. Neurogenesis is altered in adult animals that display depression-like behaviors following exposure to stressor paradigms such as CSDS or CMS.

2. Blockade of neurogenesis is sufficient to produce symptoms of depression-like behaviors in otherwise healthy adult animals.

3. Treatments that are effective in reversing depression-like behaviors in adult animals also enhance rates of neurogenesis in the hippocampus.

4. Neurogenesis is required for the effectiveness of antidepressant medications administered to adult animals displaying depression-like behaviors.

5. Boosting rates of neurogenesis through environmental manipulations or drug treatments is sufficient for improving the depression-like symptoms of adult animals.

Adapted from Miller and Hen (2015), with an emphasis on experiments with animal models of depression.

neurogenesis, but only in laboratory animals that were exposed to stressful stimulation. If neurogenesis was knocked down by exposure of animals to X-irradiation, the effectiveness of antidepressants was decreased on some but not all measures in animals that were exposed to stressful stimulation. As Liu and Howard (2018) have noted, the effects of neurogenesis in humans are likely to be context-dependent, with stressful stimulation playing a crucial role. It is also unlikely that neurogenesis is the sole target through which antidepressants exert their effects, so that some symptoms in patients with MDD would respond favorably to enhanced levels of neurogenesis, while others would not.

In the sections that follow, I will provide a brief overview of a selection of the critical experiments that have addressed the impact of neurogenesis in animal models of MDD. This section is by no means an exhaustive review of the relevant literature; rather, it provides a glimpse into some of the key experiments that have been conducted since the provocative hypothesis advanced by Jacobs et al. (2000).

Highs and lows. Experimental methods to manipulate the rate of neurogenesis in the dentate gyrus have been critical to establishing connections between stress, neurogenesis, and depression. A sample of these approaches will be described in the following subsections.

Stress in tree shrews. A comprehensive series of studies at the German Primate Center in Göttingen has been led by Professor Eberhard Fuchs and his collaborators, who have studied the impact of psychosocial stress in an unusual species, the tree shrew (*Tupaia belangeri*). Tree shrews share a close phylogenetic relationship with primates and are native to Southeast Asia. They are diurnal, and males vigorously defend their territories against invading males. Under controlled laboratory conditions, encounters between two adult male tree shrews typically end with one of the males clearly establishing his dominance over the other subordinate male. If a subordinate male lives in visual and olfactory contact with the dominant male that defeated him, he displays a host of physiological and behavioral changes that are consistent with a depression-like phenotype. These include reductions in body weight and locomotor activity, disturbances in sleep patterns and circadian rhythms, increased activity of the HPA axis and sympathetic nervous system, and reduced gonadal function. Over a 4–5-week period of sensory contact with the dominant male, subordinate male tree shrews have a pronounced decrease in neurogenesis in the dentate gyrus that is reversed following chronic treatment with a variety of antidepressants. A key advantage of working with tree shrews versus laboratory mice and rats is their greater homology (90%–98%) with humans in DNA sequences for key genes involved in the stress response (for a review, see Czéh et al., 2016).

Youth versus maturity. The ventral portion of the hippocampus plays an integral role in regulating physiological and behavioral responses to stressful stimuli.

Anacker et al. (2018) explored the impact of adult-born dentate gyrus neurons on depression-like behaviors following sub-threshold CSDS (5 minutes of social defeat per day x 5 days). The experimental approach taken was to generate a loss-of-function mouse model that included the ability to chemogenetically silence adult-born neurons in the dentate gyrus *in vivo*. Sub-threshold CSDS did not affect two measures of depression- and anxiety-like behaviors, social interaction scores and activity in the center portion of an open field arena, respectively. If a drug was infused into the dentate gyrus each day of social defeat to block neuronal activity in adult-born dentate gyrus cells, there was a significant decrease in the social interaction scores and the amount of activity in the center portion of an open field arena. These behavioral changes were accompanied by activation of neurons in the dentate gyrus as assessed by numbers of c-fos-positive cells and enhanced evoked responses of mature dentate gyrus cells to stimulation of the perforant path *in vitro*.

Further experimentation confirmed the critical role played by neurogenesis in susceptibility to social defeat stress. In mice exposed to a standard regimen of CSDS, there were significant decreases in social investigation and activity in the central portion of an open field arena. If neurogenesis was enhanced in mice by a gain-of-function approach to delete the proapoptotic gene *Bax* from adult neural stem cells and their progeny, these mice displayed control levels of social interaction and activity in the central portion of an open field arena following CSDS. In addition, mice with increased rates of neurogenesis were found to have decreases in neuronal activity of stress-responsive neurons in the dentate gyrus that were preferentially activated by social defeat or an anxiety-provoking environment such as the open field arena. These results establish a firm connection between inhibitory effects of adult-born neurons in the dentate gyrus and vulnerability to depression- and anxiety-like behaviors in mice (Anacker et al., 2018).

In an earlier study, Culig et al. (2017) also examined the effects of enhancing neurogenesis in laboratory mice using the gain-of-function approach described in the preceding. This involved ablating the pro-apoptotic gene, *Bax*, to enhance survival of adult-born neurons. Mice were handled or exposed to CMS for 10 weeks. Ablation of the *Bax* gene did not have any effect on behavioral or neuroendocrine parameters in control mice. However, if adult neurogenesis was enhanced beginning after 2 weeks of CMS, there was a significant reversal of stress-induced changes in some but not all behavioral measures and in regulation of the HPA axis. These results demonstrated that enhancing neurogenesis was a highly effective treatment for reversing symptoms of depression that were associated with exposure to chronic intermittent stressors.

Drugs that boost neurogenesis. Pieper et al. (2010) led a search for compounds that could enhance neurogenesis in the ventral dentate gyrus of adult mice. In a screen of 1,000 preselected compounds from a library of 200,000 chemicals, 8 compounds were identified that enhanced neurogenesis in the ventral dentate gyrus of mice following i.c.v. administration continuously over 7 days. One of these molecules, P7C3, could be administered orally, had a long half-life, was able to cross the blood-brain barrier, and did not produce untoward effects on embryonic or early postnatal developmental processes. P7C3 was shown to pro-tect adult-born neurons from apoptosis, thereby increasing the number of adult-born cells that were incorporated into hippocampal circuits.

Walker, Rivera, et al. (2015) examined the effects of P7C3 and a highly ac-tive analog, P7C3-A20, in ghrelin receptor (Ghsr)-null mutant mice and WT mice exposed to CSDS. The effects of CSDS were magnified in Ghsr-null mice, but were still quite evident in WT mice (Lutter et al., 2008). Exposure to CSDS resulted in greater social avoidance of a social stranger mouse in WT and Ghsr-null mice, confirming a depression-like phenotype. Using immunohisto-chemical markers of cell proliferation and apoptosis, this team of investigators demonstrated that CSDS resulted in significant reductions in cell proliferation and significant increases in cell death in the dentate gyrus compared to un-stressed controls. These effects of CSDS on rates of birth and death of neurons were greater in Ghsr-null mice compared to WT mice. Next, P7C3 (10 mg/kg i.p. twice daily) was administered to WT and Ghsr-null mice beginning 2 days before CSDS. WT and Ghsr-null mice exposed to CSDS displayed reductions in adult-born neurons and increases in apoptosis in the dentate gyrus, and both of these alterations were normalized in mice treated twice daily with P7C3. Importantly, WT and Ghsr-null mice treated with P7C3 and its more potent an-alog, P7C3-A20, were comparable to unstressed controls in levels of social inter-action with a novel test mouse. Chronic administration of P7C3-S184, a P7C3 analog that lacks neuroprotective effects, had no such effect on social interac-tion scores of CSDS-exposed WT and Ghsr-null mice, demonstrating further the specificity of the antidepressant effect of P7C3 and its more active analog. These findings provided further support for the neurogenic theory of depression and offered a new class of neuroprotective compounds for consideration as possible antidepressants (Walker et al., 2015).

Summary

The introduction of the neurogenic theory of mood disorders provided a novel and promising avenue for exploring mechanisms that underlie the development of depression. Neurogenesis in laboratory animals is exquisitely sensitive to levels of stressful stimulation, and several antidepressants stimulate rates of neurogen-esis. Carefully controlled studies in laboratory animals have also revealed a tight coupling between decreased rates of neurogenesis and increased occurrence of depression-like behaviors. A major impediment to progress in this field of inquiry is the lack of appropriate methods for measuring rates of neurogenesis in intact humans. Such a breakthrough would permit clinical assessments of neurogenesis and symptoms of depression in individual patients, resulting in a more personalized approach to therapy.

Stress, Epigenetics, and Depression

Epigenetics was introduced in Chapter 7, and in this chapter we will build upon that information and consider how stress interacts with epigenetic mechanisms to influence the development of a depression-like phenotype in various animal models. Not surprisingly, most of the research in this area has been conducted using laboratory strains of mice and rats. The vast majority of publications in this area have appeared since 2005, reflecting an intense interest in the possibility that epigenetic alterations in DNA could explain in part the highly variable nature of stress effects on humans, especially with regard to who develops depression and who doesn't (Bagot et al., 2014). Studies of stress-induced epigenetic mechanisms may also contribute to a better understanding of sex differences in depression (Hodes et al., 2016).

In the sections that follow, we will consider four types of epigenetic alterations that influence the expression of various genes, including modification of histone proteins through acetylation or methylation, methylation of DNA, and synthesis of micro RNAs.

Stress and Histone Targets

Two of the most intensively studied examples of posttranslational modification of histone proteins with relevance to the study of depression are acetylation and methylation at lysine residues (Nestler, 2014; Sun et al., 2013). Summaries of select experiments on stress effects on histone acetylation and methylation are discussed in the following subsections.

Histone acetylation. As was described earlier, the nucleus accumbens is a key limbic brain area that is altered in susceptible animals exposed to CSDS. This well-developed behavioral model provided a superb test of whether epigenetic modifications of histones might be associated with neural adaptations to chronic stress. In an initial series of experiments (Covington et al., 2009), C57BL/6J male mice were exposed to CSDS or were left undisturbed. Brains were harvested 1 hour, 1 day, or 10 days after the final social defeat and were prepared for immunohistochemical analysis of acetylated histone H3 lysine 14 (acH3K14). The lysine

14 site was selected for analysis because it had previously been associated with increases in gene transcription. One hour after CSDS, there was a 50% decrease in levels of acH3K14 relative to unstressed control mice. In contrast, beginning at 24 hours after CSDS and continuing through 10 days post-CSDS, levels of acH3K14 were elevated significantly compared to control mice. To confirm the validity of these findings, post-mortem human brain samples from controls and from depressed individuals were obtained and the nucleus accumbens isolated, sectioned, and prepared for immunohistochemical measurement of acH3K14 and HDAC2. The results were strikingly similar to the findings in CSDS-exposed mice, such that depressed individuals exhibited significant increases in acH3K14 and significant decreases in expression of HDAC2 within the nucleus accumbens relative to controls without MDD.

A second experiment explored the impact of CSDS on expression of class I histone deactylases (HDAC1, HDAC2, and HDAC3), which play an important role in regulating acetylation of H3K14. Levels of HDAC2 but not HDAC1 or HDAC3 mRNA levels were reduced significantly in C57BL/6J male mice 24 hours after CSDS and remained depressed for at least 15 days. Neither the increase in acH3K14 nor the decrease in HDAC2 within the nucleus accumbens of male mice exposed to CSDS was blocked by chronic treatment with fluoxetine.

A third experiment involved chronic infusions via subcutaneous minipumps of either of two HDAC inhibitors (MS-275 or SAHA, 100 μM) or vehicle bilaterally into the nucleus accumbens of male mice beginning the day after CSDS. Beginning 5 days after chronic infusions of drug or vehicle, control and CSDS-exposed mice were processed in a battery of behavioral tests to assess the antidepressant effects of the HDAC inhibitors. As expected, vehicle-infused mice exposed to CSDS exhibited a significant reduction in social preference, a significant decrease in preference for a 1% sucrose solution, and increased time spent immobile in a forced swim test. These drugs did not affect anxiety-like behaviors, including activity levels in an open field arena or behavior in a light-dark test chamber. Infusion of MS-375 normalized all three depression-like behaviors, while infusion of SAHA normalized the social preference and forced swim test behavioral measures. Following 10 days of continuous infusion of either HDAC inhibitor into the nucleus accumbens of CSDS-exposed mice, levels of acH3K14 in this brain region were increased significantly over vehicle-injected controls. The antidepressant-like effects of chronic infusion of HDAC inhibitors resulted from increasing histone acetylation at various gene promoters and exerting complex effects on gene expression, as was revealed in this experiment using gene arrays following chronic infusion of MS-275. These findings point to HDAC inhibitors as a new therapeutic approach to the treatment of patients with treatment-resistant depression (Fuchikami et al., 2016).

Histone methylation. Wilkinson et al. (2009) utilized the CSDS and prolonged social isolation models of depression to study the effects of stress on epigenetic modifications of chromatin in the nucleus accumbens of C57BL/6J male mice. Using chromatin immuno-precipitation (ChIP) assays, these investigators demonstrated that CSDS and chronic social isolation for 8 weeks both resulted in widespread and persistent changes in gene regulation, including changes in repressive histone methylation (H3K9meK27me) within the nucleus accumbens. For the CSDS model, there were 1,285 genes that had increased H3 methylation, while 799 genes had decreased H3 methylation. In the social isolation model, 1,448 genes displayed increased H3 methylation and 615 genes had decreased H3 methylation. In spite of the obvious differences between these two models of depression, there were 436 genes that displayed alterations in H3 methylation in animals from both models, and 75% of these changed in a similar manner. It appears that social defeat and social isolation share many similar repressive gene regulatory alterations, and this observation is consistent with the fact that similar behavioral changes (e.g., anhedonia-like and anxiety-like symptoms) were observed in both models. If CSDS mice were treated chronically with imipramine, many of the changes in gene expression were reversed, and more closely resembled the patterns seen in mice that were resilient to the effects of CSDS (Wilkinson et al., 2009).

Heller et al. (2014) directed their attention to targeted regulation of the transcription factor, ΔFosB, in the nucleus accumbens of male mice exposed to a modified CSDS protocol. Expression of ΔFosB was reduced by chronic stress, and the histone methyltransferase, G9a, which catalyzes the dimethylation of histone H3 (H3K9me2), appeared to play a pivotal role. In this experiment, H3K9me2 was artificially and selectively induced at the *Fosb* gene in the nucleus accumbens of mice exposed to sub-chronic CSDS. Compared to control mice exposed to sub-chronic CSDS, mice with induced H3K9me2 displayed reduced social interaction and increased anxiety-like behaviors in an EPM. These behavioral changes were consistent with a depression-like phenotype that resulted from targeted histone methylation at a single gene in the nucleus accumbens (Heller et al., 2014).

Taking advantage of the well-characterized system of D1- and D2-expressing MSNs in the nucleus accumbens as described earlier, Hamilton et al. (2018) examined the effects of cell-type specific targeted epigenetic modifications of the *Fosb* gene on susceptibility to a sub-threshold level of CSDS in mice. Their results revealed that histone acetylation of *Fosb* in D2-expressing MSNs, which promotes transcription, and histone methylation of *Fosb* in D1-expressing MSNs, which inhibits transcription, both resulted in a depression-like phenotype following exposure of mice to sub-threshold CSDS. Behavioral measures in these experiments included social avoidance and sucrose preference. These powerful findings for the first time revealed the potential for epigenetic editing in specific neuronal cell types to reproduce changes that occur in a social stress model of depression.

Stress and DNA Methylation

Saunderson et al. (2016) were interested in exploring behavioral adaptations following exposure to an acute stressor. For their experiments, they exposed adult male Wistar rats to forced swim stress, which has great relevance to research with animal models of depression. Of particular interest in these experiments were interrelationships among the following variables: availability of the methyl donor, S-adenosyl-L-methionine (SAMe); induction of two immediate early genes (*c-Fos* and *Erg-1*) in neurons of the dentate gyrus; DNA methylation; and behavioral responses to forced swim stress. In their first experiment, SAMe (100 mg/kg, s.c.) was administered to rats 30 minutes prior to forced swim stress (15 minutes at 25°C), and rats were exposed to the same stressor 24 hours later. Administration of SAMe did not affect scores for climbing, active swimming, and immobility during the initial 5 minutes of the first bout of swim stress compared to vehicle-injected controls. In contrast, on the second day, SAMe-treated rats displayed significantly higher active swimming scores and significantly lower immobility scores compared to controls.

To examine the mechanisms underlying this dramatic change in behavior following administration of SAMe, the first experiment was repeated, but rats were sacrificed 45 minutes after initial exposure to forced swim stress. Compared to vehicle-injected controls, rats that received a single injection of SAMe displayed significant reductions in the number of c-Fos- and Egr-1-positive neurons in the dorsal portion of the dentate gyrus. SAMe had no effect on stress-induced expression of *cFos* and Erg-1 in the CA1 and CA3 regions of the hippocampus, highlighting the specificity of the effect of SAMe on dorsal dentate gyrus neurons. Previous research demonstrated that induction of *c-Fos and Erg-1* in neurons of the dentate gyrus following forced swim stress required phosphorylation of serine 10 and acetylation of lysine 14 on histone H3 (H3S10p-K14ac). Administration of SAMe to rats 30 minutes prior to forced swim stress did not affect the formation of H3S10p-K14ac in dentate gyrus neurons. Thus, another mechanism must have been responsible for the alterations in behavior of SAMe-treated rats during their second exposure to forced swim stress (Saunderson et al., 2016).

Saunderson and colleagues next examined the methylation status of specific 5'-cytosine-phosphate-guanine-3' (CpG)s within *c-Fos* and *Egr-1* gene promoters and untranslated regions in neurons of the dentate gyrus and the CA1 and CA3 regions of the hippocampus. Their results revealed a striking anatomical precision in the effects of forced swim stress on the methylation status of *c-Fos* and *Erg-1* gene promoter regions. In the dentate gyrus, within area 2 of the *c-Fos* untranslated region, CpGs 3 and 4 showed significant hypomethylation after forced swim stress. In contrast, within the CA 1 and 3 areas, there were no significant changes in CpG methylation in the *c-Fos* gene promoter or the untranslated region after forced swim stress. Forced swim stress resulted in significantly reduced DNA methylation at CpGs 5, 11, 13, and 15 in area A of the *Egr-1* gene promoter in the dentate gyrus. In contrast, CpG methylation status of the *Erg-1* gene promoter was unaltered by forced swim stress in the CA1 and CA3 areas of the hippocampus. Administration of SAMe prior to forced swim stress resulted in significantly increased methylation of CpGs 1 and 2 in the *c-Fos* untranslated region and CpGs 4–8 and 13 in the *Egr-1* gene promoter region. Importantly, CpG methylation did not increase in SAMe-injected control animals, indicating that increased availability of the methyl donor in the absence of a stressful challenge did not result in increased CpG methylation in neurons of the dentate gyrus.

Acute swim stress also exerted highly localized effects on DNA methyltransferase (DNMT) isoforms and on Tet methylcytosine dioxygenase 1 (Tet1), a key enzyme in demethylation of DNA. Expression of *Dnmt3a* (DNA [cytosine-5-]-methyltransferase 3 alpha) was increased immediately after forced swim stress in the dentate gyrus but not in the CA1 and CA3 regions of the hippocampus. Expression of *Dnmt3b, Dnmt1*, and *Tet1* did not change in the dentate gyrus or the CA regions of the hippocampus following forced swim stress.

In summary, these experiments on acute responses to forced swim stress revealed that CpG methylation status was an important controller of immediate early gene expression in neurons in the dorsal dentate gyrus. In addition, availability of SAMe, in concert with *Dnmt3a* expression, determined in part the responsiveness of dentate gyrus neurons and the behavioral responses to acute swim stress (Saunderson et al., 2016).

In an extension of these findings, Sales and Joca (2018) were interested in the impact of antidepressants on stress-induced alterations in *Dnmt* expression in the hippocampus and PFC of rats exposed to a learned helplessness paradigm. DNA methylation and expression of *Dnmt3a* and *Dnmt3b* were elevated in the dorsal hippocampus and PFC. Chronic administration of imipramine resulted in a significant decrease in escape failures in the learned helplessness task and attenuation of the increases in DNA methylation and expression of *Dnmt3a* and *Dnmt3b* in the PFC. Regulation of DNA methylation in the PFC may be an interesting target for future antidepressant drug development.

Stress and microRNAs

Roy et al. (2017) employed a model of stress that involved chronic administration of CORT (50 mg/kg, i.p., daily for 21 days) to laboratory rats. Compared to vehicle-treated controls, CORT-treated rats displayed increased immobility in a forced swim test and reduced preference for sucrose. Using this stress-related model of depression, these investigators were interested in the role played by a neuron-specific microRNA (miRNA), miR-124-3p, on gene expression in the PFC. They reported consistent CORT-associated changes in the expression of miR-124-3p, and noted that some of the genes that were targets of this miRNA were highly dysregulated. In addition, they found that miR-124-3p was epigenetically regulated, suggesting a role for gene x environment interactions in regulation of gene expression by miRNAs. Given that down-regulation of miR-124-3p resulted in a reversal of depression-like behaviors in CORT-treated rats, this miRNA may be a target for the development of novel drugs for the treatment of depression (Roy et al., 2017).

Focusing on the nucleus accumbens, Si et al. (2018) examined miRNA profiles involved in susceptibility to depression-like behaviors in mice exposed to CUMS for 4 weeks. Relative to unstressed controls, CUMS-exposed mice displayed reduced preferences for a sucrose solution, decreased social preference, and increased immobility in the forced swim test. These behavioral changes were consistent with a depression-like phenotype. Next, using high throughput sequencing of mRNAs and miRNAs in samples from the nucleus accumbens, these investigators compared unstressed controls with CUMS-exposed mice that displayed a depression-like phenotype. Some alterations in specific mRNAs were confirmed by qRT-PCR. Down-regulated mRNAs in depressed mice included genes for 5-HT and DA synapses, calcium signaling, and circadian entrainment, whereas up-regulated genes included those regulating tyrosine metabolism, actin cytoskeleton, and inflammatory mediator regulation of transient receptor potential (TRP) ion channels. In addition, alterations in miRNAs matched well with changes in mRNAs in comparisons of unstressed controls and depressed mice. These findings provide additional support for the critical role played by stress-induced molecular alterations in the nucleus accumbens and the expression of a depression-like phenotype (Si et al., 2018).

Summary

Epigenetic regulatory mechanisms unfold in complex ways to affect the risk of depression in laboratory animals and in humans. These regulatory processes begin at conception and continue well into adulthood, necessitating a life-span developmental approach to understand vulnerability to a depression-like phenotype. Epigenetic influences on gene transcription represent a mechanism whereby stressful experiences can be translated into precise and enduring changes in gene expression in discrete areas of brain. An important methodological advance in this relatively young field has been the use of genome-wide measures of stress-related epigenetic changes. This research area is still in its early stages of development, but there are encouraging signs that epigenetic editing may emerge as a therapeutic strategy for treating, and possibly even preventing, the symptoms of depression.

Stress, Immunity, and Depression

Inflammation and Depression in Patients

Over the past two decades, an extensive body of research has developed that links stress and immune system dysregulation with symptoms of depression. Foundational to this body of research were early studies of inflammatory biomarkers in depressed patients. One such report from Maes et al. (1991) revealed that depressed patients displayed increased levels of inflammatory biomarkers, including acute phase protein and proinflammatory cytokines relative to controls. This report and others that followed from Maes and his collaborators stimulated interest from other researchers in pursuing links between inflammation and major depressive disorder. A meta-analysis was conducted by Dawlati et al. (2010) involving 24 studies of unstimulated cytokine levels in patients who met *DSM* criteria for MDD and in healthy controls. The meta-analysis revealed that circulating levels of two proinflammatory cytokines, TNF-α and IL-6, were elevated significantly in depressed patients. No differences between depressed patients and controls were noted for circulating levels of IL-1β, IL-2, IL-4, IL-8, IL-10, and interferon-γ. The design of these studies precluded a determination of whether TNF-α and IL-6 were causes or consequences of depression (Dawlati et al., 2010).

An influential clinical study by Raison et al. (2013) examined the effects of the monoclonal antibody, infliximab, an antagonist to TNFα, on symptoms of depression in a group of patients that was generally resistant to treatment with standard antidepressant medications. The placebo-controlled, double-blind, randomized trial lasted 12 weeks, with infusions of infliximab (5 mg/kg) at the start of the trial and again in weeks 2 and 6. Overall, infliximab did not improve symptoms in depressed patients compared to placebo-infused controls. However, the drug did improve symptoms of depression in patients with elevated levels of C-reactive protein (CRP, levels >5 mg/L), a peripheral biomarker of inflammation. These findings highlighted the potential benefits of peripheral blockade of the proinflammatory cytokine, TNFα, in a subgroup of depressed patients with elevated levels of CRP. These findings were also in line with a more personalized approach to treatment of depressed patients.

An additional aspect of research on immune system effects on depression lies in its relationship to sex differences in depression in patients. As noted earlier, women have a 2-fold greater risk for a diagnosis of depression compared to men. Sex differences in regulation of the immune system may explain in part these differences in risk of depression between women and men. Derry et al. (2015) noted that women experience higher levels of inflammation and greater risk of autoimmune diseases compared to men. Evidence was also presented to suggest that women may be more sensitive to the mood-altering effects of elevations in inflammatory biomarkers. Unfortunately, these sex differences in immune function and depression in patients have not been embraced broadly by scientists studying connections between the immune system and depression in animal models. There are some prominent exceptions to this general pattern, and they will be presented in the following.

IL-6 Sings the Blues

In a compelling series of experiments, Hodes et al. (2014) demonstrated that IL-6 levels, which were elevated dramatically after a single social defeat (27-fold increase above baseline), predicted whether a C57BL/6J male mouse would become susceptible or resistant to CSDS as determined by social interaction scores. In addition, IL-6 levels following the first social defeat were strongly negatively correlated with levels of social interaction following 10 days of CSDS. Finally, IL-6 levels remained significantly elevated above baseline values up to 35 days after CSDS, and chronic treatment with imipramine did not bring down IL-6 levels. In addition, plasma CORT levels were similar in susceptible and resilient mice following CSDS, suggesting that differences in HPA axis responsivity to stress did not influence the differences in IL-6 levels. Elevated levels of circulating IL-6 were also noted in two other models of stress, mice exposed to CVS for 21 days and mice that observed other mice undergoing CSDS.

Further experiments revealed that susceptible and resilient mice differed in the number of circulating monocytes prior to the first exposure to social defeat. Leukocytes collected from mice that would later display a susceptible phenotype following CSDS released more IL-6 in response to stimulation by lipopolysaccharide (LPS) ex vivo compared to leukocytes obtained from mice that would later be characterized as resilient to CSDS.

To demonstrate further the essential role of IL-6 in susceptibility to depression-like behaviors following CSDS, Hodes et al. (2014) performed two additional experiments. In the first, they transplanted bone marrow–derived hematopoietic progenitor cells from susceptible donors into irradiated host mice and found that the transplanted cells promoted susceptibility to sub-threshold social defeat stress as well as witnessing social defeat in other mice. In contrast, transplantation of IL-6-deficient bone marrow–derived hematopoietic progenitors into irradiated host mice promoted resilience to both social stressors. The degree of resilience in IL-6$^{(-/-)}$ bone marrow chimeras was similar to that observed in full body knockouts, suggesting that peripheral IL-6 was essential in regulating the expression of depression-like behaviors. In the final experiment, mice were injected i.p. with neutralizing IL-6 monoclonal antibodies, an IgG isotype control antibody, or saline just prior to each bout of CSDS. IL-6 monoclonal antibodies are too large to readily cross the blood-brain barrier, so the effects on IL-6 were mostly limited to the periphery. Administration of IL-6 antibodies, but not IgG antibodies or saline, prevented the development of social avoidance following CSDS. These results confirmed an essential role for peripheral IL-6 in predetermining the pattern of behavioral responses to various stressors. These findings suggested treatment strategies for depressed patients, especially those who are resistant to a range of antidepressants (Hodes et al., 2014).

Slipping Through the Cracks

Three studies have explored stress-induced changes in BBB permeability and the onset of depression-like behaviors. These experiments revealed the importance of periphery → brain movement of immune molecules and cells in regulating depression-like behaviors following stress exposure in mice.

IL-1β. C57BL/6J male mice treated with LPS (2.5 mg/kg, i.p.) developed depression-like behaviors and displayed increases in brain transmigrated neutrophils that persisted for several days and were reversed by administration of an anti-polymorphonuclear antibody that blocked the surge in neutrophils that accompanied administration of LPS. The energy-regulating hormone leptin was also involved in these effects, perhaps through promotion of increased permeability of the blood-brain barrier to transmigrating neutrophils (Agulair-Valles et al., 2014).

IL-6. In the first experiment (Ménard et al., 2017), using a standard CSDS paradigm as the chronic stressor, C57BL/6J mice were tested the day following the tenth social defeat and measures of social interaction were obtained. Susceptible mice had low social interaction scores relative to resilient mice and unstressed control mice. Brain samples were obtained following behavioral phenotyping, and gene expression studies were conducted in the nucleus accumbens, a brain area critically involved in the expression of depression-like behaviors. There was a significant reduction (~40%) in the expression of the endothelial cell tight junction protein, claudin-5, in susceptible mice compared to resilient and control mice. In addition, there was a significant positive correlation between claudin-5 expression and levels of social interaction on day 11. Similar results on claudin-5 expression were obtained in mice exposed to CVS for 4 weeks. Electron microscopic studies revealed ultrastructural abnormalities in the blood vessels and capillaries of the nucleus accumbens of stress-susceptible mice, including discontinuous tight junctions in the endothelial cells. Chronic administration of imipramine for 5 weeks reversed the low social interaction scores and normalized claudin-5 gene expression levels in CSDS-exposed mice.

To determine if a causal link existed between down-regulation of claudin-5 expression and a depression-like phenotype, Ménard and her colleagues employed virally mediated conditional knockdown of claudin-5 bilaterally in the nucleus accumbens of male mice. In this experiment, the stressor was a sub-threshold social defeat paradigm, which by itself did not induce a depression-like phenotype. However, following knockdown of claudin-5 in the nucleus accumbens, mice displayed a depression-like phenotype, reflected in decreased social interaction, reduced grooming of conspecifics, reduced preference for a 1% sucrose solution, and increased immobility in a forced swim test. Reversal of the down-regulation of claudin-5 expression resulted in a normalization of social interaction scores and preference for a sucrose solution. These results provided definitive support for the conclusion that claudin-5 expression was a crucial variable in the onset of a depression-like phenotype following exposure of mice to chronic stress. Further experiments confirmed the leaky nature of the blood-brain barrier in susceptible mice following CSDS and demonstrated that IL-6 passes from the circulation into the nucleus accumbens to stimulate depression-like behaviors. Taken together, these experiments revealed that maintenance of blood-brain barrier integrity in the face of stressful stimulation was essential for regulation of a normal mood state (Ménard et al., 2017).

TNF-α. Cheng et al. (2018) exposed C57BL/6 mice to a learned helplessness paradigm, and mice were later screened by exposure to escapable shocks to identify those mice that did not recover fully within 4 weeks (i.e., susceptible mice, ~30% of the total tested). Compared to mice that recovered from learned helplessness (resilient mice) and unstressed controls, susceptible mice displayed greater hippocampal activation but not expression of GSK3α and GSK3β. If susceptible mice received 3 daily injections of the GSK inhibitor, TDZD-8 (5 mg/kg, i.p.), prior to testing 4 weeks after inescapable shock, 75% of mice displayed improvements in escaping shock relative to vehicle-injected controls. Susceptible mice also exhibited increased hippocampal levels of the alarmin protein,

HMGB1, and activation of its toll-like receptor-4, as well as elevated levels of TNF-α and IL-23. Hippocampal levels of 18 other cytokines did not differ between susceptible and resilient mice. In addition, administration of TDZD-8 reduced hippocampal levels of TNF-α, IL-17a, and IL-23 in susceptible mice.

Further experiments revealed that susceptible mice displayed increased accumulation of sodium fluorescein in the hippocampus, indicating increased permeability of the blood-brain barrier. In addition, susceptible mice had reduced levels of the tight junction proteins, occludin, ZO1, and claudin-5. Treatment with the GSK3 inhibitor, TDZD-8, increased tight junction proteins and reversed escape failures in susceptible mice. In addition, administration of the sphingosine 1-phosphate receptor agonist, Fingolimod (1 mg/kg, i.p.), or the TNFα antagonist, etanercept (100 μg per mouse, i.p., every other day for 1 week) reversed the increased blood-brain barrier permeability and escape failures in susceptible mice. These results indicated that stress-induced elevations in activated GSK3 contributed to impairments in escape behavior that were mediated in part by TNFα-induced increases in BBB permeability (Cheng et al., 2018). GSK3 emerged from this report and related studies as an interesting new target for the treatment of depression (Jope et al., 2017).

Sterile Infection and the Brain

Psychological and physical stressors stimulate the release of damage-associated molecular patterns (DAMPs) in the periphery and the brain that promote sterile infection. DAMPs include ATP, heat shock proteins, high mobility group box 1 protein (HMGB1), uric acid, and S100 proteins. DAMPs activate inflammatory processes in the absence of pathogens, such as bacteria or viruses, or tissue injury by binding to pattern recognition receptors (PRRs) on innate immune cells to stimulate nuclear factor kappa beta (NFκB) signaling, followed by the production of proinflammatory cytokines. Evidence has accumulated to suggest that a bidirectional relationship exists between sterile inflammation and depression-like behaviors based upon experiments with a variety of chronic intermittent stress paradigms.

Following exposure to stressors, a sterile inflammatory response may also be stimulated by inflammasomes, including nucleotide-binding oligomerization domain, leucine-rich repeat and pyrin domain protein 3 (NLRP3). Inflammasomes are cytosolic multi-protein complexes that serve as sensors of DAMPs, and promote activation of proinflammatory caspases, resulting in cleavage and release of proinflammatory cytokines. Several inflammasomes have been characterized, and they typically include a nucleotide binding domain, an adaptor protein, and an effector caspase, often caspase-1. Formation and activation of NLRP3 require a two-step process that is initiated following ligation of pattern recognition receptors (PRRs) capable of binding DAMPS, leading to NLRP3 gene transcription, translation, and protein production. After sufficient NLRP3 protein has been formed and the cell is "primed," a second activation signal stimulates NLRP3 to cleave procaspase-1 into active caspase-1. Caspase-1 then converts pro-IL-1β into the active IL-1β molecule, which is then released from the cell (Fleshner et al., 2017; Franklin et al., 2018).

Pan et al. (2014) conducted one of the first studies on the involvement of NLRP3 in stress-induced depression-like behaviors. In their experiments, rats were exposed to 12 weeks of chronic unpredictable mild stress (CUMS). Compared to unstressed controls, CUMS-exposed rats exhibited decreased sucrose intake and increased levels of IL-1β mRNA and mature IL-1β protein in the PFC. CUMS also increased PFC levels of NLRP3 protein and mRNA. Chronic administration of fluoxetine during weeks 6–12 of CUMS significantly reduced the behavioral and immune-related molecular changes associated with stressor exposure.

Using a similar approach, Zhang et al. (2015) reported that exposure of mice to CMS for 4 weeks resulted in elevations in circulating levels of CORT and IL-1β, as well as increased concentrations of IL-1β, increased activity of caspase-1, and elevations in NLRP3 in the hippocampus. Stressed mice also displayed decreased preference for a 1% sucrose solution and increased immobility time in the tail suspension test. Treatment of mice with the NLRP3 inhibitor, VX-765 (50 mg/kg i.p. daily for 4 weeks), reversed the behavioral changes resulting from CMS and blocked the increases in circulating levels of CORT and IL-1β, as well as increases in IL-1β, caspase-1 activity, and NLRP3 levels in the hippocampus. In a second series of experiments, Su et al. (2017) examined the effects of CUMS on WT mice and NLRP3 KO mice. WT mice displayed depression-like behaviors following 4 weeks of CUMS while NLRP3 KO mice did not.

Brain microglia may enter a 'primed' state where they display phenotypic signs of activation, but they do not secrete increased levels of cytokines. However, if microglia are stimulated while in this primed state, they produce and release elevated levels of cytokines, including IL-1β. This primed activation state may be especially relevant to stress-induced priming of neuroinflammatory responses, as demonstrated in a study by Cheng et al. (2016). These investigators reported that exposure to an initial series of acute footshocks increased NLRP3 as well as mature caspase-1 in the hippocampus. However, this stressor did not result in an increase in levels of hippocampal IL-1β. If a second series of footshocks was delivered the next day, hippocampal IL-1β protein was increased, suggesting that the initial series of shocks primed the NLRP3 inflammasome in the hippocampus. A similar priming phenomenon may occur when animals are exposed to CUS.

In two earlier reports, Weber et al. (2013, 2015) combined inescapable tail shocks on day 1 to prime the neuroinflammatory response to an immune challenge on day 2 in the form of LPS (10 μg/kg, i.p.). If an antagonist to toll-like receptors 1 and 2, oxidized 1-palmitoyl-2-arachidonyl-sn-glycero-3-phosphorylcholine (OxPAPC, 150 ng), was injected into the cisterna magna prior to delivery of tail shocks, there was a significant reduction in the hippocampal pro-inflammatory response to LPS administration on the following day. Similarly, if OxPAPC was administered prior to delivery of tail shocks as described earlier, it greatly diminished the sensitized proinflammatory response of isolated microglia from hippocampus following administration of LPS *ex vivo*. In a second report, these investigators demonstrated that the CNS innate immune system responded to inescapable tail shocks in a manner that was similar to cellular damage by releasing the DAMP molecule, high mobility group box-1 (HMGB-1) protein. If an antagonist to HMGB-1 was administered into the cisterna magna prior to delivery of tail shocks, it greatly diminished the sensitized proinflammatory response of hippocampal microglia. In addition, central administration of HMGB-1 was sufficient to prime the proinflammatory response of isolated hippocampal microglia to LPS. It is possible that CORT also played a critical role in the priming of brain microglia following stressor exposure (Weber et al., 2015).

Taken together, these findings point to the NLRP3 inflammasome as a key mediator of the depression-like phenotype in mice exposed to chronic stressors (Pan et al., 2014; Su et al., 2017; Zhang et al., 2015). NLRP3 has also been linked to increased levels of circulating proinflammatory cytokines and severity of symptoms of depression in patients with MDD. In addition, anti-inflammatory interventions using pharmacological or behavioral approaches may be especially beneficial in patients with elevated levels of inflammatory biomarkers (Franklin et al., 2018; Kiecolt-Glaser et al., 2015; Miller & Raison, 2016; Wohleb et al., 2016).

Summary

Experiments with animal models of depression have established a strong link between stressful stimuli, immune system responses, and the onset of depression-like behavioral patterns. Many of the immune system responses to stress described in laboratory animals match well with immune responses noted in patients with depression. Studies of sterile infection using animal models have also revealed critical connections between HPA axis activity, circulating pro-inflammatory cytokines, and changes in blood-brain barrier permeability, brain microglia, and neuronal function. A greater understanding of the transduction of peripheral immune system activation on stress-sensitive brain circuits will open up a host of new targets for development of next-generation antidepressants.

Depression's Lasting Signature

A large-scale collaborative genetic epidemiology study involving scientists and clinicians from Oxford University, Virginia Commonwealth University, and from multiple universities and hospitals in China (CONVERGE) focused on potential biomarkers of stressful life experiences and occurrence of major depression (Cai et al., 2015). Their study population included 5,864 women who had experienced recurring episodes of major depressive disorder and 5,783 matched controls. Each study participant provided information on aggregate measures of lifetime adversities, including instances of child sexual abuse, as well as other stressful life events. In addition, DNA was extracted from saliva samples from each participant and later sequenced. This large international team of investigators reported a significant positive association between the amount of mitochrondrial DNA (mtDNA) and MDD and a significant negative association between telomere length and MDD. Although both of these molecular changes were associated with major adverse life events, they were contingent on a history of MDD.

To investigate the mechanisms underlying the associations between stressful life events, amount of mtDNA, and telomere length, this group turned to a mouse model of depression. They compared unstressed male and female C57BL/6J with male and female mice exposed to CUMS for 5 days per week for up to 4 weeks. After 4 weeks of CUMS, there were highly significant increases in amounts of mtDNA in saliva and blood samples and highly significant decreases in telomere length in saliva and blood samples relative to unstressed controls. A comparison of multiple tissues from stressed and control mice revealed a high degree of tissue specificity in the alterations in mtDNA and telomere length. If mice were permitted 4 weeks to recover from CUMS, both molecular markers returned to control levels. Daily administration of CORT to mice for 4 weeks reproduced both of these molecular changes, suggesting a connection with stress-induced activation of the HPA axis as one driver of this molecular signature. Additional experiments indicated that the efficiency of oxidative phosphorylation was compromised in stressed rats with increased levels of mtDNA in liver. These investigators concluded that alterations in levels of mtDNA and telomere length were of greater magnitude and persisted over time only in those individuals who were at higher risk of MDD. These measures may hold promise as a combined biomarker for major depression (Cai et al., 2015).

Conclusions

These two chapters on animal models of depression have emphasized the diversity of biological pathways one can follow to reach a depression-like phenotype. The one variable that connects into each of these disease-relevant pathways is stressful stimulation. Stressful experiences may exert a priming effect if exposure occurs during the prenatal period or in infancy or adolescence, or it may interact with a biological vulnerability to hasten the onset of symptoms in adulthood. Much progress has been made in developing appropriate stressor paradigms since the early work on animal models of depression that was undertaken in the 1970s. In fact, some of the earliest models of MDD later became screening tests for potential antidepressant medications. One case in point is the forced swim test, which is now one of several tools employed to assess a depression-like phenotype.

Two stressor paradigms have emerged as the most frequently employed in studies of depression in animal models. CSDS and CMS are highly effective in precipitating a depression-like pattern of behavioral changes in laboratory strains of mice and rats. These chronic intermittent stressors have been employed to understand the mechanisms responsible for symptoms of depression. Several relatively new stress-sensitive disease mechanisms have been explored in laboratory animals, and in many instances they have been informed by studies in patients with MDD. These new disease mechanisms include neurogenesis, epigenetics, and inflammation. One positive aspect of these newer lines of research is the increase in the number of novel targets that have been identified for drug discovery. Depression is clearly a psychiatric disorder that cries out for new drugs that are more effective than the ones currently approved for clinical use.

Recent research with animal models of depression has pointed to disturbances in brain reward pathways as a critical element in susceptibility to stress-induced depression. These brain reward circuits, including the VTA and the nucleus accumbens, have taken center stage in efforts to understand the underlying molecular and neural changes that are responsible for a depressed phenotype. One neurotransmitter, DA, appears to play a critical role within these reward circuits in determining susceptibility to stress and depression and should be given greater attention as a target for antidepressants.

Looking ahead to Chapter 15, many of the same experiments described in Chapters 12 and 13 have revealed molecular and neural changes following exposure to stress that are characteristic of resilient animals that do not develop depression-like phenotypes. In the years ahead, a clearer understanding of brain mechanisms of resilience to stress may lead to treatments that protect individuals at risk of developing depression from the untoward effects of life stressors.

Another potential dividend from studies of animal models of depression may derive from efforts to employ biomarkers for the identification of individuals at risk of developing depression and for tracking responses to antidepressants in patients. A major breakthrough in this work has been from experiments to identify animals that are susceptible to stress-induced depression prior to exposure to the stressor. These susceptible animals can then be compared to resilient ones with respect to blood parameters as a means of informing studies in patients at risk of developing MDD.

14

Post-Traumatic Stress Disorder

Given the critical role played by Vietnam-era veterans and their allies in advocating for post-traumatic stress disorder (PTSD) to be included in *DSM-III*, it is only appropriate to begin this chapter from their perspectives. Dr. Jonathan Shay (1994) drew on his experiences as a psychiatrist working with Vietnam veterans to situate the devastating effects of combat trauma in Vietnam with the combat trauma of Achilles nearly three millennia earlier in Homer's classic work, *Iliad*. Shay, in his moving account, emphasized the devastating impact on soldiers of betrayal by their commanders, the trauma of losing close comrades, and the long-term dangers of the berserk state, where a soldier becomes more animal than human in his conduct. The emotional scars of these traumatic experiences can, as Shay (1994, p. xx) described so vividly, persist over decades and reach the point that "[s]uch unhealed PTSD can devastate life and incapacitate its victims from participating in the domestic, economic, and political life of the nation. The painful paradox is that fighting for one's country can render one unfit to be its citizen."

From his experiences in working with Vietnam-era veterans, Shay (1994, p. 187) argues that the "essential injuries in combat PTSD are moral and social, and so the central treatment must be moral and social. The best treatment restores control to the survivor and actively encourages communalization of the trauma. Healing is done *by* survivors, not *to* survivors."

Finally, what do we owe the men and women of our armed forces when they deploy to a combat zone? Shay's response is clear and compelling (Shay, 1994, p. 195); ". . . we should *care* about how soldiers are trained, equipped, led, and welcomed home when they return from war. This is our moral duty toward those we ask to serve on our behalf, and it is in our own self-interest as well. Unhealed combat trauma blights not only the life of the veteran but the life of the family and community." He adds (Shay, 1994, p. 195, "Unhealed combat trauma diminishes democratic participation and can become a threat to democratic political institutions. Severe psychological injury originates in violation of trust and destroys the capacity for trust. When mistrust spreads widely and deeply, democratic civic discourse becomes impossible."

Clinical Overview of PTSD

As was described in Chapter 1, post-traumatic stress disorder (PTSD) was officially recognized by the psychiatric community as a mental disorder with the publication of *DSM-III* (American Psychiatric Association, 1980). This disorder stands apart from all other psychiatric disorders in that prior exposure to a highly stressful traumatic event is required for a diagnosis of PTSD (Yehuda, 2002; Yehuda et al., 2015). Other psychiatric disorders, including the disorders discussed in Chapters 8–13, include life stressors as important environmental stimuli that may contribute to the onset and/or expression of symptoms associated with these disorders, often through interaction with susceptible genotypes. But PTSD stands apart in the tight coupling between exposure to the traumatic event and the onset of symptoms of the disorder.

DSM-5 (American Psychiatric Association, 2013) includes eight criteria that are required for a diagnosis of PTSD. These criteria, summarized in Table 14.1, provide the framework for developing animal models of PTSD. Note especially that exposure to the traumatic event can be direct or indirect, the effects must persist over time, there may be marked behavioral and physiological responses to reminders of the trauma, and there are elevations in reactivity to alerting stimuli.

Epidemiological studies have shown that most individuals in the general population have been exposed to at least one traumatic event over the course of their lifetimes, but most trauma-exposed individuals do not later develop PTSD. Women have been reported to be more vulnerable to the development of PTSD than men, even after controlling for prior history of victimization or abuse. These sex differences in vulnerability to PTSD appear to reflect in part greater heritability of risk in women compared to men. However, other factors are at work, including possible sex differences in neural circuits controlling fearful memories (Ramikie & Ressler, 2018).

Rates of PTSD following a natural disaster are relatively low (less than 5%), whereas rates of PTSD following rape are very high (approximately 65%). In studies of combat veterans from the wars in Iraq and Afghanistan, levels of PTSD peaked at 25%–30% among those individuals with the highest recurring exposures to combat-related traumatic experiences. Finally, PTSD symptoms may persist in individuals for a decade or longer, especially those exposed to combat-related trauma (Keane et al., 2006; Yehuda et al., 2015).

Table 14.1 *DSM-5* Criteria Required for a Diagnosis of PTSD

Criterion A (one required): The person was exposed to: death, threatened death, actual or threatened serious injury, or actual or threatened sexual violence, in the following way(s):

- *Direct exposure*
- *Witnessing the trauma*
- Learning that a relative or close friend was exposed to a trauma
- Indirect exposure to aversive details of the trauma, usually in the course of professional duties (e.g., first responders, medics)

Criterion B (one required): The traumatic event is persistently re-experienced, in the following way(s):

- Unwanted upsetting memories
- Nightmares
- Flashbacks
- Emotional distress after exposure to traumatic reminders
- *Physical reactivity after exposure to traumatic reminders*

Criterion C (one required): Avoidance of trauma-related stimuli after the trauma, in the following way(s):

- Trauma-related thoughts or feelings
- *Trauma-related reminders*

Criterion D (two required): Negative thoughts or feelings that began or worsened after the trauma, in the following way(s):

- Inability to recall key features of the trauma
- Overly negative thoughts and assumptions about oneself or the world
- Exaggerated blame of self or others for causing the trauma
- *Negative affect*
- *Decreased interest in activities*
- Feeling isolated
- *Difficulty experiencing positive affect*

Criterion E (two required): Trauma-related arousal and reactivity that began or worsened after the trauma, in the following way(s):

- *Irritability or aggression*
- Risky or destructive behavior
- *Hyper-vigilance*

(Continued)

Table 14.1 Continued

- Heightened startle reaction

- Difficulty concentrating

- *Difficulty sleeping*

Criterion F (required): *Symptoms last for more than 1 month (adjusted for species differences in life span).*

Criterion G (required): *Symptoms create distress or functional impairment (e.g., social, occupational).*

Criterion H (required): *Symptoms are not due to medication, substance use, or other illness.*

Note: Elements of each criterion that are in italics represent symptoms that can be reasonably represented and studied in various animal models of PTSD.

Animal Models of PTSD

Challenges and Opportunities

As with any psychiatric disorder, the challenges of developing animal models of PTSD are not to be taken lightly. However, there are some features of PTSD that lend themselves to modeling in laboratory animals. First and foremost, the nature and timing of the traumatic event(s) can be specified precisely in an animal model. In addition, the brain circuitry that is involved in fear and anxiety that is so critically involved in the symptoms of PTSD has been highly conserved over evolutionary time. Finally, reasonable approximations for some of the criteria employed in the classification of PTSD can be studied in laboratory animals, including trauma reminders, negative affect, anhedonia, hypervigilance, enhanced startle reactions, and sleep disturbances (refer to italicized entries in Table 14.1). Most importantly, animal models provide an opportunity for investigators to study animals prospectively, including manipulations of early life experiences prior to the trauma, as well as careful tracking of individuals following exposure to the trauma.

As an illustration of the value of combining translational and reverse translational approaches to PTSD, Ressler et al. (2011) reported that PTSD symptoms were significantly associated with blood levels of pituitary adenylate cyclase-activating peptide (PACAP) in human females but not in males. In addition, a PTSD diagnosis in females was associated with higher blood level of PACAP. When participants were exposed to a fear conditioning paradigm, females but not males with high PACAP blood levels exhibited greater startle responses when exposed to fear cues (CS+) or safety cues (CS–) associated with the conditioned stimulus, an air blast. These differences were especially evident during the late acquisition stage when control females and male participants had habituated to the fear cues. In a study of 44 single nucleotide polymorphisms (SNPs) in the genes coding for PACAP and its PAC1 receptor, one SNP (rs2267735) associated with a putative estrogen response element of the *PAC1* gene was predictive of a PTSD diagnosis in females but not in males. Females with this SNP also displayed impaired fear discrimination late in conditioned acquisition of the fear response and enhanced startle in a darkened test area. Methylation of this same SNP in peripheral blood was also strongly associated with PTSD in females.

Based upon these findings in traumatized humans, this group of investigators moved to an animal model of PTSD, Pavlovian fear conditioning in mice in which a previously neutral tone (CS) was paired with 10 footshocks. They found that levels of the mRNA for PAC1 receptor in amygdala were increased significantly during consolidation of fear and were highly correlated with peak levels of freezing behavior. These experiments included a traumatized clinical population and were supplemented with data from an animal model and point to a possible biomarker and new drug targets to improve the diagnosis and treatment of PTSD in women (Ressler et al., 2011).

Early Models of PTSD

Beginning in the late 1980s, the first peer-reviewed publications began to appear that described early attempts to develop animal models of PTSD. Initially, there was considerable interest in exposure of laboratory rats to inescapable electric shocks as an appropriate animal model of PTSD (Ottenweller et al., 1989; van der Kolk et al., 1985). Foa et al. (1992), in a careful review of the animal and human literature relevant to PTSD to that point, proposed that exposure of laboratory animals to unpredictable and uncontrollable aversive stimuli (e.g., inescapable footshock or tail shock) resulted in behavioral and biological alterations that were similar to symptoms observed in patients with PTSD, including persistent elevations in arousal, re-experiencing of the traumatic event, numbing, and avoidance of environments that brought back memories of the traumatic event. Importantly, they argued that chronically stressed laboratory rats and patients with PTSD might share common underlying etiologies, such that studies with animal models might reveal new targets and approaches for therapeutic developments, including psychological and pharmacological interventions (Foa et al., 1992). Similar motivations guide many of the experiments with animal models of PTSD to the present time.

One issue that confronted basic scientists early on was the issue of how long PTSD-like symptoms must persist following exposure of laboratory animals to a traumatic event. As noted earlier in *DSM-5*, the persistence of symptoms in patients must be at least 1 month following the traumatic event, and in some cases, these initial symptoms of PTSD may persist for up to 6 months. How does one translate these temporal domains in human terms to a time scale for laboratory rats and mice? In one such attempt, Adamec and Swallow (1993) reasoned that 7.5 days in the life of a laboratory rat (life span = ~3 years) is equivalent to approximately 6 months for a human (life span = 72 years). In the experiments described in the following on research with two frequently utilized animal models, most studies have employed a delay of at least 7 days between trauma exposure and behavioral testing or collection of biological samples for later analysis. Such a timeline appears to comport with the temporal requirements for PTSD symptoms as contained in *DSM-5*.

One Size Does Not Fit All

In a recent review, Daskalakis and Yehuda (2014) argued that a single animal model of PTSD cannot capture the many variables associated with this disorder, especially the many unique features of deployment-related PTSD among members of the armed forces. They also offered refinements in experimental design that would distinguish between animals that were susceptible to the development of PTSD-like symptoms and those that were resilient. These issues will be discussed in greater detail in the following and again in Chapter 15.

In the sections that follow, I will present an overview and analysis of two especially well-developed animal models of PTSD. For each of these models (predator stress and single prolonged stress), I will provide key experimental findings for each model and evaluate their strengths and weaknesses. I will then conclude with suggestions for future studies based upon unexplored areas in each of the models. There are certainly other animal models of PTSD that have been developed, and the interested reader may learn more by consulting several comprehensive reviews (e.g., Deslauriers et al., 2018; Goswami et al., 2013; Schöner et al., 2017).

I Smell a Cat!

Imagine for a moment that you are a rat. Short of running into a cat in a dark alleyway, could there be anything worse than detecting the scent of a cat during your stroll around the neighborhood? Building on this possibility, early studies by Adamec and Shallow (1993) demonstrated long-lasting changes in anxiety-like behaviors of laboratory rats exposed for 5 minutes to a domestic cat in a laboratory setting. The exposure was monitored so that the cat did not injure the laboratory rats. Laboratory rats exposed briefly to this natural predator displayed increased anxiety-like behaviors that persisted over at least a 21-day period.

The PSS model of PTSD. Building upon this initial study and related ones from other laboratories, Dr. Hagit Cohen and her colleagues (Cohen & Zohar, 2004) modified this ethologically relevant animal model of PTSD by employing brief exposure (10 minutes) of individual laboratory rats to cat odors. This procedure is often referred to as the predator scent stress (PSS) model of PTSD. In some experiments, laboratory rats were exposed to clean cat litter one day after behavioral testing, a test condition which served as a reminder effect of the prior exposure to cat odors contained in soiled cat litter. When placed on the clean cat litter, those rats that displayed PTSD-like responses to behavioral testing the day before spent the vast majority of the time freezing (>75% of the test period). By replacing the real live predator with cat odors, this experimental refinement also reduced the variability associated with differences in the behavioral responses of cats to repeated pairings with test rats. In addition, a case can be made that this paradigm represents a potentially life-threatening experience for laboratory rats, and as such, is at least qualitatively similar to some traumatic experiences of humans (Cohen et al., 2014).

In contrast to the approaches of others, the Cohen research group embraced the variability of responses to the "trauma" of exposing groups of outbred Sprague-Dawley (SD) laboratory rats to cat odors by establishing cut-off behavioral scores to distinguish well-adapted from maladapted animals. When tested 7 days later, some rats previously exposed to cat odors displayed extreme behavioral alterations (approximately 22%) that were indicative of a PTSD-like response. Similar results were obtained when testing was delayed until 30 days after exposure to cat odors. Indeed, approximately 15% of all animals tested met the extreme behavioral change cut-off criteria when behavioral testing was delayed until 90 days after exposure of rats to cat odors. Other rats exhibited minimal changes in behavioral measures (approximately 7%), whereas the remaining animals (approximately 70%) displayed clear disruptions in their behaviors relative to unexposed controls, but these changes did not meet the cut-off criteria for extreme or minimal behavioral changes.

Dependent measures that made up the cut-off behavioral scores in the experiments conducted by Cohen and her group have included behaviors of rats in an elevated plus-maze (EPM) and the magnitude of the acoustic startle response (ASR) and habituation to the auditory stimulus. The EPM provided a means for assessing anxiety-like behaviors, while the ASR indicated hypervigilance as reflected by increased startle amplitude and decreased habituation to auditory stimuli, both of which are among the defining characteristics of PTSD. The heterogeneity of responses following exposure of laboratory rats to cat odors also matched well with findings from humans, where the percentage of individuals who develop PTSD following exposure to a traumatic event is highly variable and depends in part on the nature of the trauma (Matar et al., 2013) (Figure 14.1).

Evidence that the frequency of extreme behavioral responses to PSS is under at least partial genetic control was revealed in a comparative study of three strains of laboratory rats, inbred Fischer-344 (F344) and Lewis rats and outbred SD rats

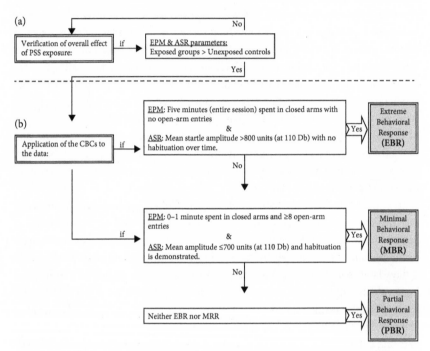

Figure 14.1. The cutoff behavioral criteria (CBC) algorithm. To situate the PSS behavioral model more closely to clinical conceptions of PTSD, the approach taken enabled the classification of test animals into groups according to degree of response to the stressor. Behavioral criteria were defined and then complemented by the definition of cutoff criteria reflecting severity of responses; this approach parallels inclusion and exclusion criteria applied in clinical research. The procedure required the following steps: A: Verification of global effect: the data must demonstrate that the stressor had a significant effect on the overall behavior of exposed versus unexposed populations at the time of assessment. B: Application of the CBCs to the data. To maximize the resolution and minimize false positives, extreme responses to both EPM and ASR paradigms, performed in sequence, were required for "inclusion" into the EBR group, whereas a negligible degree of response to both resulted in inclusion in the MBR group.

Adapted from Cohen et al. (2014) and used with permission of the publisher.

(Cohen et al., 2006). After exposure to cat odors, 50% of Lewis rats, 25% of SD rats, and only 10% of F-344 rats displayed extreme behavioral responses based upon testing in the EPM and ASR.

In an extension of this line of research, Cohen and coworkers (Cohen, Geva, et al., 2008) compared the behavioral responses of mice from six inbred strains to PSS. The results of this study revealed substantial variability between and within strains in anxiety-like behaviors, with heritability estimated at 30%. The heritability estimate decreased to 10% when considering the strain-specific behavioral responses to PSS. The BALB/cJ and 129J inbred mouse strains had the highest baseline anxiety scores, whereas the C57BL/6J had the highest levels of extreme behavioral scores following PSS.

Additional behavioral disruptions of PSS. Additional behavioral measures of rats exposed to cat odors have bolstered the validity of the PSS model of PTSD. For example, male and female rats with extreme alterations in behavior displayed significant reductions in sexually motivated behaviors as well as levels of social interaction. In addition, male rats that had extreme alterations in behavior following PSS were less attractive to unstressed females as potential partners and they had reduced circulating levels of testosterone. When presented with a choice between a familiar territory and a novel territory, male rats with extreme alterations in behavior following PSS spent significantly less time in the novel territory compared to minimally affected rats and unstressed controls. A cognitive assessment using the Morris water maze revealed that male rats with extreme alterations in behavior following PSS had difficulty learning new locations of a submerged platform compared to rats in the other groups. Finally, this laboratory did not detect differences between males and females in the prevalence of extreme alterations in behaviors following PSS. This is one measure that differs from human epidemiological studies, in which females appear to be more susceptible to PTSD than males (Cohen, Kozlovsky, Alona, et al., 2014). This issue is addressed further in the following.

Impaired formation of memories was examined in a mouse model of PTSD (El Hage et al., 2006). BALB/c mice were individually placed into contact with a cat for 5 minutes, while controls were handled. Control and predator-exposed mice were tested in a spatial learning task (8-arm radial maze) and an object recognition test beginning at 16–26 days post-stress. The results indicated that mice exposed to predator stress displayed significant long-term (up to 1 month) impairments in spatial memory relative to unstressed controls.

A key feature of PTSD in humans is the continuing response to trauma-related stimuli even when the individual is in an otherwise safe environment. A classic example of this phenomenon is a previously deployed army veteran who reacts to fireworks on a holiday as if he is still in a combat zone. Cohen et al. (2009) took a creative approach to exploring this phenomenon under controlled laboratory conditions using the PSS model. Using a contextual odor-conditioning paradigm, rats encountered the scent of cinnamon in two environments, an aversive one (exposure to footshock) and a rewarding one (access to a sucrose solution). The response to cinnamon odor was assessed in a third neutral environment. Rats that were tested in these three environments displayed freezing behavior in the aversive environment but not in the rewarding environment, and importantly, not in the neutral environment. If rats were exposed to PSS prior to or following contextual odor conditioning training, there was a dramatic increase in the freezing response of severe behaviorally affected rats to cinnamon odor in the neutral environment. The generality of these findings would be enhanced if other types of sensory stimuli (e.g., auditory or visual stimuli) were employed using this same experimental paradigm.

Peripheral stress effector systems and PSS. In an important prospective study, Danan et al. (2018) collected blood samples from venous catheters in rats at 20-minute intervals for 5 hours before and 6.5 hours after a 10-minute exposure to PSS. Blood samples were later analyzed for levels of CORT. EPM and ASR behavioral measures were obtained 7 days after exposure to cat odors. Rats with extreme behavioral responses to PSS differed from minimally or partially affected rats in several important ways that included having reduced CORT responses to PSS, as well as blunted pre-stress basal CORT pulsatility but not frequency. These investigators suggested that reductions in the amplitude of ultradian rhythms in CORT prior to a traumatic stressor may be a risk factor that conveys susceptibility to traumatic stressors in laboratory rats.

Autonomic nervous system. To examine autonomic correlates of trauma exposure in freely behaving animals, Koresh et al. (2016) surgically implanted male and female SD rats with radio telemetry devices on day 0 to measure the electrocardiogram (EKG) and locomotor activity. From days 11 to 19, basal measures of EKG and locomotor activity were captured and stored for later analyses. Rats were exposed to PSS on day 12 and EPM and ASR behavioral testing occurred on day 19. Using cutoff behavioral scores, male and female rats were characterized as extremely affected, minimally affected, or not affected by exposure to PSS.

Following exposure to PSS for 10 minutes, male and female rats exhibited significant increases in heart rate and changes in the EKG suggestive of an increase in sympathetic drive to the heart. Those male and female rats that displayed extreme behavioral disruptions were characterized by disruptions in habituation and recovery of autonomic drive to the heart. In addition, more males than females were characterized as extremely disrupted behaviorally, and females had a more rapid recovery of EKG parameters following PSS compared to males. These investigators concluded that rats that developed PTSD-like behavioral changes following PSS failed to re-establish homeostatic balance following brief exposure to the traumatic stimulus (Koresh et al., 2016).

These and other findings support the conclusion reached by Cohen and Yehuda (2011) that male rats are more susceptible to stressful stimulation and PTSD-like behaviors than females. This conclusion is clearly at odds with epidemiological findings in humans, and further studies may explain the reason for these discrepancies.

Immune system. The peripheral immune system plays a critical role in adaptive responses to stressful stimuli (refer to Chapter 4). To examine the role of immune cells in the response to PSS, Cohen et al. (2006) compared the responses of three groups of BALB/c mice: wild-type, those with severe combined immune deficiency (SCID), and immune-deficient nude mice (*nu/nu*) on a BALB/c background. Based upon the behavioral responses in the EPM and the ASR measured 7 days after PSS, significantly more SCID mice (62%) and nude mice (70%) displayed extreme behavioral responses to PSS compared to wild-type BALB/c mice (17%). These results suggested that the greater responses of SCID and nude mice to PSS were explained by an absence of mature effector T cells. Other experiments revealed that the addition of a single population of T cells reactive to CNS proteins was sufficient to rescue immune-deficient mice from the adverse behavioral effects of PSS. In contrast, naturally occurring CD4+CD25+ regulatory T cells counteracted the beneficial effect of T cells reactive to CNS proteins on behavioral responses to PSS.

Priming effects of juvenile stressors and PSS. Early life stressors have been associated with increased susceptibility to PTSD in humans. To examine further this relationship, Cohen et al. (2007) assessed the influence of "trauma" exposure during the juvenile period (PND 28) on later development of PTSD-like behaviors in adult rats (60 or 80 days of age) using the PSS paradigm. Two different juvenile trauma conditions were employed: exposure to cat odors for 10 minutes, or placement on a platform 7–10 cm above the water level in the middle of a pool. Behavioral data and autonomic control of heart rate were captured in adult animals of the various experimental groups.

The findings were quite striking in that both juvenile trauma conditions increased the PTSD-like behavioral responses (EPM and ASR) of adult animals following a second exposure to the same stimulus in adulthood. However, a dose-response relationship was noted in that the PSS condition (juvenile + adulthood) had a greater impact on behavioral responses compared to placement on the elevated platform in the pool of water (juvenile + adulthood). Exposure to the stressor in the juvenile period and in adulthood also had a greater impact on behavioral measures in adulthood compared to exposure to the stressor at one age only.

Compared to unstressed controls and rats that were minimally affected behaviorally, rats that were exposed to traumatic stressors as juveniles and as adults and that had extreme behavioral responses displayed significant disruptions in autonomic control of heart rate that did not recover toward basal values. These persistent autonomic disruptions in rats stressed during the juvenile period and in adulthood included increased heart rate responses to stressors and decreased heart rate variability, suggesting enhanced sympathetic drive to the heart. The changes in autonomic control of the heart reflect centrally mediated changes in autonomic outflow and suggest neural pathways that may be especially vulnerable to the priming effects of juvenile stressors (Cohen et al., 2007).

Neural and molecular mechanisms of PSS. Following a detailed characterization of the PSS model of PTSD, Cohen and her colleagues as well as others have employed this valuable experimental paradigm to investigate molecular mechanisms that may render animals at high risk for the development of PTSD-like symptoms. A detailed summary of all relevant studies in this area is beyond the scope of this chapter. Thus, I will be selective in providing a high-level view of research in this important area.

Changes in neuronal morphology. The traumatic experience of exposure to cat odors had an impact on the structure of individual neurons in the hippocampus and amygdala of laboratory rats. Compared to sham-PSS controls, rats that had severe disruptions in behavior 7 days after exposure to cat odors displayed alterations in neuronal morphology in the hippocampus and the amygdala. Specifically, PSS-exposed rats had significant reductions in dendritic branching, total dendritic length, and spine density of granule cells in the dentate gyrus and CA1 pyramidal neurons (Cohen, Kozlovsky, Matar, et al., 2014; S. Cohen et al., 2012). In contrast to neuronal retraction in the hippocampus, Cohen, Kozlovsky, Matar, et al. (2014) reported increased total dendritic number and spine density for pyramidal neurons in the basolateral amygdala of PSS-exposed rats with extreme behavioral responses (Figure 14.2). These alterations in neuronal morphology have been complemented by many studies that have examined molecular changes in signaling pathways that regulate synaptic plasticity and neuronal growth and function.

Brain-derived neurotrophic factor. Brain-derived neurotrophic factor (BDNF) and its intracellular kinase-activating receptor, TrkB, have been implicated in stress-related processes and neuronal plasticity. To examine the effects of a trauma-related stressor on BDNF and its receptor, SD rats were subjected to PSS, and behavioral testing occurred 7 days later. In rats that exhibited extreme disruptions in behavior following PSS, there were significant decreases in BDNF mRNA levels and significant increases in TrkB mRNA levels that were limited to the CA1 region of the hippocampus. These transcriptional alterations were not observed in other brain areas and did not occur in rats that displayed minimal behavioral alterations following PSS. It was unclear whether these highly specific changes in BDNF and its receptor were a marker for susceptibility to PSS

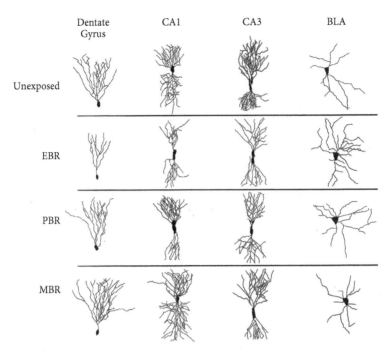

	Dentate Gyrus	CA1	CA3	BLA
Unexposed				
EBR				
PBR				
MBR				

Figure 14.2. Photomicrographs of Golgi-Cox stained brain sections enabled computer-generated plots of reconstructions of the dendritic trees of dentate granule cells from the dorsal hippocampus, CA1 pyramidal neurons, CA3 pyramidal neurons, and pyramidal cells of the basolateral amygdala (BLA) for unexposed control rats and PSS-exposed rats. PSS-exposed rats were characterized as extreme behavioral responders (EBR), partial behavioral responders (PBR), or minimal behavioral responders, as described in Figure 14.1.

Adapted from Cohen et al. (2014) and used with permission of the publisher.

or played a causal role in the disruptions in behavior following PSS (Kozlovsky et al., 2007).

Neuropeptide Y (NPY). NPY is a 36-aminoacid peptide that is found in the central nervous system as well as in the periphery (Allen et al., 1983; Zukowska-Grojec et al., 1988). The biological actions of this peptide result from activation of four distinct G-protein coupled receptors (Y1, Y2, Y4, and Y5) (Silva et al., 2002). To explore the role of NPY in trauma-related behavioral and biological responses, laboratory rats were exposed to PSS for 15 minutes, and EPM and ASR tests were administered 7 days later. On the 8th day, rats were sacrificed and levels of NPY were measured in discrete areas of the brain. Those animals that had extreme behavioral responses to PSS had significant decreases in levels of

NPY in the hippocampus, amygdala, dorsal cerebral cortex, and PAG compared to handled controls (Cohen et al., 2012).

In related experiments, 10 days before the PSS protocol, rats were implanted bilaterally with cannulae directed at the dorsal hippocampus, an area where trauma-related increases in NPY signaling appeared to occur. One hour after exposure to PSS or sham-PSS, rats received bilateral microinjections of NPY (5 or 10 μg) or artificial CSF into the dorsal hippocampus. Administration of NPY, especially the higher dose, reduced anxiety-like behaviors and startle amplitude while increasing startle habituation to levels that were similar to values for unexposed controls. The opposite effect was observed following administration of an NPY Y1 receptor antagonist, which increased anxiety-like behaviors while maintaining startle amplitude and startle habituation at levels observed in animals that received artificial CSF. Finally, administration of NPY reduced dramatically the number of rats that had extreme behavioral responses to PSS, as well as the percentage of time spent freezing when exposed to a trauma reminder on day 8 following PSS. Thus, NPY appears to play an essential role in protecting animals from the deleterious effects of exposure to traumatic experiences, perhaps through stimulation of the HPA axis (Cohen et al., 2012).

Neuropeptide S (NPS). NPS is a 20-amino acid peptide that suppresses anxiety, increases locomotor activity and wakefulness, and facilitates the extinction of conditioned fear. NPS cell bodies are found in clusters in close proximity to the locus coeruleus, while NPS receptors are found in many areas of brain, including the hypothalamus and amygdala (Xu et al., 2004; Xu et al., 2007). Cohen et al. (2018) hypothesized that NPS may play a role in the extreme behavioral responses to PSS because NPS receptors are located in high concentration in the amygdala, a brain area known to be involved in processing of fear- and anxiety-related signals, and a brain area that plays a critical role in the expression of PTSD-related behavioral responses.

These researchers tested their hypotheses relating to the pathophysiology of PTSD in an extensive series of experiments that involved the PSS paradigm. Ten days before the PSS protocol, rats were implanted bilaterally with cannulae directed at the basolateral amygdala, and were permitted to recover fully before testing. One hour after exposure to PSS or sham-PSS, rats received bilateral microinjections of NPS (1.0 nmol/0.5 μl) or an equal volume of artificial CSF. Seven days later, rats were tested in the EPM and ASR. The following day, rats were exposed to a trauma-reminder cue (clean cat litter) and freezing behavior was recorded. Microinjections of NPS into the basolateral amygdala of sham-PSS rats did not affect any of the behavioral measures relative to sham-PSS rats that received microinjections of artificial CSF. Relative to PSS rats that received vehicle injections, PSS rats that received microinjections of NPS bilaterally into the basolateral amygdala were characterized by the following: a significant reduction in anxiety-like behaviors in the EPM, a significant decrease in startle amplitude and an increase in startle habituation in the ASR test, and a reduction from 30% to 0% in the prevalence of rats that were characterized by extreme behavioral responses to PSS. In addition, there was a corresponding increase from 0% in vehicle-injected rats to 45% in NPS-injected rats that exhibited minimal behavioral responses to PSS. NPS administration also resulted in a significant and sustained increase in plasma levels of CORT for up to 40 minutes after administration. Finally, when exposed to a trauma reminder cue 8 days after PSS, NPS-injected rats displayed significantly less freezing behavior (19% of total time) compared to vehicle-injected rats (43% of total time).

The beneficial anxiolytic effects of NPS microinjected bilaterally into the basolateral amygdala of rats exposed to PSS were accompanied by increases in levels of BDNF and of NPY Y1 receptors (but not levels of NPY) in the hippocampus. Pre-injection of an NPS antagonist and/or an NPY Y1 antagonist 15 minutes after exposure of rats to cat odors blocked the protective effects of NPS on PSS-induced behavioral alterations. Thus, the actions of NPS within the basolateral amygdala appeared to involve direct interactions with NPS receptors and NPY Y1 receptors. These investigators concluded that NPS signaling in the basolateral amygdala activated three critical systems within the hippocampus that are involved in PTSD-like responses, including the HPA axis, BDNF, and NPY Y1 receptors (Cohen et al., 2018).

GR signaling pathways. Another molecular signaling pathway in the brain that has particular relevance to PTSD-like behavioral changes is the glucocorticoid receptor (GR) signaling pathway. In an important study with direct clinical implications, Daskalakis et al. (2014) performed high-throughput genome-wide expression profiling followed by quantitative polymerase chain reaction (qPCR) in blood samples and in two brain areas (amygdala and hippocampus) of male and female rats that had been characterized as extreme behavioral responders or minimal behavioral responders to PSS. Unexposed control groups of both sexes were also included in these analyses.

The differentially regulated genes that were associated with individual differences in response to PSS in males and females tended to cluster together in both brain areas. Bioinformatics analyses were then conducted to determine the transcription factors upstream of the differentially regulated genes and their canonical signaling pathways. The authors identified 73 transcription factors that were involved in extreme behavioral responses to PSS across the blood and brain samples that were assayed. Of this total, only nine transcription factors (CREB1, FOXO3, JUN, MYC, MYCN, NFE2L2, NFKBIA, NR3C1, and TP53) were common to all three of the sample types studied. Of these nine, GR signaling (NR3C1) was the only convergent pathway associated with extreme behavioral responses to PSS when using the most stringent level of statistical significance.

In addition, 19 of the 73 transcription factors were later determined to play a role in glucocorticoid signaling. Of all of the possible outcomes of this genome-wide expression assay, it is remarkable that the one gene that was identified as common to extreme behavioral responses to PSS in all three sample types and both sexes was the gene for the GR. There is a rich literature on the role of the HPA axis in the response to traumatic stress and the onset of PTSD, and this study further cemented that relationship. These findings also suggest the possibility of employing measurement of GR in blood samples as a biomarker for PTSD (Daskalakis et al., 2014).

Brain-immune interactions. Given the previous findings by Cohen et al. (2006) on immune cell-mediated effects on extreme behavioral responses to PSS in laboratory mice, Lewitus et al. (2008) extended these findings by quantifying T cell recruitment to the brain, especially the choroid plexus, in response to PSS. The choroid plexus is the main entry point into the brain for T cells, and it sits in close proximity to the hippocampus. Further, exogenous administration of CORT mimicked the effects of PSS on T cell recruitment to the choroid plexus.

To determine the impact of brain-immune interactions on trauma-related behaviors, these investigators compared the responses of C57BL/6 and BALB/c mice to PSS. C57BL/6 mice have a more extreme behavioral response to PSS compared to BALB/c mice. Two lines of evidence pointed to BDNF levels in the hippocampus as a target of trauma-related stress. Stress-induced elevations in CORT (Smith et al., 1995) and recruitment of T cells (Ziv et al., 2006) both stimulated increases in hippocampal BDNF levels. The results of this study revealed that BALB/c mice had a significant reduction in BDNF expression in the dentate gyrus within 3 hours after PSS, but levels returned to pre-stress levels by 7 days. In contrast, levels of BDNF expression in the dentate gyrus of C57BL/6 mice decreased significantly at 3 hours after PSS, but levels remained low at 7 days post-PSS.

To mitigate the adverse effects of PSS by stimulating the recruitment of auto-immune T cells, C57BL/6 mice were given a single injection to immunize them against myelin oligodendrocyte glycoprotein-derived peptide (pMOG$_{35-55}$) 7 days prior to PSS, and behavioral testing occurred 7 days after PSS. Compared to vehicle-injected controls, immunized C57BL/6 mice displayed less anxiety-like behavior in the EPM and had a significant reduction in startle amplitude in the ASR. In addition, immunized C57BL/6 mice had a reduction in BDNF expression in the dentate gyrus 24 hours after PSS, but levels were restored to control levels by 7 days post-PSS. BDNF expression remained depressed at 7 days post-PSS in vehicle-injected C57BL/6 control mice.

These investigators suggested that trafficking of immune cells to the brain was a critical component of the physiological adaptation to traumatic stress. There were also connections between the HPA axis and the immune response, as well as T cell trafficking to the brain and maintenance of BDNF expression in the dentate gyrus. A vigorous immune response to PSS was also attended by less extreme behavioral responses to exposure to cat odors. These findings also suggested that the immune system may be an appropriate target for the development of therapies to treat PTSD (Lewitus et al., 2008).

Preventing the effects of PSS. A host of experimental manipulations has been employed to block the behavioral and neurobiological effects of PSS or predator stress exposure. Several of these experimental approaches will be discussed in the following.

Administration of CORT. One approach is consistent with evidence described earlier that PSS-induced activation of the HPA axis is compromised in rats that later display extreme behavioral responses to a traumatic stressor (Danan et al., 2018). Administration of a high dose of CORT (25 mg/kg), but not lower doses, 1 hour after PSS resulted in a significant reduction in the percentage of animals that displayed extreme behavioral disruptions when tested 30 days later. In addition, animals that received the highest dose of CORT spent significantly less time freezing (24% of time) when placed on clean cat litter (reminder cue) compared to vehicle-injected controls (80% of time freezing). These investigators suggested that the high dose of CORT may have disrupted the consolidation of traumatic memories following PSS (Cohen, Matar, et al., 2008).

Inhibition of protein synthesis. Administration of a protein synthesis inhibitor soon after PSS has been employed to examine its impact on the prevalence of extreme behavioral responses. Minocycline is a broad spectrum, second-generation tetracycline that has a range of biological actions, including anti-microbial, anti-inflammatory, anti-apoptotic, and neuroprotective effects. In addition, the drug is highly lipid soluble, promotes neurogenesis, and reduces oxidative stress (Garrido-Mesa et al., 2013). Levkovitz et al. (2015) administered a single dose of minocycline (35 mg/kg) to laboratory rats 1 hour after PSS or sham PSS. Control animals exposed to PSS or sham PSS received an injection of saline. EPM and ASR tests were administered 7 days later, and a trauma reminder test (placement of rats on clean cat litter) was administered on day 8. Compared to saline-injected controls, minocycline-treated rats displayed significant increases in open-arm entries and time spent in the open arms during testing on an EPM. Minocycline-treated rats also had reduced startle amplitude and greater startle habituation in the ASR test. In addition, the prevalence of extreme behavioral responses to PSS was reduced significantly in rats treated with minocycline. With respect to the trauma reminder test on day 8, PSS rats treated with minocycline exhibited significant decreases in time spent freezing compared to PSS rats that received a saline injection. Importantly, minocycline did not alter the behaviors of sham-PSS rats compared to sham-PSS rats receiving a saline injection. The authors suggested that the effects of minocycline on elevations in levels of IL-6 and TNFα in hippocampus and PFC may have explained in part the effects of the drug on behavioral responses to PSS (Levkovitz et al., 2015).

Sleep deprivation. Interruption of sleep patterns following exposure to a traumatic stressor has been another strategy to alter the behavioral effects of PSS. S. Cohen et al. (2012) exposed rats to PSS at the end of the light phase of their 12:12 light-dark cycle. Beginning 1 hour after PSS, rats were kept awake for 6 hours by gentle handling and just enough disturbance to keep them awake, but not to add significantly to their levels of stress. Seven days later, rats were tested in the EPM and ASR, and the following day they were exposed to the trauma reminder involving placement on clean cat litter.

Six hours of sleep deprivation had a dramatic impact on behavioral responses to PSS. Sleep-deprived rats exhibited significant reductions in anxiety-like behaviors on the EPM, had decreased startle amplitudes and increased startle habituation in the ASR, and spent significantly less time freezing during the trauma reminder test. Indeed, for many of these variables, PSS rats that were sleep-deprived more closely resembled sham-PSS rats in their behaviors (S. Cohen et al., 2012).

Time-dependent intervention. The three interventions described in the preceding share in common their disruptive effects on time-dependent memory storage processes. PSS rats were given a single high dose of CORT, a single injection of minocycline to block protein synthesis (among other biological effects), or 6 hours of sleep deprivation soon after exposure to cat odors. This intervention protocol is reminiscent of post-training drug administration following an aversive event to enhance or impair memory storage processes (McGaugh, 2000; Roozendaal, 2002). These findings have great relevance to the acute treatment of some individuals exposed to traumatic experiences, as some translational studies have already been conducted in humans with promising results. These early translational research studies have tested the hypothesis that there is a golden window of time following exposure to trauma (several hours perhaps) when treatments designed to block memory consolidation would be most advantageous (Zohar et al., 2011).

Blockade of hormone receptors. Using a variety of hormonal and neurotransmitter antagonists, Adamec et al. (2007) explored the hormonal and neurobiological underpinnings of behavioral responses to a single 10-minute unmonitored exposure of laboratory rats to a cat. These investigators administered each drug 1 minute after the end of predator exposure and employed a battery of four tests to assess anxiety-like behaviors 7 days later. The following are abbreviated results from this complex study:

- Propranolol (5 or 10 mg/kg), a β-adrenergic antagonist, dose-dependently blocked the effects of traumatic stress on anxiety-like behaviors.

- Mifepristone (RU486, 20 mg/kg), a GR antagonist, did not affect the anxiogenic effects of predator exposure stress.
- Spironolactone (50 mg/kg), an MR antagonist, blocked the anxiogenic effects of predator exposure stress in three of the four tests of anxiety-like behaviors.

The conclusions from this study were that β-adrenergic receptors and MRs combined to influence the development of anxiety-like behaviors following traumatic stress. The likely neural circuits that were involved in these effects included the hippocampus and the amygdala, as well as projections to these areas from brainstem and midbrain nuclei. These findings have particular relevance to clinical studies of propranolol. If the drug is administered soon after trauma exposure and combined with behavior therapy, it appears to dampen trauma-related NE signaling in the brain and facilitates extinction learning associated with the traumatic event (Giustino et al., 2016).

To examine the role of CRF signaling in the development of behavioral responses to traumatic stress, Adamec et al. (2010) exposed C57BL/6 male mice to a cat for 10 minutes, with controls handled but not exposed to the cat. Groups of mice were injected 30 minutes before or just after predator exposure with vehicle or 2 or 20 mg/kg of a CRF_1 receptor antagonist (CRA0450). In mice exposed to predator stress, blockade of CRF_1 receptors reduced measures of anxiety-like behaviors across several tests, especially when the antagonist was administered just prior to predator exposure.

Inhibition of serotonin reuptake. Selective serotonin reuptake inhibitors (SSRIs) are utilized extensively as a first-line treatment for patients with acute and chronic symptoms of PTSD (Yehuda et al., 2015). One issue that can be addressed with an animal model of PTSD is to explore the potential benefit of administering a drug beginning immediately after exposure to trauma compared to a delay in beginning a drug treatment regimen. Using the PSS model of PTSD, Matar et al. (2006) examined the effects of immediate versus delayed administration of an SSRI, sertraline, on the pattern of behavioral responses to trauma exposure. Sertraline hydrochloride (10 mg/kg, i.p.) or saline was administered each day for 7 days beginning 1 hour after exposure of rats to PSS or the regimen of drug/saline administration was delayed until 7 days after PSS. On the 7th day of sertraline administration, sham-PSS and PSS-exposed rats were assessed in the EPM and ASR tests.

When daily sertraline administration was initiated beginning 1 hour after PSS, there was a significant decrease in anxiety-like behaviors, a reduction in startle amplitude, and an increase in startle habituation relative to saline-injected PSS rats. In addition, there was a reduction in the prevalence of extreme behavioral responses among the sertraline-treated rats. If daily administration of sertraline was delayed until 7 days after PSS, there remained a significant reduction in anxiety-like behaviors in the EPM and a decrease in startle amplitude in the ASR. However, sertraline-treated animals did not demonstrate evidence of habituation to the startle stimulus and the percentage of animals that exhibited extreme behavioral responses to PSS was not reduced compared to saline-injected PSS animals. The mechanism of action of sertraline was not investigated in this study, but the effects of the drug probably extended beyond its primary effect on reuptake of serotonin (Matar et al., 2006).

Hit Me with Your Best Shot!

This classic rock song from Pat Benatar in 1980 alluded to one best shot, but in this model of PTSD, it is actually more like hit me with your three best shots. The single prolonged stress (SPS) animal model of PTSD was first developed by Dr. Israel Liberzon and his colleagues at the University of Michigan in the late 1990s (Liberzon et al., 1999). SPS is actually a series of three different stressors to which laboratory animals are exposed sequentially as follows: restraint stress for 2 hours, followed by forced swim stress in a group for 20 minutes at 24°C, then a 15-minute recovery period to dry off, and finally, ether anesthesia until unresponsive. Following recovery from ether anesthesia, rats are returned to their home cages and left untouched for 7 days, a time which has been referred to as a period of consolidation or sensitization.

At this point, SPS-exposed animals displayed a pattern of behavioral changes that were similar to some aspects of PTSD. Exposure of rats to all three stressors was required for the behavioral and neuroendocrine changes characteristic of PTSD to occur, and some of these changes persisted for more than 40 days (Lisieski et al., 2018). The SPS paradigm, with some modifications, has also been adapted to the C57BL/6 inbred strain of laboratory mice, and the results were generally similar to findings with laboratory rats (Perrine et al., 2016). Several excellent reviews are available on various aspects of the SPS model in relation to PTSD (Lisieski et al., 2018; Souza et al., 2017; Yamamoto et al., 2009).

Neuroendocrine effects of SPS. The SPS model was developed to address the observation in PTSD patients of alterations in the regulation of the HPA axis. In the initial study, Liberzon et al. (1997) demonstrated that exposure of rats to SPS resulted in an increase in glucocorticoid fast feedback during a subsequent restraint stress session. This alteration in regulation of the HPA axis in SPS rats matched well with clinical data from patients with PTSD. In a follow-up study, Liberzon et al. (1999) noted a significant down-regulation of MR and GR mRNAs in all hippocampal subfields 1 day after SPS. In contrast, at 7 and 14 days post-SPS, levels of hippocampal GR mRNA exceeded control levels whereas MR levels remained down-regulated. This alteration in the ratio of MR:GR may explain in part the enhanced fast feedback regulation of the HPA axis observed 7 days after exposure to SPS.

These initial findings on enhanced fast-feedback regulation of the HPA axis were extended by Kohda et al. (2007) using a different experimental approach. One week after SPS, rats received an injection of dexamethasone (DEX, 0.05 mg/ kg, s.c.) or vehicle 2 hours prior to a 30-minute restraint stress session. Groups of unstressed controls also received DEX or vehicle injections and were exposed to restraint stress. Plasma CORT was elevated significantly immediately following SPS, and remained significantly higher than controls 1 day later, but only modestly. The results revealed that DEX-induced suppression of plasma CORT following restraint stress was potentiated in SPS rats, consistent with enhanced fast-feedback regulation of the HPA axis. Importantly, the effects of DEX were not observed 1 day after SPS, indicating that this alteration required the 1-week period of sensitization to develop (Kohda et al., 2007).

Behavioral changes associated with SPS. Fear-learning and fear-conditioning responses appear to play crucial roles in symptoms of PTSD. The SPS model affords an opportunity to examine trauma-related memory storage and retrieval processes and to probe their underlying neural mechanisms. In a series of experiments, Knox et al. (2012) focused on extinction of fear-related memories 1 week following exposure to SPS. Control and SPS male rats were placed individually into test chambers, and after 3.5 minutes, received 5 unsignaled footshocks, spaced 1 minute apart. Measures of time spent freezing did not differ between rats of the two groups, indicating similar patterns of acquisition of fear conditioning. The next day, rats were returned to the same test chambers for 8 minutes, but no shocks were delivered. The percentage of time spent freezing did not differ between rats of the two groups, indicating similar rates of extinction of fear conditioning. In contrast, SPS rats spent a greater percentage of time freezing than unstressed controls when re-exposed to the test chamber 2 days after footshocks were delivered. These findings suggest a disruption in retention of extinction conditioning for memories of a contextual fear paradigm. Similar differences between SPS and control groups were obtained in a separate experiment employing a cued fear paradigm. Differences between SPS and control rats were not apparent if tested only 1 day after the SPS protocol, indicating again the necessary contribution of the period of sensitization (Knox et al., 2012).

These findings were extended by Keller et al. (2015) to include evaluations of female and male rats. Consistent with their previous findings, male rats exposed to SPS exhibited cued fear extinction retention deficits. In contrast, exposure to SPS did not affect cued fear extinction retention in female rats. The authors suggested that female rats were more resistant to the traumatic effects of SPS compared to males, a conclusion consistent with earlier findings reported by Cohen and Yehuda (2011).

Using a mouse model of SPS, Aikins et al. (2017) demonstrated that a subset of stressed C57BL/6 mice displayed impaired fear discrimination in a cued-conditioning task, suggesting that this responsive group generalized conditioned fear to non-threatening stimuli more readily than less responsive mice or unstressed controls. This was a preliminary study, and further research is needed to confirm the generalizability of these findings. I should note that this is one of the rare studies to focus on individual differences in response to SPS.

In another study that took this approach, Le Dorze and Gisquet-Verrier (2016) exposed laboratory rats to SPS in the presence of a cue (tone or odor), while controls were unstressed. Using a battery of behavioral tests, PSS-exposed rats were classified as resistant or vulnerable to a trauma-related stressor. Vulnerable rats (approximately 30% of those tested) displayed increased anxiety-like behaviors, anhedonia, and avoidance of trauma-related cues. Some of these differences between controls and resilient rats versus vulnerable rats were evident up to 60 days after SPS.

PTSD patients exhibit hyper-vigilance and enhanced startle responses, and these symptoms can be studied using animal models. For example, Khan and Liberzon (2004) reported that SPS-exposed rats exhibited an enhanced mean startle amplitude in the ASR at a sound intensity level of 108 dB when testing occurred 7 days but not 1 day after the SPS stress protocol. The enhanced acoustic startle was also evident when animals were tested in a chamber that was illuminated or darkened.

Imanaka et al. (2006) compared SPS and control rats on measures of anxiety-like behavior in the EPM and analgesia in the flinch-jump and hot plate tests. Compared to unstressed controls, SPS rats spent significantly less time on the open arms and had fewer open-arm entries when tested on an EPM. In addition, SPS rats displayed significant levels of analgesia in both tests of pain thresholds. However, SPS and control rats did not differ in their behaviors during an open field test.

Sleep disturbances, including nightmares, are also core symptoms of PTSD. Few experiments have carefully examined if sleep disturbances are characteristic of trauma-exposed rats. In a comprehensive study of sleep disturbances following traumatic stress, Nedelcovych et al. (2015) surgically implanted laboratory rats with a telemetry transmitter that permitted remote recording of the electroencephalogram (EEG) prior to and following exposure to SPS. SPS resulted in significant disruption and fragmentation of REM and non-REM sleep that persisted through 2 days post-SPS. Analyses of EEG power spectra revealed PSS-induced alterations in cortical activation that persisted for several days. These findings were consistent with clinical studies of sleep disturbances in trauma patients, and provided further support for PSS as a valuable animal model of PTSD.

In a more recent study, Zhang et al. (2012) explored levels of pain sensitivity before and at timed intervals after SPS in laboratory rats. Their findings are at odds with those of Imanka et al. (2006), as they reported increased pain sensitivity in SPS rats from 7 to 28 days following the SPS protocol using thermal and mechanical stimuli. These differences in findings parallel published reports regarding pain levels in PTSD patients, with some reports suggesting decreased pain sensitivity and others enhanced levels of chronic pain following trauma exposure (Asmundson et al., 2002; Kraus et al., 2009).

Other relevant changes in behavior following SPS include decreases in social and novel object recognition (Eagle et al., 2013). In addition, Enman et al. (2015) tested SPS and control rats for sucrose intake in a two-bottle choice test with three concentrations of sucrose. SPS rats consumed significantly less sucrose, especially at the two lower concentrations, than did control rats. In addition, SPS rats displayed reduced cocaine-conditioned place preferences compared to unstressed controls. Both of these findings were consistent with greater levels of anhedonia-like behaviors in this animal model of PTSD.

Priming effects of neonatal stress and SPS. In one of the few studies that has manipulated the stress history of animals prior to exposure to the SPS protocol, Imanaka et al. (2006) employed maternal separation (MS, 1 hour per day during PNDs 2–9) as an early life stressor that also impacts the HPA axis of animals in adulthood (Meaney & Szyf, 2005ab). MS and control pups were then weaned on PND 22 and exposed to SPS or a no stress condition on PND 56. MS-exposed animals were more sensitive to the effects of SPS, with greater levels of anxiety-like behaviors in the EPM, greater levels of freezing in a contextual fear conditioning task, and further increases in the flinch-jump test of pain thresholds. MS alone did not affect any of these measures. These findings point to a potentiative interaction between early life trauma and susceptibility to PTSD in adulthood, and are consistent with findings in patients with PTSD (Yehuda et al., 2015).

Neural and molecular aspects of SPS. Several brain circuits, neurotransmitter systems, and signaling pathways have been linked to the delayed onset of the PTSD-like phenotype in rats exposed to SPS. Most studies of SPS have focused on the hippocampus, PFC, and amygdala as the brain areas most strongly associated with the behavioral changes that have been observed, including the establishment of fear-related memories. Of these, the hippocampus has taken center stage because of the disruptions in expression of MRs and GRs that were reported in the early studies of fast-feedback regulation of the HPA axis following exposure of rats to SPS. In addition, the hippocampus has been a focus of clinical research with PTSD patients, and it plays a critical role in memory for traumatic events in animals and in humans (Pitman et al., 2012; Van der Kolk, 1998).

Hippocampal synaptic plasticity. Kohda et al. (2007) examined the effects of traumatic stress on hippocampal synaptic plasticity as represented by measures of long-term potentiation (LTP) and long-term depression (LTD) in brain slices obtained from rats 7 days after exposure to SPS. LTP was significantly impaired 7 days after SPS; in contrast, LTD was reduced significantly immediately after SPS, recovered to control levels 1 day later, and then was significantly reduced at 7 days after SPS. Given this pattern of responses 1 week following SPS, the dynamic range of synaptic plasticity was severely decreased due to impairments in both LTP and LTD.

Glycine. Yamamoto et al. (2010) examined the relationship between glycinergic signaling in the hippocampus and impairments in fear extinction characteristics of SPS rats. They first confirmed that SPS-exposed rats spent significantly more time freezing during fear-extinction testing. Glycine transporter-1 (GlyT-1) mRNA levels in the hippocampus were similar between SPS and control rats under basal conditions and following fear conditioning, but were elevated significantly in SPS rats prior to and after the first context exposure session. Extracellular levels of glycine increased significantly in SPS rats but not in control rats at the time of footshock delivery during fear conditioning. At the time of the first context exposure session, extracellular levels of glycine in the hippocampus of SPS rats were reduced significantly prior to and for 2 hours after context exposure relative to controls. Levels of GlyT-1 mRNA in the SPS extinction group were decreased significantly compared with levels in the non-extinction SPS group, and GlyT-1 mRNA levels correlated with the freezing response. These results pointed to a relationship between impaired fear extinction in SPS rats and reductions in hippocampal glycinergic signaling (Yamamoto et al., 2010).

Glutamate. Levels of glutamate and glutamine were reduced significantly in the PFC but not the amygdala or hippocampus of rats 10 days after exposure to SPS. These changes may have been indicative of decreased excitatory neurotransmission in the PFC, but it was difficult to say for sure from these limited data (Knox et al., 2010).

Serotonin. In a study by Harada et al. (2008), laboratory rats served as controls or were exposed to SPS. Seven days later, animals were sacrificed and samples of the amygdala, hippocampus, and anterior cingulate cortex were removed and frozen for later analysis. RNA from brain samples was prepared for microarray analysis, and 1 gene that was significantly upregulated (2-fold) in the amygdala relative to controls was selected for further study. The over-expression of the gene for the 5-hydroxtryptamine$_{2C}$ (5-HT$_{2C}$) receptor in the amygdala was confirmed by qPCR. To examine the role of the 5-HT$_{2C}$ receptor in enhanced fear conditioning following SPS, animals received injections of vehicle or a 5-HT$_{2C}$ antagonist (FR260010) 30 minutes before fear-conditioning testing. Rats exposed to SPS exhibited enhanced freezing during fear conditioning compared to unstressed control rats. SPS-exposed rats that received injections of 1.0 or 10.0 mg/kg of FR260010 exhibited significant reductions in freezing relative to vehicle-injected SPS-exposed rats.

BDNF. BDNF and its receptor, TrkB, play a key role in the behavioral and neurobiological responses to PSS, as described earlier. One can also make a case that BDNF and TrkB are involved in the pathophysiology of SPS, especially the processes involved in the consolidation of fear memories (Lubin et al., 2008; Rosas-Vidal et al., 2014; Zovkic & Sweatt, 2013). Takei et al. (2011) quantified total and exon-specific mRNA and protein levels for BDNF and its receptor in the hippocampus following contextual fear conditioning in unstressed control rats and rats subjected to SPS. The extent of histone acetylation at the promoter of each exon of the BDNF gene as measured by chromatin immunoprecipitation was also examined in control and SPS rats.

Compared to unstressed control rats exposed to fear conditioning, SPS rats exhibited increased total BDNF mRNA (including exons I and IV) and BDNF protein levels in the hippocampus, with increased acetylation of histones H3 and H4 at the promoter of exons I and IV. In addition, TrkB protein levels in the hippocampus of SPS rats were significantly higher than those in unstressed control rats. These findings suggested that enhanced levels of BDNF and TrkB, combined with epigenetic regulation of the BDNF gene during fear memory consolidation, are critically involved in the PTSD-like effects of SPS (Takei et al., 2011).

Apoptosis. One consistent alteration that has been observed in hippocampus, PFC, and amygdala 7 days after exposure of rats to SPS is enhanced levels of apoptosis (Li et al., 2010; Li et al., 2013; Liu et al., 2010). These experiments have related changes in programmed cell death in these brain areas to the behavioral changes observed in SPS rats and to the corresponding changes in volumes of these brain areas in patients with PTSD (Karl et al., 2006).

Ghrelin impacts amygdala fear circuits. This section involves a slight detour, but I think it is an important one. Meyer et al. (2014) exposed laboratory rats to chronic daily bouts of immobilization stress (4 hours per day) for 14 consecutive days and observed enhanced fear learning following auditory Pavlovian fear conditioning relative to handled controls. This animal model differs from SPS and PSS, but the findings may be relevant to these animal models and to patients with PTSD. Circulating levels of acyl-ghrelin (AG) increased significantly over the course of repeated immobilization stress, as was noted in Chapter 4. AG appears to play a critical role in the enhanced fear learning of chronically stressed rats through an action in the amygdala involving growth hormone, and several lines of evidence support this conclusion. Chronically stressed rats also displayed a significant decrease in receptors for AG in the amygdala. Repeated peripheral administration of a ghrelin agonist enhanced fear memory, as did direct intra-amygdala infusions. In addition, peripheral administration of a ghrelin receptor antagonist blocked the effects of chronic intermittent immobilization stress on fear memory. Within the amygdala, the effects of AG appeared to require growth hormone signaling in that a growth hormone antagonist blocked the effects of ghrelin receptor stimulation on enhanced fear memory. This novel pathway from gut to amygdala involving AG and growth hormone opens up several new targets for the treatment of PTSD (Harmatz et al., 2017; Meyer et al., 2014).

Preventing the effects of SPS. Several interventions have been employed to block the behavioral and neurobiological effects of SPS. A sampling of these experimental approaches is presented in the following.

NMDA receptors. The drug D-cycloserine (D-4-amino-3-isoxazolidone; DCS), a partial agonist at the glycine recognition site of the glutamatergic N-methyl-D-aspartate (NMDA) receptor, has received considerable attention because of its cognitive-enhancing properties. In particular, evidence suggests that DCS facilitates extinction of fear learning and enhances cognitive flexibility (the ability to update and modify previously learned behaviors). To test these assertions, George et al. (2018) trained male rats to press levers for food rewards in operant chambers, and then matched the animals based upon their performances over a 10-day period and assigned them to control or SPS groups. Seven days after SPS or control treatments, rats were retrained on lever pressing and had a session for determination of left or right side bias. The next day, rats were trained to press the lever opposite their preferred side, and one day later they were trained and tested in a reversal task to again press the lever on the preferred side. DCS (15 mg/kg, i.p.) or saline was administered 30 minutes prior to the tests of reversal learning. The results indicated that administration of DCS significantly improved performance in the reversal task for SPS rats but did not affect reversal learning in unstressed controls. These results suggested that DCS enhanced cognitive flexibility in trauma-exposed rats, perhaps by boosting NMDA-mediated excitatory neurotransmission.

GR antagonist. To extend their previous findings described earlier, Kohda et al. (2007) examined the effects of a GR antagonist, RU40555 (3.2, 10, or 32 mg/kg, s.c.), administered 5 minutes prior to SPS, on contextual fear conditioning and in vitro hippocampal synaptic plasticity measured 7 days post-SPS. Their results revealed that the higher doses of RU40555 blocked the enhancement of contextual fear conditioning and 10 mg/kg RU40555 prevented the impairment of long-term potentiation (LTP) in the CA1 region of hippocampus. These findings pointed to a critical role for GR activation following traumatic stress in producing the behavioral and neurophysiological alterations observed in SPS-exposed rats.

SSRIs. The only drugs approved by the US Food and Drug Administration for treatment of symptoms of PTSD are the SSRIs sertraline (Zoloft) and paroxetine (Paxil). It is also the case that these drugs have limited effectiveness. Several experiments with laboratory rats exposed to SPS have been conducted to gain a better understanding of the effects of SSRIs on PTSD-like pathophysiology. In one such experiment (Lin et al., 2016), laboratory rats were exposed to SPS; beginning on the next day, they were given a 14-day treatment regimen with escitalopram (5 mg/kg/day, i.p.) or saline vehicle.

Chronic treatment with escitalopram did not affect body weight gain or general locomotor activity. One and 2 weeks after SPS, rats displayed a significant decrease in sucrose preference in a two-bottle choice test as a measure of anhedonia. Administration of escitalopram completely reversed the pattern of sucrose intake to control levels at the 14-day time point. In a second behavioral test, rats were placed on an elevated T-maze to assess levels of anxiety-like behaviors. SPS-induced increases in anxiety-like behaviors were completely reversed by treatment for 14 days with escitalopram. At the end of the experiment, there were significant decreases in absolute levels (mg/g) of 5-HT in PFC, amygdala, and hippocampus of saline-treated SPS rats, and these alterations were reversed by escitalopram to levels characteristic of unstressed controls. A third behavioral test measured extinction of Pavlovian fear conditioning in groups of control and SPS-treated rats beginning the day after termination of escitalopram. The results indicated that escitalopram actually impaired SPS rats further in their disrupted pattern of fear extinction relative to unstressed controls. In a final experiment, levels of 5-HT, NE, and DA were measured by placement of a microdialysis probe in the insular cortex. The results indicated that SPS rats had significant decreases in extracellular levels of 5-HT, NE, and DA, and of these decreases, escitalopram selectively reversed 5-HT levels to those of unstressed controls.

This experiment is important in that it measured the effects of an SSRI on a range of behavioral and neurochemical changes following trauma exposure in rats. Escitalopram was highly effective in reversing the effects of traumatic stress on anhedonia and anxiety-like behavior, but it did not have a beneficial effect on impaired levels of conditioned fear extinction. In addition, the drug normalized brain levels of 5-HT in fear circuits (amygdala, hippocampus, and PFC) and release of 5-HT in the insular cortex (Lin et al., 2016).

Intra-nasal infusion of NPY. NPY appears to be associated with behavioral and neural resilience to traumatic stress in laboratory animals and in humans, as noted earlier and in Chapter 15. Thus, NPY or an NPY receptor agonist delivered to the brain might be effective in reducing the symptoms associated with exposure to traumatic stressors. However, there are several hurdles that must be overcome to enhance NPY signaling in brain. Peripherally administered NPY does enter the brain, but only on a very limited basis. However, a greater concern is the undesirable effects of peripherally administered NPY on the cardiovascular system, which can lead to sustained elevations in systolic blood pressure. A breakthrough came when Serova et al. (2013) delivered NPY by intra-nasal infusion (100 µg/10 µl) into each naris of laboratory rats 30 minutes before or soon after exposure to SPS. Controls received intra-nasal infusions of water. Behavioral testing occurred 7 days later. Relative to controls, intra-nasal administration of NPY 30 minutes before SPS resulted in significantly less time spent immobile during a forced swim test, less anxiety-like behaviors in an EPM, and reduced startle amplitude, especially at 14 days after SPS. In addition, NPY-treated animals had lower plasma levels of ACTH and CORT and normalized levels of GR in the hippocampus, and down-regulated NE neurons in the locus coeruleus 7 days after SPS. Similar results were obtained in animals that received NPY intra-nasal infusions after the SPS protocol. This critical series of studies provided a proof of concept for employing intra-nasal NPY as a possible treatment for traumatic stress in humans.

This same group compared intra-nasal administration of NPY (150 µg/rat) with intra-nasal administration of an NPY Y1-preferring agonist, [Leu^{31}Pro^{34}]-NPY (132 µg/rat) delivered soon after SPS (Serova et al., 2017). NPY and the NPY Y1 agonist displayed comparable beneficial effects relative to vehicle-infused controls—reduced immobility in a forced swim test, enhanced sucrose preference, and prevention of the induction of CRF mRNA in the mediobasal hypothalamus. However, the NPY Y1 agonist did not block the SPS-induced up-regulation of GR mRNA levels in the hypothalamus. Based on this pattern of effects, these investigators expressed a preference for NPY over the NPY Y1 agonist in continued development of this potential approach to therapy in humans (Sabban et al., 2016; Serova et al., 2017).

Finally, Serova et al. (2019) reported that the proportion of animals displaying extreme anxiety-like behavior during an EPM test increased from 1 to 2 weeks following the SPS paradigm. The balance between CRF and NPY signaling in the locus coeruleus was also disrupted, with elevations in CRF$_1$ receptor gene expression and decreased gene expression for NPY and Y2 receptors. The effective dose of intranasal NPY for reducing anxiety-like behaviors also increased from 150 µg at 1 week post-SPS to 300 µg at 2 weeks post-SPS.

Physical exercise. Patki et al. (2014) employed scheduled, forced treadmill exercise as an intervention to reduce the deleterious effects of SPS in laboratory rats. Their experiment included four groups of animals: control–no exercise, control-exercise, SPS–no exercise, and SPS-exercise. Forced exercise was conducted over a 2-week period after SPS or sham-SPS, and following that, rats were subjected to a battery of tests. Rats in the SPS-exercise group displayed significantly less anxiety-like behavior in an open field arena, a light-dark box, and during an EPM test. In addition, these rats consumed greater volumes of sucrose in a two-bottle choice test and had improved memory scores compared to SPS–no exercise rats. Plasma CORT levels at the conclusion of the experiment were significantly lower in the SPS-exercise group compared to the SPS–no exercise group. These impressive findings provided strong support for further examination of this non-pharmacological intervention for the treatment of a broad array of symptoms associated with PTSD.

A Comparison of the PSS and SPS Models

Table 14.2 includes five criteria suggested by Yehuda and Antelman (1993) for an effective animal model of PTSD, and was used as a basis for comparing the PSS and SPS animal models of PTSD. Although both models stand up well to these criteria, the PSS model appears to offer somewhat greater strength across the board. For example, PSS requires very little time for exposure to the traumatic event, and the intensity of the trauma can be varied (e.g., Adamec et al., 1998). In contrast, SPS involves a rigid protocol that requires almost 3 hours for the full trauma-related protocol. Both PTSD models effected changes that persisted over time, and in the timescale of rat- or mouse-years, compared favorably to the *DSM-5* temporal requirement for humans. Most animals that were exposed to PSS displayed signs of distress within the first few days after exposure, and by 7 days post-exposure only 25% displayed extreme behavioral responses. In contrast, very few overt signs of distress were obvious in the first few days after animals were exposed to SPS. However, 7 days later, the PTSD-like symptoms were clearly evident. Thus, the two models differed in the way that trauma-related symptoms unfolded, and these differences could be exploited to answer related research questions. Finally, manipulations of experience prior to trauma exposure (PSS or SPS) or manipulations of risk genes for PTSD in animals exposed to trauma have received scant attention. These issues will be discussed in greater deal in the following.

Summary

I have highlighted experimental findings from many different laboratories that have utilized two well-described animal models of PTSD. In spite of the excellent work that has been done, several important issues remain to be addressed in basic studies of PTSD. The discrepancy between sex differences in susceptibility to PTSD in humans (females more susceptible than males) and laboratory animals (males more susceptible than females) cries out for greater attention. Unfortunately, the vast majority of studies to date with most animal models of PTSD have employed males to the exclusion of females.

Table 14.2 A Comparison of the Predator Scent Stress (PSS) and Single Prolonged Stress (SPS) Models Based upon Five Criteria Originally Proposed by Yehuda and Antelman (1993) for Evaluating Animal Models of PTSD

---

1. Even very brief stressors should be capable of inducing biological and behavioral sequelae of PTSD.

   PSS: Minimum exposure to predator scent of only 10 minutes.

   SPS: Sequence of 3 stressors requiring almost 3 hours.

2. The stressor should be capable of producing the PTSD-like sequelae in a dose-dependent manner.

   PSS: Confirmed with comparisons of direct exposure to a cat versus exposure to cat odors.

   SPS: No flexibility in the sequence of 3 stressors or their intensities or durations.

3. The stressor should produce biological alterations that persist over time or become more pronounced with the passage of time.

   PSS: Symptoms persist for up to 3 months.

   SPS: Symptoms become evident over the week following trauma exposure and persist over time.

4. The stressor should induce biobehavioral alterations that have the potential for bi-directional expression.

   PSS: This model satisfies this criterion.

   SPS: This model satisfies this criterion.

5. Inter-individual variability in response to a stressor should be present either as a function of experience (e.g., prior stress history or post-stressor adaptations), genetics, or an interaction of the two.

   PSS: A prominent feature of this model is the inter-individual variability in the behavioral responses to PSS, with some rats highly susceptible to trauma-related alterations and others highly resilient.

   SPS: Only a few studies have attempted to subdivide SPS-exposed animals into susceptible and resilient groups.

The overwhelming majority of studies to date with animal models has involved direct exposure to traumatic stressors (e.g., PSS and SPS). However, PTSD may develop in humans that witness a traumatic event, but are not themselves directly involved. In a variation of the CSDS paradigm, Warren et al. (2013) utilized mice that observed an aggressive encounter between 2 male mice from the safety of an adjacent compartment. The safety compartment was separated by a perforated clear Plexiglas partition such that the observer could see, hear, and smell the combatants but could not be harmed by them. This model, termed *vicarious social defeat stress*, provides a novel approach using animal models to understand more fully the mechanisms related to the development of PTSD in individuals who have observed a traumatic event.

A significant strength of the PSS model as implemented by Cohen's laboratory and described in detail earlier is the use of cutoff behavioral criteria to characterize individual animals based upon their behavioral responses to a trauma-related stressor. In contrast, those laboratories that have employed the SPS model of PTSD have only on rare occasions developed criteria for separating animals into susceptible and resistant groups (see, for example, Toledano & Gisquet-Verrier, 2014). This is a substantial weakness of the SPS model as discussed by Holly and Miczek (2015), and does not match well with epidemiological data on PTSD in humans, where only a percentage of those exposed to a traumatic stressor are actually diagnosed with PTSD at a later time. Future experiments that utilize the SPS model of PTSD should consider developing cutoff behavioral criteria to improve the precision with which investigators are able to characterize the animals for follow-up experiments that seek to understand more fully the pathophysiology of trauma exposure.

A continuing area of concern in the treatment of patients with PTSD is the comorbidity of this disorder with major depressive disorder and substance abuse (Yehuda et al., 2015). In particular, data from the National Comorbidity Survey suggested that approximately 29% of individuals diagnosed with PTSD also developed dependence on a drug of abuse (Kessler et al., 1995). Several research questions arise as to why some but not all individuals with PTSD go on to abuse drugs, and translational research with animal models could provide valuable mechanistic insights (Holly & Miczek, 2015).

Animal models of PTSD are especially well-suited for prospective studies that explore connections between early life exposure to stressors (prenatal or postnatal) and later life susceptibility to PTSD-like symptoms. Unfortunately, few studies of this type have been conducted (see earlier discussion). Such experiments could provide valuable insights into the observed connection between child physical and sexual abuse and increased risk of developing PTSD in adulthood (Widom, 1999). In this instance, animal models provide an opportunity to follow individuals with a history of early life stress and determine the underlying mechanisms responsible for increased vulnerability to trauma-related stressors in adulthood.

As basic research on PTSD has expanded since the late 1980s, little effort has been devoted to conducting experiments on PTSD-like responses to trauma involving manipulations of individual risk genes or of comparing inbred strains of mice with well-characterized differences in biological or behavioral measures of relevance to PTSD. This is in stark contrast to the critical role that genetic variables have played in research with animal models of other psychiatric disorders. Compare, for example, the research summarized in Chapters 8–13 with the research presented in the current chapter. It is certainly true that GWAS have not progressed in building up sample sizes as rapidly for PTSD as for other psychiatric disorders (Nievergelt et al., 2018). However, data from family and twin studies have indicated heritability estimates of 40%–50% for PTSD following trauma exposure (Sartor et al., 2011; Stein et al., 2002). Thus, research with animal models could expand its focus to include a greater emphasis on genetic contributions to PTSD-like changes following exposure to trauma.

A final basic research opportunity relates to experiments on transgenerational effects of trauma exposure. In a path-breaking study of the offspring of Holocaust survivors, Yehuda et al. (2014) examined the contributions of maternal and paternal PTSD on epigenetic modifications of the exon 1_F promoter of the GR gene in peripheral blood mononuclear leukocytes on patterns of HPA feedback regulation in offspring. Methylation of DNA inhibits gene expression, and higher levels of methylation of exon 1_F would reduce levels of transcription of the GR gene, resulting in fewer GR receptors and CORT resistance. Those offspring who had a father but not a mother with PTSD exhibited higher methylation of the exon 1_F promoter. In contrast, methylation of exon 1_F was lower in offspring where both parents had PTSD, and there was a correspondingly greater sensitivity to CORT suppression following administration of a low dose (0.5 mg) of dexamethasone. These investigators hypothesized that offspring with lower methylation of exon 1_F have a phenotype that more closely resembles PTSD, while offspring with higher methylation of exon 1_F have a phenotype that more closely resembles major depressive disorder with a history of childhood abuse.

Given these and other clinical findings relating to transgenerational transmission of risk for PTSD, one can make the case that a translational approach using animal models could provide a solid platform for delving into the mechanisms that underpin the transmission of these epigenetic signatures of trauma exposure that are separate from a pattern whereby parents who experienced trauma then abused their offspring (Yehuda & LeDoux, 2007). Breaking the cycle of transgenerational transmission of PTSD risk is an important element in reducing the incidence of PTSD in the population.

15

Resilience

Difficulties break some men but make others. No axe is sharp
enough to cut the soul of a sinner who keeps on trying, one armed
with the hope that he will rise even in the end.
A letter from Nelson Mandela to Winnie Mandela, written on
Robben Island, February 1, 1975

Nelson Mandela (1918–2013) created a lasting legacy of peace and reconcilia-
tion in his native South Africa that will continue to inspire people the world over
for many years to come. But what source of inner strength did he draw upon to
survive the brutal system of apartheid that led to his incarceration in 1962 for his
leadership of nonviolent protests by the African National Congress against the
racist policies of the South African government? In fact, in the years leading up
to his initial sentence of life imprisonment, Mandela came to believe that the only
hope for change in South Africa was through armed struggle. As late as 1985,
he refused to reject violence for the overthrow of the government. During his
27 years in prison, including 18 years on notorious Robben Island, what allowed
him to believe in the possibility of a peaceful transition from a white-minority
government to a black-majority government? In 1994, South Africa held democratic elections for the first time, and Mandela was elected its first black president, serving until 1999 (Mandela, 1994). How did he transition from political
prisoner to Nobel Peace Prize recipient and president of his country?

For much of this volume, we have focused our attention on the deleterious
effects of life stressors on mental health outcomes. But there is a flip side to this
coin—many individuals, including Nelson Mandela, are able to demonstrate resilience (physical, mental, and spiritual) in the face of exposure to even the most
traumatic and dehumanizing of stressors. In this chapter, we will explore what
is known about resilience to the adverse effects of exposure to stressful environments in humans and how we can probe the underlying mechanisms responsible for resilience by studying animal models. Some of these animal models are
the same ones we covered in chapters dealing with specific mental disorders,
especially on depression (Chapters 12–13) and PTSD (Chapter 14). However,
the focus in this chapter will be on those animals that displayed resilience to the
stressor paradigm, rather than susceptibility.

The definition of resilience has evolved over time; initially, it was considered the process by which an individual achieved a positive mental health outcome after enduring adversities earlier in life. More recently, resilience has been viewed through a multidisciplinary lens as "the capacity of a dynamic system to withstand or recover from significant challenges that threaten its stability, viability, or development" (Sapienza & Masten, 2011). This systems-level approach to resilience goes beyond a developmental perspective to include the capacity of adults to display stable mental health outcomes during and after exposure to traumatic events, or following prolonged periods of stressful life experiences (American Psychological Association, 2010; Kalisch et al., 2015).

Developmental psychologists and pediatricians have been at the forefront of research on resilience for more than 50 years (Cicchetti et al., 1993; Cowen et al., 1990; Garmezy, 1974, 1985; Luthar, 1991; Rutter, 1979, 1981, 2012). Beginning in the 1960s, longitudinal studies of children subjected to highly stressful environments or traumatic experiences early in life revealed that most, but not all, of these at-risk children developed into healthy and high-functioning adults. What became evident early on from these studies was that children who overcame adverse circumstances and exhibited positive outcomes later in life were the rule rather than the exception (Masten, 2001).

A note of caution on high rates of positive outcomes has been issued by Infurna and Luthar (2016), who challenged the assertion regarding high rates of resilience in adults undergoing stressful life experiences by reanalyzing data from studies of trajectories of change in individuals exposed to spousal loss, divorce, and unemployment. They noted that modest modifications in statistical models could lead to significant variability in trajectories of change in adults exposed to significant life events, such that resilience was the least common outcome.

An obvious next step was to ask how these positive outcomes, however frequent, were possible in the face of adverse circumstances. Armed with this information, researchers then developed strategies for promoting resilience through interventions to enhance positive life outcomes in children as well as adults (Sapienza & Masten, 2011).

Neuroscience Discovers Resilience

Looking on the Bright Side

Beginning in the first decade of the twenty-first century, neuroscientists and biological psychiatrists came to realize that basic and clinical studies involving exposure to stressful stimuli, including traumatic stressors, had been almost totally consumed with psychopathological consequences, with little interest displayed in mechanisms of resilience (Charney, 2003, 2004). With this realization came an opportunity to focus attention on resilience as a novel approach for developing new targets for drug development and as a springboard for new strategies for preventing the onset of stress-related mental illnesses. Several excellent reviews have highlighted advances in understanding the neural, neuroendocrine, and molecular genetic components of a resilient phenotype in humans and in laboratory animals (Chen, 2019; Feder et al., 2009; Hunter et al., 2018; Karatsoreos & McEwen, 2013; Murrough & Charney, 2011; Pfau & Russo, 2015; Russo et al., 2012; Southwick & Charney, 2012).

Insights from twins. What explains the variability that is so evident in individuals' responses to stressful life events? Amstadter et al. (2014) tackled this critical question by quantifying the genetic and environmental contributions to resilience in a population-based study of 7,500 twins from the Virginia Twin Registry. Data were generated in two waves, with participation rates in the twin subgroups of 72%–92%. Psychiatric resilience was defined in this study as the difference between twins' internalizing symptoms and their predicted symptoms based upon their cumulative exposure to stressful life events. Statistical modeling was performed using the residual between the actual and predicted internalizing symptom total score. It should be noted that internalizing symptoms (e.g., depressive, anxiety-related, physical symptoms) are frequently reported to be a consequence of exposure to life stressors and formed the basis of a quantitative measure of resilience for this study. Based upon their measure of resilience, Amstadter and coworkers estimated that the heritability of resilience was approximately 31% based upon analyses of both waves of data collected. When error of measurement was incorporated into the model, the heritability for resilience increased to approximately 50%. This left an equal contribution from non-shared environmental effects that were of an enduring nature.

While the study by Amstadter et al. (2014) represents an important step forward, concerns regarding the experimental design have been raised. Wertz and Pariante (2014) noted that experiencing fewer symptoms than expected may still be sufficient to categorize a given individual as in distress. In addition, the magnitude of the difference between observed and expected symptom levels varied greatly across the sample, but all individuals were classified as resilient. Finally, other relevant health data (cardiovascular, immune, or neuroendocrine measures) were not collected from this sample of twins. It is possible that individuals could be classified as resilient in one health domain, but not in others. This is an important issue that should be addressed in future studies.

Unique aspects of resilience. In a comprehensive review regarding the neurobiological underpinnings of resilience in humans and in animal models, Russo et al. (2012) emphasized that resilience includes the presence of key molecular defects in susceptible individuals, as well as the presence of distinct molecular adaptations that are part of the resilient phenotype. More recently, research on resilience has broadened considerably to include studies with animal models that address neural, endocrine, immune, and molecular aspects of resilient phenotypes (Dantzer et al., 2018; Scharf & Schmidt, 2012). In addition, epigenetic mechanisms of resilience have received increased attention (Dudley et al., 2011; Zannas & West, 2014).

Several key issues will be addressed in this chapter, including the following:

- How is resilience assessed in studies with laboratory animals?
- Are there specific neural, endocrine, immune, or molecular systems that contribute to a resilient phenotype?
- Is resilience evident across a range of stressful environments, or is it limited to one or a few of these challenges?
- Do ovarian hormones play a role in the development of a resilient phenotype?
- Is it possible to promote a resilient phenotype by exposure to stressors early in life, or even in adulthood through a process of stress inoculation?

Animal Models of Resilience

Several animal models that have been employed to study the relationship between stress and mental disorders have also been utilized to study resilience to the damaging effects of stressful stimulation (Felger et al., 2015; Liberzon & Knox, 2012; Scharf & Schmidt, 2012). For many of these model systems, a subset of animals exposed to stressful stimulation displayed later evidence of physiological or behavioral disturbances. However, some of the animals came through exposure to stressful stimulation largely unscathed, and were classified as resilient based upon one or several behavioral assessments. Let's consider what has been learned from this approach to determine if any common resilience mechanisms have emerged across model systems, and then consider their applicability to human resilience research.

Resilience to Predator Scent Stress (PSS)

Overview of PSS. The PSS model was initially developed by Cohen and her group to study biological mechanisms of PTSD, as described in the previous chapter. In this section, I will focus on the applicability of the PSS model specifically for the study of resilience (refer to Wu et al., 2013).

The basic methodology of the predator stress model is as follows. Adult male Sprague-Dawley rats were exposed to the scent of a predator (10 minutes on well-soiled cat litter) and then left undisturbed for 7 days. Controls were exposed to unsoiled cat litter for an equal amount of time. Animals were then run through a battery of tests that included an EPM and the acoustic startle response on day 7, and freezing behavior when placed on clean cat litter (the situational reminder) on day 8. Behavioral cutoff scores were employed to assign animals to the following groups: extreme behavioral response (EBR, approximately 25% of those tested); partial behavioral response (PBR, approximately 50% of those tested); or minimal behavioral response (MBR, approximately 25%). Behavioral scores for the MBR group were similar to behavioral scores for 80% of the rats in an unstressed control group (Cohen & Zohar, 2004).

NPY and resilience. A series of three experiments examined the involvement of brain neuropeptide Y (NPY) systems in resilience to the effects of predator stress (Cohen et al., 2012). NPY was of particular interest because it has been shown to dampen the negative effects of stress and has anxiolytic-like effects in brain (Heilig, 2004). In the first experiment, regional brain NPY levels were compared between controls, EBR rats, and MBR rats. NPY levels did not differ between controls and MBR rats in the anterior cortex, posterior cortex, amygdala, and periaqueductal gray (PAG), but were significantly lower in the hippocampus of MBR rats. In addition, NPY levels were significantly higher in the amygdala and PAG of MBR rats compared to EBR rats.

In a second experiment, administration of NPY (5 or 10 μg) bilaterally into the dorsal hippocampus 1 hour following exposure of rats to predator scent stress significantly reduced disruptions in behavior when testing occurred 7 days later. Specifically, rats receiving the higher dose of NPY spent significantly more time in the open arms of an elevated plus-maze (EPM), had reduced startle amplitude scores, and were less likely to engage in freezing behavior during the situational reminder test compared to rats receiving artificial cerebrospinal fluid (a-csf) injections. Administration of exogenous NPY also up-regulated expression of NPY protein and NPY-Y1 receptors as well as expression of BDNF.

In contrast, rats that received micro-injections of an NPY-Y1 receptor antagonist (20μg) bilaterally into the dorsal hippocampus 1 hour following exposure to predator scent displayed extreme disruptions in behavior when tested 7 days later. Blockade of NPY-Y1 receptors resulted in significant decreases in total time spent in the open arms and fewer open-arm and total-arm entries during EPM testing compared to controls that received a-csf injections. In addition, the percentage of drug-treated rats that had EBR scores (approximately 75%) was dramatically higher than control rats that received a-csf injections. These results provided strong evidence that brain NPY systems promote resilience in the PSS model.

The *Arc* of resilience. In a related study, Kozlovsky et al. (2008) examined the expression of activity-regulated cytoskeleton-associated protein (Arc), an immediate early gene, and its relationship to resilience in the PSS model. Those rats whose plasma CORT levels and behavioral patterns during EPM and ASR testing were most disrupted 7 days after exposure to PSS did not display up-regulation of Arc mRNA levels in areas of the hippocampus and frontal cortex. In contrast, rats that had minimal disruptions in behavior 7 days following exposure to PSS had significant increases in levels of mRNA for Arc. The investigators suggested that Arc protein may be related to resilience and/or facilitated recovery from exposure to traumatic stress.

Diet and resilience. Hoffman et al. (2015) examined the effects of dietary supplementation with β-alanine (BA, 100 mg/kg) for 30 days on the behavioral and neuroendocrine responses of laboratory rats exposed to PSS. Behavioral indices of traumatic stress were measured 7 days after exposure to PSS, and expression of BDNF and brain carnosine concentrations were analyzed on day 8.

Rats fed a normal diet that were exposed to PSS displayed significant behavioral disruptions in the EPM and the ASR tests and higher freezing scores in the situational reminder compared to controls. In contrast, BA-supplemented rats exposed to PSS had patterns of behavior that were somewhat similar to controls. BA supplementation alone did not affect behavioral patterns. Brain carnosine concentrations in the hippocampus and other brain areas were significantly greater in animals supplemented with BA compared to those receiving a control diet. BDNF expression in the CA1 and dentate gyrus subregions of the hippocampus was significantly lower in animals exposed to PSS and fed a normal diet compared to animals exposed to PSS and supplemented with BA, or to controls. Dietary supplementation with BA increased brain carnosine concentrations and reduced trauma-like behaviors, and these actions may be mediated in part by maintaining normal levels of BDNF expression in the hippocampus. The mechanism of action of brain carnosine in enhancing resilient behavior may be related to its role as an antioxidant (Kohen et al., 1988).

Resilience circuitry. Mitra and colleagues (2009) took advantage of the fact that not all animals exposed to intense stressors displayed long-lasting changes in behavior. They focused their efforts on the basolateral amygdala because of its role in affecting fear responses and modulating stress responses. Adult male Long-Evans hooded rats were used in this experiment. EPM and hole board tests were used to assess the behavioral impact of a single 10-minute exposure of rats to a cat. Behavioral tests occurred 2 weeks after exposure to the cat. Cutoff scores were used to select from a total of 71 rats tested a sample of 4 rats that were severely affected by predator exposure, 4 rats that were not significantly affected, and 4 handled controls.

Brief exposure to a cat induced long-lasting increases in anxiety in some rats, although not all animals show increased anxiety. A subset that was defined as well-adapted remained largely unaffected behaviorally by exposure to the cat. Thus, the same stress experience evoked different degrees of behavioral responses among the initial group of rats that was tested. Animals that differed in their behavioral patterns also differed in dendritic architecture of basolateral amygdala (BLA) neurons, which form part of the neural circuitry mediating stress-induced anxiety (Adamec et al., 2005). Well-adapted animals exhibited retracted dendrites and increased packing density of dendrites compared to maladapted animals with high anxiety and, surprisingly, compared to unstressed handled controls. These findings point to a putative neurobiological substrate for resilience to the anxiogenic effects of traumatic stress.

Interestingly, the resilient rats did not differ from their less resilient counterparts in their interactions with the cat. Rather, their differences were limited to the fact that the resilient rats did not generalize the fear they experienced during exposure to the cat. Two possibilities were presented to explain these findings: (1) well-adapted animals underwent dendritic retraction to counteract the effects of predator exposure, or (2) preexisting differences in dendritic morphology in BLA neurons explained the striking behavioral differences between well-adapted and maladapted animals.

Resilience to Chronic Social Defeat Stress (CSDS)

That wasn't so bad. CSDS has been employed extensively as an animal model of major depressive disorder in humans (refer to Chapters 12 and 13). Similar to studies of predator stress described earlier, there was a range of behavioral responses across animals exposed to CSDS, and this heterogeneity of responses presented an opportunity to explore mechanisms of resilience to the deleterious effects of CSDS. As with the PSS model, employing cutoff behavioral scores provided investigators with the possibility of studying susceptibility and resilience using the same stress paradigm. The following studies clearly indicate that resilience is not simply the absence of susceptibility. Rather, resilience and susceptibility to CSDS are separate and distinct categories, each with its own set of neurobiological underpinnings (e.g., Russo et al., 2012).

In a comprehensive series of experiments from the laboratory of Dr. Eric J. Nestler, C57BL/6J inbred male mice were exposed to 10 consecutive days of CSDS. Test mice were placed individually into the home cages of resident aggressive CD-1 male mice for 5 minutes, after which the resident-intruder pairs were separated by a perforated Plexiglas barrier placed in the middle of the cages for 24 hours. Each day, the C57BL/6J test mice were exposed to different CD-1 resident males. C57BL/6J control mice were housed in pairs with a perforated Plexiglas barrier present and were handled each day.

Control and defeated mice were then tested for social avoidance on day 11, and were scored based upon their tendencies to avoid (susceptible) or approach (resilient) a conspecific. Even though C57BL/6J mice are inbred and therefore genetically identical for all practical purposes, approximately 30%–50% of the males tested did not display avoidance of a social target following CSDS, while the remainder did (Figure 15.1). Social avoidance scores also correlated with other depression-like behavioral measures, including anhedonia, weight loss, and circadian amplitude in body temperature. However, resilient and susceptible mice displayed comparable elevations in plasma levels of CORT following swim stress and similar levels of stress-induced polydipsia and anxiety-like behaviors in the EPM, which are responses consistent with prior exposure of mice to chronic stress (Krishnan et al., 2007).

Reward circuits and resilience. The heterogeneity of responses to CSDS presents an opportunity to investigate neurobiological mechanisms of resilience to depression-like behaviors. Focusing on the subpopulation of mice that had low levels of social avoidance behavior, Krishnan et al. (2007) reported that resilient mice did not have an increase in levels of BDNF in the nucleus accumbens (NAc) following 10 days of CSDS. In addition, resilient mice displayed evidence of regulatory changes in a large number of genes in the ventral tegmental area (VTA) and the NAc compared to susceptible mice.

K+ to the rescue. In the VTA, three genes that were up-regulated in resilient mice but not in susceptible mice coded for voltage-gated potassium (K+) channels (*Kcnf1, Kcnh3,* and *Kcnq3*). These changes in voltage-gated K+ channels in resilient mice prevented the significant increases in firing rates of VTA DA neurons that were characteristic of susceptible mice following social defeat.

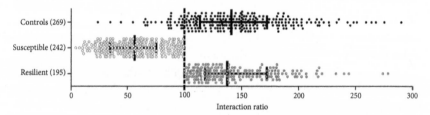

Figure 15.1. Social interaction ratios over multiple experiments of C57BL/6 male mice characterized as susceptible or resistant to the effects of CSDS. The social interaction ratio was calculated as the interaction time with conspecific present/ interaction time with conspecific absent x 100. Unstressed controls are included as a basis for comparison. Error bars represent the means ± interquartile ranges.

Adapted from Krishnan et al. (2007) and used with permission of the publisher.

Results from related experiments indicated that blunting of increases in firing rates of VTA DA neurons following CSDS also blocked release of BDNF within the NAc, resulting in a resilient phenotype (Krishnan et al., 2007) (refer to Figure 15.2).

Capitalizing on these findings, Friedman et al. (2014) targeted VTA DA neurons in susceptible mice in a novel approach for inducing resilience. Enhancing the excitatory hyperpolarization-activated cation channel current (I_h) in VTA DA neurons of susceptible mice pharmacologically or optogenetically to levels seen in resilient mice reversed the depressive-like behaviors (e.g., reduced social contact) characteristic of a susceptible phenotype. This finding may lead to novel treatment strategies for major depressive disorder based upon enhancing resilience pathways in the brain rather than repairing susceptibility pathways (Han & Nestler, 2017).

Out of the blue. Zhang et al. (2019) explored the role of locus coeruleus (LC) inputs to VTA DA neurons in development of the resilient phenotype following exposure to CSDS. They found that the firing rates of LC neurons that

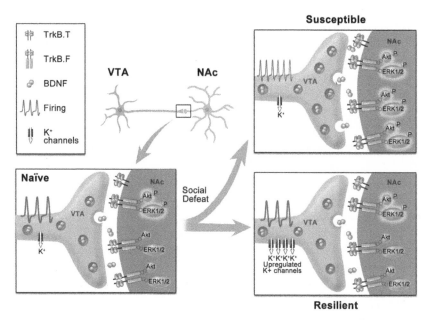

Figure 15.2. In susceptible mice, CSDS increases the firing rate of VTA DA neurons, which subsequently gives rise to heightened BDNF signaling within the nucleus accumbens (NAc). Resilient mice display a resistance to this adverse cascade of events by up-regulating various K$^+$ channels in presynaptic VTA neurons (see also Plate 8).

Adapted from Krishnan et al. (2007) and used with permission of the publisher.

projected to the VTA increased in resilient compared to susceptible mice. Using an optogenetic approach in susceptible mice, these investigators demonstrated that increasing the activity of LC neurons that projected to the VTA resulted in a resilient behavioral phenotype as well as decreased firing rates of VTA → NAc DA neurons. Finally, if α_1- and β_3-adrenergic receptors on VTA → NAc DA neurons were activated pharmacologically, this also resulted in resilient features at the level of ion channels, neuronal activity, and behavioral characteristics. If both of these receptors were selectively blocked within the VTA over a 10-day period, the effects of optogenetically driven increases in LC → VTA neurons did not result in a resilient phenotype. These exciting findings point to an LC → VTA → NAc circuit that is responsible for the emergence of a resilient phenotype following CSDS. The α_1- and β_3-adrenergic receptors that were identified as a crucial link in this pro-resilience pathway provide new therapeutic targets to enhance resilience (Zhang et al., 2019).

Delta force. Using a similar approach, Vialou et al. (2010b) measured ΔFosB in the NAc following CSDS. ΔFosB is a stable transcription factor that was induced following exposure of animals to chronic stress (Perriotti et al., 2004). Resilient mice showed the greatest induction of ΔFosB in both the core and shell subregions of the NAc compared to susceptible mice and controls. In addition, there was a significant positive correlation between amounts of ΔFosB in the NAc and social interaction scores, suggesting that the degree of ΔFosB induction in the NAc may be a critical determinant of whether a mouse displays a susceptible or a resilient pattern of behavior. In a related series of experiments, these investigators reported that induction of ΔFosB following CSDS was dependent upon expression of serum response factor, an up-stream transcriptional activator of several immediate early genes, including *c-fos* (Vialou et al., 2010a).

Using bi-transgenic mice that inducibly over-expressed ΔFosB in the adult NAc and dorsal striatum, these investigators found that these bi-transgenic mice showed significantly less social avoidance after 4 or 10 days of CSDS, suggesting that ΔFosB served a protective role against the effects of CSDS. In contrast, bi-transgenic mice that inducibly over-expressed ΔcJun, a transcriptionally inactive truncated cJun mutant that antagonizes ΔFosB activity, were more susceptible to CSDS than control littermates, and showed maximal social avoidance behavior after only 4 days of CSDS.

ΔFosB is known to regulate the transcription of many genes in the NAc. One such target gene is the AMPA glutamate receptor subunit, GluR2; mice overexpressing ΔFosB in the NAc had greater amounts of GluR2, but showed no differences in other glutamate receptor subunits. This selective up-regulation of GluR2 in the NAc appeared to play a critical role in resilience to CSDS. The induction of GluR2 seen in resilient mice appeared to reflect a direct effect of

ΔFosB on the gene encoding GluR2, as there was increased binding of ΔFosB to the GluR2 promoter.

To identify additional ΔFosB target genes that may contribute to resilience, gene expression array data sets were obtained from the NAc of both bi-transgenic mice overexpressing ΔFosB as well as C57Bl/6J mice 48 hours after CSDS that had a resilient phenotype. There was considerable (>75%) overlap between the genes induced in the NAc by ΔFosB and those induced by CSDS in resilient mice. From the population of induced genes, *Sc1* (also known as Sparc-like 1 or hevin) was selected for further study based upon the magnitude of its induction in re-silient mice and in mice over-expressing ΔFosB. SC1 is an anti-adhesive matrix molecule that is highly expressed in the adult brain, where it localizes in the postsynaptic density and has been implicated in synaptic plasticity. To assess a possible role for *Sc1* in resilience, it was reported that over-expression of *Sc1* in the NAc of susceptible mice reversed the high social avoidance scores induced by CSDS.

It's all about networking. Lorsch et al. (2019) identified a gene network that plays a unique role in the expression of a resilient phenotype following exposure to CSDS. Critical to this gene network effect on resilience is *Zfp189*, which codes for a zinc finger protein. Overexpression of *Zfp189* in PFC neurons activated this network of 281 genes and enhanced resilience. In addition, induction of *Zfp189* enhanced resilience whereas suppressing *Zfp189* resulted in susceptibility to the effects of CSDS. These exciting results open up the possibility of targeting *Zfp189* expression as a novel strategy to upregulate a resilience-related gene network as a means of treating major depressive disorder or preventing its development.

DA plays a role. Medium spiny neurons (MSNs) of the NAc play an impor-tant role in resilience to the deleterious effects of CSDS on behavioral responses. MSNs make up the majority of the NAc and come in two types, one expressing D1 receptors and playing a role in reward and the other expressing D2 receptors and playing a role in aversion. Using a variety of optogenetic and pharmacogenetic approaches, Francis et al. (2015) reported that increasing the frequency of excit-atory synaptic inputs in D1-expressing MSNs resulted in resilience to the effects of exposure to CSDS. Modulation of activity in D2-expressing MSNs did not af-fect behavioral outcomes to CSDS.

Taking further advantage of this well-characterized system of D1- and D2-expressing MSNs, Hamilton et al. (2018) examined the effects of cell-type spe-cific targeted epigenetic modifications of the *Fosb* gene on a resilient behavioral phenotype following exposure of mice to a sub-threshold level of CSDS in mice. Their results indicated that histone acetylation of *Fosb* in D1-expressing MSNs, which promotes transcription, and histone methylation of *Fosb* in D2-expressing MSNs, which inhibits transcription, both resulted in a resilient phe-notype following sub-threshold CSDS. Behavioral measures of resilience in these experiments included measures of social avoidance and sucrose preference. These powerful findings for the first time have revealed the potential for epigenetic editing in specific neuronal cell types to enhance resilience to a depression-like phenotype in a social stress-induced model of depression.

In summary, these results are consistent with a role for ΔFosB in the NAc in promoting resilience during CSDS by inducing a form of synaptic plasticity that counteracts the strong negative associative learning that occurs in susceptible mice during repeated episodes of social defeat. The dominant role of ΔFosB and its targets in promoting adaptive responses to CSDS revealed new molecular targets for the development of antidepressant treatments (Vialou et al., 2010ab). Identification of novel targets related to resilience may be facilitated by a metabolomics approach, as demonstrated in a series of experiments by Dulka et al. (2017).

Inhibition has its place. GABA$_B$ receptors may play a role in stress-related psychiatric disorders such as anxiety and depression (Ghose et al., 2011). O'Leary and colleagues (2014) explored the impact of GABA$_B$ receptor subunits on behavioral responses to CSDS in laboratory mice. Compared to wild-type (WT) mice, mice that lacked the GABA$_{B(1b)}$ subunit were resilient to the effects of CSDS, based upon their behavioral scores in tests of social withdrawal and saccharin preference. In addition, GABA$_{B(1b)}$ knockout mice had increased rates of proliferation and survival of newborn neurons in the ventral hippocampus.

Hidden in the genes. A major challenge in studies of animal models of depression is to focus in on transcriptional networks and key driver genes that regulate resilience to the depressive-like behaviors that attend CSDS. Bagot et al. (2016) took on this significant challenge by examining the NAc and its inputs from the ventral hippocampus, amygdala, and PFC in control mice and mice resilient to the effects of CSDS. Mice were tested at 2 and 28 days after the CSDS paradigm as well as at 28 days post-stress, but with an added 1-hour episode of social defeat (stress-primed).

At the 2-day post-stress time point, there were more differentially expressed genes in resilient mice versus control mice in all four brain areas compared to data for susceptible mice versus control mice. However, at 28 days post-stress, the number of differentially expressed genes remained greater in resilient mice only in the ventral hippocampus and PFC. Further analyses revealed that increased synchrony between differentially regulated genes in the PFC and NAc appeared to be especially critical for the development of the resilient phenotype following CSDS. Further analyses revealed 30 clusters of co-expressed genes in resilient mice that were non-overlapping with 52 clusters of co-expressed genes in susceptible mice. Compared to control mice, resilient mice had only two gene clusters that had a gain in connectivity and three that had a loss of connectivity. A gain in connectivity suggested a strengthening of an existing transcriptional network or the emergence of a novel one. In contrast, a loss of connectivity implied a weakening of a basal transcriptional network.

A critical aspect of this complex study was that it provided an approach to study how groups of genes were organized across brain regions into functional clusters. Changes in activity of these functional clusters appeared to underlie susceptibility or resilience to depressive-like behaviors following exposure to CSDS. By targeting hub genes within these functional clusters, it may be possible to promote resilience on the one hand, or to prevent depressive symptoms on the other hand (Bagot et al., 2016).

MRI studies. Anacker et al. (2016) identified resilient and susceptible mice following 10 days of CSDS and their brains, together with those of unstressed controls, were processed for *ex vivo* structural magnetic resonance imaging and diffusion tensor imaging to reveal any neuroanatomical differences between groups. In addition, correlations were computed for regional brain volumes versus social avoidance scores. The study was correlational and assumptions were made about fractional anisotropy reflecting the extent of dendritic branching.

Social avoidance scores correlated negatively with the local volume of the cingulate cortex, NAc, thalamus, raphe nuclei, and BNST. Social avoidance scores correlated positively with local volume of the VTA, habenula, PAG, cerebellum, hypothalamus, and hippocampal CA3 area. Fractional anisotrophy was increased in the hypothalamus and hippocampal CA3 area. Synchronized anatomical differences between the VTA and the cingulate cortex, hippocampus and VTA, hippocampus and cingulate cortex, and hippocampus and hypothalamus were observed. For resilient mice, a larger cingulate cortex volume predicted a smaller VTA volume.

The approach taken in this study offered several advantages. It revealed novel brain areas involved in resilience versus susceptibility to CSDS (e.g., thalamus, raphe nuclei, BNST) and it allowed for comparisons with complementary MRI studies in humans. Unfortunately, it was not possible to determine if these structural brain differences between resilient and susceptible mice were preexisting, or if they had changed as a result of the CSDS paradigm. This is an important question that should be addressed in the future. With these data in hand, it would be possible to detect anatomical differences in brain areas that predispose some mice to display a resilient phenotype, and others to display a susceptible phenotype following CSDS (Anacker et al., 2016).

The protein kinase connection. Experiments by Bruchas et al. (2011) focused on the family of mitogen-activated protein kinases (MAPK). p38 MAPK (also referred to as stress-activated protein kinase, SAPK) was known to block stress-induced behavioral responses. The protein kinase is widely distributed in tryptophan hydroxylase-expressing cells of the dorsal raphe nucleus (DRN). The α-isoform of p38 MAPK was selectively inactivated in 5-HT neurons and in astrocytes. A single episode of social defeat stress produced social avoidance in wild-type mice, but not in mice having the selective p38α MAPK deletion in 5-HT neurons of the DRN. Thus, mice with the p38α MAPK deletion in 5-HT neurons were resilient to the effects of acute social defeat stress. Stress-induced activation of p38α MAPK led to translocation of the serotonin transporter to the neuronal membrane, thereby increasing the rate of transmitter uptake at 5-HT nerve terminals. The results of these experiments suggested that CSDS initiated a cascade of molecular and cellular events in which p38α MAPK induced a hypo-serotonergic state underlying stress susceptibility.

Epigenetic changes. Serotonin neurons were also implicated in resilience in a series of experiments by Walsh et al. (2017). These investigators examined the role of PHF8, an X-linked histone demethylase that functions as a transcriptional activator, on depression-like and anxiety-like behaviors in mice. $Phf8^{(-/y)}$ knockout mice (KO) were generated on a mixed C57B6/129SvJae background, and behavioral patterns were assessed using a battery of tests. Compared to wild-type controls, $Phf8^{(-/y)}$ KO mice were more active and spent more time in the center portion of an open field arena and spent more time in the open arms of an EPM. Both of these tests have been used as measures of anxiety-like behaviors, and the results suggest that $Phf8^{(-/y)}$ KO mice are more resilient to anxiety-provoking environments.

$Phf8^{(-/y)}$ KO mice and wild-type controls were also exposed to CSDS each day for 10 consecutive days. Chronically stressed controls displayed high levels of social avoidance behavior following CSDS. In contrast, $Phf8^{(-/y)}$ KO mice spent as much time in social contact as did $Phf8^{(-/y)}$ KO mice and wild-type mice that were not exposed to CSDS. These findings pointed to $Phf8^{(-/y)}$ KO mice being resilient to the depressive effects of CSDS.

What connects downstream effects of *Phf8* with the resilient behavioral phenotype observed in $Phf8^{(-/y)}$ KO mice? Further experiments revealed that WT mice had high levels of expression of PHF8 in PFC, ventral striatum, and hippocampus. The absence of PHF8 in $Phf8^{(-/y)}$ KO mice was linked to increased expression of the serotonin receptors 5-HT$_{1A}$, 5-HT$_{1B}$, and 5-HT$_{2A}$, which in turn appeared to explain the increased resilience of KO mice to stressful stimulation (Walsh et al., 2017).

IL-6 looms large. As described in part in Chapter 13, Hodes et al. (2014) examined the role of the peripheral immune system in susceptibility versus resilience of C57BL/6 male mice to CSDS. They found preexisting individual differences in the sensitivity of the peripheral immune system that predicted later resilience to social stress. Cytokine profiles were quantified 20 minutes after the first exposure to social defeat. Of the cytokines regulated by stress, IL-6 was the best predictor of resilience in that levels remained comparable to handled controls, whereas IL-6 was significantly elevated in susceptible mice. In addition, prior to any physical contact in mice, there were individual differences in IL-6 levels from leukocytes stimulated ex vivo with LPS that predicted susceptibility versus resilience to a subsequent social stressor.

IL-6 knockout (IL-6$^{(-/-)}$) mice were also employed to further link low levels of IL-6 with resilience to CSDS. Bone marrow (BM) chimeras were generated by transplanting hematopoietic progenitor cells from IL-6 knockout (IL-6$^{(-/-)}$) mice. IL-6$^{(-/-)}$ BM chimeric and IL-6$^{(-/-)}$ mice, as well as mice treated with a systemic IL-6 monoclonal antibody, were resilient to CSDS. These data established that a dampened peripheral IL-6 response to CSDS was associated with a resilient behavioral phenotype (Hodes et al., 2014).

Inflammation is a pain. In a further effort to connect inflammatory responses to depressive-like behaviors, Ren et al. (2016) explored the role of soluble epoxide hydrolase (sEH) in the CSDS paradigm. sEH metabolizes epoxyeicosatrienoic acids, which have potent anti-inflammatory effects. These investigators used an inhibitor of sEH, trifluromethoxyphenyl-3(1-propionylpiperidine-4-yl) urea (TPPU), and sEH knockout (KO) mice to modify levels of inflammation following CSDS. Levels of sEH were increased significantly in brains of chronically stressed mice compared to controls. In addition, TPPU (3.0 mg/kg/day orally) given 1 hour prior to each session of CSDS resulted in a significant increase in the social interaction test compared to chronically stressed animals that received vehicle alone. Similarly, TPPU eliminated the anhedonia characteristic of mice exposed to CSDS. Consistent with these findings, sEH KO mice were resilient to the effects of CSDS, with behavioral scores comparable to unstressed control mice. sEH KO mice also had increased levels of BDNF and phosphorylation of its receptor, TrkB, in the frontal cortex and hippocampus. These investigators suggested that increased BDNF-TrkB signaling in these two brain areas may underlie the resilient phenotype of sEH KO mice (Ren et al., 2016).

Levels of sphingosine-1-phosphate receptor 3 (S1PR3) in the mPFC and in peripheral blood are associated with resilience to CSCS in laboratory rats. S1PR3 is a G protein-coupled receptor that binds to its ligand, S1P, and exerts influences on immune responsiveness, angiogenesis, and cell proliferation in the periphery. Much less is known about the role of S1PR3 signalling in the brain. S1PR3 expression in the mPFC was higher in the mPFC of resilient rats compared to susceptible and control rats. Over-expression of S1PR3 in the mPFC resulted in a resilient phenotype but knockdown of S1PR3 resulted in a susceptible phenotype following the CSDS paradigm. Anxiety- and depression-like behaviors associated with a susceptible phenotype were mediated by TNFα levels in the mPFC. Blockade of TNFα signaling in the mPFC prevented the behavioral changes observed in susceptible rats following CSDS (Corbett et al., 2019).

Small RNAs pack a big punch. Resilience to stress was explored in laboratory rats subjected to a CSDS paradigm (Pearson-Leary et al., 2017).

Latencies to display behavioral signs of defeat were employed to generate a resilient group with long latencies (LL) and a stress-susceptible group with short latencies (SL). LL rats were found to have higher levels of miR-455-3p and lower levels of miR-30e-3P in the ventral hippocampus compared to SL rats. Ingenuity Pathway Analysis (IPA) software identified inflammatory and vascular remodeling pathways associated with genes targeted by these two miRNAs. Following CSDS, resilient LL rats did not display the characteristic remodeling of the neurovascular unit within the ventral hippocampus in the way that stress-susceptible rats did. The resilient phenotype was reflected in the ventral hippocampus in a lack of new blood vessel formation, no increase in blood-brain barrier permeability, no increase in concentration of microglia with associated changes in pro-inflammatory cytokines, and no increase in neuronal activity as assessed by levels of FosB/ΔFosB positive cells. Similar changes in resilient and susceptible rats were not observed in the dorsal hippocampus or in the PFC.

To confirm this stress-resilient profile in the ventral hippocampus, these investigators found that daily i.c.v. administration of the proinflammatory cytokine vascular endothelial growth factor (VEGF164) resulted in changes in the ventral hippocampus and behavioral responses to CSDS that were characteristic of the stress-susceptible phenotype. In contrast, administration of the non-steroidal anti-inflammatory drug meloxicam (1 mg/kg, i.p.) enhanced the resilient phenotype in rats exposed to CSDS. Taken together, these findings emphasized the important role played by inflammatory processes within the ventral hippocampus in resilience to CSDS (Pearson-Leary et al., 2017).

Coping and resilience. Two studies utilized a slightly different model of CSDS in which adult male Sprague-Dawley rats were exposed to repeated resident-intruder stress (30 minutes per day for 5 consecutive days), and coping styles were determined. Long-Evans retired breeders were used as resident aggressive males. Passive coping was defined as a short latency (<300 sec) to assume a defensive posture, while active coping was defined as a longer latency to assume a defensive posture (>300 sec).

In the first experiment, Wood et al. (2010) reported that rats exhibiting longer latencies to defeat (i.e., resilient rats) did not develop depressive-like neuroendocrine or behavioral characteristics over the course of CSDS. In these resilient animals, there was habituation of HPA axis responses to CSDS. In addition, behaviors of resilient animals in a forced swim test were similar to behaviors of unstressed controls. An additional correlate of resilience to CSDS in laboratory mice, as reported by Elliott et al. (2010), related to maintenance of DNA methylation of the promoter region of the *Crf* gene.

In the second experiment (Wood et al., 2015), CSDS was reported to differentially regulate 19 genes in the locus coeruleus (LC) and 26 genes in the dorsal raphe nucleus (DR), and many of these genes coded for inflammatory factors. IL-1β expression was increased in passive coping rats and decreased in active coping rats in both the LC and the DR. Protein changes in the two brain areas were generally consistent with a proinflammatory response in passively coping rats, but not in actively coping rats. Rats that displayed passive coping styles during CSDS also exhibited anhedonia based on a sucrose preference test, and this response was blocked by i.c.v. administration of an antagonist of IL-1β. Resilience to CSDS was associated with a down-regulation of central inflammatory processes. Social stress led to up-regulated neuropeptide Y1 receptor (*Npy1r*) gene expression in the LC of active and passive coping style rats. However, only in active coping rats was *Npy2r* and *kappa opioid receptor-1* gene expression down-regulated in the LC. These latter two changes may have conferred resilience to stress in actively coping rats.

Repeated Exposure to Stress

The pioneering studies of Maier and Seligman (2016) have been adopted by many investigators to study the effects of repeated exposure to aversive stimulation on subsequent behavioral and physiological responses. An additional focus of such studies has been the differential impact of uncontrollable versus controllable delivery of aversive stimuli on adaptive behavioral and physiological responses (Lucas et al., 2014).

Taneja et al. (2011) used 100 unpredictable, inescapable tail shocks (1.2–2.0 mA, 5 seconds duration, every 25–110 seconds for 2 hours) to yield learned helpless (LH) and resilient Sprague-Dawley rats. Controls were restrained and had electrodes affixed to their tails, but no shocks were delivered. The following day, rats were tested in a shuttlebox for escape behaviors. Rats that had escape latencies within 2 standard deviations (SDs) of control rats were defined as resilient, whereas rats with escape latencies greater than 2 SDs of control rats were defined as LH. Measures taken in various brain areas were as follows: α_{2A}-adrenoceptors (α_{2A}-AR), CRF$_1$ receptors, G-protein-coupled receptor kinase 3 (GRK3, phosphorylates receptors and contributes to their down-regulation), GRK2, tyrosine hydroxylase (TH), and carbonylated protein levels.

In resilient rats, α_{2A}-AR and CRF$_1$ receptor levels were significantly down-regulated in the LC after inescapable tail shock. GRK3 was reduced in the LC of LH rats but not resilient rats. In contrast, GRK2 levels were unchanged. In the amygdala, GRK3 but not GRK2 levels were reduced in LH rats but not in resilient rats. Protein carbonylation, an index of oxidative stress, was increased in the LC and amygdala of LH rats but not of resilient rats. Resilient rats appeared to differ from LH rats in their greater ability to handle oxidative stress, maintain levels of

GRK3, and regulate receptor signaling more effectively following exposure to inescapable tail shocks (Taneja et al., 2011).

Differences in expression. A genome-wide microarray experiment tracked changes in gene expression in the hippocampus and frontal cortex of male Sprague-Dawley rats that were exposed to acute unavoidable stress (restraint for 50 minutes with 80 tail shocks, 1.5 mA, every 30 seconds) delivered through tail electrodes (Benatti et al., 2012). One day later, both groups of rats were tested for their ability to perform an active avoidance task over 30 trials. Two groups of rats emerged from those exposed to unavoidable stress—one was stress-vulnerable (fewer than 8 successful escapes/30 trials) and the other was stress-resilient (greater than 16 successful escapes/30 trials). These differences in avoidance were associated with specific changes in gene expression, with little overlap between the two groups (approximately 10% of probe sets). In the frontal cortex, there was a down-regulation of the transcripts coding for interferon-b and leukemia inhibitory factor in resilient rats and an up-regulation of the neuroendocrine-related genes coding for growth hormone and prolactin in vulnerable rats. In the hippocampus, the muscarinic M2 receptor was down-regulated in vulnerable rats but up-regulated in resilient rats. These findings demonstrated that vulnerable and resilient rats did not have opposing regulatory changes in the same genes; rather, resilience was associated with specific changes in gene expression, with little overlap, compared to the patterns detected in vulnerable rats (Benatti et al., 2012).

It's what's up front that counts. Wang et al. (2014) utilized the learned helplessness procedure in mice to examine the role of the mPFC, a brain region strongly implicated in both clinical and animal models of depression, in adaptive behavioral responses to stress. They reported that uncontrollable, inescapable stress induced changes in the excitatory synapses onto a subset of mPFC neurons that were activated as indicated by their increased levels of the immediate early gene, c-Fos. Whereas synaptic potentiation was linked to learned helplessness, a depression-like response, synaptic weakening, was associated with resilience to stress. If the activity of mPFC neurons was enhanced, it was sufficient to convert resilient mice into mice expressing the learned helplessness phenotype.

Employing the learned helpless paradigm, Yang et al. (2015) examined the roles of BDNF and dendritic spine density in various brain regions of LH and resilient Sprague-Dawley rats. BDNF levels in the mPFC and hippocampus (CA3 and dentate gyrus [DG]) were significantly lower in the LH group than in the control and resilient groups, whereas BDNF levels in the NAc in the LH group but not the resilient group were significantly higher than those in the control group. Furthermore, spine density in the prelimbic cortex, CA3, and DG was significantly lower in LH rats compared to rats in the control and resilient groups, although spine density in the NAc was significantly higher in the LH group than in the control and resilient groups. These results suggested that differential regulation of BDNF levels and spine densities, especially in the mPFC, CA1, DG, and NAc areas, may have contributed to resilience to inescapable stress.

Autoreceptors go off-line. Serotonin (5-HT) neurons in the DRN have been implicated in learned helplessness behaviors, such as poor escape responding and expression of exaggerated conditioned fear, induced by acute exposure to an uncontrollable stressor. DRN 5-HT neurons were hyperactive during exposure to an uncontrollable stressor, resulting in desensitization of $5\text{-}HT_{1A}$ inhibitory autoreceptors in the DRN. $5\text{-}HT_{1A}$ autoreceptor down-regulation was thought to induce transient sensitization of DRN 5-HT neurons, resulting in excessive 5-HT activity in brain areas that controlled the expression of learned helplessness behaviors. Regular physical activity has antidepressant/anxiolytic properties and may promote resilience to stressors, but the neurochemical mediators of these effects are not well known (Maier & Watkins, 2010).

Breaking a sweat. A study by Greenwood et al. (2003) examined the effects of 6 weeks of voluntary free wheel running on learned helpless behaviors, uncontrollable stress-induced activity of 5-HT neurons in the DRN, and basal expression of DRN $5\text{-}HT_{1A}$ autoreceptor mRNA in F344 rats. Free wheel running prevented the shuttle box escape deficits and the exaggerated conditioned fear that occurred in response to uncontrollable tail shock in sedentary rats. Furthermore, double c-Fos/5-HT immunohistochemistry revealed that running wheel activity attenuated tail shock–induced activity of 5-HT neurons in the DRN. Six weeks of free wheel running also resulted in a basal increase in $5\text{-}HT_{1A}$ inhibitory autoreceptor mRNA levels in the DRN. These results suggested that free wheel running prevented learned helpless behaviors and attenuated 5-HT neural activity in the DRN during uncontrollable stress. An increase in $5\text{-}HT_{1A}$ inhibitory autoreceptor expression may have contributed to the attenuation of DRN 5-HT activity and the prevention of learned helplessness in physically active rats (Greenwood et al., 2003).

Additional experiments, reviewed in Greenwood and Fleshner (2011), pointed to plasticity at multiple sites within the central 5-HT system that joined together to facilitate resilience to stress. These central sites included the DRN, with enhanced $5\text{-}HT_{1A}$ autoreceptor-mediated inhibition of 5-HT neurons; DRN afferent systems, such as the habenula, BNST, locus coeruleus, or mPFC, which can modulate DRN 5-HT activity during exposure to stressors; and DRN projection sites, including the basolateral nucleus of the amygdala and the striatum, with reduced expression or sensitivity of $5\text{-}HT_{2C}$ receptors in these brain regions that are critical for the expression of stress-induced behaviors. An increase in $5\text{-}HT_{1A}$ autoreceptors and a reduction in sensitivity of $5\text{-}HT_{2C}$ receptors were two prime examples of exercise-induced neuroplasticity.

Loughridge et al. (2013) extended these findings by examining changes in gene expression in the DRN following a 6-week period of voluntary wheel running and then exposure to inescapable stress. Rats that previously exercised had a greater number of genes that were differentially expressed immediately and 2 hours following exposure to inescapable stress compared to sedentary, stressed rats. In addition, modules composed of genes that were highly co-expressed were activated in a more highly coordinated manner following exposure to inescapable stress in active versus sedentary rats. There were 169 genes that were differentially regulated at both post-stressor time points in active versus sedentary rats, and these were included in further analyses. Finally, many of the stress-responsive genes in the DRN were found to be involved in immune-related pathways, including cytokine signaling and inflammatory processes. These included *transforming growth factor-β* (*tgfβ1*), the gene that codes for the cytokine TGF-β1, and *Tdo2*, a gene that codes for an enzyme, tryptophan 2,3 dioxygenase, involved in metabolism of tryptophan, the precursor of serotonin. Thus, voluntary exercise promoted the development of a resilient phenotype in rats later exposed to inescapable stress.

A natural high. In a departure from the learned helplessness model of inescapable stress, Bluett et al. (2017) explored the relationship between brain endocannabinoid (eCB) systems and resilience to chronic intermittent footshock stress. The brain eCB system consists of a presynaptic cannabinoid receptor (CB1R) and two endogenous ligands, 2-arachidonoylglycerol (2-AG) and anandamide (arachidonoylethanolamine, AEA). AEA and 2-AG are synthesized postsynaptically, and when released, travel in a retrograde fashion to bind to CB1Rs, resulting in a decrease in neurotransmitter release from the presynaptic nerve terminal; 2-AG is metabolized presynaptically by monoacylglycerol lipase (MAGL), whereas AEA is degraded postsynaptically by fatty acid amide hydrolase (FAAH). Administration of drugs that inhibit MAGL and FAAH leads to increases in 2-AG and AEA signaling, respectively.

Initially, these investigators developed a behavioral task for detection of drug treatment effects on stress resilience in outbred ICR mice. This novelty-induced feeding task involved exposing mice to a highly palatable food (vanilla-flavored Ensure) first in their home cages, and then several days later in a novel test chamber. Increased latency to feed and decreased consumption of the Ensure in the novel test chamber provided indices of anxiety-like behaviors before and after exposure to acute or repeated footshock stress.

Selective inhibition of MAGL but not FAAH resulted in a resilient phenotype as assessed following footshock stress. In addition, administration of an inhibitor of MAGL enhanced resilience in mice previously classified as stress-susceptible. In contrast, depletion of brain 2-AG levels or blockade of eCB-1Rs increased susceptibility to footshock stress in mice previously classified as stress-resilient. Stress resilience was associated with 2-AG-mediated synaptic suppression at ventral hippocampal-amygdaloid glutamatergic synapses. Finally, depletion of 2-AG selectively within the amygdala prevented the development of resilience to footshock stress. Taken together, the results of this series of experiments clearly pointed to 2-AG signaling within the amygdala as a critical component of the development of a resilient phenotype following exposure to repeated footshock stress (Bluett et al., 2017).

Stress-Enhanced Fear Learning (SEFL)

SEFL has been advanced as a valid animal model of PTSD (Maren & Holmes, 2016). This model combines acute exposure of laboratory animals to a stressor, followed by cued fear conditioning and then tests of extinction. Sillivan et al. (2017) described their exciting results of experiments with the SEFL model in which they employed inbred male and female C57BL/6 mice. Mice exposed to 2 hours of restraint stress 7 days prior to fear conditioning displayed elevated levels of freezing behavior during extinction testing, and this effect was consistently observed in females but was more variable in males. A subgroup of males was identified based upon extinction testing that appeared resilient to the effects of the SEFL paradigm. In contrast to stress-susceptible male mice, stress-resilient male mice did not display elevations in the acoustic startle response (ASR) or in plasma levels of CORT at 30 days post-testing.

To characterize further neuromolecular differences between stress-susceptible and stress-resilient male mice, animals were exposed to restraint stress for 2 hours, followed 7 days later by cued fear conditioning. Thirty days after fear conditioning, mice were exposed to a 5-tone remote memory test, and brains were processed for Fos immunohistochemistry and RNA sequence analysis. Fos was increased in the posterior infralimbic cortex of stress-resilient mice compared to stress-susceptible mice, while the opposite pattern was observed in the basolateral amygdala. These two brain areas are critically involved in the extinction of fear-related memories. The results of RNA sequence analyses in the basolateral amygdala revealed 61 differentially expressed genes between stress-susceptible and stress-resilient mice. Of this total, 9 were decreased and 52 were increased in stress-resilient male mice, including several that have previously been associated with PTSD. The SEFL paradigm and the results from these experiments with C57BL/6 male mice provide another avenue to approach the neural and molecular underpinnings of resilience to traumatic stressors (Sillivan et al., 2017).

Chronic Mild Stress (CMS)

The CMS paradigm varies slightly from laboratory to laboratory, but basic elements are shared in common. It involves exposure of laboratory mice or rats to various mildly stressful environments for extended periods of time across multiple days. Stressors include intermittent illumination, exposure to strobe lights, housing with a strange conspecific, food or water deprivation, exposure to soiled bedding, and so on.

Varying sensitivities. Delgado y Palacios et al. (2011) used a CMS paradigm with laboratory rats, and then characterized the animals as resilient or susceptible based upon their behavior in a two-bottle choice test (water versus 1.5% sucrose). Noninvasive magnetic resonance imaging and spectroscopy were employed to study structural changes in the hippocampus. The results revealed that CMS did not reduce hippocampal volume or alter glutamate metabolism in resilient mice, but did so in susceptible mice.

Bergström et al. (2007) used the CMS paradigm over a 5-week period with adult male Wistar rats. Stress-sensitive and stress-resilient rats were characterized based upon their preference for sucrose in a two-bottle choice test. Approximately 67% of animals displayed a decrease in sucrose preference, while 33% of animals had sucrose preference scores that were comparable to unstressed controls.

Resilient genes. These investigators sought to identify hippocampal gene expression pathways that were associated with resilience to CMS. Based upon microarray data, they found 155 genes that were more than 2-fold differentially regulated between stress-sensitive and stress-resilient rats. In addition, approximately 44 genes were more than 2-fold differentially regulated between unstressed controls and stress-resilient rats. From these totals, 78 of the 155 genes were deemed eligible for generating 6 networks, while 30 of the 44 genes were deemed eligible for generating 3 networks, both by using Ingenuity software. Several cellular functions were revealed by these network analyses, including signal transduction, molecular transport, growth and cellular proliferation, apoptosis, and multiple links to immune functions. The authors emphasized that the stress-resilient phenotype was associated with the capacity to maintain hippocampal neurogenesis (Bergström et al., 2007).

In an earlier study from this same group (Bisgaard et al., 2007), ventral hippocampal proteomes were compared between stress-sensitive and stress-resilient rats and unstressed controls following CMS exposure. Two forms of soluble NSF attachment protein, α-SNAP and β-SNAP, which are involved in vesicular fusion and neurotransmitter release, were not up-regulated in stress-resilient rats but were in stress-sensitive rats following CMS.

Using a 4-week CMS paradigm, Taliaz et al. (2011) examined the role of hippocampal BDNF on resilience in male Sprague-Dawley rats. Lentiviral vectors were employed to induce BDNF over-expression or knockdown within the hippocampus. The findings revealed that hippocampal BDNF expression was strongly associated with resilience to the behavioral effects of exposure to CMS, but had no effect on basal or post-CMS levels of plasma CORT.

DA joins in. Żurawek et al. (2013) compared mesolimbic DA receptors in stress-susceptible and stress-resilient rats after 2 or 5 weeks of CMS. Compared to stress-sensitive and control rats, resilient rats exhibited a down-regulation of D2 receptors as measured by ^{3}H-domperidone autoradiography in the lateral and medial aspects of the striatum, in the shell and core of the NAc, and in the lateral but not the medial portion of the VTA. In contrast, D2 receptor mRNA levels did not differ across brain areas in rats of the three groups. After 5 weeks of CMS, D2 receptor levels of resilient rats were comparable to controls, with the exception of the core of the NAc. In addition, D2 receptor mRNA levels were elevated in several brain areas of resilient rats. These results pointed to an initial blunting, followed by an up-regulation of D2 receptors in stress-resilient rats exposed to 5 weeks of CMS.

Using inbred C57BL/6 mice, Nasca et al. (2015) identified a subpopulation of mice that displayed resilience to the effects of CMS for 28 days and were also distinguishable from stress-susceptible mice after a single 2-hour period of restraint stress. Resilient mice were similar to unstressed controls in their preference for sucrose and in their behavior during a forced swim test. In addition, resilient mice had significantly higher expression of hippocampal mGlu2 metabotropic receptors compared to stress-susceptible mice. In the PFC, mGlu2 expression was reduced significantly compared to unstressed controls in both stress-susceptible and stress-resilient mice (mGlu2 is a presynaptic receptor that inhibits glutamate release and it is regulated in part by CORT signaling via hippocampal MRs). Resilient mice displayed reductions in hippocampal MRs that were key to maintaining high levels of presynaptic mGlu2 receptor signaling in the hippocampus. This hippocampal MR effect is related to inhibition of acetylation of H3K27, an epigenetic transcriptionally active mark bound to the GRM2 promoter gene, which regulates expression of the mGlu2 receptor. Taken together, the different pattern of glutamate signaling in the hippocampus of resilient mice makes possible a more adaptive coping strategy, perhaps by perceiving stressors in less threatening ways (Nasca et al. (2015).

Can you hear me now? Drugan and his collaborators (Drugan et al., 2009; Stafford et al., 2015) have raised the possibility that one can predict in advance which animals will have a resilient phenotype based upon their ultrasonic vocalizations (USVs). USVs occur under a variety of conditions, including aversive and stressful ones. In an initial study with very small sample sizes (Drugan et al., 2009), USVs were recorded from rats exposed to intermittent cold water swim (ICWS) stress, and these same rats were later evaluated for their performance in an instrumental swim escape test (SET). In the SET, rats exposed to ICWS fell into two categories, resilient or vulnerable, based upon good or poor learning, respectively. Four of 16 rats exposed to ICWS emitted far more USVs during the stressor than the remaining 12 rats. Interestingly, in the SET these USV-emitting rats appeared resilient, with escape performance scores comparable to those of controls, while on average the non-USV-emitting rats failed to learn the task.

In a follow-up study (Stafford et al., 2015), rats were tested in a social exploration test of anxiety following exposure to ICWS. The results revealed that those rats that emitted USVs during repeated swim stress were resilient to the anxiety-like behaviors in the social interaction test. Taken together, these two studies demonstrate that USVs may serve as a predictor of stress resilience.

Female Sex Hormones and Resilience

Males and females differ in their resilience profiles as a function of time of exposure to stressors during development, developmental stage when resilience is assessed, and the hormonal state of the individual at the time of assessment (Hodes & Epperson, 2019). Bredemann and McMahon (2014) explored the influence of female sex hormones on resilience to inescapable stress in adult Sprague-Dawley rats. Female rats were ovariectomized (OVX) at 6–8 weeks of age. At 14 days post-OVX, rats received 2 injections of estradiol (E2, 10 μg/250 g, s.c.), separated by 24 hours. Control rats received vehicle alone. For learned helplessness, male and female rats were exposed to 60 inescapable footshocks (0.65 mA, 25–35 sec durations and 15–35 sec intervals) on each of 2 consecutive days. On day 3, rats were placed in a novel shuttle box and tested for escape behavior. A light cued the opening of a door that allowed for escape from a shock. Helplessness was defined as failing on at least 5 of the 10 escape trials. Resilience was defined as more than 5 successful escapes out of 10 trials. Based upon these criteria, 55% of males and 56% of OVX females were "helpless." OVX rats that were not exposed to inescapable footshocks never performed so poorly in the shuttle box task as to be defined as helpless. Inescapable shock produced a significantly greater incidence of helpless behavior in vehicle-treated compared to E2-treated OVX female rats. In the vehicle-treated females, LTP was absent at CA3–CA1 synapses in hippocampal slices only from helpless rats, and spine density of neurons in CA1 was decreased compared to resilient rats. In contrast, significant LTP was observed in hippocampal slices from E2-treated helpless females. Spine density did not differ between E2-treated helpless and resilient rats, clearly dissociating spine density from magnitude of LTP. E2 replacement also reversed previously established helpless behavior in the shuttle box. These results may be especially relevant for humans, where women are at significantly greater risk of depression than men, especially following menopause.

Mahmoud et al. (2016) utilized female Sprague-Dawley rats to examine the effects of ovarian hormones on behavioral responses to chronic unpredictable stress. OVX or sham surgery was performed at 5 months of age. Four months after surgery, rats were exposed to chronic unpredictable stress (2 sessions per day) for 6 weeks. Compared to sham-operated controls, OVX rats displayed increased immobility with less struggling and swimming in the forced swim test, increased anxiety-like behavior in the novelty-suppressed feeding test, and increased anhedonia based upon a sucrose preference test. OVX also impaired glucocorticoid-dependent negative feedback on the HPA axis. Based upon these behavioral and endocrine findings, the authors concluded that ovarian hormones were key determinants of stress resilience.

Stress Inoculation and Resilience

Early efforts. As summarized in Chapter 7, Seymour Levine and his collaborators undertook a line of research to explore the long-term effects of early life stressors, including maternal separation and exposure to electric shock, on adult patterns of behavioral and physiological responses in laboratory rats (Levine, 1957, 1962; Levine et al., 1956; Levine et al., 1957). These publications and others that followed from the Levine laboratory influenced a generation of researchers and culminated in studies of mechanisms relating to mother-pup interactions and epigenetic changes in the HPA axis (Francis et al., 1999; Liu et al., 1997; Meaney & Szyf, 2005a, 2005b).

From this initial body of research with laboratory rats between birth and weaning at 21 days of age, studies have broadened to include stress inoculation paradigms with juvenile animals and with adults. A strength of these studies is the variety of stressor paradigms that have been employed, adding to the generality of the findings on stress inoculation (Ashokan et al., 2016). These studies in animal models also have great relevance for interventions that might be employed in at-risk children, adolescents, and adults to enhance levels of resilience to later life stressors (Davidson & McEwen, 2012).

Infancy. Mildly stressful stimuli during the first 10 days after birth in mice and rats have been shown to promote resilience to stressful disturbances in adulthood. Moderately increased HPA activity in lactating mothers exposed to stressful stimuli result in elevations in circulating CORT, which can in turn be transmitted to the progeny via lactation. In an experiment by Macrì et al. (2009), lactating CD-1 mice were given low (33 mg/liter) or high (100 mg/liter) doses of CORT in drinking water for the first 10 days after giving birth to their litters.

Offspring were then tested in adulthood (approximately 7 months of age). Low levels of CORT delivered to lactating mothers via the drinking water resulted in improved cognitive function and increased levels of natural auto-antibodies directed to the serotonin transporter in their adult offspring. In contrast, high levels of CORT provided to the mother resulted in reduced hippocampal BDNF levels and high levels of natural auto-antibodies directed toward the DA transporter. These results indicated that low to moderate levels of maternal CORT during the first 10 days after birth may enhance resilience in their adult offspring. In contrast, high levels of maternal CORT during the first 10 days after birth may result in greater susceptibility of adult offspring to stressful stimulation.

Match or mismatch? Branchi et al. (2013) tested the match-mismatch hypothesis relating to early life stress as described by Schmidt (2011). Briefly, early life adversity prepares animals and humans for a hostile environment in adulthood. If the early environment matches with characteristics of the adult environment, animals will be resilient. In contrast, if the early environment and the adult environment are a mismatch, then animals will be susceptible to the deleterious effects of a stressful adult environment.

C57BL/6 mice were reared under standard laboratory conditions or in a communal nest (CN) where three mothers and their litters were housed together. Communal nesting provided for increased social interactions between mothers and pups as well as between pups from different litters. In adulthood, control and CN mice were exposed for 4 weeks to either forced swim stress (10 min per day at 21°C) or a social stressor (social group disruption each day). CN mice were more resilient to the social stressor compared to control mice based upon a lack of anhedonia and lower plasma CORT levels. In contrast, mice of both groups were susceptible to the negative effects of swim stress. Resilience to the social stressor in adulthood was matched to the quality of the CN environment, which was also in the social domain (Branchi et al., 2013).

In two further tests of the match-mismatch hypothesis from Schmidt's laboratory, the first with BALB/c female mice (Santarelli et al., 2014) and the second with BALB/c male mice (Santarelli et al., 2017), a 2 × 2 experimental design was employed such that litters were reared under positive or negative conditions and adult animals from these litters experienced favorable or unfavorable environments prior to testing of behavioral, endocrine, and molecular responses to a battery of tests.

The results from these studies supported the match-mismatch hypothesis in that an impoverished early environment (limited nesting material) only exerted negative effects on stressful responses when these same male or female animals were reared in a favorable environment in adulthood. Similarly, a stressful adult environment exerted greater disruptions in male and female mice that had experienced a favorable early rearing environment (neonatal handling). Mice from these two mismatch conditions were clearly at a disadvantage compared to mice from the two matched conditions, including the group that experienced an unfavorable early rearing environment plus an unfavorable environment in adulthood (Santarelli et al., 2014, 2017).

Strained comparisons. Binder et al. (2011) took advantage of the fact that inbred mouse strains vary in their responses to early life stressors. Their experiments included litters of four inbred mouse strains (129S1/SvlmJ, C57BL/6J, DBA/2J, and FVB/NJ) that were exposed to a single 24-hour period of maternal separation beginning on PND 9 or were left undisturbed (controls). Separated litters were kept together and the temperature of the home cage was maintained with a heating pad. All animals were tested using a forced swim test and a hole board test. Despite exposure to a 24-hour period of maternal separation (MS), most animals seemed to be resilient to this early life stressor. However, one compelling finding was the long-lasting, strain-specific effect of maternal separation on 129S1/SvlmJ mice, which resulted in increased depression-like behaviors in a forced swim test and elevated anxiety-related behavior in the hole board test. In contrast, mice of the C57LB/6J, DBA/2J, and FVB/NJ strains were largely unaffected by maternal separation.

Handle with care. Stiller et al. (2011) examined the effects of early weaning or daily handling of litters on resilience to stress in adulthood. Litters of Sprague-Dawley rats were exposed to one of three rearing conditions: (1) unhandled controls, (2) early weaning at postnatal day 16, with individual housing thereafter, or (3) maternal separation for 3 hours/day from postnatal days 2 to 14. Behavioral tests included: (1) an emergence test at approximately 60 days of age, where individuals were placed into a black Plexiglas box for 1 hour the day before testing, and on the day of testing, after 15 minutes in the box, the holding box door was opened and the rat could explore an open field arena for 30 minutes; and (2) at least 2 weeks later, rats were exposed to 80 5-second swim stress bouts with water maintained at 23°C, and the following day were given swim escape trials using a warning tone, with a lever available to terminate the swim stress. After the swim escape trial, rats were decapitated and blood was collected for measurement of CORT and spleens were collected for measurement of con-A stimulation of lymphocyte proliferation in vitro. Resilient rats were defined as the top 33% of the distribution of the swim escape scores (i.e., shortest escape latencies: 30 males and 25 females) and vulnerable rats were defined as the bottom 33% of the distribution of swim escape scores (i.e., longest escape latencies: 30 males and 25 females).

Results revealed that stress-vulnerable rats were characterized by increased anxiety-like behaviors, greater post-stress plasma levels of CORT, and a higher con-A-induced T-cell proliferation response compared to resilient rats. The early weaning and social isolation treatment was a contributing factor in predicting total escape time, but maternal separation was not. Offspring that were separated from their mothers did have significantly elevated levels of plasma CORT compared to control offspring. There was no evidence that handling with maternal separation enhanced resilience when animals were tested in adulthood (Stiller et al., 2011).

Inoculating monkeys. A captive colony of squirrel monkeys (*Saimiri sciureus*) maintained at Stanford University was utilized to explore the effects of stress inoculation in a nonhuman primate species. Squirrel monkeys live in large social groups that include adult males and females as well as infants and juveniles. The gestation period in this species is 5 months and weaning occurs between 6 and 8 months of age (Zimbler-Delorenzo & Stone, 2011).

Parker et al. (2004) tested whether exposure to moderate stress in infancy produced later stress resilience in squirrel monkeys. Twenty squirrel monkeys were randomized to intermittent stress inoculation (removal from their mothers and natal group for 1 hour per week for 10 weeks) or the control condition (monkeys remained with their mothers in their natal groups throughout the 10-week period). At postnatal week 35, each mother-offspring dyad underwent testing in a moderately stressful novel environment and measures of offspring anxiety (i.e., maternal clinging, mother-offspring interactions, object exploration, and food consumption) and stress hormone concentrations were obtained. At postnatal week 50, after acclimation to an initially stressful wire-mesh box attached to the home cage, independent young monkeys underwent testing for measures of anxiety. In the novel environment, previously stressed monkeys demonstrated diminished anxiety as measured by decreased maternal clinging, enhanced exploratory behavior, and increased food consumption compared to controls. Mothers of stressed offspring accommodated offspring-initiated exploration, and served as a secure base of attachment more often than control mothers. Compared to control offspring, previously stressed offspring had lower basal plasma levels of ACTH and CORT, and both hormones remained lower following stress. In the wire-box test in the home cage, previously stressed offspring exhibited enhanced exploratory and play behaviors compared with control offspring. These results provided prospective evidence that moderately stressful early experiences strengthen socio-emotional and neuroendocrine responses to stressors later in life.

A subsequent series of experiments (Parker et al., 2006) revealed that the effects of early exposure of squirrel monkey infants to brief episodes of stress were not mediated by differences in maternal care. Taken together, these findings indicate that stress inoculation in squirrel monkeys included repeated exposure to mild stressors early in life that in turn stimulated mild levels of anxiety and activated the HPA axis. These early experiences then promoted behavioral and physiological resilience to stressors that endured well into adulthood (Lee et al., 2016; Lyons & Parker, 2007; Lyons et al., 2009, 2010).

Adolescence. Suo et al. (2013) used a predictable chronic mild stress procedure (5 minutes of restraint stress daily for 28 days) in adolescent rats (postnatal days 28–55) to assess its ability to enhance resilience to stressful stimuli in adulthood (postnatal days 63–83). Behavioral assessments in adulthood included a sucrose preference test, a novelty-suppressed feeding test, an EPM test, and a forced swim test. In addition, the role of mammalian target of rapamycin (mTOR) signaling in brain was measured during behavioral testing of adult animals. Compared to controls, rats repeatedly exposed to a mild stressor during adolescence exhibited no change in sucrose preference, a reduced latency to feed in the novelty-suppressed feeding test, increased time spent in the open arms of the EPM, and less time spent immobile in a forced swim test. Either systemic administration or intra-PFC infusion of the mTOR inhibitor, rapamycin, completely blocked the behavioral effects produced by chronic mild stress in adolescence. Finally, chronic mild stress during adolescence blocked the effects of exposure to chronic unpredictable stress in adulthood.

Kendig et al. (2011) exposed groups of four male Wistar rats (33–57 days of age) to cat fur for 30 minutes in a large arena once every other day for 24 days. Controls were placed in an empty arena without cat fur. Testing occurred from days 58 to 77. When exposed to cat fur, 3–4 rats would huddle together in the corner of the arena. This huddling behavior and suppression of activity occurred throughout the 12 exposures. In adulthood, predator-stressed rats displayed significantly less immobility in a forced swim test and exhibited increased sociability with a novel conspecific in a social interaction test. These findings suggest greater resilience in adulthood following stress exposure in adolescence.

Adulthood. The ability to control the onset, duration, intensity, frequency, or offset of a stressful stimulus may have long-lasting effects on reducing the negative impact of subsequent exposure to stressful stimuli, including those that cannot be controlled.

The illusion of control. Remarkably, as reviewed by Maier and his colleagues (Maier, 2015; Maier et al., 2006; Maier & Watkins, 2010), laboratory rats that have experienced control over electric shocks to the tail have reduced neural and behavioral responses to an uncontrollable stressor presented up to two months later. Indeed, the animals responded as if the subsequent stressor was actually controllable. It appeared that prior exposure to a controllable stressor subserved a stress inoculation function, even when the subsequent stressor was dramatically different from the initial controllable stressor, such as exposure to CSDS.

Exposure to a controllable stressor activated neurons in the ventral-medial PFC (vmPFC), which exerted inhibitory control over limbic and brainstem structures, including the dorsal raphe nucleus. In an elegant series of experiments from their laboratory, Maier and Watkins (2010) demonstrated that neural activation of the vmPFC during controllable stress was required for inhibiting activity of serotonin neurons within the DRN, and inoculation to the deleterious behavioral effects of exposure to a subsequent inescapable stressor 1 week later. Similarly, pharmacological activation of vmPFC input to the DRN during exposure of laboratory rats to inescapable tail shock resulted in an inoculation effect as if the inescapable tail shock was actually controllable. Finally, pharmacological blockade of vmPFC input to the DRN prevented the stress inoculation effect following exposure of rats to a controllable stressor. These results have far-reaching implications for understanding mechanisms of stress inoculation, particularly as it relates to resilience to the effects of traumatic stressors. Lucas et al. (2014) have made similar arguments regarding the impact of stressor controllability on enhancing stress resilience in laboratory rats. In addition, Kerr et al. (2012) supported the work of Maier and Watkins (2010) in their functional magnetic resonance imagining (fMRI) studies of the human vmPFC and anticipation of control over presentation of aversive video clips.

The social scene. Brockhurst et al. (2015) employed a stress inoculation paradigm that entailed intermittent exposure of C57BL/6 adult male mice to a mild social stressor. Mice were randomized to stress inoculation or a control treatment condition and were assessed for plasma CORT responses and behavior during open field, object-exploration, and tail-suspension tests and repeated restraint stress. Every other day for 21 days, mice in the stress inoculation condition were removed from their home cages and individually placed for 15 minutes behind a wire mesh barrier in the cage of a retired Swiss-Webster male breeder. Each subject was repeatedly exposed to the same Swiss-Webster breeder. The wire mesh barrier prevented fighting and wounding during all 11 stress inoculation sessions, but allowed visual and olfactory interactions. Mice were immediately returned to their home cages after each of the 11 sessions. Control mice remained undisturbed except for intermittent human handling during routine cage cleaning.

Stress inoculation training sessions that acutely increased plasma levels of CORT diminished subsequent immobility as a measure of behavioral despair on tail-suspension tests. Stress inoculation also decreased subsequent freezing in an open field arena despite comparable levels of thigmotaxis in mice from both treatment conditions. Stress inoculation subsequently decreased novel object exploration latencies and reduced plasma CORT responses to repeated restraint stress. These results demonstrated that stress inoculation acutely stimulated glucocorticoid signaling, and then enhanced subsequent indications of active coping behavior in mice. Stress inoculation training reflected an experience-dependent process in adulthood that resembled in part interventions designed to build resilience in humans (Brockhurst et al., 2015).

An enriched experience. Lehmann and Herkenham (2011) took a novel approach to promote resiliency in C57BL/6 male mice prior to exposure to CSDS. They housed individual mice in a standard cage (SE) or an enriched (EE) or impoverished environment (IE) for 3 weeks, followed by 2 weeks of CSDS as described previously. SE was a polycarbonate cage with bedding chips and a cardboard tunnel. An EE consisted of a polycarbonate cage with bedding chips, nest material, running wheels, and tubes of different shapes and sizes. An IE consisted of a polycarbonate cage with bedding chips. EE-housed mice but not IE- or SE-housed mice exhibited increased levels of FosB/ΔFosB immunostaining in the infralimbic, prelimbic, and anterior cingulate cortices; amygdala; and NAc following CSDS. EE mice also exhibited a resilient behavioral phenotype following CSDS. Discrete lesions of the infralimbic cortex prior to EE blocked behavioral resilience to CSDS and reduced FosB/ΔFosB expression in the NAc and amygdala while increasing expression in the paraventricular nucleus. These findings were consistent with enhanced output of neurons in the vmPFC playing a critical role in stress resilience.

Summary

Charney and his colleagues made the astute observation that resilience could be studied in laboratory animals using the tools of molecular biology and neuroscience. Prior to this, many studies of resilience had focused on psychological characteristics of children that survived and even thrived under adverse circumstances.

A consistent finding from different laboratories has been the wide range of behavioral and biological responses of laboratory animals following exposure to an acute stressor or to a chronic intermittent stressful paradigm. The variability of responses has been described in outbred as well as inbred strains of laboratory mice and rats. These findings match well with observations of humans who survived highly stressful or traumatic experiences and came through relatively unscathed psychologically.

Several stress paradigms have been employed to study neurobiological mechanisms of resilience, including two that score high on ethological validity: PSS and CSDS. Experiments employing these and other stressor paradigms have revealed a host of molecular alterations in stress-sensitive brain circuits that contribute to a resilient phenotype. A subset of these changes are not merely polar opposite changes from animals that displayed susceptibility to the stressors; rather, there are specific changes that are essential for a resilient phenotype. These studies provide new approaches to the etiology of stress-related mental disorders, especially depression and PTSD. Instead of focusing solely on the development of therapies that target stress-sensitive brain circuits, an alternative approach in the near future may be to develop therapies that up-regulate stress-resilient brain circuits.

Another major research area relates to inoculation of animals against the deleterious effects of a later intense stressor. Experiments were reviewed that included stress inoculation of animals during infancy, adolescence, or adulthood. There was compelling evidence of the positive effects of stress inoculation on the capacity of animals to adapt favorably to stressful stimulation later in life. These experiments have a direct bearing on approaches to training military personnel for deployment to combat zones and to training first-responders for the challenges of dealing effectively with casualty events following accidents or terrorist attacks.

Successful adaptation in the face of adverse circumstances involves a complex and interacting array of alterations in brain circuits, peripheral hormonal systems, innate and adaptive immune cells and signaling molecules present in the circulation, alterations in gut microbiota, and subtle alterations in the blood-brain barrier. A thorough understanding of how these stress-responsive peripheral and central systems interact in susceptible and resilient animals and humans may lead to the development of novel therapeutic strategies to treat a host of mental disorders, including depression and PTSD (Cathomus et al., 2019).

16

Thoughts for the Future

In this closing chapter, I will take a major leap of faith and suggest some issues that should be addressed in the coming years to improve the diagnosis, treatment, and prevention of mental disorders. Such a broad-based, international effort seeks to address one of the most perplexing issues in all of health care—improving outcomes for patients with psychiatric disorders and their family members. I have attempted in this book to highlight some of the bright spots in preclinical research on animal models of stress and mental disorders, and I came away with an optimistic outlook for the future. I hope you have as well. Without doubt, some of the brightest minds and most innovative thinkers in neuroscience have been attracted to these areas of basic and clinical research in psychiatry, and that fact alone bodes well for the future. Unfortunately, the brightest minds and the most innovative thinkers are not enough. Nations around the world must make long-term commitments to their people to support the translation of basic research findings into improved diagnosis, treatment, and prevention programs to reduce the disturbingly high negative impact these disorders have on quality of life and loss of productivity.

My list of seven issues for the future is a direct outgrowth of my efforts to write this book. I was not able to cover all of the major categories of mental disorders, but I made an honest attempt to deal with some of the most critical ones. I will also confess to a large measure of trepidation is compiling this list, as I am not a psychiatrist and have never been involved professionally in the care of patients with mental disorders. Some of these issues for the future are fairly obvious, while others are less so. I hope these ideas will be a stimulus for continued discussion and action that contribute to a brighter future for anyone affected by a mental disorder.

Diagnosing the Problem

The starting point for clinical or basic research studies in mental disorders is the diagnostic system. With the release of *DSM-5* in 2013 and *ICD-11* in 2019, health professionals will be dealing for the foreseeable future with diagnostic systems of mental disorders that are largely descriptive and syndromic. These diagnostic categories are based upon self-reports of symptoms by patients or their loved ones, and in some cases there is great diversity in the symptom clusters that satisfy a particular diagnosis. For example, in the *DSM-5* diagnosis of major depressive disorder, there are 681 combinations of symptoms that qualify as a diagnosis of depression. In addition, there is significant comorbidity of depressive symptoms with other psychiatric disorders. This extreme heterogeneity of symptom clusters calls into question whether major depressive disorder qualifies as a single disorder (Akil et al., 2018).

Few would agree that a current *DSM-5* or *ICD-11* diagnostic category provides an accurate representation of a given group of patients that share a similar etiology. One reason that these diagnostic systems have enjoyed such a long life is that they make possible a general agreement among clinicians regarding the diagnosis of a given patient. But this high degree of reliability of diagnosis does not come with assurances that the diagnosis has any connection to the underlying pathophysiology of the individual. In other words, the current cost of a diagnostic system with high reliability is a diagnostic system with low validity.

Results of genome-wide association studies (GWAS) also call into question the integrity of diagnostic categories featured in *DSM-5* and *ICD-11*. The impression given is that psychiatric disorders are discrete entities, when in fact, the boundaries between disorders are blurred, as are the boundaries between a given disorder and otherwise healthy individuals. It has become increasingly clear that results from GWAS, particularly in the identification of shared and syndrome-specific risk variants, can provide valuable information that has the potential to increase the validity of systems of psychiatric diagnosis (Smoller, 2013).

DSM-5 and *ICD-11* place severe limitations on future efforts to understand the etiology of psychiatric disorders or to develop new and more effective therapies (Stephan et al., 2016). The RDoC system developed by the US National Institute of Mental Health is one attempt to sever ties with *DSM/ICD* and take a distinctly dimensional approach to research in mental disorders. A guiding principle of RDoC is that mental disorders reflect disruptions in brain circuits. As such, investigators are encouraged to begin with the current state of knowledge of given brain circuits and their effects on behavior and then to relate that information to studies of carefully selected cohorts of patients. An especially valuable set of findings comes from imaging studies that have attempted to delineate circuits and neurochemical changes as they relate to behaviors. Such approaches may also provide potential biomarkers for future vulnerabilities to stressful life events (Swartz et al., 2015). This is in stark contrast to more traditional approaches to psychiatric research, where the starting point is a *DSM/ICD*-defined patient group, and efforts are then directed at discovering etiologic factors. Finally, RDoC was envisioned to be a constant work in progress, where new research findings would be incorporated into ongoing updates to the RDoC matrix (Owen, 2014).

As we look ahead, hopefully a new psychiatric diagnostic system will emerge that provides high levels of reliability and validity in the diagnosis and treatment of mental disorders. Unfortunately, the prospects for this happening quickly are not good.

Behaving

Throughout this book, I have attempted to provide a strong case for the value of animal models in the study of psychiatric disorders. In so doing, I have also tried to point out the limitations of current experimental approaches and several "best practices" that enhance the value and applicability of experimental results. One area that is in need of greater attention is the development of improved behavioral phenotyping strategies for use in animal models of specific mental disorders. Ideally, these new behavioral tests should be automated to minimize experimenter error, they should capture behavioral patterns over extended periods of time, and they should be designed to reflect to the greatest extent possible the symptoms of the patient group of interest. Many current behavioral tests are conducted during the light portion of the light-dark cycle, a time when nocturnal rodents such as laboratory strains of mice and rats are resting or asleep. Even when animals are maintained on a reversed light-dark cycle, a given test only captures behaviors during a limited period of the 24-hour cycle. Such approaches are convenient for researchers but may miss important treatment effects on the behavior of animal models.

Two examples of innovations in behavioral testing will illustrate this point. Jhuang et al. (2010) developed a trainable, automated, high-throughput computer vision system for analyzing behaviors of individual mice in their home cages. After training the system on common behaviors of mice (e.g., feeding, drinking, moving, grooming, etc.), these investigators demonstrated that the automated system was as accurate as human observers in scoring the behaviors, but the scoring occurred at a much faster rate. They estimated that 22 person-hours would be required for the detailed analysis of 1 hour of video for one mouse. In a study of four different mouse strains that was included in their report, 28 mice (7 per strain) were recorded continuously for a 24-hour period. This small-scale effort would have required more than 15,000 person-hours to analyze. In contrast, the computer system analyzed the video data in real time. This system is also capable of quantifying behaviors of two or more animals as they engage in social interactions.

In another approach, Young et al. (2007) described the behavioral pattern monitor (BPM) for use in psychopharmacological studies with laboratory rats. The BPM was later reduced in scale for use with laboratory mice with equal success. The BPM consists of a computer-monitored activity chamber provided with rearing touch plates on the walls and 10 holes in the floor and walls that allow for investigatory nose poking. This fully automated approach provides for a much richer and more nuanced analysis of exploratory behaviors compared to more typical measures of open field behavior and has been used with great success to quantify the behavioral profiles of a mouse model of mania (Kwiatkowski et al., 2018). In a prime example of a reverse translational approach, this research group also developed a scaled-up version of the BPM for use with bipolar disorder patients and unaffected controls (Young et al., 2007).

When these more nuanced measures of behaviors in animal models are combined with circuit-level experiments using optogenetic or chemogenetic techniques, they will fit nicely with the goals of the RDoC project.

In the Blood

A major challenge facing clinical psychiatrists and their patients relates to the selection of a drug that will relieve symptoms effectively and have minimal side effects. All too often, this clinical decision becomes a trial-and-error process for selection of an effective drug at an effective dose. One exciting development that may improve drug selection was reported by Stern et al. (2018). This group collected blood samples from patients with bipolar disorder (BD) and from unaffected controls that were age- and sex-matched. β-lymphocytes were immortalized with Epstein-Barr virus and the resulting induced pluripotent stem cells (iPSCs) were coaxed into differentiating into hippocampal dentate gyrus-like neurons. Whole-cell patch-clamp recordings of more than 460 of these neurons from BD patients and controls were conducted. BD patients were further subdivided into lithium responders (LRs) and lithium non-responders (NRs).

Stern et al. (2018) reported that neurons from LR and NR patients sorted into two distinct subpopulations of cells based upon their electrophysiological properties. However, LR and NR neurons did share in common a large, fast afterhyperpolarization that reflected their repetitive spiking and hyper-excitability compared to neurons from controls. LR and NR neurons differed to such an extent that a new patient's response to lithium could be predicted with 92% accuracy based upon electrophysiological properties alone. Further experiments revealed that lithium treatment of neurons from LRs exhibited reduced hyperexcitability whereas neurons from NRs did not.

These exciting findings using blood cells as a source for iPSCs open up a host of possibilities to explore with bipolar patients as well as patients with other mental disorders. As an example, one group has explored molecular mechanisms of bipolar disorder using iPSCs (Tobe et al., 2017). Could such an approach be taken with teens in an attempt to predict risk for BD before the appearance of symptoms? Would iPSCs from other patient groups exhibit distinct electro-physiological profiles that could be used to predict in advance responsiveness to specific drugs? These and many other issues await future experiments prior to playing a role in the determination of drug selection and dosage by attending physicians.

Big, Bigger, Biggest

"Big data" have become an exciting new focus within the research community, businesses, health systems, and governmental entities. Some universities have even formed new schools of data science. Psychiatry is in some ways uniquely positioned to benefit from large-scale collaborative studies with sample sizes ranging into the hundreds of thousands. This is especially true in GWAS relating to mental disorders, given the heterogeneity of the disorders and the involvement of hundreds of risk gene variants, each exerting small effects. A case in point is the report by Wray et al. (2018) that included almost 500,000 cases and controls in a GWAS of major depressive disorder. More recently, another GWAS of depression included more than 800,000 cases and controls. In addition, a replication sample included more than 1.3 million cases and controls (Howard et al., 2019). An interesting feature of these studies was the inclusion of data from 23andMe, a for-profit company that was the first to be approved by the US Food and Drug Administration to market direct-to-consumer genetic testing kits in 2015. 23andMe has a database of more than 10 million customers, and 80% have consented to participate in research studies. Health information from its customers is limited to self-reports, which may compromise the integrity of the data compared to studies where a diagnosis of depression is based upon an interview with a psychiatrist. Nonetheless, the added statistical power of including these large numbers of 23andMe customers has won the day with many researchers. Clearly, any findings from 23andMe data would need to be validated using other depression databases.

With the significant recent uptick in the use of electronic health records (EHRs), a compelling need has arisen to include behavioral, social, and psychological variables in EHRs that have been demonstrated to have an impact on individual health outcomes (Institute of Medicine [IOM], 2014a, 2014b). A challenge in developing these measures was to provide a panel of psychosocial "vital signs" that would reflect an impact on health outcomes. These vital signs could also serve to alert clinicians to the need for more thorough testing to address areas of concern (Adler & Stead, 2015; Matthews et al., 2016).

The IOM recommendations included the following: current residential address to enable geocoding to obtain neighborhood-level information, such as walkability indices and median income of the census track; race/ethnicity (2 questions), highest level and degree of education (2 questions), and financial resource strain (1 question); level of stress (1 item) and depression (2 items); social connections and isolation (4 items) as well as intimate partner violence (4 items); and physical activity (2 items) and tobacco and alcohol use (total of 5 items) (Institute of Medicine [IOM], 2014a, 2014b). With widespread adoption of these psychosocial vital signs in EHRs, one may expect improvements in patient care by facilitating access to a full range of factors that influence individual and population health management (Matthews et al., 2016).

A newer source of data comes from large-scale patient studies that link EHRs to imaging, genomic, and psychosocial data. Such efforts include the 100,000 Genomes Project of the British National Health Service, the partnership between Google and Stanford University Medical Center in precision medicine, the iPSYCH Danish birth cohort, and the US National Institutes of Health partnership with Amazon Web Services to support the Science and Technology Research Infrastructure for Discovery, Experimentation, and Sustainability (STRIDES) Initiative. Each of these efforts will be part of a larger precision medicine initiative to eventually bring decision support to the point of service for a given patient.

Simon (2019) presented a balanced view of the ways in which data science approaches in mental health settings may prove useful. He noted that algorithms developed from millions of patient health records have proven to be better predictors of suicidal behavior than clinical assessments. However, the massive numbers of EHRs available call for a different approach to statistical analyses. As Simon points out, with sample sizes in the millions, almost any comparison of interest to clinicians will be highly significant based upon standard parametric statistics. Thus, experienced clinicians will need to determine those variables that make a meaningful contribution to care of individual patients and those that don't.

Gillan and Whelan (2017) pointed out the value of using data-mining approaches to learn why some patients respond favorably to drug therapies and others do not. If data sets that typically include clinician and staff ratings and patient self-reports are further enriched with brain imaging, cognitive, and genetic data, it is possible that the sensitivity and specificity of algorithm-based predictions could be increased substantially. Finally, given the costs associated with brain imaging, data from EEG studies may represent a less expensive alternative to enhance predictive power. A major challenge going forward to enhance the predictive power of deciding which drug to prescribe for a given patient is to greatly increase the number of subjects represented in data sets and to greatly enhance the standardization and richness of phenotypic information collected (Bzdok & Meyer-Lindenberg, 2017). What is clear is the compelling need to fully incorporate a given individual's diet, behaviors, stress levels, and related vairables in determining disease risk and treatment response (Horwitz et al., 2013).

An Ounce of Prevention

In 1994, the Institute of Medicine (now the National Academy of Medicine) of the National Academies of Sciences in the United States issued a groundbreaking report on the value of early interventions to reduce the risks for developing mental disorders later in life (Institute of Medicine, 1994). The report summarized three types of preventive interventions:

Universal preventive interventions target the public at large or a population group that was not singled out based upon risk status. Examples of this type of intervention include prenatal care, childhood immunization, and school-based competence enhancement programs. Because these programs are positive and proactive and are made available independent of disease risk, their potential for singling out participants is greatly reduced and they are more likely to be embraced.

Selective interventions target individuals or subgroups whose risk of developing mental disorders is significantly higher than the population as a whole. Examples of this type of intervention includes home visitation and infant day care for low-birth-weight children, preschool programs for all children from impoverished neighborhoods, and social support groups for children who have suffered losses or traumas.

Preventive interventions are designed for individuals who have been identified based upon prodromal signs or symptoms or biological markers related to mental disorders, but who do not yet meet diagnostic criteria. Providing social skills or parent-child interaction training for children who have early behavioral problems are examples of preventive interventions that could involve partnerships between local schools, social service agencies, and public health offices.

One broad-based strategy for preventing the development of mental disorders is to be guided by the exciting findings described in Chapter 15 on resilience to stressful stimuli. Building strength and resilience in children, families, and local communities is one path that has the potential to enhance behavioral and physiological resilience to the vicissitudes of life, thereby decreasing the risk profile for development of mental disorders.

In an excellent example of a targeted preventive intervention, Garber et al. (2009) developed a group cognitive behavioral prevention program for 316 adolescents aged 13–17 years who were at high risk of developing depression. Participants were randomly assigned to the cognitive behavioral intervention that consisted of 8 weekly group sessions for 90 minutes each, followed by 6 monthly sessions, or to a control condition that included continuation of usual care. The results indicated that the cognitive behavioral prevention program exerted a significant effect through the 9-month follow-up period based upon clinical diagnoses and self-reported depressive symptoms. However, a beneficial effect of the intervention was not observed for adolescents with a currently depressed parent. A more recent study introduced the possibility of personalizing intervention programs to enhance prevention of adolescent depression based upon profiles of cognitive and interpersonal vulnerabilities of the participants (Hankin et al., 2018).

It would appear from the central thesis of this book that interventions that focused on moderating stress reactivity might also represent a promising approach to prevent depression. For example, Daches et al. (2019) reported that increased physiological reactivity to a laboratory stressor enhanced the risk of developing depression in at-risk adolescents that previously experienced a stressful life event. Might a group-based intervention that involved stress management training for at-risk adolescents be a promising approach? There is no shortage of stressors during this developmental stage, and improving the ability of adolescents to manage these stressors could reduce the trajectory of depression well into adulthood.

Another intervention strategy could involve the use of dietary supplements for pregnant women, especially those at high risk of having offspring who may go on to develop schizophrenia or ASD (Freedman et al., 2018). One such approach that has been taken involved a double-blind, placebo-controlled trial of choline supplements given to 100 healthy pregnant women beginning in the second trimester and continuing until delivery of the baby (Ross et al., 2013). In the fifth week following birth, babies were tested for inhibition of the P50 component of the cerebral evoked response to paired sounds. The criterion for suppression was a decrease in the amplitude of the second P50 response by $\geq 50\%$. Cerebral inhibition was more frequent in choline-supplemented babies compared to placebo controls (76% versus 43%, respectively). This same laboratory previously noted that a neonatal developmental delay in cerebral inhibition was associated with attentional issues as the children matured. While these results are a long way from preventing schizophrenia, the approach taken with choline supplementation is worthy of careful consideration as a possible intervention to reduce the prevalence of schizophrenia. Other strategies have also been proposed to alter the course of schizophrenia by intervening in adolescence (Millan et al., 2016).

Clear prenatal risks have been documented for the later development of schizophrenia. Unfortunately, interventions to reduce risk are complicated by the fact that the onset of symptoms of schizophrenia may not be apparent for two decades. Given the devastating effects of this disorder on quality of life, it may be time to bite the bullet and consider funding a long-term multi-site prevention study.

A Smarter Use of Cell Phones

The dramatic worldwide proliferation of smartphones and wearable digital devices such as fitness trackers has presented an opportunity for health-care providers and patients to collaborate to improve delivery of behavioral health services (Baker et al., 2018). Will it be possible, with appropriate safeguards in place to address privacy concerns and ethical issues, to measure and analyze ongoing behavioral and physiological endpoints during normal and stressful periods (locomotion, social interactions, facial expressions, vocal patterns, sleep patterns, heart rate, blood pressure, etc.) as a means of providing in real time a digital phenotype of an individual? Such information would be invaluable in predicting early warning signs of mental distress based upon past behaviors that could provide feedback to the individual as an alert to modify his or her behavior or to summon a caregiver or health-care provider to address a dire emergency.

Slavich et al. (2019) provided an overview of the technical and ethical challenges associated with measuring levels of stress by using speech parameters (e.g., pitch, jitter, energy, rate, length and number of pauses) captured from smartphones. The technology required for analysis of speech signals is currently available, but there is a need for validation of speech-related parameters of stress against various biological markers of stress, including plasma or salivary levels of cortisol, catecholamines, and cytokines, as well as electrodermal activity. Needless to say, concerns about data security and individual privacy are paramount and must be tackled before speech signals are routinely captured and analyzed by a health-care professional to guide treatment, and later stored in an individual's electronic health record (Slavich et al., 2019).

Onnela and Rauch (2016) provided a vivid summary of the normal engagement of an individual with a mental disorder (e.g., depression, bipolar disorder, schizophrenia) with the health-care system. A major psychiatric crisis is usually followed by a visit to the emergency department, followed by an assessment, and a brief in-patient hospitalization. At discharge, the patient is then encouraged to secure outpatient care if it can be afforded and is available. Not surprisingly, this pattern is frequently repeated with each subsequent crisis. Real-time digital phenotyping holds out the hope that patterns of change could be used to predict in advance which individual with depression may become suicidal, which individual with bipolar disorder is about to transition to a manic episode, or which individual with psychosis is about to de-compensate. An alert could be conveyed to the patient, to a loved one, or to a health-care provider, as appropriate. Depending on the time between the alert and the impending crisis, an effective intervention might prevent an emergency room visit and hospitalization or worse.

The technical requirements for digital phenotyping are largely in place. However, a substantial amount of experimentation and many clinical trials are required to convert real-time digital data into a framework appropriate for decisions regarding psychiatric care. A logical next step would be to fold the digital phenotyping data into databases containing brain imaging, genome, and epigenome data to inform systems of classification of mental disorders (Onnela & Rauch, 2016).

Precisely!

Most drugs used to treat mental disorders are taken by mouth and must survive in the stomach and gastrointestinal system, be absorbed into blood and survive passage through the liver, and then move across the blood-brain barrier to reach targets in various parts of the brain. But the dysfunction associated with a given mental disorder may be limited to a single brain circuit, or to one or several components of a single brain circuit. What if the beneficial effects of the drug are canceled out or diminished by its effects in other parts of the brain? In the future, how might next-generation drugs be delivered to more precisely determined sites within the brain without the need for invasive, high-risk neurosurgery?

Experiments in animal models using optogenetic and chemogenetic techniques have informed clinical trials for treating cocaine addiction in humans (Ferenczi & Deisseroth, 2016). How can the anatomical, cell-type, and temporal specificity of optogenetic and chemogenetic approaches to increase or decrease neural activity be brought from the bench to the clinic?

Szablowski et al. (2018) have developed and tested a noninvasive approach in laboratory mice termed *acoustically targeted chemogenetics* (ATAC). They employed transient opening of the blood-brain barrier by i.v. administration of microbubbles to permit the anatomically precise delivery of an adeno-associated viral vector (AAV) encoding a DREADD (hM4Di) to six different areas of the hippocampus. Blood-brain barrier opening was transient and fully reversible and was driven by microbubble cavitation at the MRI-guided ultrasound wave focal point. The damage to brain tissue was quite minimal, especially when compared to the damage that occurred during stereotaxic placement of a cannula for delivery of the DREADD. The viral construct contained a promoter that targeted expression of the DREADD within excitatory neurons and the fluorescent reporter mCherry was employed to confirm the degree of viral expression within the hippocampus. Mice were allowed 6–8 weeks after ATAC for transgene expression. Control and ATAC mice displayed high levels of freezing behavior when placed into a test chamber previously associated with delivery of electric foot shocks. However, mice that received an injection of the designer drug CNO just before fear conditioning exhibited a significant reduction in freezing behavior when re-exposed to the test chamber. These exciting findings suggest that ATAC and viral delivery of DREADDs may be employed clinically in the not-too-distant future. Stay tuned. An alternative to the use of AAV as the viral delivery vehicle may be the use of DREADDs bound to gold nanoparticles (Lee et al., 2018).

A common theme across these seven ideas is the need for a commitment to bringing greater precision to the practice of psychiatry (Fernandes et al., 2017). This includes greater precision in diagnosis, in drug selection and targeting, and in use of large data sets to enhance delivery of care. In addition, research with animal models must also increase specificity by developing more translationally relevant tests for behavioral phenotyping. Finally, there should also be a parallel commitment to explore effective therapies to prevent the onset of mental disorders in those at high risk.

Closing Comments

We have come to the end of our journey to explore the intricate web of relationships between stress and the etiology of psychiatric disorders. There were other interesting places to visit, but our page budget limited us to this set of fascinating topics. In preparation for our journey, we started with a look back at how psychiatry evolved in Europe and the United States in the 19th and 20th centuries. We also delved into the evolution of systems for the classification of mental disorders and we considered how the two principal systems of classification (*DSM* and *ICD*) have changed over time and the challenges they still present. I then attempted to make a strong case for a critical role for life stressors in the etiology of three major mental disorders: bipolar disorder, depression, and schizophrenia. If this case wasn't compelling, it would call into question the underlying motivation for our larger efforts.

Clearing that hurdle, we then considered the evolution of the stress concept across cultures and time periods and some of the key individuals who left enduring legacies on this field of inquiry. The next focus was on the nuts and bolts of our primary topic: how do individuals (animals or humans) maintain some semblance of homeostatic balance in the face of a constantly changing internal and external environment? Armed with this information, we considered how we might explore the complex relationships between stress and mental disorders in humans by studying animal models. The next eight chapters were centrally involved with looking at the impact of stressful stimulation on various animal models by using several levels of analysis: molecular, cellular, circuits, systems, and behavioral measures. We then took an exciting detour that flipped our central focus from why individuals are susceptible to stressful stimuli to why some individuals are relatively resistant to the adverse effects of stressors.

At the end of our journey, we have had time to reflect on what we learned and how we might change things for the better. You probably have a list of ideas for the future that is much better than mine. In the United States, the last decade of the 20th century was designated the *Decade of the Brain*. Since that initiative was launched, the pace of discovery in the neurosciences has accelerated, and when combined with the revolution in genomics, many of these discoveries are being applied in laboratories and clinical settings to understand the pathophysiology of mental disorders. Clearly, there is ample reason for optimism that breakthroughs in the diagnosis, treatment, and prevention of mental disorders are within sight.

Thank you for taking the time to explore some or all of these topics. It was a pleasure for me to prepare this book, and if you come away with new insights on this broad and stimulating topic, that is reward enough for my efforts.

References

Aas, M., Henry, C., Andreassen, O. A., Bellivier, F., Melle, I., & Etain, B. (2016). The role of childhood trauma in bipolar disorders. *International Journal of Bipolar Disorders, 4*, 2.

Abazyan, B., Nomura, J., Kannan, G., Ishizuka, K., Tamashiro, K. L., Nucifora, F., . . . Pletnikov, M. V. (2010). Prenatal interaction of mutant DISC1 and immune activation produces adult psychopathology. *Biological Psychiatry, 68*, 1172–1181.

Abbott, S. B. G., Stornetta, R. L., Socolovsky, C. S., West, G. H., & Guyenet, P. G. (2009). Photostimulation of channelrhodopsin-2 expressing ventrolateral medullary neurons increases sympathetic nerve activity and blood pressure in rats. *Journal of Physiology, 587*, 5613–5631.

Abdullah, C. E., Averill, L. E., & Krystal, J. H. (2017). A new journal: addressing the behavioral and biological effects of chronic stress. *Chronic Stress, 1*, 1.

Adamec, R. E., Blundell, J., & Burton, P. (2005). Neural circuit changes mediating lasting brain and behavioral response to predator stress. *Neuroscience and Biobehavioral Reviews, 29*, 1225–1241.

Adamec, R., Fougere, D., & Risbrough, V. (2010). CRF receptor blockade prevents initiation and consolidation of stress effects on affect in the predator stress model of PTSD. *International Journal of Neuropsychopharmacology, 13*, 747–757.

Adamec, R., Kent, P., Anisman, H., Shallow, T., & Merali, Z. (1998). Neural plasticity, neuropeptides and anxiety in animals: implications for understanding and treating affective disorder following traumatic stress in humans. *Neuroscience and Biobehavioral Reviews, 23*, 301–318.

Adamec, R., Muir, C., Grimes, M., & Pearcey, K. (2007). Involvement of noradrenergic and corticoid receptors in the consolidation of the lasting anxiogenic effects of predator stress. *Behavioural Brain Research, 179*, 192–207.

Adamec, R. E., & Swallow, T. (1993). Lasting effects on rodent anxiety of a single exposure to a cat. *Physiology and Behavior, 54*, 101–109.

Adams, M. D., Celniker, S. E., Holt, R. A., Evans, C. A., Gocayne, J. D., Amanatides, P. G., . . . Venter, J. C. (2000). The genome sequence of *Drosophila melanogaster. Science, 287*, 2185–2195.

Adamson, S. L., Lu, Y., Whiteley, K. J., Holmyard, D., Hemberger, M., Pfarrer, C., & Cross, J. C. (2002). Interactions between trophoblast cells and the maternal and fetal circulation in the mouse placenta. *Developmental Biology, 250*, 358–373.

Ader, R. (1980). Psychosomatic and psychoimmunologic research. *Psychosomatic Medicine, 42*, 307–321.

Ader, R., & Cohen, N. (1975). Behaviorally conditioned immunosuppression. *Psychosomatic Medicine, 37*, 333–340.

Adler, N. E., & Stead, W. W. (2015). Patients in context: EHR capture of social and behavioral determinants of health. *New England Journal of Medicine, 372*, 698–701.

Agid, Y., Buzsáki, G., Diamond, D. M., Frackowiak, R., Giedd, J., Girault, J.-A., . . . Weinberger, D. (2007). How can drug discovery for psychiatric disorders be improved? *Nature Reviews Drug Discovery, 6*, 189–201.

Agnew-Blais, J., & Danese, A. (2016). Childhood maltreatment and unfavourable clinical outcomes in bipolar disorder: a systematic review and meta-analysis. *Lancet Psychiatry*, 3, 342–349.

Agulair-Valles, A., Kim, J., Jung, S., Woodside, B., & Luheshi, G. N. (2014). Role of brain transmigrating neutrophils in depression-like behavior during systemic infection. *Molecular Psychiatry*, 19, 599–606.

Ahles, A., & Engelhardt, S. (2014). Polymorphic variants of adrenoceptors: pharmacology, physiology and role in disease. *Pharmacological Reviews*, 66, 598–637.

Aikins, D. E., Straber, J. A., Kohler, R. J., Bihani, N., & Perrine, S. A. (2017). Differences in hippocampal serotonergic activity in a mouse single prolonged stress paradigm impact discriminant fear acquisition and retention. *Neuroscience Letters*, 639, 162–166.

Ait-Ali, D., Samal, B., Mustafa, T., & Eiden, L. E. (2010). Neuropeptides, growth factors, and cytokines: a cohort of informational molecules whose expression is up-regulated by the stress-associated slow transmitter PACAP in chromaffin cells. *Cellular and Molecular Neurobiology*, 30, 1441–1449.

Akdis, M., Aab, A., Altunbulakli, C., Azkur, K., Costa, R. A., Crameri, R., . . . Akdis, C. A. (2016). Interleukins (from IL-1 to IL-38), interferons, transforming growth factor β, and TNF-α: receptors, functions, and roles in diseases. *Journal of Allergy and Clinical Immunology*, 138, 984–1010.

Akhtar, A. (2015). The flaws and human harms of animal experimentation. *Cambridge Quarterly of Healthcare Ethics*, 24, 407–419.

Akil, H., Brenner, S., Kandel, E., Kendler, K. S., King, M.-C., Scolnick, E., . . . Zoghbi, H. Y. (2010). The future of psychiatric research: genomes and circuits. *Science*, 327, 1580–1581.

Akil, H., Gordon, J., Hen, R., Javitch, J., Mayberg, H., McEwen, B., . . . Nestler, E. J. (2018). Treatment resistant depression: a multi-scale, systems biology approach. *Neuroscience and Biobehavioral Reviews*, 84, 272–288.

Akimova, E., Lanzenberger, R., & Kasper, S. (2009). The serotonin-1A receptor in anxiety disorders. *Biological Psychiatry*, 66, 627–635.

Alheid, G. F., & Heimer, L. (1988). New perspectives in basal forebrain organization of special relevance for neuropsychiatric disorders: the striatopallidal, amygdaloid, and corticopetal components of substantia innominata. *Neuroscience*, 27, 1–39.

Alisch, R. S., Chopra, P., Fox, A. S., Chen, K., White, A. T. J., Roseboom, . . . Kalin, N. H. (2014). Differentially methylated plasticity genes in the amygdala of young primates are linked to anxious temperament, an at risk phenotype for anxiety and depressive disorders. *Journal of Neuroscience*, 34, 15548–15556.

Allen, A. P., Kennedy, P. J., Cryan, J. F., Dinan, T. G., & Clarke, G. (2014). Biological and psychological markers of stress in humans: focus on the Trier Social Stress Test. *Neuroscience and Biobehavioral Reviews*, 38, 94–124.

Allen, Y. S., Adrian, T. E., Allen, J. M., Tatemoto, K., Crow, T. J., Bloom, S. R., & Polak, J. M. (1983). Neuropeptide Y distribution in rat brain. *Science*, 221, 877–879.

Allis, C. D., & Jenuwein, T. (2016). The molecular hallmarks of epigenetic control. *Nature Reviews Genetics*, 17, 487–500.

Alloy, L. B., Abramson, L. Y., Urosevic, S., Walshaw, P. D., Nusslock, R., & Neeren, A. M. (2005). The psychosocial context of bipolar disorder: environmental, cognitive, and developmental risk factors. *Clinical Psychology Review*, 25, 1043–1075.

Allsop, S. A., Vander Weele, C. M., Wichmann, R., & Tye, K. M. (2014). Optogenetic insights on the relationship between anxiety-related behaviors and social deficits. *Frontiers in Behavioral Neuroscience*, 8, 241.

Altman, J., & Das, G. D. (1965). Autoradiographic and histological evidence of postnatal hippocampal neurogenesis in rats. *Journal of Comparative Neurology, 124,* 319–336.

Altmann, S. A. (1979). Baboon progressions: order or chaos? A study of one-dimensional group geometry. *Animal Behaviour, 27,* 46–80.

Alural, B., Genc, S., & Haggarty, S. J. (2017). Diagnostic and therapeutic potential of microRNAs in neuropsychiatric disorders: past, present, and future. *Progress in Neuro-Psychopharmacology and Biological Psychiatry, 73,* 87–103.

American Psychiatric Association (1980). *Diagnostic and statistical manual of mental disorders, third edition.* Arlington, VA: American Psychiatric Association Press.

American Psychiatric Association (2013). *Diagnostic and statistical manual of mental disorders, fifth edition.* Arlington, VA: American Psychiatric Association Press.

American Psychological Association (2010). *The road to resilience.* Available at: http://www.apa.org/helpcenter/road-resilience.aspx.

Amodeo, D. A., Grospe, G., Zang, H., Dwivedi, Y., & Ragozzino, M. E. (2017). Cognitive flexibility impairment and reduced frontal cortex BDNF expression in the ouabain model of mania. *Neuroscience, 345,* 229–242.

Amstadter, A. B., Myers, J. M., & Kendler, K. S. (2014). Psychiatric resilience: longitudinal twin study. *British Journal of Psychiatry, 205,* 275–280.

Anacker, C., Luna, V. M., Stevens, G. S., Millette, A., Shores, R., Jimenez, J. C., . . . Hen, R. (2018). Hippocampal neurogenesis confers stress resilience by inhibiting the ventral dentate gyrus. *Nature, 559,* 98–102.

Anacker, C., Scholtz, J., O'Donnell, K. J., Allemang-Grand, R., Diorio, J., Bagot, R. C., . . . Meaney, M. J. (2016). Neuroanatomic differences associated with stress suscepti-bility and resilience. *Biological Psychiatry, 79,* 840–849.

Anderzhanova, E., Kirmeir, T., & Wotjak, C. T. (2017). Animal models in psychiatric re-search: the RDoC system as a new framework for endophenotype-oriented transla-tional neuroscience. *Neurobiology of Stress, 7,* 47–56.

Andreasen, N. C. (1995). Symptoms, signs, and diagnosis of schizophrenia. *Lancet, 346,* 477–481.

Andreasen, N. C. (1999). Understanding the causes of schizophrenia. *New England Journal of Medicine, 340,* 645–647.

Andreassi, J. L., Eggleston, W. B., & Stewart, J. K. (1998). Phenylethanolamine N-methyltransferase mRNA in rat spleen and thymus. *Neuroscience Letters, 241,* 75–78.

Andrews, G., Slade, T., & Peters, L. (1999). Classification in psychiatry: ICD-10 versus DSM-IV. *British Journal of Psychiatry, 174,* 3–5.

Andrews, P. W., & Thomson, J. A. (2009). The bright side of being blue: depression as an adaptation for analyzing complex problems. *Psychological Review, 116,* 620–654.

Andrus, B. M., Blizinsky, K., Vedell, P. T., Dennis, K., Shukla, P. K., Schaffer, D. J., . . . Redei, E. E. (2012). Gene expression patterns in the hippocampus and amygdala of endoge-nous depression and chronic stress models. *Molecular Psychiatry, 17,* 49–61.

Angst, J., & Sellaro, R. (2000). Historical perspectives and natural history of bipolar dis-order. *Biological Psychiatry, 48,* 445–457.

Animals (Scientific Procedures) Act (1986). www.legislation.gov.uk/ukpga/1984/14/contents.

Anonymous (1951). What is stress? *The Lancet, 257,* 277–279.

Anonymous (2017). Accounting for sex in the genome. *Nature Medicine, 23,* 1243.

Antelman, S. M., & Caggiula, A. R. (1996). Oscillation follows drug sensitiza-tion: implications. *Critical Reviews in Neurobiology, 10,* 101–117.

Antelman, S. M., Caggiula, A. R., Kiss, S., Edwards, D. J., Kocan, D., & Stiller, R. (1995). Neurochemical and physiological effects of cocaine oscillate with sequential drug treatment: possibly a major factor in drug variability. *Neuropsychopharmacology, 12*, 297–306.

Antelman, S. M., Caggiula, A. R., Knopf, S., Kocan, D. J., & Edwards, D. J. (1992). Amphetamine or haloperidol 2 weeks earlier antagonized the plasma corticosterone response to amphetamine: evidence for the stressful/foreign nature of drugs. *Psychopharmacology, 107,* 331–336.

Antelman, S. M., Caggiula, A. R., Kucinski, B. J., Fowler, H., Gershon, S., Edwards, D. J., . . . Kocan, D. (1998). The effects of lithium on a potential cycling model of bipolar disorder. *Progress in Neuro-Psychopharmacology and Biological Psychiatry, 22,* 495–510.

Antelman, S. M., Eichler, A. J., Black, C. A., & Kocan, D. (1980). Interchangeability of stress and amphetamine in sensitization. *Science, 207,* 329–331.

Antelman, S. M., Levine, J., & Gershon, S. (2000). Time-dependent sensitization: the odyssey of a scientific heresy from the laboratory to the door of the clinic. *Molecular Psychiatry, 5,* 350–356.

Antoniuk, S., Bijata, M., Ponimaskin, E., & Mlodarczyk, J. (2019). Chronic unpredictable mild stress for modeling depression in rodents: meta-analysis of model reliability. *Neuroscience and Biobehavioral Reviews, 99,* 101–116.

Anyan, J., & Amir, S. (2018). Too depressed to swim or too afraid to stop? A reinterpretation of the forced swim test as a measure of anxiety-like behavior. *Neuropsychopharmacology, 43,* 931–933.

Anzalone, A. V., Randolph, P. B., Davis, J. R., Sousa, A. A., Koblan, L. W., Levy, J. M., . . . Liu, D. R. (2019). Search-and-replace genome editing without double-strand breaks or donor DNA. *Nature, 576,* 149–157.

Aoued, H. S., Sannigrahi, S., Doshi, N., Morrison, F. G., Linsenbaum, H., Hunter, S. C., . . . Dias, B. G. (2019). Reversing behavioral, neuroanatomical, and germline influences of intergenerational stress. *Biological Psychiatry, 85,* 248–256.

Arakane, F., King, S. R., Du, Y., Kallen, C. B., Walsh, L. P., Watari, H., Stocco, D. M., Strauss, J. F., III. (1997). Phosphorylation of steroidogenic acute regulatory protein (StAR) modulates its steroidogenic activity. *Journal of Biological Chemistry, 272,* 32565–32662.

Arguello, P. A., Markx, S., Gogos, J. A., & Karayiourgou, M. (2010). Development of animal models of schizophrenia. *Disease Models and Mechanisms, 3,* 22–26.

Arling, G. L., & Harlow, H. F. (1967). Effects of social deprivation on maternal behavior in rhesus monkeys. *Journal of Comparative and Physiological Psychology, 64,* 371–377.

Armario, A., Escorihuela, R. M., & Nadal, R. (2008). Long-term neuroendocrine and behavioural effects of a single exposure to stress in adult animals. *Neuroscience and Biobehavioral Reviews, 32,* 1121–1135.

Armbruster, B. N., Li, X., Pausch, M. H., Herlitze, S., & Roth, B. L. (2007). Evolving the lock to fit the key to create a family of G protein-coupled receptors potently activated by an inert ligand. *Proceedings of the National Academy of Sciences USA, 104,* 5163–5168.

Armstadter, A. B., Myers, J. M., & Kendler, K. S. (2014). Psychiatric resilience: longitudinal twin study. *British Journal of Psychiatry, 205,* 275–280.

Arnsten, A. F. T. (2009). Stress signaling pathways that impair prefrontal cortex structure and function. *Nature Reviews Neuroscience, 10,* 410–422.

Arnsten, A. F. T. (2011). Prefrontal cortical network connections: key site of vulnerability in stress and schizophrenia. *International Journal of Developmental Neuroscience, 29,* 215–223.

Arnsten, A. F. T. (2015). Stress weakens prefrontal networks: molecular insults to higher cognition. *Nature Neuroscience, 18*, 1376–1385.

Aronsson, F., Lannebo, C., Paucar, M., Brask, J., Kristensson, K., & Karlsson, H. (2002). Persistence of viral RNA in the brain of offspring to mice infected with influenza A/WSN/33 during pregnancy. *Journal of Neurovirology, 8*, 353–357.

Ashley, E. A. (2015). The Precision Medicine Initiative: a new national effort. *Journal of the American Medical Association, 313*, 2119–2120.

Ashok, A. H., Marques, T. R., Jauhar, S., Nour, M. M., Goodwin, G. M., Young, A. H., & Howes, O. D. (2017). The dopamine hypothesis of bipolar affective disorder: the state of the art and implications for treatment. *Molecular Psychiatry, 22*, 666–679.

Ashokan, A., Sivasubramanian, M., & Mitra, R. (2016). Seeding stress resilience through inoculation. *Neural Plasticity, 2016*, 4928081.

Asmundson, G. J. G., Coons, M. J., Taylor, S., & Katz, J. (2002). PTSD and the experience of pain: research and clinical implications of shared vulnerability and mutual maintenance models. *Canadian Journal of Psychiatry, 47*, 930–937.

Atladóttir, H. Ó., Thorsen, P., Østergaard, L., Schendel, D. E., Lemcke, S., Abdallah, M., & Parner, E. T. (2010). Maternal infections requiring hospitalization during pregnancy and autism spectrum disorders. *Journal of Autism and Developmental Disorders, 40*, 1423–1430.

Auden, W. H. (1947). *The age of anxiety.* New York, NY: Random House.

Aus der Muhlen, K., & Ockenfels, H. (1969). Morphologische veranderungen im diencephalon und telencephalon nach storngen des regelkreises adenohypophysenebennierenrinde. III. ergebnisse beim meerschweinchen nach verabeichung von cortison und hydrocortison. *Zeitschrift fur Zellforschung, 93*, 126–138.

Autism Speaks, Inc. (2013). Autism advocacy in the community: a parent perspective. https://www.autismspeaks.org/sites/default/files/docs/autism_advocacy_in_the_community_-_a_parent_perspective.pdf.

Ayhan, Y., Abazyan, B., Nomura, J., Kim, R., Ladenheim, B., Krasnova, I. N., ... Pletnikov, M. V. (2011). Differential effects of prenatal and postnatal expressions of mutant human DISC1 on neurobehavioral phenotypes in transgenic mice: evidence for neurodevelopmental origin of major psychiatric disorders. *Molecular Psychiatry, 16*, 293–306.

Ayhan, Y., McFarland, R., & Pletnikov, M. V. (2016). Animal models of gene-environment interaction in schizophrenia: a dimensional perspective. *Progress in Neurobiology, 136*, 1–27.

Ayhan, Y., Sawa, A., Ross, C. A., & Pletnikov, M. V. (2009). Animal models of gene-environment interactions in schizophrenia. *Behavioural Brain Research, 204*, 274–281.

Bagot, R. C., Cates, H. M., Purushothalaman, I., Lorsch, Z. S., Walker, D. M., Wang, J., ... Nestler, E. J. (2016). Circuit-wide transcriptional profiling reveals brain region-specific gene networks regulating depression susceptibility. *Neuron, 90*, 969–983.

Bagot, R. C., Cates, H. M., Purushothalaman, I., Vialou, V., Heller, E. A., Yieh, L., ... Nestler, E. J. (2017). Ketamine and imipramine reverse transcriptional signatures of susceptibility and induce resilience-specific gene expression profiles. *Biological Psychiatry, 81*, 285–295.

Bagot, R. C., LaBonté, B., Peña, C. J., & Nestler, E. J. (2014). Epigenetic signaling in psychiatric disorders: stress and depression. *Dialogues in Clinical Neuroscience, 16*, 281–295.

Bagot, R. C., Parise, E. M., Peña, C. J., Zhang, H.-X., Maze, I., Chaudhury, D., ... Nestler, E. J. (2015). Ventral hippocampal afferents to the nucleus accumbens regulate susceptibility to depression. *Nature Communications, 6*, 7062.

Bains, J. S., Cusulin, J. I. W., & Inoue, W. (2015). Stress-related synaptic plasticity in the hypothalamus. *Nature Reviews Neuroscience, 16*, 377–388.

Baker, J. T., Germine, L. T., Ressler, K. J., Rauch, S. L., & Carlezon, W. A., Jr. (2018). Digital devices and continuous telemetry: opportunities for aligning psychiatry and neuroscience. *Neuropsychopharmacology, 43*, 2499–2503.

Baker, M. (2011). Inside the minds of mice and men. *Nature, 475*, 123–128.

Bakshi, V. P., & Kalin, N. H. (2000). Corticotropin-releasing hormone and animal models of anxiety: gene-environment interactions. *Biological Psychiatry, 48*, 1175–1198.

Bale, T. D., Abel, T., Akil, H., Carlezon, W. A., Moghaddam, B., Nestler, E. J., . . . Thompson, S. M. (2019). The critical importance of basic animal research for neuropsychiatric disorders. *Neuropsychopharmacology, 44*, 1349–1353.

Bale, T. D., Picetti, R., Contarino, A., Koob, G. F., Vale, W. W., & Lee, K.-F. (2002). Mice deficient for both corticotropin-releasing factor receptor 1 (CRFR1) and CRFR2 have an impaired stress response and display sexually dichotomous anxiety-like behavior. *Journal of Neuroscience, 22*, 193–199.

Bale, T. L., Baram, T. Z., Brown, A. S., Goldstein, J. M., Insel, T. R., McCarthy, M. M., . . . Nestler, E .J. (2010). Early life programming and neurodevelopmental disorders. *Biological Psychiatry, 68*, 314–319.

Bale, T. L., Contarino, A., Smith, G. W., Chan, R., Gold, L. H., Sawchenko, P. E., . . . Lee, K.-F. (2000). Mice deficient for corticotropin-releasing hormone receptor-2 display anxiety-like behavior and are hypersensitive to stress. *Nature Genetics, 24*, 410–414.

Bale, T. L., & Vale, W. W. (2003). Increased depression-like behaviors in corticotropin-releasing factor receptor-2-deficient mice: sexually dichotomous responses. *Journal of Neuroscience, 23*, 5295–5301.

Bale, T. L., & Vale, W. W. (2004). CRF and CRF receptors: role in stress responsivity and other behaviors. *Annual Review of Pharmacology and Toxicology, 44*, 525–557.

Ballet, G. (1903). *Traité de pathologie mentale*. Paris, France: Doin.

Balsalobre, A., Brown, S. A., Marcacci, L., Tronche, F., Kellendonk, C., Reichardt, H. M., . . . Schibler, U. (2000). Resetting circadian time in peripheral tissues by glucocorticoid signaling. *Science, 289*, 2344–2347.

Balu, D. T., & Coyle, J. T. (2018). Altered CREB binding to activity-dependent genes in serine racemase deficient mice, a mouse model of schizophrenia. *ACS Chemical Neuroscience, 9*, 2205–2209.

Balu, D. T., Li, Y., Puhl, M. D., Benneyworth, M. A., Basu, A. C., Takagi, S., . . . Coyle, J. T. (2013). Multiple risk pathways for schizophrenia converge in serine racemase knockout mice, a mouse model of NMDA receptor hypofunction. *Proceedings of the National Academy of Sciences USA, 110*, E2400–E2409.

Balusu, S., Van Wonterghem, E., De Rycke, R., Raemdonck, K., Stremersch, S., Gevaert, K., . . . Vandenbroucke, R. E. (2016). Identification of a novel mechanism of blood-brain communication during peripheral inflammation via choroid plexus-derived extracellular vesicles. *EMBO Molecular Medicine, 8*, 1162–1183.

Banerjee, S., Riordan, M., & Bhat, M. A. (2014). Genetic aspects of autism spectrum disorders: insights from animal models. *Frontiers in Cellular Neuroscience, 8*, 58.

Bangasser, D. A., Zhang, X., Garachh, V., Hanhauser, E., & Valentino, R. J. (2011). Sexual dimorphism in locus coeruleus dendritic morphology: a structural basis for sex differences in emotional arousal. *Physiology and Behavior, 103*, 342–351.

Banks, W. A., Kastin, A. J., & Broadwell, R. D. (1995). Passage of cytokines across the blood-brain barrier. *Neuroimmunomodulation, 2*, 241–248.

Barker, D. J. P. (1990). The fetal and infant origins of adult disease. *British Medical Journal*, *301*, 1111.

Barker, D. J. P. (1995). Fetal origins of coronary heart disease. *British Medical Journal*, *311*, 171–174.

Barlow, D. H. (2002). *Anxiety and its disorders: the nature and treatment of anxiety and panic* (2nd ed.). New York, NY: Guilford Press.

Barros, V. G., Rodríguez, P., Martijena, I. D., Pérez, A., Molina, V. A., & Antonelli, M. C. (2006). Prenatal stress and early adoption effects on benzodiazepine receptors and anxiogenic behavior in the adult rat brain. *Synapse*, *60*, 609–618.

Bauman, M. D., Iosif, A.-M., Smith, S. E. P., Bregere, C., Amaral, D. G., & Patterson, P. H. (2014). Activation of the maternal immune system during pregnancy alters behavioral development of rhesus monkey offspring. *Biological Psychiatry*, *75*, 332–341.

Baxter, A. J., Vos, T., Scott, K. M., & Ferrari, A. J. (2014). The global burden of anxiety disorders in 2010. *Psychological Medicine*, *44*, 2363–2374.

Beards, S., Gayer-Anderson, C., Borges, S., Dewey, M. E., Fisher, H. L., & Morgan, C. (2013). Life events and psychosis: a review and meta-analysis. *Schizophrenia Bulletin*, *39*, 740–747.

Beas, B. S., Wright, B. J., Skirzewski, M., Leng, Y., Hyun, J. H., Koita, O., . . . Penzo, M. A. (2018). The locus coeruleus drives disinhibition in the midline thalamus via a dopaminergic mechanism. *Nature Neuroscience*, *21*, 963–973.

Beaulieu, J.-M., & Gainetdinov, R. R. (2011). The physiology, signaling, and pharmacology of dopamine receptors. *Pharmacological Reviews*, *63*, 182–217.

Beaulieu, J.-M., Zhang, X., Rodriguiz, R. M., Sotnikova, T. D., Cools, M. J., Wetsel, W. C., . . . Caron, M. G. (2008). Role of GSK3 beta in behavioral abnormalities induced by serotonin deficiency. *Proceedings of the National Academy of Sciences USA*, *105*, 1333–1338.

Beck, A. T., & Bredemeier, K. (2016). A unified model of depression: integrating clinical, cognitive, biological, and evolutionary perspectives. *Clinical Psychological Science*, *4*, 596–619.

Becker, E. B. E., & Stoodley, C. J. (2013). Autism spectrum disorder and the cerebellum. *International Review of Neurobiology*, *113*, 1–34.

Beery, A. K., & Zucker, I. (2011). Sex bias in neuroscience and biomedical research. *Neuroscience and Biobehavioral Reviews*, *35*, 565–572.

Behringer, R., Gertsenstein, M., Nagy, K. V., & Nagy, A. (2014). *Manipulating the mouse embryo: a laboratory manual* (4th ed.). New York, NY: Cold Spring Harbor Laboratory Press.

Bekelman, J. E., Li, Y., & Gross, C. P. (2003). Scope and impact of financial conflicts of interest in biomedical research: a systematic review. *Journal of the American Medical Association*, *289*, 454–465.

Belmaker, R. H. (2004). Bipolar disorder. *New England Journal of Medicine*, *351*, 476–486.

Belujon, P., & Grace, A. A. (2015). Regulation of dopamine system responsivity and its adaptive and pathological response to stress. *Proceedings of the Royal Society B*, *282*, 2014–2516.

Belzung, C. (2014). Innovative drugs to treat depression: did animal models fail to be predictive or did clinical trials fail to detect effects? *Neuropsychopharmacology*, *39*, 1041–1051.

Belzung, C., & Griebel, G. (2001). Measuring normal and pathological anxiety-like behavior in mice: a review. *Behavioural Brain Research*, *125*, 141–149.

Belzung, C., & Lemoine, M. (2011). Criteria of validity for animal models of psychiatric disorders: focus on anxiety disorders and depression. *Biology of Mood and Anxiety Disorders, 1,* 9.

Ben-Ari, Y. (2015). Is birth a critical period in the pathogenesis of autism spectrum disorders? *Nature Reviews Neuroscience, 16,* 498–505.

Ben-Ari, Y. (2017). NKCC1 chloride importer antagonists attenuate many neurological and psychiatric disorders. *Trends in Neurosciences, 40,* 536–554.

Benarroch, E. E. (2012). Periaqueductal gray: an interface for behavioral control. *Neurology, 78,* 210–217.

Benatti, C., Valensisi, C., Blom, J. M. C., Alboni, S., Montanari, C., Ferrari, F., . . . Tascedda, F. (2012). Transcriptional profiles underlying vulnerability and resilience in rats exposed to an acute unavoidable stress. *Journal of Neuroscience Research, 90,* 2103–2115.

Bender, R. E., & Alloy, L. B. (2011). Life stress and kindling in bipolar disorder: review of evidence and integration with emerging biopsychosocial theories. *Clinical Psychology Review, 31,* 383–398.

Benison, S., & Barger, A. C. (1987). *Walter B. Cannon: the life and times of a young scientist.* Cambridge, MA: Belknap Press.

Benno, R., Smirnova, Y., Vera, S., Liggett, A., & Schanz, N. (2009). Exaggerated responses to stress in the BTBR T+tf/J mouse: an unusual behavioral phenotype. *Behavioural Brain Research, 197,* 462–465.

Bennur, S., Shankaranarayana Rao, B. S., Pawlak, R., Strickland, S., McEwen, B. S., & Chattarji, S. (2007). Stress-induced spine loss in the medial amygdala is mediated by tissue-plasminogen activator. *Neuroscience, 144,* 8–16.

Benzer, S. (1967). Behavioral mutants of *Drosophila* isolated by countercurrent distribution. *Proceedings of the National Academy of Sciences USA, 58,* 1112–1119.

Berenbaum, H. (2013). Classification and psychopathology research. *Journal of Abnormal Psychology, 122,* 894–901.

Bergink, V., Larsen, J. T., Hillegers, M. H. J., Dahl, S. K., Stevens, H., Mortensen, P. B., . . . Munk-Olsen, T. (2016). Childhood adverse life events and parental psychopathology as risk factors for bipolar disorder. *Translational Psychiatry, 6,* e929.

Bergström, A., Jayatissa, M. N., Thykjaer, T., & Wiborg, O. (2007). Molecular pathways associated with stress resilience and drug resistance in the chronic mild stress rat model of depression: a gene expression study. *Journal of Molecular Neuroscience, 33,* 201–215.

Bernard, C. (1974). *Lectures on the phenomena of life common to animals and plants.* H. E. Hoff, R. Guillemin, & L. Guillemin (Trans.). Springfield, IL: Charles C. Thomas (original work published in 1878).

Bertocchi, I., Oberto, A., Longo, A., Mele, P., Sabetta, M., Bartolomucci, A., . . . Eva, C. (2011). Regulatory functions of limbic Y1 receptors in body weight and anxiety uncovered by conditional knockout and maternal care. *Proceedings of the National Academy of Sciences USA, 108,* 19395–19400.

Berton, O., Hahn, C.-G., & Thase, M. E. (2012). Are we getting closer to valid translational models for major depression? *Science, 338,* 75–79.

Berton, O., McClung, C. A., DiLeone, R. J., Krishnan, V., Renthal, W., Russo, S. J., . . . Nestler, E. J. (2006). Essential role of BDNF in the mesolimbic dopamine pathway in social defeat stress. *Science, 311,* 864–868.

Besedovsky, H. O., del Rey, A. E., & Sorkin, E. (1981). Lymphokine-containing supernatants from Con A-stimulated cells increase corticosterone blood levels. *Journal of Immunology*, *126*, 385–389.

Besedovsky, H. O., del Rey, A. E., Sorkin, E., Da Prada, M., Burri, R., & Honegger, C. (1983). The immune response evokes changes in brain noradrenergic neurons. *Science*, *221*, 564–566.

Besedovsky, H. O., del Rey, A., Sorkin, E., Da Prada, M., & Keller, H. H. (1979). Immunoregulation mediated by the sympathetic nervous system. *Cellular Immunology*, *48*, 346–355.

Besedovsky, H. O., del Rey, A., Sorkin, E., & Dinarello, C. A. (1986). Immunoregulatory feedback between interleukin-1 and glucocorticoid hormones. *Science*, *233*, 652–654.

Beutler, B., & Rietschel, E. T. (2003). Innate immune sensing and its roots: the story of endotoxin. *Nature Reviews Immunology*, *3*, 169–176.

Beversdorf, D. Q., Manning, S. E., Hillier, A., Anderson, S. L., Nordgren, R. E., Walters, S. E., ... Bauman, M. L. (2005). Timing of prenatal stressors and autism. *Journal of Autism and Developmental Disorders*, *35*, 471–479.

Beyer, D. K. E., & Freund, N. (2017). Animal models for bipolar disorder: from bedside to the cage. *International Journal of Bipolar Disorders*, *5*, 35.

Bhatnagar, S., & Dallman, M. (1998). Neuroanatomical basis for facilitation of hypothalamic-pituitary-adrenal responses to a novel stressor after chronic stress. *Neuroscience*, *84*, 1025–1039.

Bhatnagar, S., Huber, R., Nowak, N., & Trotter, P. (2002). Lesions of the posterior paraventricular thalamus block habituation of hypothalamic-pituitary-adrenal responses to repeated restraint. *Journal of Neuroendocrinology*, *14*, 403–410.

Biaggioni, I., & Robertson, D. (2018). Adrenoceptor agonists and sympathomimetic drugs. In B. G. Katzung (Ed.), *Basic and clinical pharmacology* (14th ed.) (online). New York, NY: McGraw-Hill.

Bilder, R. M., Howe, A. S., Sabb, F. W., & Parker, D. S. (2013). Multilevel models from biology to psychology: mission impossible? *Journal of Abnormal Psychology*, *122*, 917–927.

Binder, E., Malki, K., Paya-Cano, J. L., Fernandes, C., Aitchison, K. J., Mathé, A. A., Sluyter, F., & Schalkwyk, L. C. (2011). Antidepressants and the resilience to early-life stress in inbred mouse strains. *Pharmacogenetics and Genomics*, *21*, 779–789.

Binder, E. B., & Nemeroff, C. B. (2010). The CRF system, stress, depression and anxiety: insights from human genetic studies. *Molecular Psychiatry*, *15*, 574–588.

Binkerd, P. E., Rowland, J. M., Nau, H., & Hendrickx, A. G. (1988). Evaluation of valproic acid (VPA) developmental toxicity and pharmacokinetics in Sprague-Dawley rats. *Fundamental and Applied Toxicology*, *11*, 485–493.

Bipolar Disorder and Schizophrenia Working Group of the Psychiatric Genomics Consortium (2018). Genomic dissection of bipolar disorder and schizophrenia, including 28 subphenotypes. *Cell*, *173*, 1705–1715.

Birley, J., & Brown, G. W. (1970). Crisis and life changes preceding the onset of relapse of acute schizophrenia: clinical aspects. *British Journal of Psychiatry*, *16*, 327–333.

Bisgaard, C. F., Jayatissa, M. N., Enghild, J. J., Sanchéz, C., Artemychyn, R., & Wiborg, O. (2007). Proteomic investigation of the ventral rat hippocampus links DRP-2 to escitalopram treatment resistance and SNAP to stress resilience in the chronic mild stress model of depression. *Journal of Molecular Neuroscience*, *32*, 132–144.

Blalock, A. (1930). Experimental shock: the cause of the low blood pressure produced by muscle injury. *Archives of Surgery, 20,* 959–996.

Blaze, J., & Roth, T. L. (2015). Evidence from clinical and animal model studies of the long-term and transgenerational impact of stress on DNA methylation. *Seminars in Cell and Developmental Biology, 43,* 76–84.

Blechert, J., Michael, T., Grossman, P., Lajtman, M., & Wilhelm, F. H. (2007). Autonomic and respiratory characteristics of posttraumatic stress disorder and panic disorder. *Psychosomatic Medicine, 69,* 935–943.

Bleuler, M. (1963). Conception of schizophrenia within the last fifty years and today. *Proceedings of the Royal Society of Medicine, 56,* 945–952.

Bloom, D. (2002). *Love at Goon Park: Harry Harlow and the science of affection.* New York, NY: Perseus Press.

Bluett, R. J., Báldi, R., Haymer, A., Gaulden, A. D., Hartley, N. D., Parrish, W. P., ... Patel, S. (2017). Endocannabinoid signalling modulates susceptibility to traumatic stress exposure. *Nature Communications, 8,* 14782.

Blum, I. D., Lamont, E. W., & Abizaid, A. (2012). Competing clocks: metabolic status moderates signals from the master circadian pacemaker. *Neuroscience and Biobehavioral Reviews, 36,* 254–270.

Bock, J., Wainstock, T., Braun, K., & Segal, M. (2015). Stress in utero: prenatal programming of brain plasticity and cognition. *Biological Psychiatry, 78,* 315–326.

Boksa, P. (2004). Animal models of obstetric complications in relation to schizophrenia. *Brain Research Reviews, 45,* 1–17.

Boksa, P. (2010). Effects of prenatal infection on brain development and behavior: a review of findings from animal models. *Brain, Behavior, and Immunity, 24,* 881–897.

Boksa, P., & El-Khodor, B. F. (2003). Birth insult interacts with stress at adulthood to alter dopaminergic function in animal models: possible implications for schizophrenia and other disorders. *Neuroscience and Biobehavioral Reviews, 27,* 91–101.

Bolivar, V. J., Walters, S. R., & Phoenix, J. L. (2007). Assessing autism-like behavior in mice: variations in social interactions among inbred strains. *Behavioural Brain Research, 176,* 21–26.

Bolon, B., & Ward, J. M. (2015). Anatomy and physiology of the developing mouse and placenta. In B. Bolon (Ed.), *Pathology of the developing mouse: a systematic approach* (pp. 39–98). Boca Raton, FL: Chapman and Hall/CRC Press.

Bolton, J. L., Molet, J., Ivy, A., & Baram, T. Z. (2017). New insights into early-life stress and behavioral outcomes. *Current Opinion in Behavioral Sciences, 14,* 133–139.

Borges, R., Gandia, L., & Carbone, E. (2018). Old and emerging concepts on adrenal chromaffin cell stimulus-secretion coupling. *Pflugers Archiv – European Journal of Physiology, 470,* 1–6.

Bosch, O. J., Krömer, S. A., & Neumann, I. D. (2006). Prenatal stress: opposite effects on anxiety and hypothalamic expression of vasopressin and corticotropin-releasing hormone in rats selectively bred for high and low emotionality. *European Journal of Neuroscience, 23,* 541–551.

Boullerne, A. I. (2011). Neurophysiology to neuroanatomy: the transition from Claude Bernard to Louis Antoine Ranvier. *Archives Italiennes de Biologie, 149* (Suppl.), 38–46.

Bourgeron, T. (2015). From the genetic architecture to synaptic plasticity in autism spectrum disorder. *Nature Reviews Neuroscience, 16,* 551–563.

Bourin, M. (2015). Animal models for screening anxiolytic-like drugs: a perspective. *Dialogues in Clinical Neuroscience, 17,* 295–303.

Bourin, M., & Hascoët, M. (2003). The mouse light/dark box test. *European Journal of Pharmacology, 463,* 55–65.

Bourin, M., Masse, F., Dailly, E., & Hascoët, M. (2005). Anxiolytic-like effect of milnacipran in the four-plate test in mice: mechanism of action. *Pharmacology, Biochemistry and Behavior, 81,* 645–656.

Bousman, C. A., Forbes, M., Jayaram, M., Eyre, H., Reynolds, C. F., Berk, M., . . . Ng, C. (2017). Antidepressant prescribing in the precision medicine era: a prescriber's primer on pharmacogenetic tools. *BMC Psychiatry, 17,* 60.

Bousman, C. A., & Hopwood, M. (2016). Commercial pharmacogenetic-based decision-support tools in psychiatry. *Lancet Psychiatry, 3,* 585–590.

Bouton, M. E., Mineka, S., & Barlow, D. H. (2001). A modern learning theory perspective on the etiology of panic disorder. *Psychological Review, 108,* 4–32.

Bowlby, J. (1951). Maternal care and mental health. *Bulletin of the World Health Organization, 3,* 355–534.

Bradley, A. J., & Dinan, T. G. (2010). A systematic review of hypothalamic-pituitary-adrenal axis function in schizophrenia: implications for mortality. *Journal of Psychopharmacology, 24* (Suppl. 4), 91–118.

Braff, D. L., & Geyer, M. A. (1990). Sensorimotor gating and schizophrenia: human and animal studies. *Archives of General Psychiatry, 47,* 181–188.

Braff, D. L., Grillon, C., & Geyer, M. (1992). Gating and habituation of the startle reflex in schizophrenic patients. *Archives of General Psychiatry, 49,* 206–215.

Branchi, I., Santarelli, S., D'Andrea, I., & Alleva, E. (2013). Not all stressors are equal: early social enrichment favors resilience to social but not physical stress in male mice. *Hormones and Behavior, 63,* 503–509.

Bräunig, P., & Krüger, S. (1999). Karl Ludwig Kahlbaum, M.D. 1828–1899. *American Journal of Psychiatry, 156,* 989.

Bredemann, T. M., & McMahon, L. L. (2014). 17ß estradiol increases resilience and improves hippocampal synaptic function in helpless ovariectomized rats. *Psychoneuroendocrinology, 42,* 77–88.

Breslow, M. J. (1992). Regulation of adrenal medullary and cortical blood flow. *American Journal of Physiology, 262,* H1317–H1330.

Brielmaier, J., Matteson, P. G., Silverman, J. L., Senerth, J. M., Kelly, S., Genestine, M., . . . Crawley, J. N. (2012). Autism-relevant social abnormalities and cognitive deficits in Engrailed-2 knockout mice. *PLoS ONE, 7,* e40914.

Brindley, R. L., Bauer, M. B., Blakely, R. D., & Currie, K. P. M. (2016). An interplay between the serotonin transporter (SERT) and 5-HT receptors controls stimulus-secretion coupling in sympathoadrenal chromaffin cells. *Neuropharmacology, 110,* 438–448.

Brockhurst, J., Cheleuitte-Nieves, C., Buckmaster, C. L., Schatzberg, A. F., & Lyons, D. M. (2015). Stress inoculation modeled in mice. *Translational Psychiatry, 5,* e537.

Brodkin, E. S. (2007). BALB/c mice: low sociability and other phenotypes that may be relevant to autism. *Behavioural Brain Research, 176,* 53–65.

Bromley, R. L., Mawer, G., Clayton-Smith, J., & Baker, G. A. (2008). Autism spectrum disorders following in utero exposure to antiepileptic drugs. *Neurology, 71,* 1923–1924.

Bronson, S. L., & Bale, T. L. (2014). Prenatal stress-induced increases in placental inflammation and offspring hyperactivity are male-specific and ameliorated by maternal anti-inflammatory treatment. *Endocrinology, 155,* 2635–2646.

Bronson, S. L., & Bale, T. L. (2016). The placenta as a mediator of stress effects on neurodevelopmental programming. *Neuropsychopharmacology Reviews, 41,* 207–218.

Bronstein, P. M., Levine, M. J., & Marcus, M. (1975). A rat's first bite: the nongenetic, cross-generational transfer of information. *Journal of Comparative and Physiological Psychology, 89*, 295–298.

Brown, A. S. (2011). Exposure to prenatal infection and risk of schizophrenia. *Frontiers in Psychiatry, 2*, 63.

Brown, A. S., Begg, M. D., Gravenstein, S., Schaefer, C. A, Wyatt, R. J., Bresnahan, M. A., . . . Susser, E. S. (2004). Serologic evidence for prenatal influenza in the etiology of schizophrenia. *Archives of General Psychiatry, 61*, 774–780.

Brown, A. S., & Derkits, E. J. (2010). Prenatal infection and schizophrenia: a review of epidemiological and translational studies. *American Journal of Psychiatry, 167*, 261–280.

Brown, A. S., Schaefer, C. A., Quesenberry, C. P., Jr., Liu, L., Babulas, V. P., & Susser, E. S. (2005). Maternal exposure to toxoplasmosis and risk of schizophrenia in adult offspring. *American Journal of Psychiatry, 162*, 767–773.

Brown, A. S., Schaefer, C. A., Wyatt, R. J., Goetz, R., Begg, M. D., Gorman, J. M., & Susser, E. S. (2000). Maternal exposure to respiratory infections and adult schizophrenia spectrum disorders: a prospective birth cohort study. *Schizophrenia Bulletin, 26*, 287–295.

Brown, G. W., & Birley, J. (1968). Crisis and life changes and the onset of schizophrenia. *Journal of Health and Social Behavior, 9*, 203–214.

Bruchas, M. R., Schindler, A. G., Shankar, H., Messinger, D. I., Miyatake, M., Land, B. B., . . . Chavkin, C. (2011). Selective p38α MAPK deletion in serotonergic neurons produces stress resilience in models of depression and addiction. *Neuron, 71*, 498–511.

Buckingham, J. C., & Flower, R. J. (2017). Annexin A1. In G. Fink (Ed.), *Stress: neuroendocrinology and neurobiology. Handbook of stress*, Vol. 2 (pp. 257–264). London, UK: Academic Press.

Buckingham, J. C., John, C. D., Solito, E., Tierney, T., Flower, R. J., Christian, H., & Morris, J. (2006). Annexin 1, glucocorticoids, and the neuroendocrine-immune interface. *Annals of the New York Academy of Sciences, 1088*, 396–409.

Buckley, P. F., & Miller, B. J. (2017). Personalized medicine for schizophrenia. *NPJ Schizophrenia, 3*, 2.

Buijs, R. M. (2013). The autonomic nervous system: a balancing act. In R. M. Buijs & D. F. Swaab (Eds.), *Handbook of clinical neurology*, Vol. 117 (pp. 1–11). Amsterdam, The Netherlands: Elsevier.

Buijs, R. M., La Fleur, S. E., Wortel, J., van Heyningen, C., Zuiddam, L., Mettenleiter, T. C., . . . Niijima, A. (2003). The suprachiasmatic nucleus balances sympathetic and parasympathetic output to peripheral organs through separate preautonomic neurons. *Journal of Comparative Neurology, 464*, 36–48.

Buijs, R. M., Wortel, J., Van Heerikhuize, J. J., Feenstra, M. G. P., Ter Horst, G. J., Romijn, H. J., & Kalsbeek, A. (1999). Anatomical and functional demonstration of a multisynaptic suprachiasmatic nucleus adrenal (cortex) pathway. *European Journal of Neuroscience, 11*, 1535–1544.

Buka, S. L., Cannon, T. D., Torrey, E. F., & Yolken, R. H. (2008). Maternal exposure to herpes simplex virus and risk of psychosis among adult offspring. *Biological Psychiatry, 63*, 809–815.

Bulik-Sullivan, B., Finucane, H. K., Anttila, V., Gusev, A., Day, F. R., Loh, P.-R., . . . Neale, B. M. (2015). An atlas of genetic correlations across human diseases and traits. *Nature Genetics, 47*, 1236–1241.

Burgdorf, J., Moskal, J. R., Brudzynski, S. M., & Panksepp, J. (2013). Rats selectively bred for low levels of play-induced 50 KHz vocalizations as a model of autism spectrum disorders: a role for NMDA receptors. *Behavioural Brain Research, 251*, 18–24.

Burgdorf, K. S., Trabjerg, B. B., Pedersen, M. G., Nissen, J., Banasik, K., Pedersen, O. B., . . . Ullum, H. (2019). Large-scale study of *Toxoplasma* and cytomegalovirus shows an association between infection and serious psychiatric disorders. *Brain, Behavior, and Immunity, 79*, 152–158. https://doi.org/10.1016/j.bbi.2019.01.026.

Burne, T., Scott, E., van Swinderen, B., Hilliard, M., Reinhard, J., Claudianos, C., . . . McGrath, J. (2011). Big ideas for small brains: what can psychiatry learn from worms, flies, bees and fish? *Molecular Psychiatry, 16*, 7–16.

Bzdok, D., & Meyer-Lindenberg, A. (2017). Machine learning for precision psychiatry: opportunities and challenges. *Biological Psychiatry: Cognitive Neuroscience and Neuroimaging, 3*, 223–230.

Caggiula, A. R., Antelman, S. M., Palmer, A. M., Kiss, S., Edwards, D. J., & Kocan, D. (1996). The effects of ethanol on striatal dopamine and frontal cortical D-[3H] aspartate efflux oscillate with repeated treatment: relevance to individual differences in drug responsiveness. *Neuropsychopharmacology, 15*, 125–132.

Cai, N., Chang, S., Li, Y., Li, Q., Hu, J., Liang, J., . . . Flint, J. (2015). Molecular signatures of major depression. *Current Biology, 25*, 1146–1156.

Calcia, M. A., Bonsall, D. R., Bloomfield, P. S., Selvaraj, S., Barichello, T., & Howes, O. D. (2016). Stress and neuroinflammation: a systematic review of the effects of stress on microglia and the implications for mental health. *Psychopharmacology, 233*, 1637–1650.

Caldji, C., Tannenbaum, B., Sharma, S., Francis, D., Plotsky, P. M., & Meaney, M. J. (1998). Maternal care during infancy regulates the development of neural systems mediating the expression of fearfulness in the rat. *Proceedings of the National Academy of Sciences USA, 95*, 5335–5340.

Cameron, N., Del Corpo, A., Diorio, J., McAllister, K., Sharma, S., & Meaney, M. J. (2008). Maternal programming of sexual behavior and hypothalamic-pituitary-gonadal function in the female rat. *PLoS One, 3*, e2210.

Campos, C. A., Bowen, A. J., Roman, C. W., & Palmiter, R. D. (2018). Encoding of danger by parabrachial CGRP neurons. *Nature, 555*, 617–622.

Canetta, S. E., Bao, Y., Co, M. D. T., Ennis, F. A., Cruz, J., Terajima, M., . . . Brown, A. S. (2014). Serological documentation of maternal influenza exposure and bipolar disorder in adult offspring. *American Journal of Psychiatry, 171*, 557–563.

Cannon, B. (1994). Walter Bradford Cannon: reflections on the man and his contributions. *International Journal of Stress Management, 1*, 145–158.

Cannon, W. B. (1902). Movements of the intestines studied by means of the Röentgen rays. *Journal of Medical Research, 7*, 72–75.

Cannon, W. B. (1914a). The emergency function of the adrenal medulla in pain and the major emotions. *American Journal of Physiology, 33*, 356–372.

Cannon, W. B. (1914b). The interrelations of emotions as suggested by recent physiological researches. *American Journal of Psychology, 25*, 256–282.

Cannon, W. B. (1915). *Bodily changes in pain, hunger, fear and rage*. New York, NY: Appleton-Century.

Cannon, W. B. (1919). Studies on the conditions of activity of adrenal glands. V. The isolated heart as an indicator of adrenal secretion induced by pain, asphyxia and excitement. *American Journal of Physiology, 50*, 399–432.

Cannon, W. B. (1922). Studies in experimental traumatic shock: evidence of a toxic factor in wound shock. *Archives of Surgery, 4,* 1–22.

Cannon, W. B. (1927). The James-Lange theory of emotions: a critical examination and an alternative theory. *American Journal of Psychology, 39,* 106–124.

Cannon, W. B. (1928). The mechanisms of emotional disturbance of bodily functions. *New England Journal of Medicine, 198,* 877–884.

Cannon, W. B. (1932). *The wisdom of the body.* New York, NY: W. W. Norton.

Cannon, W. B. (1935). Stresses and strains of homeostasis. *American Journal of Medical Science, 189,* 1–14.

Cannon, W. B. (1940). The adrenal medulla. *Bulletin of the New York Academy of Medicine, 16,* 3–13.

Cannon, W. B. (1941). The body physiologic and the body politic. *Science, 93,* 1–10.

Cannon, W. B. (1942). Voodoo death. *American Anthropologist, 44,* 169–181.

Cannon, W. B. (1945). *The way of an investigator.* New York, NY: Hafner (reprinted in 1968 for the XXIV International Congress of Physiological Sciences).

Cannon, W. B., & de la Paz, D. (1911). Emotional stimulation of adrenal secretion. *American Journal of Physiology, 28,* 64–70.

Cannon, W. B., & Lissak, K. (1939). Evidence for adrenaline in adrenergic neurons. *American Journal of Physiology, 125,* 765–777.

Cannon, W. B., & Rosenblueth, A. (1933). Studies on conditions of activity in endocrine organs. XXIX. Sympathin E and sympathin I. *American Journal of Physiology, 104,* 557–574.

Cappeliez, P., & Moore, E. (1990). Effects of lithium on an amphetamine animal model of bipolar disorder. *Progress in Neuro-Psychopharmacology and Biological Psychiatry, 14,* 347–358.

Caramillo, E. M., Khan, K. M., Collier, A. D., & Echevarria, D. J. (2015). Modeling PTSD in the zebrafish: are we there yet? *Behavioural Brain Research, 276,* 151–160.

Caramona, M. M., & Soares da Silva, P. (1985). The effects of chemical sympathectomy on dopamine, noradrenaline and adrenaline content in some peripheral tissues. *British Journal of Pharmacology, 86,* 351–356.

Careaga, M., Murai, T., & Bauman, M. D. (2017). Maternal immune activation and autism spectrum disorder: from rodents to nonhuman and human primates. *Biological Psychiatry, 81,* 391–401.

Carnevali, L., Trombini, M., Graiani, G., Madeddu, D., Quaini, F., Landgraf, R., . . . Sgoifo, A. (2014). Low vagally-mediated heart rate variability and increased susceptibility to ventricular arrhythmias in rats bred for high anxiety. *Physiology and Behavior, 128,* 16–25.

Carobrez, A. P., & Bertoglio, L. J. (2005). Ethological and temporal analyses of anxiety-like behavior: the elevated plus-maze 20 years on. *Neuroscience and Biobehavioral Reviews, 29,* 1193–1205.

Carter, C. S. (2007). Sex differences in oxytocin and vasopressin: implications for autism spectrum disorders? *Behavioural Brain Research, 176,* 170–186.

Casey, B. J., Craddock, N., Cuthbert, B. N., Hyman, S. E., Lee, F. S., & Ressler, K. J. (2013). DSM-5 and RDoC: progress in psychiatry research? *Nature Reviews Neuroscience, 14,* 810–814.

Caspi, A., & Moffitt, T. E. (2018). All for one and one for all: mental disorders in one dimension. *American Journal of Psychiatry, 175,* 831–844.

Caspi, A., Sugden, K., Moffitt, T. E., Taylor, A., Craig, I. W., Harrington, H., . . . Poulton, R. (2003). Influence of life stress on depression: moderation by a polymorphism in the 5-HTT gene. *Science, 301*, 386–389.

Castagné, V., Porsolt, R. D., & Moser, P. (2009). Use of latency to immobility improves detection of antidepressant-like activity in the behavioral despair test in the mouse. *European Journal of Pharmacology, 616*, 128–133.

Castro, J. E., Diessler, S., Varea, E., Márquez, C., Larsen, M. H., Cordero, M. I., & Sandi, C. (2012). Personality traits in rats predict vulnerability and resilience to developing stress-induced depression-like behaviors, HPA axis hyper-reactivity and brain changes in pERK 1-2 activity. *Psychoneuroendocrinology, 37*, 1209–1223.

Cathomas, F., Murrough, J. W., Nestler, E. J., Han, M.-H., & Russo, S. J. (2019). Neurobiology of resilience: interface between mind and body. *Biological Psychiatry, 86*, 410–420.

Ceccato, F., Scaroni, C., & Boscaro, M. (2018). The adrenal glands. In A. Belfiore & D. LeRoith (Eds.), *Principles of endocrinology and hormone action* (pp. 387–421). New York, NY: Springer.

Cerqueira, J. J., Mailliet, F., Almeida, O. F. X., Jay, T. M., & Sousa, N. (2007). The prefrontal cortex as a key target of the maladaptive response to stress. *Journal of Neuroscience, 27*, 2781–2787.

Chadman, K. K., Yang, M., & Crawley, J. N. (2009). Criteria for validating mouse models of psychiatric disorders. *American Journal of Medical Genetics Part B, 150B*, 1–11.

Chambers, N. K., & Buchman, T. G. (2000). Shock at the millennium. I. Walter B. Cannon and Alfred Blalock. *Shock, 13*, 497–504.

Chambers, N. K., & Buchman, T. G. (2001). Shock at the millennium. II. Walter B. Cannon and Lawrence J. Henderson. *Shock, 16*, 278–284.

Chambers, R. A., & Lipska, B. K. (2011). A method to the madness: producing the neonatal ventral hippocampal lesion rat model of schizophrenia. In W. Walz (Series Ed.) & P. O'Donnell (Vol. Ed.) *Neuromethods: Vol. 59. Animal models of schizophrenia and related disorders* (pp. 1–24). New York, NY: Humana Press.

Champagne, F. A., & Meaney, M. J. (2007). Transgenerational effects of social environment on variations in maternal care and behavioral response to novelty. *Behavioral Neuroscience, 121*, 1353–1363.

Champagne, F. A., Weaver, I. C., Diorio, J., Dymov, S., Szyf, M., & Meaney, M. J. (2006). Maternal care associated with methylation of the estrogen receptor-alpha1b promoter and estrogen receptor-alpha expression in the medial preoptic area of female offspring. *Endocrinology, 147*, 2909–2915.

Chan, J. C., Nugent, B. M., & Bale, T. L. (2018). Parental advisory: maternal and paternal stress can impact offspring neurodevelopment. *Biological Psychiatry, 83*, 886–894.

Chang, S., Bok, P., Tsai, C.-Y., Sun, C.-P., Liu, H., Deussing, J. M., & Huang, G.-J. (2018). NPTX2 is a key component in the regulation of anxiety. *Neuropsychopharmacology, 43*, 1943–1953.

Charney, D. S. (2003). The psychobiology of resilience and vulnerability to anxiety disorders: implications for prevention and treatment. *Dialogues in Clinical Neuroscience, 5*, 207–221.

Charney, D. S. (2004). Psychobiological mechanisms of resilience and vulnerability: implications for successful adaptation to extreme stress. *American Journal of Psychiatry, 161*, 195–216.

Chaste, P., & Leboyer, M. (2012). Autism risk factors: genes, environment, and gene-environment interactions. *Dialogues in Clinical Neuroscience, 14*, 281–292.

Chaudhury, D., Walsh, J. J., Friedman, A. K., Juarez, B., Ku, S. M., Koo, J. W., . . . Han, M.-H. (2013). Rapid regulation of depression-related behaviours by control of midbrain dopamine neurons. *Nature, 493*, 532–553.

Chekmareva, N. Y., Slotnikov, S. V., Diepold, R. P., Naik, R. R., Landgraf, R., & Czibere, L. (2014). Environmental manipulations generate bidirectional shifts in both behavior and gene regulation in a crossbred mouse model of extremes in trait anxiety. *Frontiers in Behavioral Neuroscience, 8*, 87.

Chen, A., Editor (2019). *Stress resilience: molecular and behavioral aspects*. San Diego, CA: Academic Press.

Chen, G. Y., & Nuñez, G. (2010). Sterile inflammation: sensing and reacting to damage. *Nature Reviews Immunology, 10*, 826–837.

Chen, Q., Yan, W., & Duan, E. (2016). Epigenetic inheritance of acquired traits through sperm RNAs and sperm RNA modifications. *Nature Reviews Genetics, 17*, 733–743.

Chen, X., Choo, H., Huang, X.-P., Yang, X., Stone, O., Roth, B. L., & Jin, J. (2015). The first structure-activity relationship studies for designer receptors exclusively activated by designer drugs. *ACS Chemical Neuroscience, 6*, 476–484.

Chen, Z., Yoo, S.-H., & Takahashi, J. S. (2018). Development and therapeutic potential of small-molecule modulators of circadian systems. *Annual Review of Pharmacology and Toxicology, 58*, 231–252.

Chen, Z.-Y., Jing, D., Bath, K. G., Ieraci, A., Khan, T., Siao, C.-J., . . . Lee, F. S. (2006). Genetic variant BDNF (Val66Met) polymorphism alters anxiety-related behavior. *Science, 314*, 140–143.

Cheng, Y., Desse, S., Martinez, A., Worthen, R. J., Jope, R. S., & Beurel, E. (2018). TNFα disrupts blood brain barrier integrity to maintain prolonged depressive-like behavior in mice. *Brain, Behavior and Immunity, 69*, 556–567.

Cheng, Y., Pardo, M., de Souza Armini, R., Martinez, A., Mouhsine, H., Zagury, J.-F., . . . Beurel, E. (2016). Stress-induced inflammation is mediated by GSK3-dependent TLR4 signaling that promotes susceptibility to depression-like behavior. *Brain, Behavior and Immunity, 53*, 207–222.

Cheslack-Postava, K., Cremers, S., Bao, Y., Shen, L., Schaefer, C. A., & Brown, A. S. (2017). Maternal serum cytokine levels and risk of bipolar disorder. *Brain, Behavior, and Immunity, 63*, 108–114.

Chiueh, C. C., & Kopin, I. J. (1978). Hyperresponsivitiy of spontaneously hypertensive rat to indirect measurement of blood pressure. *American Journal of Physiology, 234*, H690–H695.

Choi, G. B., Yim, Y. S., Wong, H., Kim, S., Kim, H., Kim, S. V., . . . Huh, J. R. (2016). The maternal interleukin-17a pathway in mice promotes autism-like phenotypes in offspring. *Science, 351*, 933–939.

Chorpita, B. F., & Barlow, D. H. (1998). The development of anxiety: the role of control in the early environment. *Psychological Bulletin, 124*, 3–21.

Choy, K. H. C., & van den Buuse, M. (2008). Attenuated disruption of prepulse inhibition by dopaminergic stimulation after maternal deprivation and adolescent corticosterone treatment in rats. *European Neuropsychopharmacology, 18*, 1–13.

Christian, K. M., Miracle, A. D., Wellman, C. L., & Nakazawa, K. (2011). Chronic stress-induced hippocampal dendritic retraction requires CA3 NMDA receptors. *Neuroscience, 174*, 26–36.

Chrousos, G. P. (2009). Stress and disorders of the stress system. *Nature Reviews Endocrinology, 5,* 374–381.

Chrousos, G. P., & Gold, P. W. (1992). The concepts of stress and stress system disorders. Overview of physical and behavioral homeostasis. *Journal of the American Medical Association, 267,* 1244–1252.

Chung, C., Ha, S., Kang, H., Lee, J., Um, S. M., Yan, H., . . . Kim, E. (2019). Early correction of N-methyl-D-aspartate receptor function improves autistic-like social behaviors in adult Shank2-/- mice. *Biological Psychiatry, 85,* 534–543.

Cicchetti, D., Fogosch, F. A., Lynch, M., & Holt, K. D. (1993). Resilience in maltreated children: processes leading to adaptive outcome. *Developmental Psychopathology, 5,* 629–648.

Clancy, B., Darlington, R. B., & Finlay, B. L. (2001). Translating developmental time across mammalian species. *Neuroscience, 105,* 7–17.

Clapcote, S. J., Duffy, S., Xie, G., Kirshenbaum, G., Bechard, A. R., Schack, V. R., . . . Roder, J. C. (2009). Mutation I810N in the α3 isoform of Na,K-ATPase causes impairments in the sodium pump and hyperexcitability in the CNS. *Proceedings of the National Academy of Sciences USA, 106,* 14085–14090.

Clapier, C. R., & Cairns, B. R. (2009). The biology of chromatin remodeling complexes. *Annual Review of Biochemistry, 78,* 273–304.

Clark, F. M., & Proudfit, H. K. (1993). The projections of noradrenergic neurons in the A5 catecholamine cell group to the spinal cord in the rat: anatomical evidence that A5 neurons modulate nociception. *Brain Research, 616,* 200–210.

Clarke, D. J., Stuart, J., McGregor, I. S., & Arnold, J. C. (2017). Endocannabinoid dysregulation in cognitive and stress-related brain regions in the *Nrg1* mouse model of schizophrenia. *Progress in Neuro-Psychopharmacology and Biological Psychiatry, 72,* 9–15.

Clayton, J. A., & Collins, F. S. (2014). NIH to balance sex in cell and animal studies. *Nature, 509,* 282–283.

Clinton, S. M. (2015). Maternal style selectively shapes amygdalar development and social behavior in rats genetically prone to high anxiety. *Developmental Neuroscience, 37,* 203–214.

Clinton, S. M., Bedrosian, T. A., Abraham, A. D., Watson, S. J., & Akil, H. (2010). Neural and environmental factors impacting maternal behavior differences in high- versus low-novelty-seeking rats. *Hormones and Behavior, 57,* 463–473.

Clinton, S. M., Vazquez, D. M., Kabbaj, M., Kabbaj, M. H., Watson, S. J., & Akil, H. (2007). Individual differences in novelty-seeking and emotional reactivity correlate with variation in maternal behavior. *Hormones and Behavior, 51,* 655–664.

CNV and Schizophrenia Working Groups of the Psychiatric Genomics Consortium (2017). Contribution of copy number variants to schizophrenia from a genome-wide study of 41,321 subjects. *Nature Genetics, 49,* 27–35.

Cohen, H., Geva, A. B., Matar, M. A., Zohar, J., & Kaplan, Z. (2008). Post-traumatic stress behavioural responses in inbred mouse strains: can genetic predisposition explain phenotypic vulnerability? *International Journal of Neuropsychopharmacology, 11,* 331–349.

Cohen, H., Kaplan, Z., Matar, M. A., Loewenthal, U., Zohar, J., & Richter-Levin, G. (2007). Long-lasting behavioral effects of juvenile trauma in an animal model of PTSD associated with a failure of the autonomic nervous system to recover. *European Neuropsychopharmacology, 17,* 464–477.

Cohen, H., Kozlovsky, N., Alona, C., Matar, M. A., & Zohar, J. (2014). Animal model for PTSD: from clinical concept to translational research. *Neuropharmacology, 62,* 715–724.

Cohen, H., Kozlovsky, N., Matar, M. A., Zohar, J., & Kaplan, Z. (2014). Distinctive hippocampal and amygdalar cytoarchitectural changes underlie specific patterns of behavioral disruption following stress exposure in an animal model of PTSD. *European Neuropsychopharamcology, 24,* 1925–1944.

Cohen, H., Liberzon, I., & Richter-Levin, G. (2009). Exposure to extreme stress impairs contextual odour discrimination in an animal model of PTSD. *International Journal of Neuropsychopharmacology, 12,* 291–303.

Cohen, H., Liu, T., Kozlovsky, N., Kaplan, Z., Zohar, J., & Mathé, A. A. (2012). The neuropeptide Y (NPY)-ergic system is associated with behavioral resilience to stress exposure in an animal model of post-traumatic stress disorder. *Neuropsychopharmacology, 37,* 350–363.

Cohen, H., Matar, M. A., Buskila, D., Kaplan, Z., & Zohar, J. (2008). Early post-stressor intervention with high-dose corticosterone attenuates posttraumatic stress response in an animal model of posttraumatic stress disorder. *Biological Psychiatry, 64,* 708–717.

Cohen, H., Matar, M. A., Richter-Levin, G., & Zohar, J. (2006). Contributions of an animal model toward uncovering biological risk factors for PTSD. *Annals of the New York Academy of Sciences, 1071,* 335–350.

Cohen, H., Vainer, E., Kaplan, Z., Zohar, J., & Mathé, A. A. (2018). Neuropeptide S in the basolateral amygdala mediates an adaptive behavioral stress response in a rat model of posttraumatic stress disorder by increasing the expression of BDNF and the neuropeptide YY1 receptor. *European Neuropsychopharmacology, 28,* 159–170.

Cohen, H., & Yehuda, R. (2011). Gender differences in animal models of posttraumatic stress disorder. *Disease Markers, 30,* 141–150.

Cohen, H., Ziv, Y., Cardon, M., Kaplan, Z., Matar, M. A., Gidron, Y., . . . Kipnis, J. (2006). Maladaptation to mental stress mitigated by the adaptive immune system via depletion of naturally occurring regulatory CD4+CD25+ cells. *Journal of Neurobiology, 66,* 552–563.

Cohen, H., & Zohar, J. (2004). An animal model of posttraumatic stress disorder: the use of cut-off behavioral criteria. *Annals of the New York Academy of Sciences, 1032,* 167–178.

Cohen, J. L., Glover, M. E., Pugh, P. C., Fant, A. D., Simmons, R. K., Akil, H., . . . Clinton, S. M. (2015). Maternal style selectively shapes amygdalar development and social behavior in rats genetically prone to high anxiety. *Developmental Neuroscience, 37,* 203–214.

Cohen, S., Kozkovsky, N., Matar, M. A., Kaplan, Z., Zohar, J., & Cohen, H. (2012). Post-exposure sleep deprivation facilitates correctly timed interactions between glucocorticoid and adrenergic systems, which attenuate traumatic stress responses. *Neuropsychopharmacology, 37,* 2388–2404.

Cole, S. W., Arevalo, J. M. G., Takahashi, R., Sloan, E. K., Lutgendorf, S. K., Sood, A. K., . . . Seeman, T. E. (2010). Computational identification of gene–social environment interaction at the human *IL6* locus. *Proceedings of the National Academy of Sciences USA, 107,* 5681–5686.

Cole, S. W., Korin, Y. D., Fahey, J. L., & Zack, J. A. (1998). Norepinephrine accelerates HIV replication via protein kinase A-dependent effects on cytokine production. *Journal of Immunology, 161,* 610–616.

Coleman, W. (1985). The cognitive basis of the discipline: Claude Bernard on physiology. *Isis, 76,* 49–70.

Collins, F. S., & Varmus, H. (2015). A new initiative on precision medicine. *New England Journal of Medicine, 372,* 793–795.

Collins, P. Y., Patel, V., Joestl, S. S., March, D., Insel, T. R., Daar, A. S., . . . Walport, M. (2011). Grand challenges in global mental health. *Nature, 475,* 27–30.

Colman, I., Jones, P. B., Kuh, D., Weeks, M., Maicker, K., Richards, M., & Croudace, T. J. (2014). Early development, stress and depression across the life course: pathways to depression in a national British birth cohort. *Psychological Medicine, 44,* 2845–2854.

Colvert, E., Tick, B., McEwen, F., Stewart, C., Curran, S. R., Woodhouse, E., . . . Bolton, P. (2015). Heritability of autism spectrum disorder in a UK population-based twin sample. *JAMA Psychiatry, 72,* 415–423.

Committee on Statistics of the American Medico-Psychological Association in collaboration with the Bureau for Statistics of the National Committee for Mental Hygiene (1918). *Statistical manual for the use of institutions for the insane.* New York, NY: National Committee for Mental Hygiene.

Conway, C. C., Forbes, M. K., Forbush, K. T., Fried, E. I., Hallquist, M. N., Kotov, R., . . . Eaton, N. R. (2019). A hierarchical taxonomy of psychopathology can transform mental health research. *Perspectives on Psychological Science, 14,* 419–436.

Cooney, G. M., Dwan, K., Greig, C. A., Lawlor, D. A., Rimer, J., Waugh, F. R., . . . Mead, G. E. (2013). Exercise for depression. *Cochrane Database of Systematic Reviews, 9,* CD004366.

Cooper, S. J. (2008). From Claude Bernard to Walter Cannon: emergence of the concept of homeostasis. *Appetite, 51,* 419–427.

Corbett, B. A., Schupp, C. W., Simon, D., Ryan, N., & Mendoza, S. (2010). Elevated cortisol during play is associated with age and social engagement in children with autism. *Molecular Autism, 1,* 13.

Corbett, B. F., Luz, S., Arner, J., Pearson-Leary, J., Sengupta, A., Taylor, D., . . . Bhatnagar, S. (2019). Spingosine-1-phosphate receptor 3 in the medial prefrontal cortex promotes stress resilience by reducing inflammatory processes. *Nature Communications, 10,* 3146.

Corcoran, C., Walker, E., Huot, R., Mittal, V., Tessner, K., Kestler, L., & Malaspina, D. (2003). The stress cascade and schizophrenia: etiology and onset. *Schizophrenia Bulletin, 29,* 671–692.

Corradini, I., Focchi, E., Rasile, M., Morini, R., Desiato, G., Tomasoni, R., . . . Matteoli, M. (2018). Maternal immune activation delays excitatory-to-inhibitory gamma-aminobutyric acid switch in offspring. *Biological Psychiatry, 83,* 680–691.

Corvin, A., Craddock, N., & Sullivan, P. F. (2010). Genome-wide association studies: a primer. *Psychological Medicine, 40,* 1063–1077.

Costa, E., Davis, J., Pesold, C., Tueting, P., & Guidotti, A. (2002). The heterozygote reeler mouse as a model for the development of a new generation of antipsychotics. *Current Opinion in Pharmacology, 2,* 56–62.

Costall, B., Jones, B. J., Kelly, M. E., Naylor, R. J., & Tomkins, D. M. (1989). Exploration of mice in a black and white test box: validation as a model of anxiety. *Pharmacology, Biochemistry and Behavior, 32,* 777–785.

Cotecchia, S. (2010). The α1-adrenergic receptors: diversity of signaling networks and regulation. *Journal of Receptors and Signal Transduction, 30,* 410–419.

Covington, H. E., III, Maze, I., LaPlant, Q. C., Vialou, V. F., Ohnishi, Y. N., Berton, O., . . . Nestler, E. J. (2009). Antidepressant actions of histone deacetylase inhibitors. *Journal of Neuroscience, 29,* 11451–11460.

Cowan, W. M., Konisky, K. L., & Hyman, S. E. (2002). The human genome project and its impact on psychiatry. *Annual Review of Neuroscience, 25,* 1–50.

Cowen, E. L., Wyman, P. A., Work, W. C, & Parker, G. R. (1990). The Rochester Child Resilience Project: overview and summary of first year findings. *Development and Psychopathology, 2,* 193–212.

Coyle, J. T., & Balu, D. T. (2018). The role of serine racemase in the pathophysiology of brain disorders. *Advances in Pharmacology, 82,* 35–56.

Crabbe, J. C., Wahlsten, D., & Dudek, B. C. (1999). Genetics of mouse behavior: interactions with laboratory environment. *Science, 284,* 1670–1672.

Craske, M. G., Rauch, S. L., Ursano, R., Prenoveau, J., Pine, D. S., & Zinbarg, R. E. (2009). What is an anxiety disorder? *Depression and Anxiety, 26,* 1066–1085.

Craske, M. G., Stein, M. B., Eley, T. C., Milad, M. R., Holmes, A., Rapee, R. M., & Wittchen, H.-U. (2017). Anxiety disorders. *Nature Reviews Disease Primers, 3,* 17024.

Crawley, J. N. (1981). Neuropharmacologic specificity of a simple animal model for the behavioral actions of benzodiazepines. *Pharmacology, Biochemistry and Behavior, 15,* 695–699.

Crawley, J. N. (1985). Exploratory behavior models of anxiety in mice. *Neuroscience and Biobehavioral Reviews, 9,* 37–44.

Crawley, J. N. (2012). Translational animal models of autism and neurodevelopmental disorders. *Dialogues in Clinical Neuroscience, 14,* 293–305.

Crawley, J., & Goodwin, F. K. (1980). Preliminary report of a simple animal behavior model for the anxiolytic effects of benzodiazepines. *Pharmacology, Biochemistry and Behavior, 13,* 167–170.

Crestani, C. C., Alves, F. H. F., Gomes, F. V., Resstel, L. B. M., Correa, F. M. A., & Herman, J. P. (2013). Mechanisms in the bed nucleus of the stria terminalis involved in control of autonomic and neuroendocrine functions: a review. *Current Neuropharmacology, 11,* 141–159.

Crile, G. W. (1915). *The origin and nature of the emotions: miscellaneous papers.* Philadelphia, PA: W. B. Saunders.

Crile, G. W. (1922). *The thyroid gland.* Philadelphia, PA: W. B. Saunders.

Cross, S. J., & Albury, W. R. (1987). Walter B. Cannon, L. J. Henderson, and the organic analogy. *Osiris, 3,* 165–192.

Cross-Disorder Group of the Psychiatric Genetics Consortium (2013). Identification of risk loci with shared effects on five major psychiatric disorders: a genome-wide analysis. *Lancet, 381,* 1371–1379.

Crow, T. J. (2000). Schizophrenia as the price that Homo sapiens pays for language: a resolution of the central paradox in the origin of the species. *Brain Research Reviews, 31,* 118–129.

Cryan, J. F., & Holmes, A. (2005). The ascent of mouse: advances in modeling human depression and anxiety. *Nature Reviews Drug Discovery, 4,* 775–790.

Cryan, J. F., & O'Mahoney, S. M. (2011). The microbiome-gut-brain axis: from bowel to behavior. *Neurogastroenterology and Motility, 23,* 187–192.

Cryan, J. F., & Sweeney, F. F. (2011). The age of anxiety: role of animal models of anxiolytic action in drug discovery. *British Journal of Pharmacology, 164,* 1129–1161.

Culig, L., Surget, A., Bourdey, M., Khemissi, W., Le Guisquet, A.-M., Vogel, E., . . . Belzung, C. (2017). Increasing adult hippocampal neurogenesis in mice after exposure to unpredictable chronic mild stress may counteract some of the effects of stress. *Neuropharmacology, 126,* 179–189.

Culverhouse, R. C., Saccone, N. L., Horton, A. C., Ma, Y., Anstey, K. J., Banaschewski, T., . . . Bierut, L. J. (2018). Collaborative meta-analysis finds no evidence of a strong interaction between stress and 5-HTTLPR genotype contributing to the development of depression. *Molecular Psychiatry, 23,* 133–142.

Cuthbert, B. N. (2014). The RDoC framework: facilitating transition from ICD/DSM to dimensional approaches that integrate neuroscience and psychopathology. *World Psychiatry, 13,* 28–35.

Cuthbert, B. N., & Insel, T. R. (2013). Toward the future of psychiatric diagnosis: the seven pillars of RDoC. *BMC Medicine, 11,* 126.

Cuthbert, B. N., & Kozak, M. J. (2013). Constructing constructs for psychopathology: the NIMH Research Domain Criteria. *Journal of Abnormal Psychology, 122,* 928–937.

Czéh, B., Fuchs, E., Wiborg, O., & Simon, M. (2016). Animal models of major depression and their clinical implications. *Progress in Neuro-Psychopharmacology and Biological Psychiatry, 64,* 293–310.

Daar, A. S., Singer, P. A., Persad, D. L., Pramming, S. K., Matthews, D. R., Beaglehole, R., . . . Bell, J. (2007). Grand challenges in chronic, non-communicable diseases. *Nature, 450,* 494–496.

Daches, S., Vine, V., George, C. J., & Kovacs, M. (2019). Adversity and depression: the moderating role of stress reactivity among high and low risk youth. *Journal of Abnormal Child Psychology, 47,* 1391–1399.

Dallman, M. F., Akana, S. F., Cascio, C. S., Darlington, D. N., Jacobson, L., & Levin, N. (1987). Regulation of ACTH secretion: variations on a theme of B. *Recent Progress in Hormone Research, 43,* 113–173.

Daly, M. J., Robinson, E. B., & Neale, B. M. (2016). Natural selection and neuropsychiatric disease: theory, observation, and emerging genetic findings. In T. Lehner, B. L. Miller, & M. W. State (Eds.), *Genomics, circuits, and pathways in clinical neuropsychiatry* (pp. 51–61). Amsterdam, The Netherlands: Elsevier.

Dampney, R. A. L. (2011). The hypothalamus and autonomic regulation: an overview. In I. J. Lewellyn-Smith and A. J. M. Verberne (Eds.), *Central regulation of autonomic functions* (2nd ed.) (pp. 47–61). New York, NY: Oxford University Press.

Danan, D., Matar, M. A., Kaplan, Z., Zohar, J., & Cohen, H. (2018). Blunted basal corticosterone pulsatility predicts post-exposure susceptibility to PTSD phenotype in rats. *Psychoneuroendocrinology, 87,* 35–42.

Dantzer, R. (2001). Cytokine-induced sickness behavior: where do we stand? *Brain, Behavior and Immunity, 15,* 7–24.

Dantzer, R. (2018). Neuroimmune interactions: from the brain to the immune system and vice versa. *Physiological Reviews, 98,* 477–504.

Dantzer, R., Cohen, S., Russo, S. J., & Dinan, T. G. (2018). Resilience and immunity. *Brain, Behavior, and Immunity, 74,* 28–42.

Dantzer, R., O'Connor, J. C., Freund, G. G., Johnson, R. W., & Kelley, K. W. (2008). From inflammation to sickness and depression: when the immune system subjugates the brain. *Nature Reviews Neuroscience, 9,* 46–57.

Dao, D. T., Mahon, P. B., Cai, X., Kovacsics, C. E., Blackwell, R. A., Arad, M., . . . Gould, T. D. (2010). Mood disorder susceptibility gene CACNA1C modifies mood-related behaviors in mice and interacts with sex to influence behavior in mice and diagnosis in humans. *Biological Psychiatry, 68,* 801–810.

Darwin, C. (1859). *On the origin of species by means of natural selection, or the preservation of favoured races in the struggle for survival.* London, England: John Murray.

Darwin, C. (1871). *The descent of man, and selection in relation to sex.* London, England: John Murray.

Darwin, C. (1872). *The expression of the emotions in man and animals.* London, England: John Murray.

Daskalakis, N. P., Bagot, R. C., Parker, K. J., Vinkers, C. H., & de Kloet, E. R. (2013). The three-hit concept of vulnerability and resilience: toward understanding adaptation to early-life adversity outcome. *Psychoneuroendocrinology, 38,* 1858–1873.

Daskalakis, N. P., & Binder, E. B. (2015). Schizophrenia in the spectrum of gene-stress interactions: the FKBP5 example. *Schizophrenia Bulletin, 41,* 323–329.

Daskalakis, N. P., Cohen, H., Cai, G., Buxbaum, J. D., & Yehuda, R. (2014). Expression profiling associates blood and brain glucocorticoid receptor signaling with trauma-related individual differences in both sexes. *Proceedings of the National Academy of Sciences USA, 111,* 13529–13534.

Daskalakis, N. P., & Yehuda, R. (2014). Principles for developing animal models of military PTSD. *European Journal of Psychotraumatology, 5,* 23825.

Dautzenberg, F. M., & Hauger, R. L. (2002). The CRF peptide family and their receptors: yet more partners discovered. *Trends in Pharmacological Sciences, 23,* 71–77.

Davidson, R. J., & McEwen, B. S. (2012). Social influences on neuroplasticity: stress and interventions to promote well-being. *Nature Neuroscience, 15,* 689–695.

Davies, A. G., Pierce-Shimomura, J. T., Kim, H., VanHoven, M. K., Thiele, T. R., Bonci, A., . . . McIntire, S. L. (2003). A central role of the BK potassium channel in behavioral responses to ethanol in *C. elegans. Cell, 116,* 655–666.

Davies, C., Danger, D. J., Steinberg, H., Tomkiewicz, M., & U'Prichard, D. C. (1974). Lithium and α-methyl-p-tyrosine prevent "manic" activity in rodents. *Psychopharmacologia, 36,* 263–274.

Davis, J., Maes, M., McGrath, J. J., Tye, S. J., & Berk, M. (2015). Towards a classification of biomarkers of neuropsychiatric disease: from encompass to compass. *Molecular Psychiatry, 20,* 152–153.

Davis, M. (2006). Neural systems involved in fear and anxiety measured with fear-potentiated startle. *American Psychologist, 61,* 741–756.

Davis, M., Falls, W. A., Campeau, S., & Kim, M. (1993). Fear-potentiated startle: a neural and pharmacological analysis. *Behavioural Brain Research, 58,* 175–198.

Davis, R. L., & Dauwalder, B. (1991). The *Drosophila* dunce locus: learning and memory genes in the fly. *Trends in Genetics, 7,* 224–229.

Dawlati, Y., Herrmann, N., Swardfager, W., Liu, H., Sham, L., Reim, E. K., & Lanctôt, K. L. (2010). A meta-analysis of cytokines in major depression. *Biological Psychiatry, 67,* 446–457.

Day, R., Nielsen, J. A., Korten, A., Ernberg, G., Dube, K. C., Gebhart, J., . . . Wynne, L. C. (1987). Stressful life events preceding the acute onset of schizophrenia: a cross-national study from the World Health Organization. *Culture, Medicine and Psychiatry, 11,* 123–205.

Debnath, M., Venkatasubramanian, G., & Berk, M. (2015). Fetal programming of schizophrenia: select mechanisms. *Neuroscience and Biobehavioral Reviews, 49,* 90–104.

De Boer, S. F., & Koolhaas, J. M. (2003). Defensive burying in rodents: ethology, neurobiology and psychopharmacology. *European Journal of Pharmacology, 463,* 146–161.

De Boer, S. F., Koopmans, S. J., Slangen, J. L., & Van der Gugten, J. (1990). Plasma catecholamine, corticosterone and glucose responses to repeated stress in rats: effect of interstressor interval length. *Physiology and Behavior, 47*, 1117–1124.

De Boer, S. F., Van Der Gugten, J., & Slangen, J. L. (1989). Plasma catecholamine and corticosterone responses to predictable and unpredictable noise stress in rats. *Physiology and Behavior, 45*, 789–795.

Decavel, C., & van den Pol, A. N. (1992). Converging GABA- and glutamate-immunoreactive axons make synaptic contact with identified hypothalamic neurosecretory neurons. *Journal of Comparative Neurology, 316*, 104–116.

DeFelippis, M., & Wagner, K. D. (2016). Treatment of autism spectrum disorder in children and adolescents. *Psychopharmacology Bulletin, 46*, 18–41.

Defensor, E. B., Pearson, B. L., Pobbe, R. L. H., Bolivar, V. J., Blanchard, D. C., & Blanchard, R. J. (2011). A novel social proximity test suggests patterns of social avoidance and gaze aversion-like behavior in BTBR T+tf/J mice. *Behavioural Brain Research, 217*, 302–308.

Deisseroth, K. (2015). Optogenetics: 10 years of microbial opsins in neuroscience. *Nature Neuroscience, 18*, 1213–1225.

de Kloet, E. R., Joëls, M., & Holsboer, F. (2005). Stress and the brain: from adaptation to disease. *Nature Reviews Neuroscience, 6*, 463–475.

De La Garza, R., II, & Mahoney, J. J., III (2004). A distinct neurochemical profile in WKY rats at baseline and in response to acute stress: implications for animal models of anxiety and depression. *Brain Research, 1021*, 209–218.

Delgado y Palacios, R., Campo, A., Henningsen, K., Verhoye, M., Poot, D., Dijkstra, J., . . . Van der Linden, A. (2011). Magnetic resonance imaging and spectroscopy reveal differential hippocampal changes in anhedonic and resilient subtypes of the chronic mild stress rat model. *Biological Psychiatry, 70*, 449–457.

Del Giudice, M. (2017). Mating, sexual selection, and the evolution of schizophrenia. *World Psychiatry, 16*, 141–142.

Demontis, D., Walters, R. K., Martin, J., Mattheisen, M., Als, T. D., Agerbo, A., . . . Neale, B. M. (2019). Discovery of the first genome-wide significant risk loci for attention deficit/hyperactivity disorder. *Nature Genetics, 51*, 63–75.

De Moore, G., & Westmore, A. (2016). *Finding sanity: John Cade, lithium and the taming of bipolar disorder.* Crow's Nest, NSW, Australia: Allen & Unwin.

Denenberg, V. H., 1999. Commentary: is maternal stimulation the mediator of the handling effect in infancy? *Developmental Psychobiology, 34*, 1–3.

Denenberg, V. H., & Rosenberg, K. M. (1967). Nongenetic transmission of information. *Nature, 216*, 549–550.

Denenberg, V. H., & Whimby, A. E. (1963). Behavior of adult rats is modified by the experiences their mothers had as infants. *Science, 142*, 1192–1193.

De Pablo, J. M., Parra, A., Segovia, S., & Guillamón, A. (1989). Learning immobility explains the behavior of rats in the forced swimming task. *Physiology and Behavior, 46*, 229–237.

Derry, H. M., Padin, A. C., Kuo, J. L., Hughes, S., & Kiecolt-Glaser, J. K. (2015). Sex differences in depression: does inflammation play a role? *Current Psychiatry Reports, 17*, 78.

De Rubeis, S., & Buxbaum, J. D. (2015). Genetics and genomics of autism spectrum disorder: embracing complexity. *Human Molecular Genetics, 24*, R24–R31.

Desbonnet, L., O'Tuathaigh, C., Clarke, G., O'Leary, C., Petit, E., Clarke, N., . . . Waddington, J. L. (2012). Phenotypic effects of repeated psychosocial stress during adolescence in mice mutant for the schizophrenia risk gene neuregulin-1: a putative model of gene x environment interaction. *Brain, Behavior, and Immunity, 26,* 660–671.

Deslauriers, J., Toth, M., Der-Avakian, A., & Risbrough, V. B. (2018). Current status of animal models of posttraumatic stress disorder: behavioral and biological phenotypes, and future challenges in improving translation. *Biological Psychiatry, 83,* 895–907.

DeVore, I, & Washburn, S. L. (1992). An interview with Sherwood Washburn. *Current Anthropology, 33,* 411–423.

Dewing, P., Shi, T., Horvath, S., & Vilain, E. (2003). Sexually dimorphic gene expression in mouse brain precedes gonadal differentiation. *Molecular Brain Research, 118,* 82–90.

Dhabhar, F. S., McEwen, B. S., & Spencer, R. L. (1993). Stress response, adrenal steroid receptor levels and corticosteroid-binding globulin levels: a comparison between Sprague-Dawley, Fischer 344 and Lewis rats. *Brain Research, 616,* 89–98.

Dias, B. G., & Ressler, K. J. (2014a). Experimental evidence needed to demonstrate inter- and trans-generational effects of ancestral experiences in mammals. *Bioessays, 36,* 919–923.

Dias, B. G., & Ressler, K. J. (2014b). Parental olfactory experience influences behavior and neural structure in subsequent generations. *Nature Neuroscience, 17,* 89–95.

DiCarlo, G. E., Aguilar, J. I., Matthies, H. J. G., Harrison, F. E., Bundschuh, K. E., West, A., ... Galli, A. (2019). Autism-linked dopamine transporter mutation alters striatal dopamine neurotransmission and dopamine-dependent behaviors. *Journal of Clinical Investigation, 129,* 3407–3419.

Dickmeis, T. (2009). Glucocorticoids and the circadian clock. *Journal of Endocrinology, 200,* 3–22.

Dickson, D. A., Paulus, J. K., Mensah, V., Lem, J., Saavedra-Rodriguez, L., Gentry, A., ... Feig, L. A. (2018). Reduced levels of miRNAs 449 and 34 in sperm of mice and men exposed to early life stress. *Translational Psychiatry, 8,* 101.

Dienes, K. A., Hammen, C., Henry, R. M., Cohen, A. N., & Daley, S. E. (2006). The stress sensitization hypothesis: understanding the course of bipolar disorder. *Journal of Affective Disorders, 95,* 43–49.

Dietz, D. M., LaPlant, Q., Watts, E. L., Hodes, G. E., Russo, S. J., Feng, J., ... Nestler, E. J. (2011). Paternal transmission of stress-induced pathologies. *Biological Psychiatry, 70,* 408–414.

Dinarello, C. A., Renfer, L., & Wolff, S. M. (1977). Human leukocytic pyrogen: purification and development of a radioimmunoassay. *Proceedings of the National Academy of Sciences USA, 74,* 4624–4627.

Domschke, K., Dannlowski, U., Hohoff, C., Ohrmann, P., Bauer, J., Kugel, H., ... Baune, B. T. (2010). Neuropeptide Y (NPY) gene, impact on emotional processing and treatment response in anxious depression. *European Neuropsychopharmacology, 20,* 301–309.

Domschke, K., Reif, A., Weber, H., Richter, J., Hohoff, C., Ohrmann, P., ... Deckert, J. (2011). Neuropeptide S receptor gene: converging evidence for a role in panic disorder. *Molecular Psychiatry, 16,* 938–948.

Donaldson, Z. R., & Hen, R. (2015). From psychiatric disorders to animal models: a bidirectional and dimensional approach. *Biological Psychiatry, 77,* 15–21.

Donegan, J. J., Tyson, J. A., Branch, S. Y., Bechstead, M. J., Anderson, S. A., & Lodge, D. J. (2017). Stem cell-derived interneuron transplants as a treatment for schizophrenia: preclinical validation in a rodent model. *Molecular Psychiatry, 22,* 1492–1501.

Dong, E., Dzitoyeva, S. G., Matrisciano, F., Tueting, P., Grayson, D. R., & Guidotti, A. (2015). Brain-derived neurotrophic factor epigenetic modifications associated with schizophrenia-like phenotype induced by prenatal stress in mice. *Biological Psychiatry, 77*, 589–596.

Donner, J., Haapakoski, R., Ezer, S., Melén, E., Pirkola, S., Gratacòs, M., . . . Hovatta, I. (2010). Assessment of the neuropeptide S system in anxiety disorders. *Biological Psychiatry, 68*, 474–483.

Driscoll, C. A., & Barr, C. S. (2016). Studying longitudinal trajectories in animal models of psychiatric illness and their translation to the human condition. *Neuroscience Research, 102*, 67–77.

Drugan, R. C., Christianson, J. P., Stine, W. W., & Soucy, D. P. (2009). Swim stress-induced ultrasonic vocalizations forecast resilience in rats. *Behavioural Brain Research, 202*, 142–145.

Du, Y., & Grace, A. A. (2013). Peripubertal diazepam administration prevents the emergence of dopamine system hyperresponsivity in the MAM developmental disruption model of schizophrenia. *Neuropsychopharmacology, 38*, 1881–1888.

Duangdao, D. M., Clark, S. D., Okamura, N., & Reinscheid, R. K. (2009). Behavioral phenotyping of neuropeptide S receptor knockout mice. *Behavioural Brain Research, 205*, 1–9.

Dudley, K. J., Li, X., Kobor, M. S., Kippin, T. E., & Bredy, T. W. (2011). Epigenetic mechanisms mediating vulnerability and resilience to psychiatric disorders. *Neuroscience and Biobehavioral Reviews, 35*, 1544–1551.

Dufour, S., & De Koninck, Y. (2015). Optrodes for combined optogenetics and electrophysiology in live animals. *Neurophotonics, 2*, 031205.

Dulawa, S. C., & Hen, R. (2005). Recent advances in animal models of chronic antidepressant effects: the novelty-induced hypophagia test. *Neuroscience and Biobehavioral Reviews, 29*, 771–783.

Dulawa, S. C., & Janowsky, D. S. (2019). Cholinergic regulation of mood: from basic and clinical studies to emerging therapeutics. *Molecular Psychiatry, 24*, 694–709.

Dulka, B. N., Bourdon, A. K., Clinard, C. T., Muvvala, M. B. K., Campagna, S. R., & Cooper, M. A. (2017). Metabolomics reveals distinct neurochemical profiles associated with stress resilience. *Neurobiology of Stress, 7*, 103–112.

Duman, R. S. (2004). Depression: a case of neuronal life and death? *Biological Psychiatry, 56*, 140–145.

Duman, R. S., & Monteggia, L. M. (2006). A neurotrophic model for stress-related mood disorders. *Biological Psychiatry, 59*, 1116–1127.

Duncan, P. J., Tabak, J., Ruth, P., Bertram, R., & Shipston, M. J. (2016). Glucocorticoids inhibit CRH/AVP-evoked bursting activity of male murine anterior pituitary corticotrophs. *Endocrinology, 157*, 3108–3121.

Duplan, S. M., Boucher, F., Anexandrov, L., & Michaud, J. L. (2009). Impact of Sim1 gene dosage on the development of the paraventricular and supraoptic nuclei of the hypothalamus. *European Journal of Neuroscience, 30*, 2239–2249.

Eagle, A. L., Fitzpatrick, C. J., & Perrine, S. A. (2013). Single prolonged stress impairs social and object novelty recognition in rats. *Behavioural Brain Research, 256*, 591–597.

Eells, J. B., Varela-Stokes, A., Guo-Ross, S. X., Kummari, E., Smith, H. M., Cox, E., & Lindsay, D. S. (2015). Chronic *Toxoplasma gondii* in Nurr1-null heterozygous mice exacerbates elevated open field activity. *PLoS ONE, 10*, e0119280.

Egan, M. F., Kojima, M., Callicott, J. H., Goldberg, T. E., Kolachana, B. S., Bertolino, A., . . . Weinberger, D. R. (2003). The BDNF val66met polymorphism affects activity-dependent secretion of BDNF and human memory and hippocampal function. *Cell, 112,* 257–269.

Egerton, A., Howes, O. D., Houle, S., McKenzie, K., Valmaggia, L. R., Bagby, M. R., . . . Mizrahi, R. (2017). Elevated striatal dopamine function in immigrants and their children: a risk mechanism for psychosis. *Schizophrenia Bulletin, 43,* 293–301.

Ehrhart-Bornstein, M., Hinson, J. P., Bornstein, S. R., Scherbaum, W. A., & Vinson, G. P. (1998). Intraadrenal interactions in the regulation of adrenocortical steroidogenesis. *Endocrine Reviews, 19,* 101–143.

Eiden, L. E., & Jiang, S. Z. (2018). What's new in endocrinology: the chromaffin cell. *Frontiers in Endocrinology, 9,* 711.

Einer-Jensen, N., & Carter, A. M. (1995). Local transfer of hormones between blood vessels within the adrenal gland may explain the functional interaction between the adrenal cortex and medulla. *Medical Hypotheses, 44,* 471–474.

Eisch, A. J., & Petrik, D. (2012). Depression and hippocampal neurogenesis: a road to remission? *Science, 338,* 72–75.

Elenkov, I. J., Wilder, R. L., Chrousos, G. P., & Vizi, E. S. (2000). The sympathetic nerve: an integrative interface between two supersystems: the brain and the immune system. *Pharmacological Reviews, 52,* 595–638.

El Hage, W., Griebel, G., & Belzung, C. (2006). Long-term impaired memory following predatory stress in mice. *Physiology and Behavior, 87,* 45–50.

El-Kordi, A., Winkler, D., Hammerschmidt, K., Kästner, A., Krueger, D., Ronnenberg, A., . . . Ehrenreich, H. (2013). Development of an autism severity score for mice using NLGN4 null mutants as a construct-valid model of heritable monogenic autism. *Behavioural Brain Research, 251,* 41–49.

Ellenbroek, B. A., & Cools, A. R. (2000). The long-term effects of maternal deprivation depend on the genetic background. *Neuropsychopharmacology, 23,* 99–106.

Ellenbroek, B. A., & Cools, A. R. (2002). Apomorphine susceptibility and animal models for psychopathology: genes and environment. *Behavior Genetics, 32,* 349–361.

Ellenbroek, B. A., Geyer, M. A., & Cools, A. R. (1995). The behavior of APO-SUS rats in animal models with construct validity for schizophrenia. *Journal of Neuroscience, 15,* 7604–7611.

Ellenbroek, B. A., & Riva, M. A. (2003). Early maternal deprivation as an animal model for schizophrenia. *Clinical Neuroscience Research, 3,* 297–302.

Ellenbroek, B. A., Sluyter, F., & Cools, A. R. (2000). The role of genetic and early environmental factors in determining apomorphine susceptibility. *Psychopharmacology (Berlin), 148,* 124–131.

Ellenbroek, B., & Youn, J. (2016). Rodent models in neuroscience research: is it a rat race? *Disease Models and Mechanisms, 9,* 1079–1087.

Ellicott, A., Hammen, C., Gitlin, M., Brown, G., & Jamison, K. (1990). Life events and the course of bipolar disorder. *American Journal of Psychiatry, 147,* 1194–1198.

Elliott, E., Ezra-Nevo, G., Regev, L., Neufeld-Cohen, A., & Chen, A. (2010). Resilience to social stress coincides with functional DNA methylation of the *Crf* gene in adult mice. *Nature Neuroscience, 13,* 1351–1353.

Elliott, G. R., & Eisdorfer, C. (1982). *Stress and human health: analysis and implications of research.* New York, NY: Springer.

El-Mallakh, R. S. (1983). The Na,K-ATPase hypothesis for manic-depression. I. General considerations. *Medical Hypotheses, 12,* 253–268.

El-Mallakh, R. S., Harrison, L. T., Li, R., Changaris, D. G., & Levy, R. S. (1995). An animal model for mania: preliminary results. *Progress in Neuro-Psychopharmacology and Biological Psychiatry, 19,* 955–962.

Engel, B. T. (1985). Stress is a noun! No, a verb! No, an adjective! In T. M. Field, P. M. McCabe, & N. Schneiderman (Eds.), *Stress and coping* (pp. 3–12). Hillsdale, NJ: Lawrence Erlbaum.

English, J. G., & Roth, B. L. (2015). Chemogenetics: a transformational and translational platform. *JAMA Neurology, 72,* 1361–1366.

Engstrom, E. J., & Kendler, K. S. (2015). Emil Kraepelin: icon and reality. *American Journal of Psychiatry, 172,* 1190–1196.

Enkel, T., Spanagel, R., Vollmayr, B., & Schneider, M. (2010). Stress triggers anhedonia in rats bred for learned helplessness. *Behavioural Brain Research, 209,* 183–186.

Enman, N. M., Arthur, K., Ward, S. J., Perrine, S. A., & Unterwald, E. M. (2015). Anhedonia, reduced cocaine reward, and dopamine dysfunction in a rat model of post-traumatic stress disorder. *Biological Psychiatry, 78,* 871–879.

Entringer, S., Buss, C., & Wadhwa, P. D. (2015). Prenatal stress, development, health and disease risk: a psychobiological perspective—2015 Curt Richter Award paper. *Psychoneuroendocrinology, 62,* 366–375.

Erhardt, A., Czibere, L., Roeske, D., Lucae, S., Unschuld, P. G., Ripke, S., . . . Binder, E. B. (2011). TMEM132D, a new candidate for anxiety phenotypes: evidence from human and mouse studies. *Molecular Psychiatry, 16,* 647–663.

Ericsson, A. C., Crim, M. J., & Franklin, C. L. (2013). A brief history of animal modeling. *Missouri Medicine, 110,* 201–205.

Estes, M. L., & McAllister, A. K. (2015). Immune mediators in the brain and peripheral tissues in autism spectrum disorder. *Nature Reviews Neuroscience, 16,* 468–486.

Estes, M. L., & McAllister, A. K. (2016). Maternal immune activation: implications for neuropsychiatric disorders. *Science, 353,* 772–777.

Etain, B., Mathieu, F., Henry, C., Raust, A., Roy, I., Germain, A., . . . Bellivier, F. (2010). Preferential association between childhood emotional abuse and bipolar disorder. *Journal of Traumatic Stress, 23,* 376–383.

Evanson, N. K., Tasker, J. G., Hill, M. N., Hillard, C. J., & Herman, J. P. (2010). Fast feedback inhibition of the HPA axis by glucocorticoids is mediated by endocannabinoid signaling. *Endocrinology, 151,* 4811–4819.

Fatemi, S. H., Pearce, D. A., Brooks, A. I., & Sidwell, R. W. (2005). Prenatal viral infection in mouse causes differential expression of genes in brain of mouse progeny: a potential animal model for schizophrenia and autism. *Synapse, 57,* 91–99.

Fava, G. A. (2007). Financial conflicts of interest in psychiatry. *World Psychiatry, 6,* 19–24.

Favre, M., La Mendola, D., Meystre, J., Christodoulou, D., Cochrane, M. J., Markram, H., and Markram, K. (2015). Predictable enriched environment prevents development of hyper-emotionality in the VPA rat model of autism. *Frontiers in Neuroscience, 9,* 127.

Feder, A., Nestler, E. J., & Charney, D. S. (2009). Psychobiology and molecular genetics of resilience. *Nature Reviews Neuroscience, 10,* 446–457.

Feighner, J. P., Robins, E., Guze, S. B., Woodruff, R. A., Jr., Winokur, G., & Munoz, R. (1972). Diagnostic criteria for use in psychiatric research. *Archives of General Psychiatry, 26,* 57–63.

Felger, J. C., Haroon, E., & Miller, A. H. (2015). Risk and resilience: animal models shed light on the pivotal role of inflammation in individual differences in stress-induced depression. *Biological Psychiatry, 78,* 7–9.

Fendt, M., Imobersteg, S., Bürki, H., McAllister, K. H., & Sailer, A. W. (2010). Intra-amygdala injections of neuropeptide S block fear-potentiated startle. *Neuroscience Letters, 474*, 154–157.

Ferenczi, E., & Deisseroth, K. (2016). Illuminating next-generation brain therapies. *Nature Neuroscience, 19*, 414–416.

Fernandes, B. S., Williams, L. M., Steiner, J., Leboyer, M., Carvalho, A. F., & Berk, M. (2017). The new field of "precision psychiatry." *BMC Medicine, 15*, 80.

File, S. E. (1980). The use of social interaction as a method for detecting anxiolytic activity of chlordiazepoxide-like drugs. *Journal of Neuroscience Methods, 2*, 219–238.

File, S. E., & Seth, P. (2003). A review of 25 years of the social interaction test. *European Journal of Pharmacology, 463*, 35–53.

Fink, G. (2016). Eighty years of stress. *Nature, 539*, 175–176.

Flaisher-Grinberg, S., & Einat, H. (2010). Strain-specific battery of tests for domains of mania: effects of valproate, lithium and imipramine. *Frontiers in Psychiatry, 1*, 10.

Flak, J. N., Solomon, M. B., Jankord, R., Krause, E. G., & Herman, J. P. (2012). Identification of chronic stress-activated regions reveals a potential recruited circuit in rat brain. *European Journal of Neuroscience, 36*, 2447–2455.

Fleming, D. (1984). Walter B. Cannon and homeostasis. *Social Research, 51*, 609–640.

Flint, A. J., Jr. (1878). Claude Bernard and his physiological works. *American Journal of the Medical Sciences, 76*, 161–173.

Fleshner, M., Frank, M., & Maier, S. F. (2017). Danger signals and inflammasomes: stress-evoked sterile inflammation in mood disorders. *Neuropsychopharmacology Reviews, 42*, 36–45.

Foa, E. B., Zinbarg, R., & Rothbaum, B. O. (1992). Uncontrollability and unpredictability in post-traumatic stress disorder: an animal model. *Psychological Bulletin, 112*, 218–238.

Folsom, T. D., & Fatemi, S. H. (2013). The involvement of Reelin in neurodevelopmental disorders. *Neuropharmacology, 68*, 122–135.

Fontes, M. A. P., Xavier, C. H., De Menezes, R. C. A., & Dimicco, J. A. (2011). The dorsomedial hypothalamus and the central pathways involved in the cardiovascular response to emotional stress. *Neuroscience, 184*, 64–74.

Fox, A. S., & Kalin, N. H. (2014). A translational neuroscience approach to understanding the development of social anxiety disorder and its pathophysiology. *American Journal of Psychiatry, 171*, 1162–1173.

Fox, A. S., Oler, J. A., Shackman, A. J., Shelton, S. E., Raveendram, M., McKay, D. R., . . . Kalin, N. H. (2015). Intergenerational neural mediators of early-life anxious temperament. *Proceedings of the National Academy of Sciences USA, 112*, 9118–9122.

Fox, A. S., Oler, J. A., Shelton, S. E., Nanda, S. A., Davidson, R. J., Roseboom, P. H., & Kalin, N. H. (2012). Central amygdala nucleus (Ce) gene expression linked to increased trait-like Ce metabolism and anxious temperament in young primates. *Proceedings of the National Academy of Sciences USA, 109*, 18108–18113.

Fox-Edmiston, E., & Van de Water, J. (2015). Maternal anti-fetal brain IgG autoantibodies and autism spectrum disorder: current knowledge and its implications for potential therapeutics. *CNS Drugs, 29*, 715–724.

Frances, A. (2014). RDoC is necessary, but very oversold. *World Psychiatry, 13*, 47–49.

Francis, D., Diorio, J., Liu, D., & Meaney, M. J. (1999). Nongenomic transmission across generations of maternal behavior and stress responses in the rat. *Science, 286*, 1155–1158.

Francis, D. D., Szegda, K., Campbell, G., Martin, W. D., & Insel, T. R. (2003). Epigenetic sources of behavioral differences in mice. *Nature Neuroscience, 6*, 445–446.

Francis, T. C., Chandra, R., Friend, D. M., Finkel, E., Dayrit, G., Miranda, J., . . . Lobo, M. K. (2015). Nucleus accumbens medium spiny neuron subtypes mediate depression-related outcomes to social defeat stress. *Biological Psychiatry, 77*, 212–222.

Francis, T. C., Chandra, R., Gaynor, A., Konkalmatt, P., Metzbower, S. R., Evans, B., . . . Lobo, M. K. (2017). Molecular basis of dendritic atrophy and activity in stress susceptibility. *Molecular Psychiatry, 22*, 1512–1519.

Frank, E., Salchner, P., Aldag, J. M., Salomé, N., Singewald, N., Landgraf, R., & Migger, A. (2006). Genetic predisposition to anxiety-related behavior determines coping style, neuroendocrine responses, and neuronal activation during social defeat. *Behavioral Neuroscience, 120*, 60–71.

Frank, M. G., Baratta, M. V., Sprunger, D. B., Watkins, L. R., & Maier, S. F. (2007). Microglia serve as a neuroimmune substrate for stress-induced potentiation of CNS pro-inflammatory cytokine responses. *Brain, Behavior and Immunity, 21*, 47–59.

Frank, M. G., Fonken, L. K., Annis, J. L., Watkins, L. R., & Maier, S. F. (2018). Stress disinhibits microglia via down-regulation of CD200R: a mechanism of neuroinflammatory priming. *Brain, Behavior, and Immunity, 69*, 62–73.

Frank, M. G., Fonken, L. K., Watkins, L. R., & Maier, S. F. (2019). Microglia: neuroimmune-sensors of stress. *Seminars in Cell and Developmental Biology, 94*, 176–185.

Frank, M. G., Watkins, L. R., & Maier, S. F. (2013). Stress-induced glucocorticoids as a neuroendocrine alarm signal of danger. *Brain, Behavior and Immunity, 33*, 1–6.

Frank, M. G., Weber, M. D., Watkins, L. R., & Maier, S. F. (2015). Stress sounds the alarmin: the role of the danger-associated molecular pattern HMGB1 in stress-induced neuroinflammatory priming. *Brain, Behavior and Immunity, 48*, 1–7.

Franklin, T. B., & Mansuy, I. M. (2009). Epigenetic inheritance in mammals: evidence for the impact of adverse environmental effects. *Neurobiology of Disease, 39*, 61–65.

Franklin, T. B., Russig, H., Weiss, I. C., Gräff, J., Linder, N., Michalon, A., . . . Mansuy, I. M. (2010). Epigenetic transmission of the impact of early stress across generations. *Biological Psychiatry, 68*, 408–415.

Franklin, T. C., Xu, C., & Duman, R. S. (2018). Depression and sterile inflammation: essential role of danger associated molecular patterns. *Brain, Behavior and Immunity, 72*, 2–13.

Freedman, R., Hunter, S. K., & Hoffman, M. C. (2018). Prenatal primary prevention of mental illness by micronutrient supplements in pregnancy. *American Journal of Psychiatry, 175*, 607–619.

Frey, B. N., Andreazza, A. C., Cereser, K. M. M., Martins, M. R., Valvassori, S. S., Réus, G. Z., . . . Kapczinski, F. (2006). Effects of mood stabilizers on hippocampus BDNF levels in an animal model of mania. *Life Sciences, 79*, 281–286.

Friedman, A. K., Walsch, J. J., Juarez, B., Ku, S. M., Chaudhury, D., Wang, J., . . . Han, M.-H. (2014). Enhancing depression mechanisms in midbrain dopamine neurons achieves homeostatic resilience. *Science, 344*, 313–319.

Friedman, E., Berman, M., & Overstreet, D. (2006). Swim test immobility in a genetic rat model of depression is modified by maternal environment: a cross-foster study. *Developmental Psychobiology, 48*, 169–177.

Fries, G. R., Quevedo, J., Zeni, C. P., Kazimi, I. F., Zunta-Soares, G., Spiker, D. E., . . . Soares, J. C. (2017). Integrated transcriptome and methylome analysis in youth at high risk for bipolar disorder: a preliminary analysis. *Translational Psychiatry, 7*, e1059.

Fries, G. R., Walss-Bass, C., Soares, J. C., & Quevedo, J. (2016). Non-genetic transgenerational transmission of bipolar disorder: targeting DNA methyltransferases. *Molecular Psychiatry, 21*, 1653–1654.

Frye, C. A., & Llaneza, D. C. (2010). Corticosteroid and neurosteroid dysregulation in an animal model of autism, BTBR mice. *Physiology and Behavior, 100*, 264–267.

Fuchikami, M., Yamamoto, S., Morinobu, S., Okada, S., Yamawaki, Y., & Yamawaki, S. (2016). The potential use of histone deacetylase inhibitors in the treatment of depression. *Progress in Neuro-Psychopharmacology and Biological Psychiatry, 64*, 320–324.

Füger, P., Hefendehl, J. K., Veeraraghavalu, K., Wendeln, A.-C., Schlosser, C., Obermüller, U., . . . Juncker, M. (2017). Microglia turnover with aging and in Alzheimer's model via long-term in vivo single-cell imaging. *Nature Neuroscience, 20*, 1371–1376.

Furukubo-Tokunaga, K. (2009). Modeling schizophrenia in flies. *Progress in Brain Research, 179*, 107–115.

Gainetdinov, R. R., Wetsel, W. C., Jones, S. R., Levin, E. D., Jaber, M., & Caron, M. G. (1999). Role of serotonin in the paradoxical calming effect of psychstimulants on hyperactivity. *Science, 283*, 397–401.

Galea, I., Bechmann, I., & Perry, V. H. (2007). What is immune privilege (not)? *Trends in Immunology, 28*, 12–18.

Gallitano-Mendel, A., Izumi, Y., Tokuda, K., Zorumski, C. F., Howell, M. P., Muglia, L. J., . . . Milbrandt, J. (2007). The immediate early gene early growth response gene 3 mediates adaptation to stress and novelty. *Neuroscience, 148*, 633–643.

Gallitano-Mendel, A., Wozniak, D. F., Pehek, E. A., & Milbrandt, J. (2008). Mice lacking the immediate early gene Egr3 respond to the anti-aggressive effects of clozapine yet are relatively resistant to its sedating effects. *Neuropsychopharmacology, 33*, 1266–1275.

Gapp, K., Jawaid, A., Sarkies, P., Bohacek, J., Pelczar, P., Prados, J., . . . Mansuy, I. M. (2014). Implication of sperm RNAs in transgenerational inheritance of the effects of early trauma in mice. *Nature Neuroscience, 17*, 667–669.

Garay, P. A., Hsiao, E. Y., Patterson, P. H., & McAllister, A. K. (2013). Maternal immune activation causes age- and region-specific changes in brain cytokines in offspring throughout development. *Brain, Behavior and Immunity, 31*, 54–68.

Garber, J., Clarke, G. N., Weersing, V. R., Beardslee, W. R., Brent, D. A., Gladstone, T. R. G., . . . Iyengar, S. (2009). Prevention of depression in at-risk adolescents: a randomized controlled trial. *Journal of the American Medical Association, 301*, 2215–2224.

Garmezy, N. (1974). The study of competence in children at risk for severe psychopathology. In E. J. Anthony & C. Koupernik (Eds.), *The child in his family: children at psychiatric risk*, Vol. 3 (pp. 77–97). New York, NY: Wiley.

Garmezy, N. (1985). Stress-resistant children: the search for protective factors. In A. Davids (Ed.), *Recent research in developmental psychopathology* (pp. 213–233). Elmsford, NY: Pergamon Press.

Garner, J. P. (2014). The significance of meaning: why do over 90% of behavioral neuroscience results fail to translate to humans and what can we do to fix it? *ILAR Journal, 55*, 438–456.

Garrido-Mesa, N., Zarzuelo, A., & Gálvez, J. (2013). Minocycline: far beyond an antibiotic. *British Journal of Pharmacology, 169*, 337–352.

Garzón-Niño, J., Rodriguez-Muñoz, M., Cortés-Montero, E., & Sánchez-Blázquez, P. (2017). Increased PKC activity and altered GSK3β/NMDAR function drive behavior cycling in HINT1-deficient mice: bipolarity or opposing forces. *Scientific Reports, 7*, 43468.

Gass, N., Becker, R., Schwarz, A. J., Weber-Fahr, W., von Hohenberg, C. C., Vollmayr, B., & Sartorius, A. (2016). Brain network reorganization differs in response to stress in rats genetically predisposed to depression and stress-resilient rats. *Translational Psychiatry, 6,* e970.

Gass, N., Cleppien, D., Zheng, L., Schwarz, A. J., Meyer-Lindenberg, A., Vollmayr, B., . . . Sartorius, A. (2014). Functionally altered neurocircuits in a rat model of treatment-resistant depression show prominent role of the habenula. *European Neuropsychopharmacology, 24,* 381–390.

Gass, P., & Wotjak, C. (2013). Rodent models of psychiatric disorders—practical considerations. *Cell and Tissue Research, 354,* 1–7.

Geaghan, M., & Cairns, M. J. (2015). MicroRNA and posttranscriptional dysregulation in psychiatry. *Biological Psychiatry, 78,* 231–239.

Geddes, J. R., & Miklowitz, D. J. (2013). Treatment of bipolar disorder. *Lancet, 381,* 1672–1682.

Geller, I., & Seifter, S. (1960). The effects of meprobamate, barbiturate, D-amphetamine and promazine on experimentally induced conflict in the rat. *Psychopharmacologia, 1,* 482–492.

George, S. A., Rodriguez-Santiago, M., Riley, J., Abelson, J. L., Floresco, S. B., & Liberzon, I. (2018). D-cycloserine facilitates reversal in an animal model of post-traumatic stress disorder. *Behavioural Brain Research, 347,* 332–338.

Gerlach, J. L., & McEwen, B. S. (1972). Rat brain binds adrenal steroid hormone: radioautography of hippocampus with corticosterone. *Science, 175,* 1133–1136.

Gerlai, R., Lahav, M., Guo, S., & Rosenthal, A. (2000). Drink like a fish: zebra fish (*Danio rerio*) as a behavior genetic model to study alcohol effects. *Pharmacology, Biochemistry and Behavior, 67,* 773–782.

Geschwind, D. H., & Flint, J. (2015). Genetics and genomics of psychiatric disease. *Science, 349,* 1489–1494.

Geschwind, D. H., & State, M. W. (2015). Gene hunting in autism spectrum disorder: on the path to precision medicine. *Lancet Neurology, 14,* 1109–1120.

Geyer, M. A., Wilkinson, L. S., Humby, T., & Robbins, T. W. (1993). Isolation rearing of rats produces a deficit in prepulse inhibition of acoustic startle similar to that in schizophrenia. *Biological Psychiatry, 34,* 361–372.

Gheorghe, C. P., Goyal, R., Mittal, A., & Longo, L. D. (2010). Gene expression in the placenta: maternal stress and epigenetic responses. *International Journal of Developmental Biology, 54,* 507–523.

Ghose, S., Winter, M. K., McCarson, K. E., Tamminga, C. A., & Enna, S. J. (2011). The GABAB receptor as a target for antidepressant drug action. *British Journal of Pharmacology, 162,* 1–17.

Giardino, W. J., Eban-Rothschild, A., Christoffel, D. J., Li, S.-B., Malenka. R. C., & de Lecea, L. (2018). Parallel circuits from the bed nuclei of stria terminalis to the lateral hypothalamus circuits drive opposing emotional states. *Nature Neuroscience, 21,* 1084–1095.

Gillan, C. M., & Whelan, R. (2017). What big data can do for treatment in psychiatry. *Current Opinion in Behavioral Sciences, 18,* 34–42.

Giovanoli, S., Engler, H., Engler, A., Richetto, J., Voget, M., Willi, R., . . . Meyer, U. (2013). Stress in puberty unmasks latent neuropathological consequences of prenatal immune activation in mice. *Science, 339,* 1095–1099.

Giovanoli, S., Weber, L., & Meyer, U. (2014). Single and combined effects of prenatal immune activation and peripubertal stress on parvalbumin and reelin expression in the hippocampal formation. *Brain, Behavior and Immunity, 40,* 48–54.

Girardi, C. E. N., Zanta, N. C., & Suchecki, D. (2014). Neonatal stress-induced affective changes in adolescent Wistar rats: early signs of schizophrenia-like behavior. *Frontiers in Behavioral Neuroscience, 8*, 319.

Girotti, M., Weinberg, M. S., & Spencer, R. L. (2009). Diurnal expression of functional and clock-related genes throughout the rat HPA axis: system-wide shifts in response to a restricted feeding schedule. *American Journal of Physiology, 296*, E888–E897.

Giustino, T. F., Fitzgerald, P. J., & Maren, S. (2016). Revisiting propranolol and PTSD: memory erasure or extinction enhancement? *Neurobiology of Learning and Memory, 130*, 26–33.

Gjerstad, J. K., Lightman, S. L., & Spiga, F. (2018). Role of glucocorticoid negative feedback in the regulation of HPA axis pulsatility. *Stress, 21*, 403–416.

Glassner, B., and Haldipur, C. V. (1983). Life events and early and late onset of bipolar disorder. *American Journal of Psychiatry, 140*, 215–217.

Gleason, G., Liu, B., Bruening, S., Zupan, B., Auerbach, A., Mark, W., . . . Toth, M. (2010). The serotonin1A receptor gene as a genetic and prenatal maternal environmental factor in anxiety. *Proceedings of the National Academy of Sciences USA, 107*, 7592–7597.

Gleason, G., Zupan, B., & Toth, M. (2011). Maternal genetic mutations as gestational and early life influences in producing psychiatric disease-like phenotypes in mice. *Frontiers in Psychiatry, 2*, 25.

Goddard, G. V., McIntyre, D. C., & Leech, C. K. (1969). A permanent change in brain function resulting from daily electrical stimulation. *Experimental Neurology, 25*, 295–330.

Goehler, L. E., Gaykema, R. P. A., Hansen, M. K., Anderson, K., Maier, S. F., & Watkins, L. R. (2000). Vagal immune-to-brain communication: a visceral chemosensory pathway. *Autonomic Neuroscience: Basic and Clinical, 85*, 49–59.

Goines, P., & Ashwood, P. (2013). Cytokine dysregulation in autism spectrum disorders (ASD): possible role of the environment. *Neurotoxicology and Teratology, 36*, 67–81.

Goines, P., & Van de Water, J. (2010). The immune system's role in the biology of autism. *Current Opinion in Neurology, 23*, 111–117.

Gold, P. W. (2015). The organization of the stress system and its dysregulation in depressive illness. *Molecular Psychiatry, 20*, 32–47.

Goldstein, D. S. (2006). *Adrenaline and the inner world.* Baltimore, MD: The Johns Hopkins University Press.

Goldstein, D. S., & Kopin, I. J. (2007). Evolution of concepts of stress. *Stress, 10*, 109–120.

Goldstein, D. S., McCarty, R., Polinsky, R. J., & Kopin, I. J. (1983). Relationship between plasma norepinephrine and sympathetic neural activity. *Hypertension, 5*, 552–559.

Gomes, F. V., & Grace, A. A. (2017a). Adolescent stress as a driving factor for schizophrenia development: a basic science perspective. *Schizophrenia Bulletin, 43*, 486–489.

Gomes, F. V., & Grace, A. A. (2017b). Prefrontal cortex dysfunction increases susceptibility to schizophrenia-like changes induced by adolescent stress exposure. *Schizophrenia Bulletin, 43*, 592–600.

Gomes, F. V., Rincón-Cortés, M., & Grace, A. A. (2016). Adolescence as a period of vulnerability and intervention in schizophrenia: insights from the MAM model. *Neuroscience and Biobehavioral Reviews, 70*, 260–270.

Gomez, J. L., Bonaventura, J., Lesniak, W., Mathews, W. B., Sysa-Shah, P., Rodriguez, L. A., . . . Michaelides, M. (2017). Chemogenetics revealed: DREADD occupancy and activation via converted clozapine. *Science, 357*, 503–507.

Gómez-Galán, M., Femenía, T., Aberg, E., Graae, L., Van eeckhaut, A., Smolders, I., . . . Lindskog, M. (2016). Running opposes the effects of social isolation on synaptic plasticity and transmission in a rat model of depression. *PLoS ONE*, *11*, e0165071.

Goncalvesova, E., Micutkova, L., Mravec, B., Ksinantova, L., Krizanova, O., Fabian, J., & Kvetnansky, R. (2004). Changes in gene expression of phenylethanolamine N-methyltransferase in the transplanted human heart. *Annals of the New York Academy of Sciences*, *1018*, 430–436.

Gong, Q., Scarpazza, C., Dai, J., He, M., Xu, X., Shi, Y., . . . Mechelli, A. (2019). A transdiagnostic neuroanatomical signature of psychiatric illness. *Neuropsychopharmacology*, *44*, 869–875.

Gong, S., Doughty, M., Harbaugh, C. R., Cummins, A., Hatten, M. E., Heintz, N., & Gerfen, C. R. (2007). Targeting CRE recombinase to specific neuron populations with Bacterial Artificial Chromosome constructs. *Journal of Neuroscience*, *27*, 9817–9823.

Goodall, J. (2010). *In the shadow of man*. London, England: Orion.

Goodwill, H. L., Manzano-Nieves, G., Gallo, M., Lee, H.-I., Oyerinde, E., Serre, T., & Bath, K. G. (2019). Early life stress leads to sex differences in development of depressive-like outcomes in a mouse model. *Neuropsychopharmacology*, *44*, 711–720.

Gordon, J. (2017). The future of RDoC. Posted June 5, 2017, as Director's Message. https://www.nimh.nih.gov/about/director/messages/2017/the-future-of-rdoc.shtml.

Gordon, J. A. (2019). From neurobiology to novel medications: a principled approach to translation. *American Journal of Psychiatry*, *176*, 425–427.

Goswami, S., Rodríguez-Sierra, O., Cascardi, M., & Paré, D. (2013). Animal models of post-traumatic stress disorder: face validity. *Frontiers in Neuroscience*, *7*, 89.

Gotlib, I. H., Joormann, J., Minor, K. L., & Hallmayer, J. (2008). HPA axis reactivity: a mechanism underlying the associations among 5-HTTLPR, stress, and depression. *Biological Psychiatry*, *63*, 847–851.

Gottesman, I. I., & Gould, T. D. (2003). The endophenotype concept in psychiatry: etymology and strategic intentions. *American Journal of Psychiatry*, *160*, 636–645.

Gottesman, I. I., & Shields, J. (1967). A polygenic theory of schizophrenia. *Proceedings of the National Academy of Sciences USA*, *58*, 199–205.

Gottesman, I. I., & Shields, J. (1982). *Schizophrenia: the epigenetic puzzle*. New York, NY: Cambridge University Press.

Gould, G. G., Burke, T. F., Osorio, M. D., Smolik, C. M., Zhang, W. Q., Onaivi, E. S., . . . Hensler, J. G. (2014). Enhanced novety-induced corticosterone spike and upregulated serotonin 5-HT1A and cannabinoid CB1 receptors in adolescent BTBR mice. *Psychoneuroendocrinology*, *39*, 158–169.

Gould, T. D., & Gottesman, I. I. (2006). Psychiatric endophenotypes and the development of valid animal models. *Genes, Brain and Behavior*, *5*, 113–119.

Grace, A. A. (2016). Dysregulation of the dopamine system in the pathophysiology of schizophrenia and depression. *Nature Reviews Neuroscience*, *17*, 524–532.

Grace, A. A. (2017). Dopamine system dysregulation and the pathophysiology of schizophrenia: insights from the methylazoxymethanol acetate model. *Biological Psychiatry*, *81*, 5–8.

Greco, B., Managò, F., Tucci, V., Kao, H.-T., Valtorta, F., & Benfenati, F. (2013). Autism-related behavioral abnormalities in synapsin knockout mice. *Behavioural Brain Research*, *251*, 65–74.

Greek, R., Menache, A., & Rice, M. J. (2012). Animal models in an age of personalized medicine. *Personalized Medicine*, *9*, 47–64.

Green, R. E., Krause, J., Briggs, A. W., Maricic, T., Stenzel, U., Kircher, M., . . . Pääbo, S. (2010). A draft sequence of the Neanderthal genome. *Science, 328,* 710–722.

Greenwood, B. N., & Fleshner, M. (2011). Exercise, stress resistance, and central serotonergic systems. *Exercise and Sport Sciences Reviews, 39,* 140–149.

Greenwood, B. N., Foley, T. E., Day, H. E. W., Campisi, J., Hammack, S. H., Campeau, S., . . . Fleshner, M. (2003). Free wheel running prevents learned helplessness/behavioral depression: role of dorsal raphe serotonergic neurons. *Journal of Neuroscience, 23,* 2889–2898.

Grillon, C., Ameli, R., Goddard, A., Woods, S. W., & Davis, M. (1994). Baseline and fear-potentiated startle in panic disorder patients. *Biological Psychiatry, 35,* 431–439.

Grippo, A. J., & Johnson, A. K. (2002). Biological mechanisms in the relationship between depression and heart disease. *Neuroscience and Biobehavioral Reviews, 26,* 941–962.

Grob, G. N. (1991). Origins of *DSM-I:* a study in appearance and reality. *American Journal of Psychiatry, 148,* 421–431.

Gross, C., Zhuang, X., Stark, K., Ramboz, S., Oosting, R., Kirby, L., . . . Hen, R. (2002). Serotonin1A receptor acts during development to establish normal anxiety-like behavior in the adult. *Nature, 416,* 396–400.

Gross, C. G. (1998). Claude Bernard and the constancy of the internal environment. *The Neuroscientist, 4,* 380–385.

Gross, C. G. (2000). Neurogenesis in the adult brain: death of a dogma. *Nature Reviews Neuroscience, 1,* 67–73.

Grouzmann, E., Cavadas, C., Grand, D., Moratel, M., Aubert, J.-F., Brunner, H. R., & Mazzolai, L. (2003). Blood sampling methodology is crucial for precise measurement of plasma catecholamines concentrations in mice. *Pflügers Archiv – European Journal of Physiology, 447,* 254–258.

Gruenberg, E. M. (1968). Foreword. In *Diagnostic and statistical manual of mental disorders, second edition* (pp. vii–x). Washington, DC: American Psychiatric Association.

Grupe, D. W., & Nitschke, J. B. (2013). Uncertainty and anticipation in anxiety: an integrated neurobiological and psychological perspective. *Nature Reviews Neuroscience, 14,* 488–501.

Guidotti, A., Dong, E., Tueting, P., & Grayson, D. R. (2014). Modeling the molecular epigenetic profile of psychosis in prenatally stressed mice. *Progress in Molecular Biology and Translational Science, 128,* 89–101.

Guillemin, R. (1985). A personal reminiscence of Hans Selye. *Experientia, 41,* 560–561.

Gumusoglu, S. B., & Stevens, H. E. (2019). Maternal inflammation and neurodevelopmental programming: a review of preclinical outcomes and implications for translational psychiatry. *Biological Psychiatry, 85,* 107–121.

Gupta, D., Chuang, J.-C., Mani, B. K., Shankar, K., Rodriguez, J. A., Osborne-Lawrence, S., . . . Zigman, J. M. (2019). ß1-adrenergic receptors mediate plasma acyl-ghrelin elevation and depressive-like behavior induced by chronic psychosocial stress. *Neuropsychopharmacology, 44,* 1319–1327.

Guyenet, P. G. (2006). The sympathetic control of blood pressure. *Nature Reviews Neuroscience, 7,* 335–346.

Guyenet, P. G., Stornetta, R. L., Bochorishvili, G., DePuy, S. D., Burke, P. G. R., & Abbott, S. B. G. (2013). C1 neurons: the body's EMTs. *American Journal of Physiology, 305,* R187–R204.

Haenisch, B., Bilkei-Gorzo, A., Caron, M. G., & Bönisch, H. (2009). Knockout of the norepinephrine transporter and pharmacologically diverse antidepressants prevent behavioral and brain neurotraophin alterations in two chronic stress models of depression. *Journal of Neurochemistry, 111*, 403–416.

Hagen, E. H. (2011). Evolutionary theories of depression: a critical review. *Canadian Journal of Psychiatry, 56*, 716–726.

Haig, D. (2012). Commentary: the epidemiology of epigenetics. *International Journal of Epidemiology, 41*, 13–16.

Hallmayer, J., Cleveland, S., Torres, A., Phillips, J., Cohen, B., Torigoe, T., . . . Risch, N. (2011). Genetic heritability and shared environmental factors among twin pairs with autism. *Archives of General Psychiatry, 68*, 1095–1102.

Hamilton, P. J., Burek, D. J., Lombrosos, S. I., Neve, R. L., Robison, A. J., Nestler, E. J., & Heller, E. A. (2018). Cell-type-specific epigenetic editing at the *Fosb* gene controls susceptibility to social defeat stress. *Neuropsychopharmacology, 43*, 272–284.

Hammen, C., & Gitlin, M. (1997). Stress reactivity in bipolar patients and its relation to prior history of disorder. *American Journal of Psychiatry, 154*, 856–857.

Hammond, G. L. (2016). Plasma steroid-binding proteins: primary gatekeepers of steroid hormone action. *Journal of Endocrinology, 230*, R13–R25.

Han, M.-H., & Nestler, E. J. (2017). Neural substrates of depression and resilience. *Neurotherapeutics, 14*, 677–686.

Hankin, B. L., Young, J. F., Gallop, R., & Garber, J. (2018). Cognitive and interpersonal vulnerabilities to adolescent depression: classification of risk profiles for a personalized prevention approach. *Journal of Abnormal Child Psychology, 46*, 1521–1533.

Hansen, C., & Spuhler, K. (1984). Development of the National Institutes of Health genetically heterogeneous rat stock. *Alcoholism: Clinical and Experimental Research, 8*, 477–479.

Haque, F. N., Lipina, T. V., Roder, J. C., & Wong, A. H. C. (2012). Social defeat interacts with *Disc1* mutations in the mouse to affect behavior. *Behavioural Brain Research, 233*, 337–344.

Harada, K., Yamaji, T., & Matsuoka, N. (2008). Activation of the serotonin 5-HT2C receptor is involved in the enhanced anxiety in rats after single-prolonged stress. *Pharmacology, Biochemistry and Behavior, 89*, 11–16.

Harding, J. D., Van Hoosier, G. L., Jr., & Grieder, F. B. (2010). The contribution of laboratory animals to medical progress: past, present, and future. In J. Hann & S. J. Shapiro (Eds.), *Handbook of laboratory animal science, Vol. 1. Essential principles and practices* (3rd ed.) (pp. 1–20). New York, NY: CRC Press.

Hariri, A. R., & Holmes, A. (2015). Finding translation in stress research. *Nature Neuroscience, 18*, 1347–1352.

Harlow, H. F. (1949). The formation of learning sets. *Psychological Review, 56*, 51–65.

Harlow, H. F. (1958). The nature of love. *American Psychologist, 13*, 673–685.

Harlow, H. F., Harlow, M. K., & Suomi, S. J. (1971). From thought to therapy: lessons from a primate laboratory. *American Scientist, 59*, 538–549.

Harlow, H. R., & Suomi, S. J. (1971). Social recovery by isolation-reared monkeys. *Proceedings of the National Academy of Sciences USA, 68*, 1534–1538.

Harlow, H. R., & Suomi, S. J. (1974). Induced depression in monkeys. *Behavioral Biology, 12*, 273–296.

Harmatz, E. S., Stone, L., Lim, S. H., Lee, G., McGrath, A., Gisabella, B., . . . Goosens, K. A. (2017). Central ghrelin resistance permits the overconsolidation of fear memory. *Biological Psychiatry, 81*, 1003–1013.

Harrison, P. J., & Eastwood, S. L. (2001). Neuropathological studies of synaptic connectivity in the hippocampal formation in schizophrenia. *Hippocampus, 11*, 508–519.

Hartl, D. L., & Orel, V. (1992). What did Gregor Mendel think he discovered? *Genetics*, *131*, 245–253.

Harvey, L., & Boksa, P. (2012). Prenatal and postnatal animal models of immune activation: relevance to a range of neurodevelopmental disorders. *Developmental Neurobiology*, *72*, 1335–1348.

Hascoët, M., Bourin, M., Colombel, M. C., Fiocco, A. J., & Baker, G. B. (2000). Anxiolytic-like effects of antidepressants after acute administration in a four-plate test in mice. *Pharmacology, Biochemistry and Behavior*, *65*, 339–344.

Hasler, G., Drevets, W. C., Gould, T. D., Gottesman, I. I., & Manji, H. K. (2006). Toward constructing an endophenotype strategy for bipolar disorders. *Biological Psychiatry*, *60*, 93–105.

Hauger, R. L., Grigoriadis, D. E., Dallman, M. F., Plotsky, P. M., Vale, W. W., & Dautzenberg, F. M. (2003). International Union of Pharmacology. XXXVI. Current status of the nomenclature for receptors for corticotropin-releasing factor and their ligands. *Pharmacological Reviews*, *55*, 21–26.

Haukka, J., Suvisaari, J., & Lönnqvist, J. (2003). Fertility of patients with schizophrenia, their siblings, and the general population: a cohort study from 1950 to 1959 in Finland. *American Journal of Psychiatry*, *160*, 460–463.

Hausdorff, W. P. (1990). Turning off the signal: desensitization of β-adrenergic receptor function. *FASEB Journal*, *4*, 2881–2889.

Heckers, S. (2015). The value of psychiatric diagnoses. *JAMA Psychiatry*, *72*, 1165–1166.

Heidenreich, M., & Zhang, F. (2016). Applications of CRISPR–Cas systems in neuroscience. *Nature Reviews Neuroscience*, *17*, 36–44.

Heilig, M. (2004). The NPY system in stress, anxiety and depression. *Neuropeptides*, *38*, 213–224.

Heilig, M., MacLeod, S., Koob, G. K., & Britton, K. T. (1992). Anxiolytic-like effect of neuropeptide Y (NPY), but not other peptides in an operant conflict task. *Regulatory Peptides*, *41*, 61–69.

Heim, C., & Bender, E. B. (2012). Current research trends in early life stress and depression: review of human studies on sensitive periods, gene-environment interactions, and epigenetics. *Experimental Neurology*, *233*, 102–111.

Helle, K. B., Metz-Boutigue, M.-H., Cerra, M. C., & Angelone, T. (2018). Chromogranins: from discovery to current times. *Pflugers Archiv – European Journal of Physiology*, *470*, 143–154.

Heller, E. A., Cates, H. M., Peña, C. J., Sun, H., Shao, N., Feng, J., . . . Nestler, E. J. (2014). Locus-specific epigenetic remodeling controls addiction- and depression-related behaviors. *Nature Neuroscience*, *17*, 1720–1727.

Hemmerle, A. M., Ahlbrand, R., Bronson, S. L., Lundgren, K. H., Richtand, N. M., & Seroogy, K. B. (2015). Modulation of schizophrenia-related genes in the forebrain of adolescent and adult rats exposed to maternal immune activation. *Schizophrenia Research*, *168*, 411–420.

Henckens, M. J. A. G., Deussing, J. M., & Chen, A. (2016). Region-specific roles of the corticotropin-releasing factor-urocortin system in stress. *Nature Reviews Neuroscience*, *17*, 636–651.

Henckens, M. J. A. G., Printz, Y., Shamgar, U., Lebow, M., Drori, Y., Kuehne, C., . . . Chen, A. (2017). CRF receptor type 2 neurons in the posterior bed nucleus of the stria terminalis critically contribute to stress recovery. *Molecular Psychiatry*, *22*, 1691–1700.

Henderson, L. J. (1927). Introduction. In C. Bernard, *Introduction to the study of experimental medicine*. New York, NY: Henry Schuman.

Henley, D. E., & Lightman, S. L. (2011). New insights into corticosteroid-binging globulin and glucocorticoid delivery. *Neuroscience, 180*, 1–8.

Henley, D. E., Lightman, S. L., & Carrell, R. (2016). Cortisol and CBG: getting cortisol to the right place at the right time. *Pharmacology and Therapeutics, 166*, 128–135.

Henn, F. A., & Vollmayr, B. (2005). Stress models of depression: forming genetically vulnerable strains. *Neuroscience and Biobehavioral Reviews, 29*, 799–804.

Henry, B. L., Minassian, A., Young, J. W., Paulus, M. P., Geyer, M. A., & Perry, W. (2010). Cross-species assessments of motor and exploratory behavior related to bipolar disorder. *Neuroscience and Biobehavioral Reviews, 34*, 1296–1306.

Herman, J. P. (2013). Neural control of chronic stress adaptation. *Frontiers in Behavioral Neuroscience, 7*, 61.

Herman, J. P. (2018). Regulation of hypothalamo-pituitary-adrenocortical responses to stressors by the nucleus of the solitary tract/dorsal vagal complex. *Cellular and Molecular Neurobiology, 38*, 25–35.

Herman, J. P., Figueiredo, H., Mueller, N. K., Ulrich-Lai, Y., Ostrander, M. M., Choi, D. C., & Cullinan, W. E. (2003). Central mechanisms of stress integration: hierarchical circuitry controlling hypothalmo-pituitary-adrenocortical responsiveness. *Frontiers in Neuroendocrinology, 24*, 151–180.

Herman, L., Hougland, T., & El-Mallakh, R. S. (2007). Mimicking human bipolar ion dysregulation models mania in rats. *Neuroscience and Biobehavioral Reviews, 31*, 874–881.

Herzog, C. J., Czéh, B., Corbach, S., Wuttke, W., Schulte-Herbrüggen, O., Hellweg, R., . . . Fuchs, E. (2009). Chronic social instability stress in female rats: a potential animal model for female depression. *Neuroscience, 159*, 982–992.

Hettema, J. M., Neale, M. C., & Kendler, K. S. (2001). A review and meta-analysis of the genetic epidemiology of anxiety disorders. *American Journal of Psychiatry, 158*, 1568–1578.

Hicks, J. K., Swen, J. J., Thorn, C. F., Sangkuhl, K., Karasch, E. D., Ellingrod, V. L., . . . Stingl, J. C. (2013). Clinical pharmacogenetics implementation consortium guideline for CYP2D6 and CYP2C19 genotypes and dosing of tricyclic antidepressants. *Clinical Pharmacology and Therapeutics, 93*, 402–408.

Hikosaka, O. (2010). The habenula: from stress evasion to value-based decision-making. *Nature Reviews Neuroscience, 11*, 503–513.

Hill, R. A., Wu, Y. W., Kwek, P., & van den Buuse, M. (2012). Modulatory effects of sex steroid hormones on brain-derived neurotrophic factor-tyrosine kinase B expression during adolescent development in C57Bl/6 mice. *Journal of Neuroendocrinology, 24*, 774–788.

Hiramoto, Y., Kang, G., Suzuki, G., Satoh, Y., Kucherlapati, R., Watanabe, Y., & Hiroi, N. (2011). Tbx1: identification of a 22q11.2 gene as a risk factor for autism spectrum disorder in a mouse model. *Human Molecular Genetics, 20*, 4775–4785.

Hlastala, S. A., Frank, E., Kowalski, J., Sherrill, J. T., Tu, X. M., Anderson, B., & Kupfer, D. J. (2000). Stressful life events, bipolar disorder, and the "kindling model." *Journal of Abnormal Psychology, 109*, 777–786.

Hodes, G. E., & Epperson, C. N. (2019). Sex differences in vulnerability and resilience to stress across the life span. *Biological Psychiatry, 86*, 421–432.

Hodes, G. E., Pfau, M. L., Leboeuf, M., Golden, S. A., Christoffel, D. J., Bregman, D., . . . Russo, S. J. (2014). Individual differences in the peripheral immune system promote resilience versus susceptibility to social stress. *Proceedings of the National Academy of Sciences USA*, *111*, 16136–16141.

Hodes, G. E., Pfau, M. L., Purushothaman, I., Ahn, H. F., Golden, S. A., Christoffel, D. J., . . . Russo, S. J. (2015). Sex differences in nucleus accumbens transcriptome profiles associated with susceptibility versus resilience to subchronic variable stress. *Journal of Neuroscience*, *35*, 16362–16376.

Hodes, G. E., Walker, D. M., LaBonté, B., Nestler, E. J., & Russo, S. J. (2016). Understanding the epigenetic basis of sex differences in depression. *Journal of Neuroscience Research*, *95*, 692–702.

Hoffman, J. R., Ostfeld, I., Stout, J. R., Harris, R. C., Kaplan, Z., & Cohen, H. (2015). ß-alanine supplemented diets enhance behavioral resilience to stress exposure in an animal model of PTSD. *Amino Acids*, *47*, 1247–1257.

Hogg, S. (1996). A review of the validity and variability of the elevated plus-maze as an animal model of anxiety. *Pharmacology, Biochemistry and Behavior*, *54*, 21–30.

Holl, K., He, H., Wedemeyer, M., Clopton, L., Wert, S., Meckes, J. K., . . . Solberg Woods, L. C. (2018). Heterogeneous stock rats: a model to study the genetics of despair-like behavior in adolescence. *Genes, Brain and Behavior*, *17*, 139–148.

Hollingshead, A. B., & Redlich, F. C. (1958). *Social class and mental illness*. New York, NY: Wiley.

Hollis, F., & Kabbaj, M. (2014). Social defeat as an animal model for depression. *ILAR Journal*, *55*, 221–232.

Holloway, T., Moreno, J. L., Umali, A., Rayannavar, V., Hodes, G. E., Russo, S. J., & González-Maeso, J. (2013). Prenatal stress induces schizophrenia-like alterations of serotonin 2A and metabotropic glutamate 2 receptors in the adult offspring: role of maternal immune system. *Journal of Neuroscience*, *33*, 1088–1098.

Holly, E. N., & Miczek, K. A. (2015). Capturing individual differences: challenges in animal models of posttraumatic stress disorder and drug abuse. *Biological Psychiatry*, *78*, 816–818.

Holmes, A., Yang, R. J., Lesch, K.-P., Crawley, J. N., & Murphy, D. L. (2003). Mice lacking the serotonin transporter exhibit 5-HT1A receptor-mediated abnormalities in tests for anxiety-like behavior. *Neuropsychopharmacology*, *28*, 2077–2088.

Holmes, C., Eisenhofer, G., & Goldstein, D. S. (1994). Improved assay for plasma dihydroxyphenylacetic acid and other catechols using high performance liquid chromatography with electrochemical detection. *Journal of Chromatography B Biomedical Science Applications*, *653*, 131–138.

Holmes, F. L. (1986). Claude Bernard, the *milieu intérieur* and regulatory physiology. *History and Philosophy of the Life Sciences*, *8*, 3–25.

Horan, W. P., Ventura, J., Nuechterlein, K. H., Subotnik, K. L., Hwang, S. S., & Mintz, J. (2005). Stressful life events in recent-onset schizophrenia: reduced frequencies and altered subjective appraisals. *Schizophrenia Research*, *75*, 363–374.

Horiuchi, J., McDowell, L. M., & Dampney, R. A. L. (2006). Differential control of cardiac and sympathetic vasomotor activity from the dorsomedial hypothalamus. *Clinical and Experimental Pharmacology and Physiology*, *33*, 1265–1268.

Hornig, M., Bresnahan, M. A., Che, X., Schultz, A. F., Ukaigwe, J. E., Eddy, M. L., . . . Lipkin, W. I. (2018). Prenatal fever and autism risk. *Molecular Psychiatry*, *23*, 759–766.

Horváth, S., & Kirnics, K. (2014). Immune system disturbances in schizophrenia. *Biological Psychiatry, 75,* 316–323.

Horwitz, R. I., Cullen, M. R., Abell, J., & Christian, J. B. (2013). (De)personalized medicine. *Science, 339,* 1155–1156.

Hosang, G. M., Fisher, H. L., Cohen-Woods, S., McGuffin, P., & Farmer, A. E. (2016). Stressful life events and catechol-O-methyl-transferase (COMT) gene in bipolar disorder. *Depression and Anxiety, 34,* 419–426.

Hosang, G. M., Uher, R., Keers, R., Cohen-Woods, S., Craig, I., Korszun, A., . . . Farmer, A. E. (2010). Stressful life events and the brain-derived neurotrophic factor gene in bipolar disorder. *Journal of Affective Disorders, 125,* 345–349.

Howard, D. M., Adams, M. J., Clarke, T.-K., Hafferty, J. D., Gibson, J., Shirali, M., . . . McIntosh, A. M. (2019). Genome-wide meta-analysis of depression in 807,553 individuals identifies 102 independent variants with replication in a further 1,507,153 individuals. *Nature Neuroscience, 22,* 343–352.

Howe, K., Clark, M. D., Torroja, C. F., Berthelot, C., Muffato, M., Collins, J. E., . . . Stemple, D. L. (2013). The zebrafish reference genome sequence and its relationship to the human genome. *Nature, 496,* 498–503.

Howell, K. R., & Pillai, A. (2014). Effects of prenatal hypoxia on schizophrenia-related phenotypes in heterozygous reeler mice: a gene x environment interaction study. *European Neuropsychopharmacology, 24,* 1324–1336.

Howerton, C. L., & Bale, T. L. (2014). Targeted placental deletion of OGT recapitulates the prenatal stress phenotype including hypothalamic mitochondrial dysfunction. *Proceedings of the National Academy of Sciences USA, 111,* 9639–9644.

Howerton, C. L., Morgan, C. P., Fischer, D. B., & Bale, T. L. (2013). O-GlcNAc transferase (OGT) as a placental biomarker of maternal stress and reprogramming of CNS gene transcription in development. *Proceedings of the National Academy of Sciences USA, 110,* 5169–5174.

Howes, O. D., & McCutcheon, R. (2017). Inflammation and the neural diathesis-stress hypothesis of schizophrenia: a reconceptualization. *Translational Psychiatry, 7,* e1024.

Howes, O. D., McCutcheon, R., Owen, M. J., & Murray, R. M. (2016). The role of genes, stress, and dopamine in the development of schizophrenia. *Biological Psychiatry, 81,* 9–20.

Hsiao, E. Y., McBride, S. W., Chow, J., Mazmanian, S. K., & Patterson, P. H. (2012). Modeling an autism risk factor in mice leads to permanent immune dysregulation. *Proceedings of the National Academy of Sciences USA, 109,* 12776–12781.

Hsu, D. T., Kirouac, G. J., Zubieta, J.-K., & Bhatnagar, S. (2014). Contributions of the paraventricular thalamic nucleus in the regulation of stress, motivation, and mood. *Frontiers in Behavioral Neuroscience, 8,* 73.

Hsu, S. Y., & Hsueh, A .J. W. (2001). Human stresscopin and stresscopin-related peptide are selective ligands for the type 2 corticotropin-releasing hormone receptor. *Nature Medicine, 7,* 605–611.

Huang, H.-J., Zhu, X.-C., Han, Q.-Q., Wang, Y.-L., Yue, N., Wang, J., . . . Yu, J. (2017). Ghrelin alleviates anxiety- and depression-like behaviors induced by chronic unpredictable mild stress in rodents. *Behavioural Brain Research, 326,* 33–43.

Hultman, R., Ulrich, K., Sachs, B. D., Blount, C., Carlson, D. E., Ndubuizu, N., . . . Dzirasa, K. (2018). Brain-wide electrical spatiotemporal dynamics encode depression vulnerability. *Cell, 173,* 166–180.

Hunter, R. G., Gray, J. D., & McEwen, B. S. (2018). The neuroscience of resilience. *Journal of the Society for Social Work and Research, 9,* 305–339.

Huxley, J., Mayr, E., Osmond, H., & Hoffer, A. (1964). Schizophrenia as a genetic morphism. *Nature, 204,* 220–221.

Hyman, S. E. (2007). Can neuroscience be integrated into the DSM-V? *Nature Reviews Neuroscience, 8,* 725–732.

Hyman, S. E. (2012). Revolution stalled. *Science Translational Medicine, 4,* 155cm11.

Hyman, S. E. (2014). How far can mice carry autism research? *Cell, 158,* 13–14.

Hyman, S. E. (2018). The daunting polygenicity of mental illness: making a new map. *Philosophical Transactions of the Royal Society B, 373,* 20170031.

Ikeda, M., Takahashi, A., Kamatani, Y., Okahisa, Y., Kunugi, H., Mori, N., . . . Iwata, N., for the advanced Collaborative Study of Mood Disorder (COSMO) team (2018). A genome-wide association study identifies two novel susceptibility loci and trans population polygenicity associated with bipolar disorder. *Molecular Psychiatry, 23,* 639–647.

Imanaka, A., Morinobu, S., Toki, S., & Yamawaki, S. (2006). Importance of early environment in the development of post-traumatic stress disorder-like behaviors. *Behavioural Brain Research, 173,* 129–137.

Impagnatiello, F., Guidotti, A. R., Pesold, C., Dwivedi, Y., Caruncho, H., Pisu, M. G., . . . Costa, E. (1998). A decrease in reelin expression as a putative vulnerability factor in schizophrenia. *Proceedings of the National Academy of Sciences USA, 95,* 15718–15723.

Infurna, F. J., & Luthar, S. S. (2016). Resilience to major life stressors is not as common as thought. *Perspectives on Psychological Science, 11,* 175–194.

Iñiguez, S. D., Riggs, L. M., Nieto, S. J., Dayrit, G., Zamora, N. N., Shawhan, K. L., . . . Warren, B. L. (2014). Social defeat stress induces a depression-like phenotype in adolescent male c57BL/6 mice. *Stress, 17,* 247–255.

Insel, T. R. (2007). From animal models to model animals. *Biological Psychiatry, 62,* 1337–1339.

Insel, T. R. (2012). Next-generation treatments for mental disorders. *Science Translational Medicine, 4,* 155ps19.

Insel, T. R. (2014). The NIMH Research Domain Criteria (RDoC) Project: precision medicine for psychiatry. *American Journal of Psychiatry, 171,* 395–397.

Insel, T. R., & Cuthbert, B. N. (2015). Brain disorders? Precisely. Precision medicine comes to psychiatry. *Science, 348,* 499–500.

Insel, T. R., Cuthbert, B., Garvey, M., Heinssen, R., Pine, D. S., Quinn, K., . . . Wang, P. (2010). Research domain criteria (RDoC): toward a new classification framework for research on mental disorders. *American Journal of Psychiatry, 167,* 748–751.

Insel, T. R., & Young, L. J. (2001). The neurobiology of attachment. *Nature Reviews Neuroscience, 2,* 129–136.

Institute of Medicine (IOM). (1994). *Reducing risks for mental disorders: frontiers for preventive intervention research.* Washington, DC: National Academy Press.

Institute of Medicine (IOM). (2014a). *Capturing social and behavioral domains in electronic health records: Phase 1.* Washington, DC: National Academies Press.

Institute of Medicine (IOM). (2014b). *Capturing social and behavioral domains and measures in electronic health records: Phase 2.* Washington, DC: National Academies Press.

International Advisory Group for the Revision of ICD-10 Mental and Behavioural Disorders (2011). A conceptual framework for the revision of the ICD-10 classification of mental and behavioural disorders. *World Psychiatry, 10*, 86–92.

Irwin, M. R., & Cole, S. W. (2011). Reciprocal regulation of the neural and innate immune systems. *Nature Reviews Immunology, 11*, 625–632.

Issler, O, & Nestler, E. J. (2018). The molecular basis for sex differences in depression susceptibility. *Current Opinion in Behavioral Sciences, 23*, 1–6.

Iwata, K., Matsuzaki, H., Takei, N., Manabe, T., & Mori, N. (2010). Animal models of autism: an epigenetic and environmental viewpoint. *Journal of Central Nervous System Disease, 2*, 37–44.

Jackson, M. (2013). *The age of stress; science and the search for stability*. Oxford, UK: Oxford University Press.

Jackson, M. (2014a). *The history of medicine: a beginner's guide*. New York, NY: Oneworld Publications.

Jackson, M. (2014b). Evaluating the role of Hans Selye in the modern history of stress. In D. Cantor & E. Ramsden (Eds.), *Stress, shock and adaptation in the twentieth century* (pp. 21–48). Rochester, NY: Boydell and Brewer.

Jacobs, B. L., von Praag, H., & Gage, F. H. (2000). Adult brain neurogenesis and psychiatry: a novel theory of depression. *Molecular Psychiatry, 5*, 262–269.

Jacobsen, J. P. R., Medvedev, I. O., & Caron, M. G. (2012). The 5-HT deficiency theory of depression: perspectives from a naturalistic 5-HT deficiency model, the tryptophan hydroxylase 2Arg439His knockin mouse. *Philospohical Transactions of the Royal Society B, 367*, 2444–2459.

Jacome, L. F., Burket, J. A., Herndon, A. L., & Deutsch, S. I. (2011). Genetically inbred Balb/c mice differ from outbred Swiss Webster mice on discrete measures of sociability: relevance to a genetic mouse model of autism spectrum disorders. *Autism Research, 4*, 393–400.

Jamain, S., Radyushkin, K., Hammerschmidt, K., Granon, S., Boretius, S., Varoqueaux, F., . . . Brose, N. (2008). Reduced social interaction and ultrasonic communication in a mouse model of monogenic heritable autism. *Proceedings of the National Academy of Sciences USA, 105*, 1710–1715.

Jamison, K. R. (1996). *An unquiet mind: a memoir of moods and madness*. New York, NY: Vintage.

Janeway, C. A. (1989). Approaching the asymptote? Evolution and revolution in immunology. *Cold Spring Harbor Symposia on Quantitative Biology, 54*, 1–13.

Jänig, W., & McLachlan, E. M. (2013). Neurobiology of the autonomic system. In C. J. Mathias & R. Bannister (Eds.), *Autonomic failure: a textbook of clinical disorders of the autonomic nervous system* (pp. 21–34). Oxford, UK: Oxford University Press.

Jansen, A. S. P., Nguyen, X. V., Karpitskiy, V., Mettenleiter, T. C., & Loewy, A. D. (1995). Central command neurons of the sympathetic nervous system: basis of the flight-or-flight response. *Science, 270*, 644–646.

Jarrard, L. E. (1989). On the use of ibotenic acid to lesion selectively different components of the hippocampal formation. *Journal of Neuroscience Methods, 29*, 251–259.

Jenkins, D. E., Sreenivasan, D., Carman, F., Samal, B., Eiden, L. E., & Bunn, S. J. (2016). Interleukin-6-mediated signaling in adrenal medullary chromaffin cells. *Journal of Neurochemistry, 139*, 1138–1150.

Jenuwein, T., & Allis, C. D. (2001). Translating the histone code. *Science, 293*, 1074–1080.

Jessberger, S., & Gage, F. H. (2014). Adult neurogenesis: bridging the gap between mice and humans. *Trends in Cell Biology, 24,* 558–563.

Jhuang, H., Garrote, E., Mutch, J., Yu, X., Khilnani, V., Poggio, T., . . . Serre, T. (2010). Automated home-cage behavioural phenotyping of mice. *Nature Communications, 1,* 68.

Jiao, X., Pare, W. P., & Tejani-Butt, S. (2003). Strain differences in the distribution of dopamine transporter sites in rat brain. *Progress in Neuro-Psychopharmacology and Biological Psychiatry, 27,* 913–919.

Joel, D., & McCarthy, M. M. (2017). Incorporating sex as a biological variable in neuropsychiatric research: where are we now and where should we be? *Neuropsychopharmacology, 42,* 379–385.

Joëls, M., & Baram, T. Z. (2009). The neuro-symphony of stress. *Nature Reviews Neuroscience, 10,* 459–466.

Joëls, M., Karst, H., Alfarez, D., Heine, V. M., Qin, Y., Van Riel, E., . . . Krugers, H. J. (2004). Effects of chronic stress on structure and cell function in rat hippocampus and hypothalamus. *Stress, 7,* 221–231.

Johnson, J. W., & Asher, P. (1987). Glycine potentiates the NMDA response in cultured mouse brain neurons. *Nature, 325,* 529–531.

Johnson, S. L. (2005). Life events in bipolar disorder: towards more specific models. *Clinical Psychology Review, 25,* 1008–1027.

Johnson, S. L., & Miller, I. (1997). Negative life events and time to recovery from episodes of bipolar disorder. *Journal of Abnormal Psychology, 106,* 449–457.

Johnson, S. L., & Roberts, J. E. (1995). Life events and bipolar disorder: implications from biological theories. *Psychological Bulletin, 117,* 434–449.

Jones, C. A., Watson, D. J. G., & Fone, K. C. F. (2011). Animal models of schizophrenia. *British Journal of Pharmacology, 164,* 1162–1194.

Jones, J., & Hunter, D. (1995). Consensus methods for medical and health services research. *British Medical Journal, 311,* 376–380.

Jones, K. L., Smith, R. M., Edwards, K. S., Givens, B., Tilley, M. R., & Beversdorf, D. Q. (2010). Combined effect of maternal serotonin transporter genotype and prenatal stress in modulating offspring social interaction in mice. *International Journal of Developmental Neuroscience, 28,* 529–536.

Jope, R. S., Cheng, Y., Lowell, J. A., Worthen, R. J., Sitbon, Y. H., & Beurel, E. (2017). Stressed and inflamed, can GSK3 be blamed? *Trends in Biochemical Sciences, 42,* 180–192.

Jouroukhin, Y., McFarland, R., Ayhan, Y., & Pletnikov, M. V. (2016). Modeling gene–environment interaction in schizophrenia. *Handbook of Behavioral Neuroscience, 23,* 345–360.

Juetten, J., & Einat, H. (2012). Behavioral differences in black Swiss mice from separate colonies: implications for modeling domains of mania. *Behavioural Pharmacology, 23,* 211–214.

Jüngling, K., Liu, X., Lesting, J., Coulon, P., Sosulina, L., Reinscheid, R. K., & Pape, H.-C. (2012). Activation of neuropeptide S-expressing neurons in the locus coeruleus by corticotropin-releasing factor. *Journal of Physiology, 590,* 3701–3717.

Junyent, F., & Kremer, E. J. (2015). CAV-2: why a canine virus is a neurobiologist's best friend. *Current Opinion in Phamacology, 24,* 86–93.

Kabbaj, M., Devine, D. P., Savage, V. R., & Akil, H. (2000). Neurobiological correlates of individual differences in novelty-seeking behavior in the rat: differential expression of stress-related molecules. *Journal of Neuroscience, 20,* 6983–6988.

Kaffman, A., & Krystal, J. J. (2012). New frontiers in animal research of psychiatric illness. In F. Kobeissy (Ed.), *Psychiatric disorders: methods in molecular biology (methods and protocols)*, Vol. 829 (pp. 3–30). New York, NY: Humana Press.

Kafkafi, N., Agassi, J., Chesler, E. J., Crabbe, J. C., Crusio, W. E., Eilam, D., . . . Benjamini, Y. (2018). Reproducibility and replicability of rodent phenotyping in preclinical studies. *Neuroscience and Biobehavioral Reviews, 87*, 218–232.

Kahn, R. S., Sommer, I. E., Murray, R. M., Meyer-Lindenberg, A., Weinberger, D. R., Cannon, T. D., . . . Insel, T. R. (2015). Schizophrenia. *Nature Reviews Disease Primers, 1*, 15067.

Kalin, N. H., Fox, A. S., Kovner, R., Riedel, M. K., Fekete, E. M., Roseboom, P. H., . . . Oler, J. A. (2016). Overexpressing corticotropin-releasing factor in the primate amygdala increases anxious temperament and alters its neural circuit. *Biological Psychiatry, 80*, 345–355.

Kalin, N. H., & Shelton, S. E. (1989). Defensive behaviors in infant rhesus monkeys: environmental cues and neurochemical regulation. *Science, 243*, 1718–1721.

Kalisch, R., Müller, M. B., & Tüscher, O. (2015). A conceptual framework for the neurobiological study of resilience. *Behavioral and Brain Sciences, 38*, e92.

Kalivas, P. W., & Stewart, J. (1991). Dopamine transmission in the initiation and expression of drug- and stress-induced sensitization of motor activity. *Brain Research Reviews, 16*, 223–244.

Kalsbeek, A. van der Spek, R., Lei, J., Endert, E., Buijs, R. M., & Fliers, E. (2012). Circadian rhythms in the hypothalamo-pituitary-adrenal (HPA) axis. *Molecular and Cellular Endocrinology, 349*, 20–29.

Kalueff, A. V., Stewart, A. M., Song, C., Berridge, K. C., Graybiel, A. M., & Fentress, J. C. (2016). Neurobiology of rodent self-grooming and its value for translational neuroscience. *Nature Reviews Neuroscience, 17*, 45–59.

Kalueff, A. V., Wheaton, M., & Murphy, D. L. (2007). What's wrong with my mouse model? Advances and strategies in animal modeling of anxiety and depression. *Behavioural Brain Research, 179*, 1–18.

Kannan, G., Sawa, A., & Pletnikov, M. V. (2013). Mouse models of gene-environment interactions in schizophrenia. *Neurobiology of Disease, 57*, 5–11.

Kanner, L. (1943). Autistic disturbances of affective contact. *Nervous Child: Journal of Psychopathology, Psychotherapy, Mental Hygiene, and Guidance of the Child, 2*, 217–250.

Kapczinski, F., Vieta, E., Andreazza, A. C., Frey, B. N., Gomes, F. A., Tramontina, J., . . . Post, R. M. (2008). Allostatic load in bipolar disorder: implications for pathophysiology and treatment. *Neuroscience and Biobehavioral Reviews, 32*, 675–692.

Kapur, S., Phillips, A. G., & Insel, T. R. (2012). Why has it taken so long for biological psychiatry to develop clinical tests and what to do about it? *Molecular Psychiatry, 17*, 1174–1179.

Kara, N. Z., Stukalin, Y., & Einat, H. (2018). Revisiting the validity of the mouse forced swim test: systematic review and meta-analysis of the effects of prototypic antidepressants. *Neuroscience and Biobehavioral Reviews, 84*, 1–11.

Karatsoreos, I. N., & McEwen, B. S. (2013). Annual research review: the neurobiology and physiology of resilience and adaptation across the life course. *Journal of Child Psychology and Psychiatry, 54*, 337–347.

Karayiorgou, M., Flint, J., Gogos, J. A., Malenka, R. C., & the Genetic and Neural Complexity in Psychiatry 2011 Working Group (2012). The best of times, the worst of times for psychiatric disease. *Nature Neuroscience, 15*, 811–812.

Karg, K., Burmeister, M., Shedden, K., & Sen, S. (2011). The serotonin transporter promoter variant (5-HTTLPR), stress, and depression meta-analysis revisited. *Archives of General Psychiatry, 68*, 444–454.

Karl, A., Schaefer, M., Malta, L. S., Dörfel, D., Rohleder, N., & Werner, A. (2006). A meta-analysis of structural brain abnormalities in PTSD. *Neuroscience and Biobehavioral Reviews, 30*, 1004–1031.

Karl, T., & Arnold, J. C. (2014). Schizophrenia: a consequence of gene-environment interactions? *Frontiers in Behavioral Neuroscience, 8*, 435.

Karl, T., Duffy, L., Scimone, A., Harvey, R. P., & Schofield, P. R. (2007). Altered motor activity, exploration and anxiety in heterozygous neuregulin 1 mutant mice: implications for understanding schizophrenia. *Genes, Brain and Behavior, 6*, 677–687.

Karst, H., Berger, S., Turiault, M., Tronche, F., Schütz, G., & Joëls, M. (2005). Mineralocorticoid receptors are indispensible for nongenomic modulation of hippocampal glutamate transmission by corticosterone. *Proceedings of the National Academy of Sciences USA, 102*, 19204–19207.

Kataoka, S., Takuma, K., Hara, Y., Maeda, Y., Ago, Y., & Matsuda, T. (2013). Autism-like behaviours with transient histone hyperacetylation in mice treated prenatally with valproic acid. *International Journal of Neuropsychopharmacology, 16*, 91–103.

Kato, T. M., Fujimori-Tonou, N., Mizukami, H., Ozawa, K., Fujisawa, S., & Kata, T. (2019). Presynaptic dysregulation of the paraventricular thalamic nucleus causes depression-like behavior. *Scientific Reports, 9*, 16506.

Katz, R. J. (1981). Acute and chronic stress effects on open field activity in the rat: implications for a model of depression. *Neuroscience and Biobehavioral Reviews, 5*, 247–251.

Kauer-Sant'Anna, M., Tramontina, J., Andreazza, A. C., Cereser, K., da Costa, S., Santin, A., & Kapczinski, F. (2007). Traumatic life events in bipolar disorder: impact on BDNF levels and psychopathology. *Bipolar Disorders, 9* (Suppl. 1), 128–135.

Kaufman, J., Wymbs, N. F., Montalvo-Ortiz, J. L., Orr, C., Albaugh, M. D., Althoff, R., . . . Hudziak, J. (2018). Methylation in OTX2 and related genes, maltreatment, and depression in children. *Neuropsychopharmacology, 43*, 2204–2211.

Keane, T. M., Marshall, A. D., & Taft, C. T. (2006). Posttraumatic stress disorder: etiology, epidemiology, and treatment outcome. *Annual Review of Clinical Psychology, 2*, 161–197.

Keane, T. M., Wolfe, J., & Taylor, K. I. (1987). Post-traumatic stress disorder: evidence for diagnostic validity and methods of psychological assessment. *Journal of Clinical Psychology, 43*, 32–43.

Kearns, R. R., & Spencer, R. L. (2013). An unexpected increase in restraint duration alters the expression of stress response habituation. *Physiology and Behavior, 122*, 193–200.

Kebir, O., Chaumette, B., Rivollier, F., Miozzo, F., Lemieux Perreault, L. P., . . . Krebs, M.-O. (2017). Methylomic changes during conversion to psychosis. *Molecular Psychiatry, 22*, 512–518.

Kekesi, G., Petrovszki, Z., Benedek, G., & Horvath, G. (2015). Sex-specific alterations in behavioral and cognitive functions in a "three hit" animal model of schizophrenia. *Behavioural Brain Research, 284*, 85–93.

Kellendonk, C., Simpson, E. H., & Kandel, E. R. (2009). Modeling cognitive endophenotypes of schizophrenia in mice. *Trends in Neurosciences, 32*, 347–358.

Keller, M. C., & Visscher, P. M. (2015). Genetic variation links creativity to psychiatric disorders. *Nature Neuroscience, 18*, 928–929.

Keller, S. M., & Roth, T. L. (2016). Environmental influences on the female epigenome and behavior. *Environmental Epigenetics, 2016*, 1–10.

Keller, S. M., Schreiber, W. B., Staib, J. M., & Knox, D. (2015). Sex differences in the single prolonged stress model. *Behavioural Brain Research, 286*, 29–32.

Kempermann, G., Gage, F. H., Aigner, L., Song, H., Curtis, M. A., Thuret, S., . . . Frisén, J. (2018). Human adult neurogenesis: evidence and remaining questions. *Cell Stem Cell, 22*, 25–30.

Kendig, M. D., Bowen, M. T., Kemp, A. H., & McGregor, I. S. (2011). Predatory threat induces huddling in adolescent rats and residual changes in early adulthood suggestive of increased resilience. *Behavioural Brain Research, 225*, 405–414.

Kendler, K. S. (2016). The transformation of American psychiatric nosology at the dawn of the twentieth century. *Molecular Psychiatry, 21*, 152–158.

Kendler, K. S., & Engstrom, E. J. (2017). Kahlbaum, Hecker, and Kraepelin and the transition from psychiatric symptom complexes to empirical disease forms. *American Journal of Psychiatry, 174*, 102–109.

Kendler, K. S., Gardner, C. O., & Prescott, C. A. (2002). Toward a comprehensive developmental model for major depression in women. *American Journal of Psychiatry, 159*, 1133–1145.

Kendler, K. S., Gardner, C. O., & Prescott, C. A. (2006). Toward a comprehensive developmental model for major depression in men. *American Journal of Psychiatry, 163*, 115–124.

Kendler, K. S., & Greenspan, R. J. (2006). The nature of genetic influences on behavior: lessions from "simpler" organisms. *American Journal of Psychiatry, 163*, 1683–1694.

Kendler, K. S., Karkowski, L. M., & Prescott, C. A. (1999). Causal relationship between stressful life events and the onset of major depression. *American Journal of Psychiatry, 156*, 837–841.

Kendler, K. S., Kuhn, J. W., Vittum, J., Prescott, C. A., & Riley, B. (2005). The interaction of stressful life events and a serotonin transporter polymorphism in the prediction of episodes of major depression. *Archives of General Psychiatry, 62*, 529–535.

Kendler, K. S., Muñoz, R. A., & Murphy, G. (2010). The development of the Feighner criteria: a historical perspective. *American Journal of Psychiatry, 167*, 134–142.

Kendler, K. S., Neale, M., Kessler, R., Health, A., & Eaves, L. (1993). A twin study of recent life events and difficulties. *Archives of General Psychiatry, 50*, 789–796.

Kendler, K. S., Thornton, L. M., & Gardner, C. O. (2000). Stressful life events and previous episodes in the etiology of major depression in women: an evaluation of the "kindling" hypothesis. *American Journal of Psychiatry, 157*, 1243–1251.

Kendler, K. S., Thornton, L. M., & Gardner, C. O. (2001). Genetic risk, number of previous depressive episodes, and stressful life events in predicting onset of major depression. *American Journal of Psychiatry, 158*, 582–586.

Kendler, K. S., Thornton, L. M., & Prescott, C. A. (2001). Gender differences in the rates of exposure to stressful life events and sensitivity to their depressogenic effects. *American Journal of Psychiatry, 158*, 587–593.

Kennett, G. A., Chaouloff, F., Marcou, M., & Curzon, G. (1986). Female rats are more vulnerable than males in an animal model of depression: the possible role of serotonin. *Brain Research, 382*, 416–421.

Kerr, D. L., McLaren, D. G., Mathy, R. M., & Nitschke, J. B. (2012). Controllability modulates the anticipatory response in the human ventromedial prefrontal cortex. *Frontiers in Psychology, 3*, 557.

Kesby, J. P., Eyles, D. W., McGrath, J. J., & Scott, J. G. (2018). Dopamine, psychosis and schizophrenia: the widening gap between basic and clinical neuroscience. *Translational Psychiatry, 8*, 30.

Kessing, L. V., Agerbo, E., & Mortensen, P. B. (2004). Major stressful life events and other risk factors for first admission with mania. *Bipolar Disorders, 6*, 122–129.

Kessler, M. S., Bosch, O. J., Bunck, M., Landgraf, R., & Neumann, I. D. (2011). Maternal care differs in mice bred for high vs. low trait anxiety: impact of brain vasopressin and cross-fostering. *Social Neuroscience, 6*, 156–168.

Kessler, R. C., McGonagle, K. A., Swartz, M., Blazer, D. G., & Nelson, C. B. (1993). Sex and depression in the National Comorbidity Survey I: lifetime prevalence, chronicity and recurrence. *Journal of Affective Disorders, 29*, 85–96.

Kessler, R. C., Ruscio, A. M., Shear, K., & Wittchen, H.-U. (2009). Epidemiology of anxiety disorders. In M. B. Stein and T. Teckler (Eds.), *Behavioral neurobiology of anxiety and its treatment* (pp. 21–35). Berlin, Germany: Springer-Verlag.

Kessler, R. C., Sonnega, A., Bromet, E., Hughes, M., & Nelson, C. B. (1995). Posttraumatic stress disorder in the National Comorbidity Survey. *Archives of General Psychiatry, 52*, 1048–1060.

Kety, S. S. (1974). From rationalization to reason. *American Journal of Psychiatry, 131*, 957–963.

Khan, S., & Liberzon, I. (2004). Topiramate attenuates exaggerated acoustic startle in an animal model of PTSD. *Psychopharmacology, 172*, 225–229.

Kiecker, C. (2018). The origins of the circumventricular organs. *Journal of Anatomy, 232*, 540–553.

Kiekolt-Glaser, J. K., Derry, H. M., & Fagundes, C. P. (2015). Inflammation: depression fans the flames and feasts on the heat. *American Journal of Psychiatry, 172*, 1075–1091.

Kiening, K., & Sartorius, A. (2013). A new translational target for deep brain stimulation to treat depression. *EMBO Molecular Medicine, 5*, 1151–1153.

Kikuta, A., & Murakami, T. (1982). Microcirculation of the rat adrenal gland: a scanning electron microscope study of vascular casts. *American Journal of Anatomy, 164*, 19–28.

Kim, D. R., Bale, T. L., & Epperson, C. N. (2015). Prenatal programming of mental illness: current understanding of relationship and mechanisms. *Current Psychiatry Reports, 17*, 5.

Kim, J., Lee, S., Fang, Y.-Y., Shin, A., Park, S., Hashikawa, K., . . . Suh, G. S. B. (2019). Rapid, biphasic CRF neuronal responses encode positive and negative valence. *Nature Neuroscience, 22*, 576–585.

Kim, J. S., Han, S. Y., & Iremonger, K. J. (2019). Stress experience and hormone feedback tune distinct components of hypothalamic CRH neuron activity. *Nature Communications, 10*, 5696.

Kim, J.-W., Park, K., Kang, R. J., Gonzales, E. L. T., Kim, D. G., Oh, H. A., . . . Shin, C. Y. (2019). Pharmacological modulation of AMPA receptor rescues social impairments in animal models of autism. *Neuropsychopharmacology, 44*, 314–323.

Kim, J.-W., Seung, H., Kwon, K. J., Ko, M. J., Lee, E. J., Oh, H. A., . . . Bahn, G. H. (2014). Subchronic treatment of donepezil rescues impaired social, hyperactive, and stereotypic behavior in valproic acid-induced animal model of autism. *PLoS ONE, 9*, e104927.

Kim, K. C., Kim, P., Go, H. S., Choi, C. S., Yang, S.-I., Cheong, J. H., . . . Ko, K. H. (2011). The critical period of valproate exposure to induce autistic symptoms in Sprague-Dawley rats. *Toxicology Letters, 201*, 137–142.

Kim, S., Kim, H., Yim, Y. S., Ha, S., Atarashi, K., Tan, T. G., . . . Huh, J. R. (2017). Maternal gut bacteria promote neurodevelopmental abnormalities in mouse offspring. *Nature, 549*, 528–532.

Kimmel, C.B ., Ballard, W. W., Kimmel, S. R., Ullmann, B., & Schilling, T. F. (1995). Stages of embryonic development of the zebrafish. *Developmental Dynamics, 203*, 253–310.

King, D. P., Zhao, Y., Sangoram, A. M., Wilsbacher, L. D., Tanaka, M., Antoch, M. P., . . . Takahashi, J. S. (1997). Positional cloning of the mouse circadian clock gene. *Cell, 89*, 641–653.

King, L. S. (1968). Signs and symptoms. *Journal of the American Medical Association, 206*, 1063–1065.

Kirshenbaum, G. S., Burgess, C. R., Déry, N., Fahnestock, M., Peever, J. H., & Roder, J. C. (2014). Attenuation of mania-like behavior in Na+, K+-ATPase α3 mutant mice by prospective therapies for bipolar disorder: melatonin and exercise. *Neuroscience, 260*, 195–204.

Kirshenbaum, G. S., Clapcote, S. J., Duffy, S., Burgess, C. R., Petersen, J., Jarowek, K. J., . . . Roder, J. C. (2011). Mania-like behavior induced by genetic dysfunction of the neuron-specific Na+,K+-ATPase α3 sodium pump. *Proceedings of the National Academy of Sciences USA, 108*, 18144–18149.

Kirshenbaum, G. S., Clapcote, S. J., Petersen, J., Vilsen, B., Ralph, M. R., & Roder, J. C. (2012). Genetic suppression of agrin reduces mania-like behavior in Na+,K+-ATPase α3 mutant mice. *Genes, Brain and Behavior, 11*, 436–443.

Kirsten, T. B., Chaves-Kirsten, G. P., Chaible, L. M., Silva, A. C., Martins, D. O., Britto, L. R. G., . . . Bernardi, M. M. (2012). Hypoactivity of the central dopaminergic system and autistic-like behavior induced by a single early prenatal exposure to lipopolysaccharide. *Journal of Neuroscience Research, 90*, 1903–1912.

Kirsten, T. B., Taricano, M., Maiorka, P. C., Palermo-Neto, J., & Bernardi, M. M. (2010). Prenatal lipopolysaccharide reduces social behavior in male offspring. *Neuroimmunomodulation, 17*, 240–251.

Kiselycznyk, C., & Holmes, A. (2011). All (C57BL/6) mice are not created equal. *Frontiers in Neuroscience, 5*, 10.

Kleckner, N. W., & Dingledine, R. (1988). Requirement for glycine in activation of NMDA-receptors expressed in *Xenopus* oocytes. *Science, 241*, 835–837.

Klengel, T., & Binder, E. B. (2015). Epigenetics of stress-related psychiatric disorders and gene x environment interactions. *Neuron, 86*, 1343–1357.

Klengel, T., Pape, J., Binder, E. B., & Mehta, D. (2014). The role of DNA methylation in stress-related psychiatric disorders. *Neuropharmacology, 80*, 115–132.

Klimeš, I., Weston, K., Gašperíková, D., Kovács, P., Kvetňansky, R., Ježová, D., . . . Samani, N. J. (2005). Mapping of genetic determinants of the sympathoneural response to stress. *Physiological Genomics, 20*, 183–187.

Klug, M., Hill, R. A., Choy, K. H., Kyrios, M., Hannan, A. J., & van den Buuse, M. (2012). Long-term behavioral and NMDA receptor effects of young-adult corticosterone treatment in BDNF heterozygous mice. *Neurobiology of Disease, 46*, 722–731.

Knowland, D., Lilascharoen, V., Pacia, C. P., Shin, S., Wang, E. H.-J., & Lim, B. K. (2017). Distinct ventral pallidal neural populations mediate separate symptoms of depression. *Cell, 170*, 284–297.

Knox, D., George, S. A., Fitzpatrick, C. J., Rabinak, C. A., Maren, S., & Liberzon, I. (2012). Single prolonged stress disrupts retention of extinguished fear in rats. *Learning and Memory, 19*, 43–49.

Knox, D., Perrine, S. A., George, S. A., Galloway, M. P., & Liberzon, I. (2010). Single pro-longed stress decreases glutamate, glutamine, and creatine concentrations in the rat medial prefrontal cortex. *Neuroscience Letters, 480,* 16–20.

Koenig, J. I., Elmer, G. I., Shepard, P. D., Lee, P. R., Mayo, C., Joy, B., . . . Brady, D. L. (2005). Prenatal exposure to a repeated variable stress paradigm elicits behavioral and neuro-endocrinological changes in the adult offspring: potential relevance to schizophrenia. *Behavioural Brain Research, 156,* 251–261.

Koester, S. E., & Insel, T. R. (2016). Understanding how non-coding genomic polymorphisms affect gene expression. *Molecular Psychiatry, 21,* 448–449.

Kohane, I. S. (2015). Ten things we have to do to achieve precision medicine. *Science, 349,* 37–38.

Kohda, K., Harada, K., Kato, K., Hoshino, A., Motohashi, J., Yamaji, T., . . . Kato, N. (2007). Glucocorticoid receptor activation is involved in producing abnormal phenotypes of single prolonged stress rats: a putative post-traumatic stress disorder model. *Neuroscience, 148,* 22–33.

Kohen, R., Yamamoto, Y., Cundy, K. C., & Ames, B. N. (1988). Antioxidant activity of carnosine, homocarnosine, and anserine present in muscle and brain. *Proceedings of the National Academy of Sciences USA, 85,* 3175–3179.

Kohli, M. A., Lucae, S., Saemann, P. G., Schmidt, M. V., Demirkan, A., Hek, K., . . . Binder, E. B. (2011). The neuronal transporter gene SLC6A15 confers risk to major depression. *Neuron, 70,* 252–265.

Kole, M. H. P., & Stewart, G. J. (2012). Signal processing in the axon initial segment. *Neuron, 73,* 235–247.

Kolvin, I. (1971). Studies in the childhood psychoses. I. Diagnostic criteria and classifica-tion. *British Journal of Psychiatry, 118,* 381–384.

Konradi, C., & Heckers, S. (2003). Molecular aspects of glutamate dysregulation: implications for schizophrenia and its treatment. *Pharmacology and Therapeutics, 97,* 153–179.

Koo, J. W., Chaudhury, D., Han, M.-H., & Nestler, E. J. (2019). Role of mesolimbic brain-derived neurotrophic factor in depression. *Biological Psychiatry, 86,* 738–748.

Koolhaas, J. M., Bartolomucci, A., Buwalda, B., de Boer, S. F., Flügge, G., Korte, S. M., . . . Fuchs, E. (2011). Stress revisited: a critical evaluation of the stress concept. *Neuroscience and Biobehavioral Reviews, 35,* 1291–1301.

Koolhaas, J. M., de Boer, S. F., Buwalda, B., & Meerlo, P. (2017). Social stress models in rodents: towards enhanced validity. *Neurobiology of Stress, 6,* 104–112.

Koresh, O., Kaplan, Z., Zohar, J., Matar, M. A., Greva, A. B., & Cohen, H. (2016). Distinctive cardiac autonomic dysfunction following stress exposure in both sexes in an animal model of PTSD. *Behavioural Brain Research, 308,* 128–142.

Kourrich, S., Su, T.-P., Fujimoto, M., & Bonci, A. (2012). The sigma-1 receptor: roles in neuronal plasticity and disease. *Trends in Neurosciences, 35,* 762–771.

Kozicz, T. (2007). On the role of urocortin 1 in the non-preganglionic Edinger-Westphal nucleus in stress adaptation. *General and Comparative Endocrinology, 153,* 235–240.

Kozicz, T., Bittencourt, J. C., May, P. J., Reiner, A., Gamlin, P. D. R., Palkovits, M., . . . Ryabinin, A. E. (2011). The Edinger-Westphal nucleus: a historical, structural and functional perspective on a dichotomous terminology. *Journal of Comparative Neurology, 519,* 1413–1434.

Kozikowski, A. P., Gaisina, I. N., Yuan, H., Petukhov, P. A., Blond, S. Y., Fedolak, A., . . . McGonigle, P. (2007). Structure-based design leads to the identification of lithium mimetics that block mania-like effects in rodents. Possible new GSK-3β therapies for bipolar disorders. *Journal of the American Chemical Society, 129,* 8328–8332.

Kozlovsky, N., Matar, M. A., Kaplan, Z., Kotler, M., Zohar, J., & Cohen, H. (2007). Long-term down-regulation of BDNF mRNA in rat hippocampal CA1 subregion correlates with PTSD-like behavioural stress response. *International Journal of Neuropsychopharmacology, 10,* 741–758.

Kozlovsky, N., Matar, M. A., Kaplan, Z., Kotler, M., Zohar, J., & Cohen, H. (2008). The immediate early gene *Arc* is associated with behavioral resilience to stress exposure in an animal model of posttraumatic stress disorder. *European Neuropsychopharmacology, 18,* 107–116.

Kraemer, H. C. (2015). Research Domain Criteria (RDoC) and the *DSM*: two methodological approaches to mental health diagnosis. *JAMA Psychiatry, 72,* 1163–1164.

Kraepelin, E. (1899). *Psychiatrie. Ein Lehrbuch für Studierende und Ärzte* (6th ed.), Vol. 2. Leipzig, Germany: Barth.

Kraepelin, E. (2002). *Manic-depressive insanity and paranoia.* Chicago, IL: University of Chicago Press (original work published 1927).

Kraus, A., Geuze, E., Schmahl, C., Greffrath, W., Treede, R.-D., Bohus, M., & Vermetten, E. (2009). Differentiation of pain ratings in combat-related posttraumatic stress disorder. *Pain, 143,* 179–185.

Krishnan, V., Han, M.-H., Graham, D. L., Berton, O., Renthal, W., Russo, S. J., . . . Nestler, E. J. (2007). Molecular adaptations underlying susceptibility and resistance to social defeat in brain reward regions. *Cell, 131,* 391–404.

Kristensen, M., Nierenberg, A. A., & Østergaard, S. D. (2018). Face and predictive validity of the *Clock*Δ19 mouse as an animal model for bipolar disorder: a systematic review. *Molecular Psychiatry, 23,* 70–80.

Krizanova, O., Micutkova, L., Jelokova, J., Filipenko, M., Sabban, E., & Kvetnansky, R. (2001). Existence of cardiac PNMT mRNA in adult rats: elevation by stress in a glucocorticoid-dependent manner. *American Journal of Physiology, 281,* H1372–H1379.

Krömer, S. A., Keßler, M. S., Milfay, D., Birg, I. N., Bunck, M., Czibere, L., . . . Turck, C. W. (2005). Identification of glyoxylase-I as a protein marker in a mouse model of extremes in trait anxiety. *Journal of Neuroscience, 25,* 4375–4384.

Krout, K. E., Mettenleiter, T. C., & Loewy, A. D. (2003). Single CNS neurons link both central motor and cardiosympathetic systems: a double-virus tracing study. *Neuroscience, 118,* 853–866.

Krystal, J. H., & State, M. W. (2014). Psychiatric disorders: diagnosis to therapy. *Cell, 157,* 201–214.

Kubovcakova, L., Micutkova, L., Bartosova, Z., Sabban, E. L., Krizanova, O., & Kvetnansky, R. (2006). Identification of phenylethanolamine N-methyltransferase gene expression in stellate ganglia and its modulation by stress. *Journal of Neurochemistry, 97,* 1419–1430.

Kuemerle, B., Gulden, F., Cherosky, N., Williams, E., & Herrup, K. (2007). The mouse *Engrailed* genes: a window into autism. *Behavioural Brain Research, 176,* 121.

Kundakovic, M., & Champagne, F. A. (2015). Early-life experience, epigenetics, and the developing brain. *Neuropsychopharmacology, 40,* 141–153.

Kuo, L. E., & Zukowska, Z. (2007). Stress, NPY and vascular remodeling: implications for stress-related diseases. *Peptides, 28,* 435–440.

Kupfer, D. J. (2015). Anxiety and DSM-5. *Dialogues in Clinical Neuroscience, 17,* 245–246.

Kuzmin, A. I., Pogorelov, V. M., Zaretsky, D. V., Medvedev, O. S., & Chazov, E. I. (1995). Comparison of the effects of 2-deoxyglucose and immobilization on secretion and synthesis rate of catecholamines in the adrenal gland: a microdialysis study in conscious rats. *Acta Physiologica Scandanavica, 155,* 147–155.

Kuzmin, A. I., Selivanovv, N., Anisimovs, P., & Medvedevo, S. (1990). Catecholamine secretion during hypovolemic hypotension as measured by microdialysis in the rat adrenal gland (in Russian). *Fiziologicheskii Zhurnal SSSR, 76,* 227–232.

Kuzmiski, J. B., Marty, V., Baimoukhametova, D. V., & Bains, J. S. (2010). Stress-induced priming of glutamate synapses unmasks associative short-term plasticity. *Nature Neuroscience, 13,* 1257–1264.

Kvetnansky, R., Fukuhara, K., Pacak, K., Cizza, G., Goldstein, D. S., & Kopin, I. J. (1993). Endogenous glucocorticoids restrain catecholamine synthesis and release at rest and during immobilization stress in rats. *Endocrinology, 133,* 1411–1419.

Kvetnansky, R., Kubovcakova, L., Tillinger, A., Micutkova, L., Krizanova, O., & Sabban, E. L. (2006). Gene expression of phenylethanolamine N-methyltransferase in corticotropin-releasing hormone knockout mice during stress exposure. *Cellular and Molecular Neurobiology, 26,* 733–752.

Kvetnansky, R., Sabban, E. L., & Palkovits, M. (2009). Catecholaminergic systems in stress: structural and molecular genetic approaches. *Physiological Reviews, 89,* 535–606.

Kvetnansky, R., Sun, C. L., Lake, C. R., Thoa, N., Torda, T., & Kopin, I. J. (1978). Effect of handling and forced immobilization on rat plasma levels of epinephrine, norepinephrine, and dopamine-beta-hydroxylase. *Endocrinology, 103,* 1868–1874.

Kvetnansky, R., Weise, V. K., Thoa, N. B., & Kopin, I. J. (1979). Effects of chronic guanethidine treatment and adrenal medullectomy on plasma levels of catecholamines and corticosterone in forcibly immobilized rats. *Journal of Pharmacology and Experimental Therapeutics, 209,* 287–291.

Kwiatkowski, M. A., Hellemann, G., Sugar, C. A., Cope, Z. A., Minassian, A., Perry, W., . . . Young, J. W. (2019). Dopamine transporter knockdown mice in the behavioral pattern monitor: a robust, reproducible model for mania-relevant behaviors. *Pharmacology, Biochemistry and Behavior, 178,* 42–50.

Kwon, C.-H., Luikart, B. W., Powell, C. M., Zhou, J., Matheny, S. A., Zhang, W., . . . Parada, L. F. (2006). Pten regulates neuronal arborization and social interaction in mice. *Neuron, 50,* 377–388.

Laas, K., Reif, A., Akkermann, K., Kiive, E., Domschke, K., Lesch, K.-P., . . . Harro, J. (2014). Interaction of the neuropeptide S receptor gene Asn107Ile variant and environment: contribution to affective and anxiety disorders, and suicidal behavior. *International Journal of Neuropsychopharmacology, 17,* 541–552.

Labonté, B., Engmann, O., Purushothaman, I., Menard, C., Wang, J., Tan, C., . . . Nestler, E. J. (2017). Sex-specific transcriptional signatures in human depression. *Nature Medicine, 23,* 1102–1111.

Labrie, V., Fukumura, R., Rastogi, A., Fick, L. J., Wang, W., Boutros, P. C., . . . Roder, J. C. (2009). Serine racemase is associated with schizophrenia susceptibility in humans and in a mouse model. *Human Molecular Genetics, 18,* 3227–3243.

Labrie, V., Wong, A. H. C., & Roder, J. C. (2012). Contributions of the D-serine pathway to schizophrenia. *Neuropharmacology, 62,* 1484–1503.

Lahmame, A., del Arco, C., Pazos, A., Yritia, M., & Armario, A. (1997). Are Wistar-Kyoto rats a genetic animal model of depression resistant to antidepressants? *European Journal of Pharmacology, 337,* 115–123.

Laitinen, T., Polvi, A., Rydman, P., Vendelin, J., Pulkkinen, V., Salmikangas, P., . . . Kere, J. (2004). Characterization of a common susceptibility locus for asthma-related traits. *Science, 304,* 300–304.

Lancaster, K., Dietz, D. M., Moran, T. H., & Pletnikov, M. V. (2007). Abnormal social behaviors in young and adult rats neonatally infected with Borna disease virus. *Behavioural Brain Research, 176,* 141–148.

Landgraf, R., Keßler, M. S., Bunck, M., Murgatroyd, C., Spengler, D., Zimbelmann, M., M., . . . Frank, E. (2007). Candidate genes of anxiety-related behavior in HAB/LAB rats and mice: focus on vasopressin and glyoxalase-I. *Neuroscience and Biobehavioral Reviews, 31,* 89–102.

Landgraf, R., & Wigger, A. (2002). High vs low anxiety-related behavior rats: an animal model of extremes in trait anxiety. *Behavior Genetics, 32,* 301–314.

Landgraf, R., & Wigger, A. (2003). Born to be anxious: neuroendocrine and genetic correlates of trait anxiety in HAB rats. *Stress, 6,* 111–119.

Landman, O. E. (1991). The inheritance of acquired characteristics. *Annual Review of Genetics, 25,* 1–20.

Lane, M., Robker, R. L., & Robertson, S. A. (2014). Parenting from before conception. *Science, 345,* 756–760.

Lange, M., Norton, W., Coolen, M., Chaminade, M., Merker, S., Proft, F., . . . Bally-Cuif, L. (2012). The ADHD-susceptibility gene lphn3.1 modulates dopaminergic neuron formation and locomotor activity during zebrafish development. *Molecular Psychiatry, 17,* 946–954.

Langley, W. N. (1987). Specializations in the predatory behavior of grasshopper mice (*Onychomys leucogaster* and *O. torridus*): a comparison with the golden hamster (*Mesocricetus auratus*). *Journal of Comparative Psychology, 101,* 322–327.

Lao, L., Xu, L., & Xu, S. (2012). Traditional Chinese medicine. In A. Längler, P. J. Mansky, & G. Seifert (Eds.), *Integrative pediatric oncology* (pp. 125–135). Berlin, Germany: Springer-Verlag.

Law, S. W., Conneely, O. M., DeMayo, F. J., & O'Malley, B. W. (1992). Identification of a new brain-specific transcription factor, NURR1. *Molecular Endocrinology, 6,* 2129–2135.

Lebow, M. A., & Chen, A. (2016). Overshadowed by the amygdala: the bed nucleus of the stria terminalis emerges as key to psychiatric disorders. *Molecular Psychiatry, 21,* 450–463.

Le Dorze, C., & Gisquet-Verrier, P. (2016). Sensitivity to trauma-associated cues is restricted to vulnerable traumatized rats and reinstated after extinction by yohimbine. *Behavioural Brain Research, 313,* 120–134.

Lee, A. G., Nechvatal, J. M., Shen, B., Buckmaster, C. L., Levy, M. J., Chin, F. T., Lyons, D. M. (2016). Striatal dopamine D2/3 receptor regulation by stress inoculation in squirrel monkeys. *Neurobiology of Stress, 3,* 68–73.

Lee, B., Lee, K., Panda, S., Gonzales-Rojas, R., Chong, A., Bugay, V., . . . Lee, H. Y. (2018). Nanoparticle delivery of CRISPR into the brain rescues a mouse model of fragile X syndrome from exaggerated repetitive behaviours. *Nature Biomedical Engineering, 2,* 497–507.

Lee, E., Lee, J., & Kim, E. (2017). Excitation/inhibition imbalance in animal models of autism spectrum disorders. *Biological Psychiatry, 81,* 838–847.

Lee, R. C., Feinbaum, R. L., and Ambros, V. (1993). The *C. elegans* heterochronic gene *lin-4* encodes small RNAs with antisense complementarity to *lin-14. Cell, 75,* 843–854.

Lehmann, M. L., & Herkenham, M. (2011). Environmental enrichment confers stress resiliency to social defeat through an infralimbic cortex-dependent neuroanatomical pathway. *Journal of Neuroscience, 31,* 6159–6173.

Le Moal, M. (2007). Historical approach and evolution of the stress concept: a personal account. *Psychoneuroendocrinology, 32,* 53–59.

Lemonnier, E., Villeneuve, N., Sonie, S., Serret, S., Rosier, A., Roue, M., . . . Ben-Ari, Y. (2017). Effects of bumetanide on neurobehavioral function in children and adolescents with autism spectrum disorder. *Translational Psychiatry, 7,* e1056.

Le-Niculescu, H., McFarland, M. J., Ogden, C. A., Balaraman, Y., Patel, S., Tan, J., . . . Niculescu, A. B. (2008). Phenomic, convergent functional genomic, and bio-marker studies in a stress-reactive genetic animal model of bipolar disorder and co-morbid alcoholism. *American Journal of Medical Genetics B, 147B,* 134–166.

Leussis, M. P., & Andersen, S. L. (2008). Is adolescence a sensitive period for depres-sion? Behavioral and neuroanatomical findings from a social stress model. *Synapse, 62,* 22–30.

Leussis, M. P., Berry-Scott, E. M., Saito, M., Jhuang, H., de Haan, G., Alkan, O., . . . Petryshen, T. L. (2013). The *ANK3* bipolar disorder gene regulates psychiatric-related behaviors that are modulated by lithium and stress. *Biological Psychiatry, 73,* 683–690.

Leverich, G. S., & Post, R. M. (2006). Course of bipolar illness after history of childhood trauma. *Lancet, 367,* 1040–1042.

Levine, S., 1957. Infantile experience and resistance to physiological stress. *Science, 126,* 405.

Levine, S., 1962. Plasma-free corticosteroid response to electric shock in rats stimulated in infancy. *Science, 135,* 795–796.

Levine, S. (2005). Stress: an historical perspective. In J. Steckler, N. H. Kalin, & J. M. Reul (Eds.), *Handbook of stress and the brain* (pp. 3–24). Amsterdam, The Netherlands: Elsevier.

Levine, S., Alpert, M., & Lewis, G. W. (1957). Infantile experience and the maturation of the pituitary adrenal axis. *Science, 126,* 1347.

Levine, S., Chevalier, J. A., & Korchin, S. J. (1956). The effects of early shock and handling on later avoidance learning. *Journal of Personality, 24,* 475–493.

Levine, S., & Ursin, H. (1991). What is stress? In M. R. Brown, G. F. Koob, & C. Rivier, (Eds.), *Stress: neurobiology and neuroendocrinology* (pp. 3–21). New York, NY: Marcel Dekker.

Levinson, D. F., Mostafavi, S., Milaneschi, Y., Rivera, M., Ripke, S., Wray, N. R., & Sullivan, P. F. (2014). Genetic studies of major depressive disorder: why are there no GWAS findings, and what can we do about it? *Biological Psychiatry, 76,* 510–512.

Levkovitz, Y., Fenchel, D., Kaplan, Z., Zohar, J., & Cohen, H. (2015). Early post-stressor intervention with minocycline, a second-generation tetracycline, attenuates post-traumatic stress response in an animal model of PTSD. *European Neuropsycho-pharmacology, 25,* 124–132.

Levy, N. (2012). The use of animals as models: ethical considerations. *International Journal of Stroke, 7,* 440–442.

Lewinsohn, P. M., Joiner, T. E., & Rohde, P. (2001). Evaluation of cognitive diathesis-stress models in predicting major depressive disorder in adolescents. *Journal of Abnormal Psychology, 110,* 203–215.

Lewis, D. A., Hasimoto, T., & Volk, D. W. (2005). Cortical inhibitory neurons and schizo-phrenia. *Nature Reviews Neuroscience, 6,* 312–324.

Lewis, K., Perrin, M. H., Blount, A., Kunitake, K., Donaldson, C., Vaughn, J., . . . Vale, W. W. (2001). Identification of urocortins III, and additional family member of the corticotropin-releasing factor (CRF) family with high affinity for the CRF2 receptor. *Proceedings of the National Academy of Sciences USA, 98*, 7570–7575.

Lewitus, G. M., Cohen, H., & Schwartz, M. (2008). Reducing post-traumatic anxiety by immunization. *Brain, Behavior, and Immunity, 22*, 1108–1114.

Lewontin, R. C. (1979). Sociobiology as an adaptationist program. *Systems Research and Behavioral Science, 24*, 5–14.

Lex, C., Bäzner, E., & Meyer, T. D. (2017). Does stress play a significant role in bipolar disorder: a meta-analysis. *Journal of Affective Disorders, 208*, 298–308.

Li, B., Piriz, J., Mirrione, M., Chung, C., Proulx, C. D., Schulz, D., Henn, F., & Malinow, R. (2011). Synaptic potentiation onto habenula neurons in the learned helplessness model of depression. *Nature, 470*, 535–539.

Li, J., Vestergaard, M., Obel, C., Christensen, J., Precht, D. H., Lu, M., & Olsen, J. (2009). A nationwide study on the risk of autism after prenatal stress exposure to maternal bereavement. *Pediatrics, 123*, 1102–1107.

Li, L., Hu, S., & Chen, X. (2018). Non-viral delivery systems for CRISPR/Cas9-based genome editing: challenges and opportunities. *Biomaterials, 171*, 207–218.

Li, Q., & Barres, B. A. (2018). Microglia and macrophages in brain homeostasis and disease. *Nature Reviews Immunology, 18*, 225–242.

Li, W., Zhou, Y., Jentsch, J. D., Brown, R. A. M., Tian, X., Ehninger, D., . . . Cannon, T. D. (2007). Specific developmental disruption of disrupted-in-schizophrenia-1 function results in schizophrenia-related phenotypes in mice. *Proceedings of the National Academy of Sciences USA, 104*, 18280–18285.

Li, X. M., Han, F., Liu, D. J., & Shi, Y. X. (2010). Single-prolonged stress induced mitochondrial-dependent apoptosis in hippocampus in the rat model of posttraumatic stress disorder. *Journal of Chemical Neuroanatomy, 40*, 248–255.

Li, Y., Han, F., & Shi, Y. (2013). Increased neuronal apoptosis in medial prefrontal cortex is accompanied with changes of Bcl-2 and Bax in a rat model of posttraumatic stress disorder. *Journal of Molecular Neuroscience, 51*, 127–137.

Liberzon, I., & Knox, D. (2012). Expanding our understanding of neurobiological mechanisms of resilience by using animal models. *Neuropsychopharmacology, 37*, 317–318.

Liberzon, I., Krstov, M., & Young, E. A. (1997). Stress-restress: effects on ACTH and fast feedback. *Psychoneuroendocrinology, 22*, 443–453.

Liberzon, I., López, J. F., Flagel, S. B., Vázquez, D. M., & Young, E. A. (1999). Differential regulation of hippocampal glucocorticoid receptors mRNA and fast feedback: relevance to post-traumatic stress disorder. *Journal of Neuroendocrinology, 11*, 11–17.

Lin, C.-C., Tung, C.-S., & Liu, Y.-P. (2016). Escitalopram reversed the traumatic stress-induced depressed and anxiety-like symptoms but not the deficits of fear memory. *Psychopharmacology, 233*, 1135–1146.

Lindholm, J. S. O., & Castrén, E. (2014). Mice with altered BDNF signaling as models for mood disorders and antidepressant effects. *Frontiers in Behavioral Neuroscience, 8*, 143.

Lipina, T. V., Zai, C., Hlousek, D., Roder, J. C., & Wong, A. H. C. (2013). Maternal immune activation during gestation interacts with *Disc-1* point mutation to exacerbate schizophrenia-related behaviors in mice. *Journal of Neuroscience, 33*, 7654–7666.

Lipska, B. K. (2002). Neonatal disconnection of the rat hippocampus: a neurodevelopmental model of schizophrenia. *Dialogues in Clinical Neuroscience, 4*, 361–367.

Lipska, B. K., Halim, N. D., Segal, P. N., & Weinberger, D. R. (2002). Effects of reversible inactivation of the neonatal ventral hippocampus on behavior in the adult rat. *Journal of Neuroscience, 22,* 2835–2842.

Lipska, B. K., Jaskiw, G. E., Chrapusta, S., Karoum, F., & Weinberger, D. R. (1992). Ibotenic acid lesion of the ventral hippocampus differentially affects dopamine and its metabolites in the nucleus accumbens and prefrontal cortex in the rat. *Brain Research, 585,* 1–6.

Lipska, B. K., Jaskiw, G. E., & Weinberger, D. R. (1993). Postpubertal emergence of hyperresponsiveness to stress and to amphetamine after neonatal excitotoxic hippocampal damage: a potential animal model of schizophrenia. *Neuropsychopharmacology, 9,* 67–75.

Lipska, B. K., & Weinberger, D. R. (1995). Genetic variation in vulnerability to the behavioral effects of neonatal hippocampal damage in rats. *Proceedings of the National Academy of Sciences USA, 92,* 8906–8910.

Lipska, B. K., & Weinberger, D. R. (2000). To model a psychiatric disorder in animals: schizophrenia as a reality test. *Neuropsychopharmacology, 23,* 223–239.

Lipska, B. K., & Weinberger, D. R. (2002). A neurodevelopmental model of schizophrenia: neonatal disconnection of the hippocampus. *Neurotoxicity Research, 4,* 469–475.

Lisieski, M. J., Eagle, A. L., Conti, A. C., Liberzon, I., & Perrine, S. A. (2018). Single-prolonged stress: a review of two decades of progress in a rodent model of posttraumatic stress disorder. *Frontiers in Psychiatry, 9,* 196.

Lisman, J. E., Coyle, J. T., Green, R. W., Javitt, D. C., Benes, F. M., Heckers, S., & Grace, A. A. (2008). Circuit-based framework for understanding neurotransmitter and risk gene interactions in schizophrenia. *Trends in Neurosciences, 31,* 234–242.

Lister, R. G. (1987). The use of a plus-maze to measure anxiety in the mouse. *Psychopharmacology, 92,* 180–185.

Lister, R. G. (1990). Ethologically-based animal models of anxiety disorders. *Pharmacology and Therapeutics, 46,* 321–340.

Liu, D., Diorio, J., Tannenbaum, B., Caldki, C., Francis, D., Freedman, A., . . . Meaney, M. J. (1997). Maternal care, hippocampal glucocorticoid receptors, and hypothalamic-pituitary-adrenal responses to stress. *Science, 277,* 1659–1662.

Liu, H., Li, H., Xu, A., Kan, Q., & Liu, B. (2010). Role of phosphorylated ERK in amygdala neuronal apoptosis in single-prolonged stress rats. *Molecular Medicine Reports, 3,* 1059–1063.

Liu, K. Y., & Howard, R. (2018). Why has adult hippocampal neurogenesis had so little impact on psychiatry? *British Journal of Psychiatry, 212,* 193–194.

Liu, L., Foroud, T., Xuei, X., Berrettini, W., Byerley, W., Coryell, W., . . . Nurnberger, J. I. (2008). Evidence of association between brain-derived neurotrophic factor (*BDNF*) gene and bipolar disorder. *Psychiatric Genetics, 18,* 267–274.

Liu, Y., Blackwood, D. H., Caesar, S., de Geus, E. J. C., Farmer, A., Ferreira, M. A. R., . . . Sullivan, P. F. (2011). Meta-analysis of genome-wide association data of bipolar disorder and major depressive disorder. *Molecular Psychiatry, 16,* 2–6.

Llewellyn-Smith, I. J. (2009). Anatomy of synaptic circuits controlling the activity of sympathetic preganglionic neurons. *Journal of Chemical Anatomy, 38,* 231–239.

Llorente-Berzal, A., Fuentes, S., Gagliano, H., López-Gallardo, M., Armario, A., Viveros, M.-P., & Nadal, R. (2011). Sex-dependent effects of maternal deprivation and adolescent cannabinoid treatment on adult rat behavior. *Addiction Biology, 16,* 624–637.

Lobo-Silva, D., Carriche, G. M., Castro, A. G., Roque, S., & Saraiva, M. (2016). Balancing the immune response in the brain: IL-10 and its regulation. *Journal of Neuroinflammation, 13,* 297.

Lodge, D. J., & Grace, A. A. (2007). Aberrant hippocampal activity underlies the dopamine dysregulation in an animal model of schizophrenia. *Journal of Neuroscience, 27,* 11424–11430.

Lodge, D. J., & Grace, A. A. (2009). Gestational methylazoxymethanol acetate administration: a developmental disruption model of schizophrenia. *Behavioural Brain Research, 204,* 306–312.

Lodge, D. J., & Grace, A. A. (2011). Developmental pathology, dopamine, stress and schizophrenia. *International Journal of Developmental Neuroscience, 29,* 207–2013.

Loewy, A. D. (1991). Forebrain nuclei involved in autonomic control. *Progress in Brain Research, 87,* 253–268.

Logan, C. A. (1999). The altered rationale for the choice of a standard animal in experimental psychology: Henry H. Donaldson, Adolph Meyer, and "the" albino rat. *History of Psychology, 2,* 3–24.

Logan, C. A. (2005). The legacy of Adolph Meyer's comparative approach: Worcester rats and the strange birth of the animal model. *Integrative Physiological and Behavioral Science, 40,* 169–181.

Logan, R. W., & McClung, C. A. (2016). Animal models of bipolar mania: the past, present and future. *Neuroscience, 321,* 163–188.

Logue, M. W., Amstader, A. B., Baker, D. G., Duncan, L., Koenen, K. C., Liberzon, I., ... Uddin, M. (2015). The Psychiatric Genomics Consortium Posttraumatic Stress Disorder Workgroup: posttraumatic stress disorder enters the age of large-scale genomic collaboration. *Neuropsychopharmacology, 40,* 2287–2297.

Logue, M. W., Vieland, V. J., Goedken, R. J., & Crowe, R. R. (2003). Bayesian analysis of a previously published genome screen for panic disorder reveals new, compelling evidence for linkage to chromosome 7. *American Journal of Medical Genetics Part B Neuropsychiatric Genetics, 121B,* 95–99.

London, E., & Etzel, R. A. (2000). The environment as an etiologic factor in autism: a new direction for research. *Environmental Health Perspectives, 108* (suppl. 3), 401–404.

Longo, A., Mele, P., Bertocchi, I., Oberto, A., Bachmann, A., Bartolomucci, A., ... Eva, C. (2014). Conditional inactivation of neuropeptide Y Y1 receptors unravels the role of Y1 and Y5 receptors coexpressing neurons in anxiety. *Biological Psychiatry, 76,* 840–849.

Lorsch, Z. S., Hamilton, P. J., Ramakrishnan, A., Parise, E. M., Salery, M., Wright, W. J., ... Nestler, E. J. (2019). Stress resilience is promoted by a *Zfp189*-driven transcriptional network in prefrontal cortex. *Nature Neuroscience, 22,* 1413–1423.

Loughridge, A. B., Greenwood, B. N., Day, H. E. W., McQueen, M. B., & Fleshner, M. (2013). Microarray analyses reveal novel targets of exercise-induced stress resistance in the dorsal raphe nucleus. *Frontiers in Behavioral Neuroscience, 7,* 37.

Louveau, A., Plog, B. A., Antila, S., Alitalo, K., Nedergaard, M., & Kipnis, J. (2017). Understanding the functions and relationships of the glymphatic system and meningeal lymphatics. *Journal of Clinical Investigation, 127,* 3210–3219.

Louveau, A., Smirnov, I., Keyes, T. J., Eccles, J. D., Rouhani, S. J., Peske, J. D., ... Kipnis, J. (2015). Structural and functional features of central nervous system lymphatic vessels. *Nature, 523,* 337–341.

Lowry, P. (2016). 60 years of POMC: purification and biological characterisation of melanotropins and corticotropins. *Journal of Molecular Endocrinology, 56,* T1–T12.

Lu, H., Zou, Q., Gu, H., Raichle, M. E., Stein, E. A., & Yang, Y. (2012). Rat brains also have a default mode network. *Proceedings of the National Academy of Sciences USA, 109,* 3979–3984.

Lu, L., Mamiya, T., Koseki, T., Mouri, A., & Nabeshima, T. (2011). Genetic animal models of schizophrenia related with the hypothesis of abnormal neurodevelopment. *Biological and Pharmaceutical Bulletin, 34,* 1358–1363.

Lubin, F. D., Roth, T. L., & Sweatt, J. D. (2008). Epigenetic regulation of *bdnf* gene transcription in the consolidation of fear memory. *Journal of Neuroscience, 28,* 10576–10586.

Lucas, M., Ilin, Y., Anunu, R., Kehat, O., Xu, L., Desmedt, A., & Richter-Levin, G. (2014). Long-term effects of controllability or the lack of it on coping abilities and stress resilience in the rat. *Stress, 17,* 423–430.

Lucassen, P. J., Bosch, O. J., Jousma, E., Krömer, S. A., Andrew, R., Seckl, J. R., & Neumann, I. D. (2009). Prenatal stress reduced postnatal neurogenesis in rats relectively bred for high, but not low, anxiety: possible key role of placental 11β-hydroxysteroid dehydrogenase type 2. *European Journal of Neuroscience, 29,* 97–103.

Lugo, J. N., Smith, G. D., Arbuckle, E. P., White, J., Holly, A. J., Flouta, C. M., . . . Okonkwo, O. (2014). Deletion of PTEN produces autism-like behavioral deficits and alterations in synaptic proteins. *Frontiers in Molecular Neuroscience, 7,* 27.

Lukas, M., & Neumann, I. D. (2012). Nasal application of neuropeptide S reduces anxiety and prolongs memory in rats: social versus non-social effects. *Neuropsychopharmacology, 62,* 398–405.

Lukas, M., & Neumann, I. D. (2013). Oxytocin and vasopressin in rodent behaviors related to social dysfunctions in autism spectrum disorders. *Behavioural Brain Research, 251,* 85–94.

Lupien, S. J., Sasseville, M., François, N., Giguère, C. E., Boissonneault, J., Plusquellec, P., . . . the Signature Consortium (2017). The DSM5/RDoC debate on the future of mental health research: implication for studies on human stress and presentation of the signature bank. *Stress, 20,* 2–18.

Luthar, S. S. (1991). Vulnerability and resilience: a study of high-risk adolescents. *Child Development, 62,* 600–616.

Lutter, M., Sakata, I., Osborne-Lawrence, S., Rovinsky, S. A., Anderson, J. G., Jung, S., . . . Zigman, J. M. (2008). The orexigenic hormone ghrelin defends against depressive symptoms of chronic stress. *Nature Neuroscience, 11,* 752–753.

Lydholm, C. N., Köhler-Forsberg, O., Nordentoft, M., Yolken, R. H., Mortensen, P. B., Petersen, L., & Benros, M. E. (2019). Parental infections before, during, and after pregnancy as risk factors for mental disorders in childhood and adolescence: a nationwide Danish study. *Biological Psychiatry, 85,* 317–325.

Lyons, D. M., & Parker, K. J. (2007). Stress inoculation-induced indications of resilience in monkeys. *Journal of Traumatic Stress, 20,* 423–433.

Lyons, D. M., Parker, K. J., Katz, M., & Schatzberg, A. F. (2009). Developmental cascades linking stress inoculation, arousal regulation, and resilience. *Frontiers in Behavioral Neuroscience, 3,* 32.

Lyons, D. M., Parker, K. J., & Schatzberg, A. F. (2010). Animal models of early life stress: implications for understanding resilience. *Developmental Psychobiology, 52,* 616–624.

MacDonald, M. L., Alhassan, J., Newman, J. T., Richard, M., Gu, H., Kelly, R. M., . . . Sweet, R. A. (2017). Selective loss of smaller spines in schizophrenia. *American Journal of Psychiatry, 174,* 586–594.

Machado, C. J., Whitaker, A. M., Smith, S. E. P., Patterson, P. H., & Bauman, M. D. (2015). Maternal immune activation in nonhuman primates alters social attention in juvenile offspring. *Biological Psychiatry, 77*, 823–832.

Mack, A. H., Forman, L., Brown, R., & Frances, A. (1994). A brief history of psychiatric classification: from the ancients to DSM-IV. *Psychiatric Clinics of North America, 17*, 515–523.

Macrì, S., Granstrem, O., Shumilina, M., Gomes dos Santos, F. J. A., Berry, A., Saso, L., & Laviola, G. (2009). Resilience and vulnerability are dose-dependently related to neonatal stressors in mice. *Hormones and Behavior, 56*, 391–398.

Madden, K. S., & Felten, D. L. (1995). Experimental basis for neural-immune interactions. *Physiological Reviews, 75*, 77–106.

Maeng, L. Y., & Milad, M. R. (2015). Sex differences in anxiety disorders: interactions between fear, stress, and gonadal hormones. *Hormones and Behavior, 76*, 106–117.

Maes, M., Bosmans, E., Suy, E., Vandervorst, C., DeJonckheere, C., & Raus, J. (1991). Depression-related disturbances in mitogen-induced lymphocyte responses and interleukin-1β and soluable interleukin-2 receptor production. *Acta Psychiatrica Scandinavica, 84*, 379–386.

Magariños, A. M., & McEwen, B. S. (1995). Stress-induced atrophy of apical dendrites of hippocampal CA3c neurons: involvement of glucocorticoid secretion and excitatory amino acid receptors. *Neuroscience, 69*, 89–98.

Magariños, A. M., Verdugo, J. M. G., & McEwen, B. S. (1997). Chronic stress alters synaptic terminal structure in hippocampus. *Proceedings of the National Academy of Sciences USA, 94*, 14002–14008.

Magnus, C. J., Lee, P. H., Bonaventura, J., Zemla, R., Gomez, J. L., Ramirez, M. H., . . . Sternson, S. M. (2019). Ultrapotent chemogenetics for research and potential clinical applications. *Science, 364*, eaav5282.

Mahmoud, R., Wainwright, S. R., Chaiton, J. A., Lieblich, S. E., & Galea, L. A. M. (2016). Ovarian hormones, but not fluoxetine, impart resilience within a chronic unpredictable stress model in middle-aged female rats. *Neuropharmacology, 107*, 278–293.

Maier, S. F. (2015). Behavioral control blunts reactions to contemporaneous and future adverse events: medial prefrontal cortex plasticity and a corticostriatal network. *Neurobiology of Stress, 1*, 12–22.

Maier, S. F., Amat, J., Baratta, M. V., Paul, E., & Watkins, L. R. (2006). Behavioral control, the medial prefrontal cortex, and resilience. *Dialogues in Clinical Neuroscience, 8*, 397–406.

Maier, S. F., Peterson, C., & Schwartz, B. (2000). From helplessness to hope: the seminal career of Martin Seligman. In J. E. Gillham (Ed.), *The science of optimism and hope: research essays in honor of Martin E. P. Seligman* (pp. 11–37). Philadelphia, PA: Templeton Foundation Press.

Maier, S. F., & Seligman, M. E. P. (1976). Learned helplessness: theory and evidence. *Journal of Experimental Psychology: General, 105*, 3–46.

Maier, S. F., & Seligman, M. E. P. (2016). Learned helplessness at fifty: insights from neuroscience. *Psychological Review, 123*, 349–367.

Maier, S. F., & Watkins, L. R. (1998). Cytokines for psychologists: implications of bidirectional immune-to-brain communication for understanding behavior, mood, and cognition. *Psychological Review, 105*, 83–107.

Maier, S. F., & Watkins, L. R. (2010). Role of the medial prefrontal cortex in coping and resilience. *Brain Research, 1355*, 52–60.

Mairesse, J., Lesage, J., Breton, C., Bréant, B., Hahn, T., Darnaudéry, M., . . . Viltart, O. (2007). Maternal stress alters endocrine function of the feto-placental unit in rats. *American Journal of Physiology, 292*, E1526–E1533.

Major Depressive Disorder Working Group of the Psychiatric GWAS Consortium (2013). A mega-analysis of genome-wide association studies for major depressive disorder. *Molecular Psychiatry, 18*, 497–511.

Malaspina, D., Corcoran, C., Kleinhaus, K. R., Perrin, M. C., Fennig, S., Nahon, D., . . . Harlap, S. (2008). Acute maternal stress in pregnancy and schizophrenia in offspring: a cohort prospective study. *BMC Psychiatry, 8*, 71.

Malkesman, O., Austin, D. R., Chen, G., & Manji, H. (2009). Reverse translational strategies for developing animal models of bipolar disorder. *Disease Models and Mechanisms, 2*, 238–245.

Malkesman, O., Braw, Y., Maayan, R., Weizman, A., Overstreet, D. H., Shabat-Simon, M., . . . Weller, A. (2006). Two different putative genetic animal models of childhood depression. *Biological Psychiatry, 59*, 17–23.

Malkova, N. V., Yu, C. Z., Hsiao, E. Y., Moore, M. J., & Patterson, P. H. (2012). Maternal immune activation yields offspring displaying mouse versions of the three core symptoms of autism. *Brain, Behavior and Immunity, 26*, 607–616.

Mandela, N. (1994). *Long walk to freedom: the autobiography of Nelson Mandela.* Philadelphia, PA: Little, Brown.

Maple, A. M., Zhao, X., Elizalde, D. I., McBride, A. K., & Gallitano, A. L. (2015). *Htr2a* expression responds rapidly to environmental stimuli in an *Egr3*-dependent manner. *ACS Chemical Neuroscience, 6*, 1137–1142.

Marangoni, C., Hernandez, M., & Faedda, G. L. (2016). The role of environmental exposures as risk factors for bipolar disorder: a systematic review of longitudinal studies. *Journal of Affective Disorders, 193*, 165–174.

Marco, E. M., Llorente, R., López-Gallardo, M., Mela, V., Llorente-Berzal, Á., Prada, C., & Viveros, M.-P. (2015). The maternal deprivation animal model revisited. *Neuroscience and Biobehavioral Reviews, 51*, 151–163.

Maren, S., & Holmes, A. (2016). Stress and fear extinction. *Neuropsychopharmacology, 41*, 58–79.

Markram, K., & Markram, H. (2010). The Intense World Theory: a unifying theory of the neurobiology of autism. *Frontiers in Human Neuroscience, 4*, 224.

Markram, K., Rinaldi, T., La Mendola, D., Sandi, C., & Markram, H. (2008). Abnormal fear conditioning and amygdala processing in an animal model of autism. *Neuropsychopharmacology, 33*, 901–912.

Marques, F., Sousa, J. C., Correia-Neves, M., Oliveira, P., Sousa, N., & Palha, J. A. (2007). The choroid plexus response to peripheral inflammatory stimulus. *Neuroscience, 144*, 424–430.

Martin, L. A., Ashwood, P., Braunschweig, D., Cabanlit, M., Van de Water, J., & Amaral, D. G. (2008). Sterotypies and hyperactivity in rhesus monkeys exposed to IgG from mothers of children with autism. *Brain, Behavior, and Immunity, 22*, 806–816.

Martin, S. J. (2016). Cell death and inflammation: the case of IL-1 family cytokines as the canonical DAMPs of the immune system. *FEBS Journal, 283*, 2599–2615.

Martinon, F., Burns, K., & Tschopp, J. (2002). The inflammasome: a molecular platform triggering activation of inflammatory caspases and processing of proIL-β. *Molecular Cell, 10*, 417–426.

Mason, J. W. (1971). A re-evaluation of the concept of "nonspecificity" in stress theory. *Journal of Psychiatric Research, 8*, 323–333.

Mason, J. W. (1975a). A historical view of the stress field: Part I. *Journal of Human Stress, 1*, 6–12.

Mason, J. W. (1975b). A historical view of the stress field: Part II. *Journal of Human Stress, 1*, 22–36.

Masten, A. S. (2001). Ordinary magic: resilience processes in development. *American Psychologist, 56*, 227–238.

Matar, M. A., Cohen, H., Kaplan, Z., & Zohar, J. (2006). The effect of early poststressor intervention with sertraline on behavioral responses in an animal model of post-traumatic stress disorder. *Neuropsychopharmacology, 31*, 2610–2618.

Matar, M. A., Zohar, J., & Cohen, H. (2013). Translationally relevant modeling of PTSD in rodents. *Cell and Tissue Research, 354*, 127–139.

Mathies, L. D., Blackwell, G. G., Austin, M. K., Edwards, A. C., Riley, B. P., Davies, A. G., & Bettinger, J. C. (2015). SWI/SNF chromatin remodeling regulates alcohol response behaviors in *Caenorhabditis elegans* and is associated with alcohol dependence in humans. *Proceedings of the National Academy of Sciences USA, 112*, 3032–3037.

Mathur, P., & Guo, S. (2010). Use of zebrafish as a model to understand mechanisms of addiction and complex neurobehavioral phenotypes. *Neurobiology of Disease, 40*, 66–72.

Matrisciano, F., Tueting, P., Dalal, I., Kadriu, B., Grayson, D. R., Davis, J. M., Nicoletti, F., & Guidotti, A. (2013). Epigenetic modifications of GABAergic interneurons are associated with the schizophrenia-like phenotype induced by prenatal stress in mice. *Neuropharmacology, 68*, 184–194.

Matrisciano, F., Tueting, P., Maccari, S., Nicoletti, F., & Guidotti, A. (2012). Pharmacological activation of group-II metabotropic glutamate receptors corrects a schizophrenia-like phenotype induced by prenatal stress in mice. *Neuropsychopharmacology, 37*, 929–938.

Matsuo, N., Takao, K., Nakanishi, K., Yamasaki, N., Tanda, K., & Miyakawa, T. (2010). Behavioral profiles of three C57BL/6 substrains. *Frontiers in Behavioral Neuroscience, 4*, 29.

Matthews, K., Christmas, D., Swan, J., & Sorrel, E. (2005). Animal models of depression: navigating through the clinical fog. *Neuroscience and Biobehavioral Reviews, 29*, 503–513.

Matthews, K. A., Adler, N. E., Forrest, C. B., & Stead, W. W. (2016). Collecting psychosocial "vital signs" in electronic health records: why now? what are they? what's new for psychology? *American Psychologist, 71*, 497–504.

Matzinger, P. (1994). Tolerance, danger, and the extended family. *Annual Review of Immunology, 12*, 991–1045.

Matzinger, P. (2002). The danger model: a renewed sense of self. *Science, 296*, 301–305.

Maurano, M. T., Humbert, R., Rynes, E., Thurman, R. E., Haugen, E., Wang, H., . . . Stamatoyannopoulos, J. A. (2012). Systematic localization of common disease-associated variation in regulatory DNA. *Science, 337*, 1190–1195.

McCall, J. G., Al-Hasani, R., Siuda, E. R., Hong, D. Y., Norris, A. J., Ford, C. P., & Bruchas, M. R. (2015). CRH engagement of the locus coeruleus noradrenergic system mediates stress-induced anxiety. *Neuron, 87*, 605–620.

McCarty, R. (1975). *Onychomys torridus. Mammalian Species, 59*, 1–5.

McCarty, R. (1978). *Onychomys leucogaster. Mammalian Species, 87*, 1–6.

McCarty, R. (2016). Learning about stress: neural, endocrine and behavioral adaptations. *Stress, 19*, 449–475.

McCarty, R. (2017). Cross-fostering: elucidating the effects of gene x environment interactions on phenotypic development. *Neuroscience and Biobehavioral Reviews, 73*, 219–254.

McCarty, R., & Kirby, R. F. (1982). Spontaneous hypertension and open-field behavior. *Behavioral and Neural Biology, 34,* 450–452.

McCarty, R., & Kopin, I. J. (1978). Sympatho-adrenal medullary activity and behavior during exposure to stress: a comparison of seven rat strains. *Physiology and Behavior, 21,* 567–572.

McCarty, R., & Kopin, I. J. (1979). Stress-induced alterations in plasma catecholamines and behavior of rats: effects of chlorisondamine and bretylium. *Behavioral and Neural Biology, 27,* 249–265.

McClung, C. A. (2013). How might circadian rhythms control mood? Let me count the ways. . . . *Biological Psychiatry, 74,* 2420–249.

McCormick, C. M., & Green, M. R. (2013). From the stressed adolescent to the anxious and depressed adult: investigations in rodent models. *Neuroscience, 249,* 242–257.

McEwen, B. S. (1998). Protective and damaging effects of stress mediators. *New England Journal of Medicine, 338,* 171–179.

McEwen, B. S. (2002a). *The end of stress as we know it.* Washington, DC: Joseph Henry Press.

McEwen, B. S. (2002b). The neurobiology and neuroendocrinology of stress: implications for post-traumatic stress disorder from a basic science perspective. *Psychiatric Clinics of North America, 25,* 469–494.

McEwen, B. S. (2007). Physiology and neurobiology of stress and adaptation: central role of the brain. *Physiological Reviews, 87,* 873–904.

McEwen, B. S. (2010). Stress, sex, and neural adaptation to a changing environment: mechanisms of neuronal remodeling. *Annals of the New York Academy of Sciences, 1204,* E38–E59.

McEwen, B. S. (2012). Brain on stress: how the social environment gets under the skin. *Proceedings of the National Academy of Sciences USA, 109* (Suppl. 2), 17180–17185.

McEwen, B. S., Nasca, C., & Gray, J. D. (2016). Stress effects on neuronal structure: hippocampus, amygdala, and prefrontal cortex. *Neuropsychopharmacology Reviews, 41,* 3–23.

McEwen, B. S., & Stellar, E. (1993). Stress and the individual: mechanisms leading to disease. *Archives of Internal Medicine, 153,* 2093–2101.

McEwen, B. S., & Wingfield, J. C. (2003). The concept of allostasis in biology and biomedicine. *Hormones and Behavior, 43,* 2–15.

McGaugh, J. L. (2000). Memory: a century of consolidation. *Science, 287,* 248–251.

McGhie, A., & Chapman, J. (1961). Disorders of attention and perception in early schizophrenia. *British Journal of Medical Psychology, 34,* 103–116.

McGorry, P. D. (2013). The next stage for diagnosis: validity through utility. *World Psychiatry, 12,* 3.

McGowan, P. O., Meaney, M. J., & Szyf, M. (2008). Diet and the epigenetic (re)programming of phenotypic differences in behavior. *Brain Research, 1237,* 12–24.

McGowan, P. O., Suderman, M., Sasaki, A., Huang, T. C., Hallett, M., Meaney, M. J., & Szyf, M. (2011). Broad epigenetic signature of maternal care in the brain of adult rats. *PLoS One, 6,* e14739.

McGrath, J. J. (2005). Myths and plain truths about schizophrenia epidemiology: the NAPE lecture 2004. *Acta Psychiatrica Scandinavica, 111,* 4–11.

McKim, D. B., Weber, M. D., Niraula, A., Sawicki, C. M., Liu, X., Jarrett, B. L., . . . Gosbout, J. P. (2018). Microglial recruitment of IL-1β-producing monocytes to brain endothelium causes stress-induced anxiety. *Molecular Psychiatry, 23,* 1421–1431.

McKinney, W. T. (1984). Animal models of depression: an overview. *Psychiatric Developments, 2,* 77–96.

McKinney, W. T. (1988). *Models of mental disorder: a new comparative psychiatry.* New York, NY: Plenum.

McKinney, W. T. (2001). Overview of the past contributions of animal models and their changing place in psychiatry. *Seminars in Clinical Neuropsychiatry, 6,* 68–78.

McKinney, W. T., Suomi, S. J., & Harlow, H. F. (1971). Depression in primates. *American Journal of Psychiatry, 127,* 1313–1320.

McKlveen, J. M., Myers, B., & Herman, J. P. (2015). The medial prefrontal cortex: coordinator of autonomic, neuroendocrine and behavioural responses to stress. *Journal of Neuroendocrinology, 27,* 446–456.

McKlveen, J. M., Moloney, R. D., Scheimann, J. R., Myers, B., & Herman, J. P. (2019). "Braking" the prefrontal cortex: the role of glucocorticoids and interneurons in stress adaptation and pathology. *Biological Psychiatry, 86,* 669–681.

McLaughlin, K. A., Conron, K. J., Koenen, K. C., & Gilman, S. E. (2010). Childhood adversity, adult stressful life events, and risk of past-year psychiatric disorder: a test of the stress sensitization hypothesis in a population-based sample of adults. *Psychological Medicine, 40,* 1647–1658.

McLeod, J., Sinal, C. J., & Perrot-Sinal, T. S. (2007). Evidence for non-genomic transmission of ecological information via maternal behavior in female rats. *Genes, Brain and Behavior, 6,* 19–29.

McTighe, S. M., Neal, S. J., Lin, Q., Hughes, Z. A., & Smith, D. G. (2013). The BTBR mouse model of autism spectrum disorders has learning and attentional impairments and alterations in acetylchoine and kynurenic acid in prefrontal cortex. *PLoS ONE, 8,* e62189.

Meador, K., Reynolds, M. W., Crean, S., Fahrbach. K., & Probst, C. (2008). Pregnancy outcomes in women with epilepsy: a systematic review and meta-analysis of published pregnancy registries and cohorts. *Epilepsy Research, 81,* 1–13.

Meaney, M. J., & Szyf, M. (2005a). Maternal care as a model for experience-dependent chromatin plasticity? *Trends in Neuroscience, 28,* 456–463.

Meaney, M. J., & Szyf, M. (2005b). Environmental programming of stress responses through DNA methylation: life at the interface between a dynamic environment and a fixed genome. *Dialogues in Clinical Neuroscience, 7,* 103–123.

Medawar, P. B. (1946). Immunity to homologous grafted skin: the relationship between the antigens of blood and skin. *British Journal of Experimental Pathology, 27,* 15–24.

Meehan, T. F., Conte, N., West, D. B., Jacobsen, J. O., Mason, J., Warren, J., . . . Smedley, D. (2017). Disease model discovery from 3,328 gene knockouts by the International Mouse Phenotyping Consortium. *Nature Genetics, 49,* 1231–1238.

Mehta, D., & Binder, E. B. (2012). Gene x environment vulnerability factors for PTSD: the HPA-axis. *Neuropharmacology, 62,* 654–662.

Mehta, M. V., Gandal, M. J., & Siegel, S. J. (2011). mGluR5-antagonist mediated reversal of elevated stereotyped, repetitive behaviors in the VPA model of autism. *PLoS ONE, 6,* e26077.

Mehta-Raghavan, N. S., Wert, S. L., Morley, C., Graf, E. N., & Redei, E. E. (2016). Nature and nurture: environmental influences on a genetic rat model of depression. *Translational Psychiatry, 6,* e770.

Mei, L., & Xiong, W.-C. (2008). Neuregulin 1 in neural development, synaptic plasticity and schizophrenia. *Nature Reviews Neuroscience, 9,* 437–452.

Meltzer, A., & Van de Water, J. (2017). The role of the immune system in autism spectrum disorder. *Neuropsychopharmacology Reviews, 42*, 284–298.

Ménard, C., Hodes, G. E., & Russo, S. J. (2016). Pathogenesis of depression: insights from human and rodent studies. *Neuroscience, 321*, 138–162.

Ménard, C., Pfau, M. L., Hodes, G. E., Kana, V., Wang, V. X., Bouchard, S., . . . Russo, S. J. (2017). Social stress induces neurovascular pathology promoting depression. *Nature Neuroscience, 20*, 1752–1760.

Mendel, C. M. (1989). The free hormone hypothesis: a physiologically based mathematical model. *Endocrine Reviews, 10*, 232–274.

Mendell, J. T., & Olson, E. N. (2012). MicroRNAs in stress signaling and human disease. *Cell, 148*, 1172–1187.

Metalnikov, S., & Chorine, V. (1926). Rôle des réflexes conditionnels dans l'immunité. *Annales de l' Institut Pasteur (Paris), 40*, 893–900.

Meyer, A. (1896). Book review. *American Journal of Insanity, 53*, 298–302.

Meyer, E. J., Nenke, M. A., Rankin, W., Lewis, J. G., & Torpy, D. J. (2016). Corticosteroid-binding globulin: a review of basic and clinical advances. *Hormone and Metabolic Research, 48*, 359–371.

Meyer, F., & Louilot, A. (2014). Consequences at adulthood of transient inactivation of the parahippocampal and prefrontal regions during early development: new insights from a disconnection animal model for schizophrenia. *Frontiers in Behavioral Neuroscience, 8*, 118.

Meyer, R. M., Burgos-Robles, A., Liu, E., Correia, S. S., & Goosens, K. A. (2014). A ghrelin-growth hormone axis drives stress-induced vulnerability to enhanced fear. *Molecular Psychiatry, 19*, 1284–1294.

Meyer, U. (2014). Prenatal poly(I:C) exposure and other developmental immune activation models in rodent systems. *Biological Psychiatry, 75*, 307–315.

Meyer, U., & Feldon, J. (2010). Epidemiology-driven neurodevelopmental animal models of schizophrenia. *Progress in Neurobiology, 90*, 285–326.

Meyer, U., & Feldon, J. (2012). To poly(I:C) or not to poly(I:C): advancing preclinical schizophrenia research through the use of prenatal immune activation models. *Neuropharmacology, 62*, 1308–1321.

Meyer, U., Feldon, J., & Dammann, O. (2011). Schizophrenia and autism: both shared and disorder-specific pathogenesis *via* perinatal inflammation? *Pediatric Research, 69*, 26R-33R.

Meyer, U., Feldon, J., & Fatemi, S. H. (2009). In-vivo rodent models for the experimental investigation of prenatal immune activation effects in neurodevelopmental brain disorders. *Neuroscience and Biobehavioral Reviews, 33*, 1061–1079.

Meyer, U., Feldon, J., Schwendener, S., & Yee, B. K. (2005). Towards an immuno-precipitated neurodevelopmental animal model of schizophrenia. *Neuroscience and Biobehavioral Reviews, 29*, 913–947.

Meyer, U., Nyffeler, M., Schwendener, S., Knuesel, I., Yee, B. K., & Feldon, J. (2008a). Relative prenatal and postnatal maternal contributions to schizophrenia-related neurochemical dysfunction after in *utero* immune challenge. *Neuropsychopharmacology, 33*, 441–456.

Meyer, U., Nyffeler, M., Yee, B. K., Knuesel, I., & Feldon, J. (2008b). Adult brain and behavioral pathological markers of prenatal immune challenge during early/middle and late fetal development in mice. *Brain, Behavior, and Immunity, 22*, 469–486.

Meyer, U., Schwendener, S., Feldon, J., & Yee, B. K. (2006). Prenatal and postnatal maternal contributions in the infection model of schizophrenia. *Experimental Brain Research, 173,* 243–257.

Meyza, K. Z., & Blanchard, D. C. (2017). The BTBR mouse model of idiopathic autism: current view on mechanisms. *Neuroscience and Biobehavioral Reviews, 76,* 99–110.

Meyza, K. Z., Defensor, E. B., Jensen, A. L., Corley, M. J., Pearson, B. L., Pobbe, R. L. H., . . . Blanchard, R. J. (2013). The BTBR mouse model for autism spectrum disorders: in search of biomarkers. *Behavioural Brain Research, 251,* 25–34.

Milekic, M. H., O'Donnell, A., Kumar, K. K., Bradley-Moore, M., Malaspina, D., Moore, H., . . . Gingrich, J. A. (2015). Age-related sperm DNA methylation changes are transmitted to offspring and associated with abnormal behavior and dysregulated gene expression. *Molecular Psychiatry, 20,* 995–1001.

Milienne-Petiot, M., Kesby, J. P., Graves, M., van Enkhuizen, J., Semenova, S., Minassian, A., . . . Young, J. W. (2017). The effects of reduced dopamine transporter function and chronic lithium on motivation, probabilistic learning, and neurochemistry in mice: modeling bipolar mania. *Neuropharmacology, 113,* 260–270.

Millan, M. J., Andrieux, A., Bartzokis, G., Cadenhead, K., Dazzan, P., Fusar-Poli, P., . . . Weinberger, D. (2016). Altering the course of schizophrenia: progress and perspectives. *Nature Reviews Drug Discovery, 15,* 485–515.

Miller, A. H., & Raison, C. L. (2016). The role of inflammation in depression: from evolutionary imperative to modern treatment target. *Nature Reviews Immunology, 16,* 22–34.

Miller, B. R., & Hen, R. (2015). The current state of the neurogenic theory of depression and anxiety. *Current Opinion in Neurobiology, 30,* 51–58.

Miller, D., Brinkworth, M., & Iles, D. (2010). Paternal DNA packaging in spermatozoa: more than the sum of its parts? DNA, histones, protamines and epigenetics. *Reproduction, 139,* 287–301.

Miller, D. B., & O'Callaghan, J. P. (2013). Personalized medicine in major depressive disorder- opportunities and pitfalls. *Metabolism Clinical and Experimental, 62* (Suppl. 1), S34–S39.

Miller, R., Wankerl, M., Stalder, T., Kirschbaum, C., & Alexander, N. (2013). The serotonin transporter gene-linked polymorphic region (5-HTTLPR) and cortisol stress reactivity: a meta-analysis. *Molecular Psychiatry, 18,* 1018–1024.

Mineka, S., & Oehlberg, K. (2007). The relevance of recent developments in classical conditioning to understanding the etiology and maintenance of anxiety disorders. *Acta Psychologica, 127,* 567–580.

Mineur, Y. S., Obayemi, A., Wigestrand, M. B., Fote, G. M., Calarco, C. A., Li, A. M., & Picciotto, M. R. (2013). Cholinergic signaling in the hippocampus regulates social stress resilience and anxiety- and depression-like behavior. *Proceedings of the National Academy of Sciences USA, 110,* 3573–3578.

Mitra, R., Adamec, R., & Sapolsky, R. (2009). Resilience against predator stress and dendritic morphology of amygdala neurons. *Behavioural Brain Research, 205,* 535–543.

Mitra, R., Jadhav, S., McEwen, B. S., Vyas, A., & Chattarji, S. (2005). Stress duration modulates the spatiotemporal patterns of spine formation in the basolateral amygdala. *Proceedings of the National Academy of Sciences USA, 102,* 9371–9376.

Mittal, V. A., Ellman, L. M., & Cannon, T. D. (2008). Gene-environment interaction and covariation in schizophrenia: the role of obstetric complications. *Schizophrenia Bulletin, 34,* 1083–1094.

Miyata, A., Arimura, A., Dahl, R. R., Minamino, N., Uehara, A., Jiang, L., . . . Coy, D. H. (1989). Isolation of a novel 38 residue-hypothalamic polypeptide which stimulates adenylate cyclase in pituitary cells. *Biochemical and Biophysical Research Communications, 164,* 567–574.

Modi, M. E., & Young, L. J. (2012). The oxytocin system in drug discovery for autism: animal models and novel therapeutic strategies. *Hormones and Behavior, 61,* 340–350.

Modinos, G., Allen, P., Grace, A. A., & McGuire, P. (2015). Translating the MAM model of psychosis to humans. *Trends in Neurosciences, 38,* 129–138.

Moffat, J. J., Jung, E.-M., Ka, M., Smith, A. L., Jeon, B. T., Santen, G. W. E., & Kim, W.-Y. (2019). The role of ARID1B, a BAF chromatin remodeling complex subunit, in neural development and behavior. *Progress in Neuropsychopharmacology and Biological Psychiatry, 89,* 30–38.

Moghaddam, B. (2002). Stress activation of glutamate neurotransmission in the prefrontal cortex: implications for dopamine-associated psychiatric disorders. *Biological Psychiatry, 51,* 775–787.

Molendijk, M. L., & de Kloet, E. R. (2015). Immobility in the forced swim test is adaptive and does not reflect depression. *Psychoneuroendocrinology, 62,* 389–391.

Molteni, R., Lipska, B. K., Weinberger, D. R., Racagni, G., & Riva, M. A. (2001). Developmental and stress-related changes of neurotrophic factor gene expression in an animal model of schizophrenia. *Molecular Psychiatry, 6,* 285–292.

Mondelli, V. (2014). From stress to psychosis: whom, how, when and why? *Epidemiology and Psychiatric Sciences, 23,* 215–218.

Monroe, S. M., & Harkness, K. L. (2005). Life stress, the "kindling" hypothesis, and the recurrence of depression: considerations from a life stress perspective. *Psychological Review, 112,* 417–445.

Monroe, S. M., & Simons, A. D. (1991). Diathesis-stress theories in the context of life stress research: implications for the depressive disorders. *Psychological Bulletin, 110,* 406–425.

Monteggia, L. M., Heimer, H., & Nestler, E. J. (2018). Meeting report: can we make animal models of human mental illness? *Biological Psychiatry, 84,* 542–545.

Moore, H., Jentsch, J. D., Ghajarnia, M., Geyer, M. A., & Grace, A. A. (2006). A neurobehavioral systems analysis of adult rats exposed to methylazoxymethanol acetate on E17: implications for the neuropathology of schizophrenia. *Biological Psychiatry, 60,* 253–264.

Moran, P., Stokes, J., Marr, J., Bock, G., Desbonnet, L., Waddington, J., & O'Tuathaigh, C. (2016). Gene x environment interactions in schizophrenia: evidence from genetic mouse models. *Neural Plasticity, 2016,* 2173748.

Moreira, F. A., Aguiar, D. C., & Guimarães, F. S. (2006). Anxiolytic-like effect of cannabidiol in the rat Vogel conflict test. *Progress in Neuro-Psychopharmacology and Biological Psychiatry, 30,* 1466–1471.

Moreno-Jiménez, E. P., Flor-García, M., Terreros-Roncal, J., Rábana, A., Cafini, F., Pallas-Bazarra, N., . . . Llorens-Martin, M. (2019). Adult hippocampal neurogenesis is abundant in neurologically healthy subjects and drops sharply in patients with Alzheimer's disease. *Nature Medicine, 25,* 554–560.

Morgan, C. P., & Bale, T. L. (2011). Early prenatal stress epigenetically programs dysmasculinization in second-generation offspring via the paternal lineage. *Journal of Neuroscience, 31,* 11748–11755.

Morgan, C. P., Chan, J. C., & Bale, T. L. (2019). Driving the next generation: paternal life-time experiences transmitted via extracellular vesicles and their small RNA cargo. *Biological Psychiatry, 85,* 164–171.

Moriyama, I. M., Loy, R. M., & Robb-Smith, A. H. T. (2011). *History of the statistical classification of diseases and causes of death.* Hyattsville, MD: National Center for Health Statistics.

Morris, S. E., & Cuthbert, B. N. (2012). Research domain criteria: cognitive systems, neural circuits, and dimensions of behavior. *Dialogues in Clinical Neuroscience, 14,* 1429–1437.

Morrison, S. F. (2001). Differential control of sympathetic outflow. *American Journal of Physiology, 281,* R683–R698.

Moskal, J. R., Burgdorf, J., Kroes, R. A., Brudzynski, S. M., & Panksepp, J. (2011). A novel NMDA receptor glycine-site partial agonist, GLYX-13, has therapeutic potential for the treatment of autism. *Neuroscience and Biobehavioral Reviews, 35,* 1982–1988.

Motta, V., Soares, F., Sun, T., & Philpott, D. J. (2015). NOD-like receptors: versatile cytosolic sentinels. *Physiological Reviews, 95,* 149–178.

Moy, S. S., & Nadler, J. J. (2008). Advances in behavioral genetics: mouse models of autism. *Molecular Psychiatry, 13,* 4–26.

Moy, S. S., Nadler, J. J., Perez, A., Barbaro, R. P., Johns, J. M., Magnuson, T. R., ... Crawley, J. N. (2004). Sociability and preference for social novelty in five inbred strains: an approach to assess autistic-like behavior in mice. *Genes, Brain and Behavior, 3,* 287–302.

Moy, S. S., Nadler, J. J., Young, N. B., Perez, A., Holloway, L. P., Barbaro, R. P., ... Crawley, J. N. (2007). Mouse behavioral tasks relevant to autism: phenotypes of 10 inbred strains. *Behavioural Brain Research, 176,* 4–20.

Moy, S. S., Nadler, J. J., Young, N. B., Nonneman, R. J., Segall, S. K., Andrade, G. M., ... Magnuson, T. R. (2008). Social approach and repetitive behavior in eleven inbred mouse strains. *Behavioural Brain Research, 191,* 118–129.

Mtui, E. P., Anwar, M., Gomez, R., Reis, D. J., & Ruggiero, D. A. (1993). Projections from the nucleus tractus solitarii to the spinal cord. *Journal of Comparative Neurology, 337,* 231–252.

Muir, J., Lopez, J., & Bagot, R. C. (2019). Wiring the depressed brain: optogenetic and chemogenetic circuit interrogation in animal models of depression. *Neuropsychopharmacology, 44,* 1013–1026.

Muir, J., Lorsch, Z. S., Ramakrishnan, C., Deisseroth, K., Nestler, E. J., Calipari, E. S., & Bagot, R. C. (2018). *In vivo* fiber photometry reveals signature of future stress susceptibility in nucleus accumbens. *Neuropsychopharmacology, 43,* 255–263.

Mukherjee, S. (2016). *The gene: an intimate history.* New York, NY: Scribner.

Mukherjee, S., Coque, L., Cao, J.-L., Kumar, J., Chakravarty, S., Asaithamby, A., ... McClung, C. A. (2010). Knockdown of *Clock* in the ventral tegmental area through RNA interference results in a mixed state of mania and depression-like behavior. *Biological Psychiatry, 68,* 503–511.

Mulders, P. C., van Eijndhoven, P. F., Schene, A. H., Beckmann, C. F., & Tendolkar, I. (2015). Resting-state functional connectivity in major depressive disorder: a review. *Neuroscience and Biobehavioral Reviews, 56,* 330–344.

Mulle, J. G., Sharp, W. G., & Cubells, J. F. (2013). The gut microbiome: a new frontier in autism research. *Current Psychiatry Reports, 15,* 337.

Munck, A., Guyre, P. M., & Holbrook, N. J. (1984). Physiological functions of glucocorticoids in stress and their relation to pharmacological action. *Endocrine Reviews, 5,* 25–44.

Mundinger, T. O., Cummings, D. E., & Taborsky, G. J., Jr. (2006). Direct stimulation of ghrelin secretion by sympathetic nerves. *Endocrinology, 147,* 2893–2901.

Murgatroyd, C., Wigger, A., Frank, E., Singewald, N., Bunck, M., Holsboer, F., . . . Spengler, D. (2004). Impaired repression at a vasopressin promoter polymorphism underlies overexpression of vasopressin in a rat model of trait anxiety. *Journal of Neuroscience, 24,* 7762–7770.

Murgatroyd, C., Wu, Y., Bockmühl, Y., & Spengler, D. (2010). Genes learn from stress: how infantile trauma programs us for depression. *Epigenetics, 5,* 194–199.

Murray, C. J. L. (1994). Quantifying the burden of disease: the technical basis for disability adjusted life years. *Bulletin of the World Health Organization, 72,* 429–445.

Murray, C. J. L., & Lopez, A. D. (Eds.). (1996). *The global burden of disease: a comprehensive assessment of mortality and disability from diseases, injuries and risk factors in 1990 and projected to 2020* (GBD Series Vol. I). Cambridge, MA: Harvard School of Public Health on behalf of the World Health Organization and the World Bank.

Murrough, J. W., & Charney, D. S. (2011). The serotonin transporter and emotionality: risk, resilience, and new therapeutic opportunities. *Biological Psychiatry, 69,* 510–512.

Myers, B., Scheimann, J. R., Franco-Villanueva, A., & Herman, J. P. (2017). Ascending mechanisms of stress integration: implications for brainstem regulation of neuroendocrine and behavioral stress responses. *Neuroscience and Biobehavioral Reviews, 74,* 366–375.

Nadeem, A., Ahmad, S. F., El-Sherbeeny, A. M., Al-Harbi, N. O., Bakheet, S. A., & Attia, S. M. (2018). Systemic inflammation in asocial BTBR T+ tf/J mice predisposes them to increased psoriatic inflammation. *Progress in Neuro-Psychopharmacology and Biological Psychiatry, 83,* 8–17.

Nagata, Y., & Matsumoto, H. (1969). Studies on methylazoxymethanol: methylation of nucleic acids in the fetal rat brain. *Proceedings of the Society for Experimental Biology and Medicine, 132,* 383–385.

Nahar, J., Haam, J., Chen, C., Jiang, Z., Glatzer, N. R., Muglia, L. J., . . . Tasker, J. G. (2015). Rapid nongenomic glucocorticoid actions in male mouse hypothalamic neuroendocrine cells are dependent on the nuclear glucocorticoid receptor. *Endocrinology, 156,* 2831–2842.

Nahar, J., Rainville, J. R., Dohanich, G. P., & Tasker, J. G. (2016). Further evidence for a membrane receptor that binds glucocorticoids in the rodent hypothalamus. *Steroids, 114,* 33–40.

Naik, R. R., Sotnikov, S. V., Diepold, R. P., Iurato, S., Markt, P. O., Bultmann, A., . . . Czibere, L. (2018). Polymorphism in Tmem132d regulates expression and anxiety-related behavior through binding of RNA polymerase II complex. *Translational Psychiatry, 8,* 1.

Nakatani, J., Tamada, K., Hatanaka, F., Ise, S., Ohta, H., Inoue, K., . . . Takumi, T. (2009). Abnormal behavior in a chromosome-engineered mouse model for human 15q11-13 duplication seen in autism. *Cell, 137,* 1235–1246.

Nasca, C., Bigio, B., Zelli, D., Nicoletti, F., & McEwen, B. S. (2015). Mind the gap: glucocorticoids modulate hippocampal glutamate tone underlying individual differences in stress susceptibility. *Molecular Psychiatry, 20,* 755–763.

Natelson, B. H. (1983). Stress, predisposition and the onset of serious disease: implications about psychosomatic etiology. *Neuroscience and Biobehavioral Reviews, 7*, 511–527.

Natelson, B. H., Creighton, D., McCarty, R., Tapp, W. N., Pitman, D., & Ottenweller, J. E. (1987). Adrenal hormonal indices of stress in laboratory rats. *Physiology and Behavior, 39*, 117–125.

Natelson, B. H., Tapp, W. N., Adamus, J. E., Mittler, J. C., & Levin, B. E. (1981). Humoral indices of stress in rats. *Physiology and Behavior, 26*, 1049–1054.

National Institute of Mental Health (2008). *National Institute of Mental Health Strategic Plan*. U.S. Department of Health and Human Services, National Institute of Health. NIH Publication No. 08-6368.

National Research Council (2011). *Toward precision medicine: building a knowledge network for biomedical research and a new taxonomy of disease*. Washington, DC: National Academies Press.

Nedelcovych, M. T., Gould, R. W., Zhan, X., Bubser, M., Gong, X., Grannan, M., . . . Jones, C. K. (2015). A rodent model of traumatic stress induces lasting sleep and quantitative electroencephalographic disturbances. *ACS Chemical Neuroscience, 6*, 485–493.

Nemeroff, C. B., Weinberger, D., Rutter, M., Macmillan, H. L., Bryant, R. A., Wessely, S., . . . Lysaker, P. (2013). DSM-5: a collection of psychiatrist views on the changes, controversies, and future directions. *BMC Medicine, 11*, 202.

Nesse, R. M. (2000). Is depression an adaptation? *Archives of General Psychiatry, 57*, 14–20.

Nesse, R. M., & Stein, D. J. (2012). Towards a genuinely medical model for psychiatric nosology. *BMC Medicine, 10*, 5.

Nestler, E. J. (2014). Epigenetic mechanisms of depression. *JAMA Psychiatry, 71*, 454–456.

Nestler, E. J. (2016). Transgenerational epigenetic contributions to stress responses: fact or fiction? *PLoS Biology, 14*, e1002426.

Nestler, E. J., Gould, E., Manji, H., Bucan, M., Duman, R. S., Gershenfeld, H. K., . . . Zalcman, S. (2002). Preclinical models: status of basic research in depression. *Biological Psychiatry, 52*, 503–528.

Nestler, E. J., & Hyman, S. E. (2010). Animal models of neuropsychiatric disorders. *Nature Neuroscience, 13*, 1161–1169.

Network and Pathway Analysis Subgroup of Psychiatric Genomics Consortium (2015). Psychiatric genome-wide association study analyses implicate neuronal, immune and histone pathways. *Nature Neuroscience, 18*, 199–209.

Neufeld-Cohen, A., Evans, A. K., Getselter, D., Spyroglou, A., Hill, A., Gil, S., Tsoory, M., Beuschlein, F., Lowry, C. A., Vale, W., & Chen, A. (2010). Urocortin-1 and -2 double-deficient mice show robust anxiolytic phenotype and modified serotonergic activity in anxiety circuits. *Molecular Psychiatry, 15*, 426–441.

Neumann, I. D., Wigger, A., Krömer, S., Frank, E., Landgraf, R., & Bosch, O. J. (2005). Differential effects of periodic maternal separation on adult stress coping in a rat model of extremes in trait anxiety. *Neuroscience, 132*, 867–877.

Newman, E. L., Covington, H. E., Suh, J., Bicakci, M. B., Ressler, K. J., DeBold, J. F., & Miczek, K. A. (2019). Fighting females: neural and behavioral consequences of social defeat stress in female mice. *Biological Psychiatry, 86*, 657–668.

Newsom, R.J., Garcia, R.J., Stafford, J., Osterland, C., O'Neill, C.E., Day, H.E.W., & Campeau, S. (2020). Remote CB1 antagonist administration reveals multiple sites of tonic and phasic endocannabinoid neuroendocrine regulation. Psychoneuroendocrinology, in press. doi:10.1016/j.psyneuen.2019.104549

Neylan, T. C. (1998). Hans Selye and the field of stress research. *Journal of Neuropsychiatry*, *10*, 230–231.

Niculescu, A. B., III, Segal, D. S., Kuczenski, R., Barrett, T., Hauger, R. L., & Kelsoe, J. R. (2000). Identifying a series of candidate genes for mania and psychosis: a convergent functional genomics approach. *Physiological Genomics*, *4*, 83–91.

Nievergelt, C. M., Ashley-Koch, A. E., Dalvie, S., Hauser, M. A., Morey, R. A., Smith, A. K., & Uddin, M. (2018). Genomic approaches to posttraumatic stress disorder: the Psychiatric Genomic Consortium Initiative. *Biological Psychiatry*, *83*, 831–839.

Nimgaonkar, V. L., Prasad, K. M., Chowdari, K. V., Severance, E. G., & Yolken, R. H. (2017). The complement system: a gateway to gene-environment interactions in schizophrenia pathogenesis. *Molecular Psychiatry*, *22*, 1554–1561.

Nimmerjahn, A., Kirchodd, F., & Helmchen, F. (2005). Resting microglial cells are highly dynamic surveillants of brain parenchyma in vivo. *Science*, *308*, 1314–1318.

Niraula, A., Witcher, K. G., Sheridan, J. F., & Godbout, J. P. (2019). Interleukin-6 induced by social stress promotes a unique transcriptional signature in the monocytes that facilitate anxiety. *Biological Psychiatry*, *85*, 679–689.

Njung'e, K., & Handley, S. L. (1981). Evaluation of marble-burying behavior as a model of anxiety. *Pharmacology, Biochemistry and Behavior*, *38*, 63–67.

Nojima, M., Hosoda, H., Date, Y., Nakazato, M., Matsuo, H., & Kangawa, K. (1999). Ghrelin is a growth-hormone-releasing acylated peptide from stomach. *Nature*, *402*, 656–660.

Nolan, N. A., & Parkes, M. W. (1973). The effects of benzodiazepines on the behavior of mice on a hole-board. *Psychopharmacologia*, *29*, 277–288.

Norman, R. M. G., & Malla, A. K. (1993). Stressful life events and schizophrenia I. A review of the research. *British Journal of Psychiatry*, *162*, 161–166.

Norton, W. H. J., Stumpenhorst, K., Faus-Kessler, T., Folchert, A., Rohner, N., Harris, M. P., . . . Bally-Cuif, L. (2011). Modulation of Fgfr1a signaling in zebrafish reveals a genetic basis for the aggression–boldness syndrome. *Journal of Neuroscience*, *31*, 13796–13807.

Notaras, M., Hill, R., Gogos, J. A., & van den Buuse, M. (2017). BDNF Val66Met genotype interacts with a history of simulated stress exposure to regulate sensorimotor gating and startle reactivity. *Schizophrenia Bulletin*, *43*, 665–672.

Notaras, M., Hill, R., & van den Buuse, M. (2015a). A role for the BDNF gene Val66Met polymorphism as a modifier of psychiatric disorder susceptibility: progress and controversy. *Molecular Psychiatry*, *20*, 916–930.

Notaras, M., Hill, R., & van den Buuse, M. (2015b). A role for the BDNF gene Val66Met polymorphism in schizophrenia? A comprehensive review. *Neuroscience and Biobehavioral Reviews*, *51*, 15–30.

Novak, G., Fan, T., O'Dowd, B. F., & George, S. R. (2013). Postnatal maternal deprivation and pubertal stress have additive effects on dopamine D2 receptor and CaMKII beta expression in the striatum. *International Journal of Developmental Neuroscience*, *31*, 189–195.

Nuechterlein, K. H., & Dawson, M. E. (1984). A heuristic vulnerability/stress model of schizophrenic episodes. *Schizophrenia Bulletin*, *10*, 300–312.

Nuechterlein, K. H., Dawson, M. E., Ventura, J., Gitlin, M., Subotnik, K. L., Snyder, K. S., . . . Bartzokis, G. (1994). The vulnerability/stress model of schizophrenic relapse: a longitudinal study. *Acta Psychiatrica Scandinavica*, *89* (Supplement 382), 58–64.

Nugent, B. M., O'Donnell, C. M., Epperson, C. N., & Bale, T. L. (2018). Placental H3K27me3 establishes female resilience to prenatal insults. *Nature Communications, 9*, 2555.

Nyhuis, T. J., Masini, C. V., Taufer, K. L., Day, H. E. W., & Campeau, S. (2016). Reversible inactivation of rostral nucleus raphe pallidus attenuates acute autonomic responses but not their habituation to repeated audiogenic stress in rats. *Stress, 19*, 248–259.

O'Callaghan, E., Sham, P. C., Takei, N., Murray, G., Glover, G., Hare, E. H., & Murray, R. M. (1994). The relationship of schizophrenic births to 16 infectious diseases. *British Journal of Psychiatry, 165*, 353–356.

O'Donnell, K., O'Connor, T. G., & Glover, V. (2009). Prenatal stress and neurodevelopment of the child: focus on the HPA axis and role of the placenta. *Developmental Neuroscience, 31*, 285–292.

O'Donnell, K. J., & Meaney, M. J. (2017). Fetal origins of mental health: the developmental origins of health and disease hypothesis. *American Journal of Psychiatry, 174*, 319–328.

O'Donnell, P. (2011). Adolescent onset of cortical disinhibition in schizophrenia: insights from animal models. *Schizophrenia Bulletin, 37*, 484–492.

O'Donovan, M. C. (2015). What we have learned from the Psychiatric Genomics Consortium. *World Psychiatry, 14*, 291–293.

O'Donovan, M. C., & Owen, M. J. (2016). The implications of the shared genetics of psychiatric disorders. *Nature Medicine, 22*, 1214–1219.

Okamoto, K., & Aoki, K. (1963). Development of a strain of spontaneously hypertensive rats. *Japanese Circulation Journal, 27*, 282–293.

O'Leary, C., Desbonnet, L., Clarke, N., Petit, E., Tighe, O., Lai, D., . . . O'Tuathaigh, C. (2014). Phenotypic effects of maternal immune activation and early postnatal milieu in mice mutant for the schizophrenia risk gene neuregulin-1. *Neuroscience, 277*, 294–305.

O'Leary, O. F., Felice, D., Galimberti, S., Savifnac, H. M., Bravo, J. A., Crowley, T., . . . Cryan, J. F. (2014). GABAB(1) receptor subunit isoforms differentially regulate stress resilience. *Proceedings of the National Academy of Sciences USA, 111*, 15232–15237.

Oler, J. A., Fox, A. S., Shelton, S. E., Rodgers, J., Dyer, T. Y. D., Davidson, R. J., . . . Kalin, N. H. (2010). Amygdalar and hippocampal substrates of anxious temperament differ in their heritability. *Nature, 466*, 864–868.

Oliver, P. L. (2011). Challenges of analyzing gene-environment interactions in mouse models of schizophrenia. *Scientific World Journal, 11*, 1411–1420.

Olivier, B., Zethof, T., Pattij, T., van Boogaert, M., van Oorschot, R., Leahy, C., . . . Groenink, L. (2003). Stress-induced hyperthermia and anxiety: pharmacological validation. *European Journal of Pharmacology, 463*, 117–132.

Olivier, J. D. A., van der Hart, M. G. C., van Swelm, R. P. L., Cremers, T., Deen, P. M. T., Cuppen, E., . . . Ellenbroek, B. A. (2008). A study in male and female 5-HT transporter knockout rats: an animal model for anxiety and depression disorders. *Neuroscience, 152*, 573–584.

Onnela, J. P., & Rauch, S. L. (2016). Harnessing smartphone-based digital phenotyping to enhance behavioral and mental health. *Neuropsychopharmacology, 41*, 1691–1696.

Ornoy, A., Weinstein-Fudim, L., & Ergaz, Z. (2019). Prevention or amelioration of autism-like symptoms in animal models: will it bring us closer to treating human ASD? *International Journal of Molecular Sciences, 20*, 1074.

Ostiguy, C. S., Ellenbogen, M. A., Walker, C.-D., Walker, E. F., & Hodgins, S. (2011). Sensitivity to stress among the offspring of parents with bipolar disorder: a study of daytime cortisol levels. *Psychological Medicine, 41*, 2447–2457.

Otowa, T., Hek, K., Lee, M., Byrne, E. M., Mizra, S. S., Nivard, M. G., . . . Hettema, J. M. (2016). Meta-analysis of genome-wide association studies of anxiety disorders. *Molecular Psychiatry, 21*, 1391–1399.

Otte, C., Gold, S. M., Penninx, B. W., Pariante, C. M., Etkin, A., Fava, M., . . . Schatzberg, A. F. (2016). Major depressive disorder. *Nature Reviews Disease Primers, 2*, 16065.

Ottenweller, J. E., Natelson, B. H., Pitman, D. L., & Drastal, S. D. (1989). Adrenocortical and behavioral responses to repeated stressors: toward an animal model of chronic stress and stress-related mental illness. *Biological Psychiatry, 26*, 829–841.

Overall, K. L. (2000). Natural animal models of human psychiatric conditions: assessment of mechanism and validity. *Progress in Neuro-Psychopharmacology and Biological Psychiatry, 24*, 727–776.

Overmier, J. B., & Leaf, R. C. (1965). Effects of discriminative Pavlovian fear conditioning upon previously or subsequently acquired avoidance responding. *Journal of Comparative and Physiological Psychology, 60*, 213–217.

Overmier, J. B., & Seligman, M. E. (1967). Effects of inescapable shock upon subsequent escape and avoidance responding. *Journal of Comparative and Physiological Psychology, 63*, 28–33.

Overstreet, D. H., Friedman, E., Mathé, A. A., & Yadid, G. (2005). The Flinders Sensitive Line rat: a selectively bred putative animal model of depression. *Neuroscience and Biobehavioral Reviews, 29*, 739–759.

Overstreet, D. H., & Rezvani, A. H. (1996). Behavioral differences between two inbred strains of Fawn-Hooded rat: a model of serotonin dysfunction. *Psychopharmacology, 128*, 328–330.

Overstreet, D. H., and Wegener, G. (2013). The Flinders sensitive line rat model of depression: 25 years and still producing. *Pharmacological Reviews, 65*, 143–155.

Owen, M. J. (2014). New approaches to psychiatric diagnostic classification. *Neuron, 84*, 564–571.

Owens, M., Overstreet, D. H., Knight, D. L., Rezvani, A. H., Ritchie, J. C., Bissette, G., . . . Nemeroff, C. B. (1991). Alterations in the hypothalamic-pituitary-adrenal axis in a proposed animal model of depression with genetic muscarinic supersensitivity. *Neuropsychopharmacology, 4*, 87–94.

Pacak, K., & Palkovits, M. (2001). Stressor specificity of central neuroendocrine responses: implications for stress-related disorders. *Endocrine Reviews, 22*, 502–548.

Pacak, K., Palkovits, M., Kopin, I. J., & Goldstein, D. S. (1995). Stress-induced norepinephrine release in the hypothalamic paraventricular nucleus and pituitary-adrenocortical and sympathoadrenal activity: in vivo microdialysis studies. *Frontiers in Neuroendocrinology, 16*, 89–150.

Pacak, K., Palkovits, M., Yadid, G., Kvetnansky, R., Kopin, I. J., & Goldstein, D. S. (1998). Heterogeneous neurochemical responses to different stressors: a test of Selye's doctrine of nonspecificity. *American Journal of Physiology, 275*, R1247–R1255.

Pajer, K., Andrus, B. M., Gardner, W., Lourie, A., Strange, B., Campo, J., . . . Redei, E. E. (2012). Discovery of blood transcriptomic markers for depression in animal models and pilot validation in subjects with early-onset major depression. *Translational Psychiatry, 2*, e101.

Palermo, M. T., & Curatolo, P. (2004). Pharmacologic treatment of autism. *Journal of Child Neurology, 19*, 155–164.

Pan, Y., Chen, X.-Y., Zhang, Q.-Y., & Kong, L.-D. (2014). Microglial NLRP inflammasome activation mediates IL-1β-related inflammation in prefrontal cortex of depressed rats. *Brain, Behavior and Immunity, 41*, 90–100.

Paré, W. P. (1989). Stress ulcer susceptibility and depression in Wistar Kyoto (WKY) rats. *Physiology and Behavior, 46*, 993–998.

Paré, W. P. (1994). Open field, learned helplessness, conditioned defensive burying, and forced-swim tests in WKY rats. *Physiology and Behavior, 55*, 433–439.

Pariante, C. M., & Lightman, S. L. (2008). The HPA axis in major depression: classical theories and new developments. *Trends in Neurosciences, 31*, 464–468.

Parker, K. J., Buckmaster, C. L., Schatzberg, A. F., & Lyons, D. M. (2004). Prospective investigation of stress inoculation in young monkeys. *Archives of General Psychiatry, 61*, 933–941.

Parker, K. J., Buckmaster, C. L., Sundlass, K., Schatzberg, A. F., & Lyons, D. M. (2006). Maternal mediation, stress inoculation, and the development of neuroendocrine stress resistance in primates. *Proceedings of the National Academy of Sciences USA, 103*, 3000–3005.

Pathak, G., Ibrahim, B. A., McCarthy, S. A., Baker, K., & Kelly, M. P. (2015). Amphetamine sensitization in mice is sufficient to produce both manic- and depressive-related behaviors as well as changes in the functional connectivity of corticolimbic circuits. *Neuropharmacology, 95*, 434–447.

Patki, G., Li, L., Allam, F., Solanki, N., Dao, A. T., Alkadhi, K., & Salim, S. (2014). Moderate treadmill exercise rescues anxiety and depression-like behavior as well as memory impairment in a rat model of posttraumatic stress disorder. *Physiology and Behavior, 130*, 47–53.

Paton, J. A., & Nottebohm, F. N. (1984). Neurons generated in the adult brain are recruited into functional circuits. *Science, 225*, 1046–1048.

Patrick, C. J., Venables, N. C., Yancey, J. R., Hicks, B. M., Nelson, L. D., & Kramer, M. D. (2013). A construct-network approach to bridging diagnostic and physiological domains: application to assessment of externalizing psychopathology. *Journal of Abnormal Psychology, 122*, 902–916.

Patterson, P. H. (2011). Modeling autistic features in animals. *Pediatric Research, 69*, 34R–40R.

Paulose, C. S., & Dakshinamurti, K. (1987). Chronic catheterization using vascular-access-port in rats: blood sampling with minimal stress for plasma catecholamine determination. *Journal of Neuroscience Methods, 22*, 141–146.

Pavlov, I. P. (1928). *Lectures on conditioned reflexes: twenty-five years of objective study of the higher nervous activity (behaviour) of animals* (W. H. Gantt, Trans.). New York, NY: Liverwright.

Pavlov, I. P. (1941). *Lectures on conditioned reflexes: Vol. 2. Conditioned reflexes and psychiatry* (W. H. Gantt, Trans.). London, England: Lawrence and Wishart.

Paykel, E. S., Myers, J. K., Dienelt, M. N., Klerman, G. L., Lindenthal, J. J., & Pepper, M. P. (1969). Life events and depression: a controlled study. *Archives of General Psychiatry, 21*, 753–760.

Pearce, B. D., Kruszon-Moran, D., & Jones, J. L. (2012). The relationship between Toxoplasma gondii infection and mood disorders in the Third National Health and Nutrition Survey. *Biological Psychiatry, 72*, 290–295.

Pearson, B. L., Pobbe, R. L. H., Defensor, E. B., Oasay, L., Bolivar, V. J., Blanchard, D. C., & Blanchard, R. J. (2011). Motor and cognitive stereotypies in the BTBR T+tf/J mouse model of autism. *Genes, Brain and Behavior, 10*, 228–235.

Pearson-Leary, J., Eacret, D., Chen, R., Takano, H., Nicholas, B., & Bhatnagar, S. (2017). Inflammation and vascular remodeling in the ventral hippocampus contributes to vulnerability to stress. *Translational Psychiatry, 7*, e1160.

Pedroso, I., Lourdasamy, A., Rietschel, M., Nöthen, M. N., Cichon, S., McGuffin, P., . . . Warnich, L. (2018). The genetic architecture of schizophrenia, bipolar disorder, obsessive compulsive disorder and autism spectrum disorder. *Molecular and Cellular Neuroscience, 88*, 300–307.

Pellow, S., Chopin, P., File, S. E., & Briley, M. (1985). Validation of open:closed arm entries in an elevated plus-maze as a measure of anxiety in the rat. *Journal of Neuroscience Methods, 14*, 149–167.

Peña, C. J., Kronman, H. G., Walker, D. W., Cates, H. M., Bagot, R. C., Purushothaman, I., . . . Nestler, E. J. (2017). Early life stress confers lifelong stress susceptibility in mice via ventral tegmental area OTX2. *Science, 356*, 1185–1188.

Peña, C. J., Monk, C., & Champagne, F. A. (2012). Epigenetic effects of prenatal stress on 11β-hydroxysteroid dehydrogenase-2 in the placenta and fetal brain. *PLoS ONE, 7*, e39791.

Peña, C. J., Neugut, Y. D., & Champagne, F. A. (2013). Developmental timing of the effects of maternal care on gene expression and epigenetic regulation of hormone receptor levels in female rats. *Endocrinology, 154*, 4340–4351.

Peñagarikano, O., Abrahams, B. S., Herman, E. I., Winden, K. D., Gdalyahu, A., Dong, H., . . . Geschwind, D. H. (2011). Absence of CNTNAP2 leads to epilepsy, neuronal migration abnormalities, and core autism-related deficits. *Cell, 147*, 235–246.

Perez, J. A., Clinton, S. M., Turner, C. A., Watson, S. J., & Akil, H. (2009). A new role for FGF2 as an endogenous inhibitor of anxiety. *Journal of Neuroscience, 29*, 6379–6387.

Perez, S. M., Aguilar, D. D., Neary, J. L., Carless, M. A., Giuffrida, A., & Lodge, D. J. (2016). Schizophrenia-like phenotype inherited by the F2 generation of a gestational disruption model of schizophrenia. *Neuropsychopharmacology, 41*, 477–486.

Perona, M. T. G., Waters, S., Hall, F. S., Sora, I., Lesch, K.-P., Murphy, D. L., . . . Uhl, G. R. (2008). Animal models of depression in dopamine, serotonin, and norepinephrine transporter knockout mice: prominent effects of dopamine transporter deletions. *Behavioural Pharmacology, 19*, 566–574.

Perrine, S. A., Eagle, A. L., George, S. A., Kulo, K., Kohler, R. J., Gerard, J., . . . Conti, A. C. (2016). Severe, multimodal stress exposure induces PTSD-like characteristics in a mouse model of single prolonged stress. *Behavioural Brain Research, 303*, 228–237.

Perriotti, L. I., Hadeishi, Y., Ulery, P. G., Barrot, M., Monteggia, M., Duman, R. S., & Nestler, E. J. (2004). Induction of ΔFosB in reward-related brain structures after chronic stress. *Journal of Neuroscience, 24*, 10594–10602.

Persico, A. M., & Napolioni, V. (2013). Autism genetics. *Behavioural Brain Research, 251*, 95–112.

Petersen, H. H., Andreassen, T. K., Breiderhoff, T., Bräsen, J. H., Schulz, H., Gross, V., . . . Willnow, T. E. (2006). Hyporesponsiveness to glucocorticoids in mice genetically deficient for the corticosterone binding globulin. *Molecular and Cellular Biology, 26*, 7236–7245.

Petronis, A., & Gottesman, I. I. (2000). Psychiatric epigenetics: a new focus for the new century. *Molecular Genetics, 5*, 342–346.

Petrovszki, Z., Adam, G., Tuboly, G., Kekesi, G., Benedek, G., Keri, S., & Horvath, G. (2013). Characterization of gene-environment interactions by behavioral profiling of selectively bred rats: the effect of NMDA receptor inhibition and social isolation. *Behavioural Brain Research, 240*, 134–145.

Petticrew, M. P., & Lee, K. (2011). The "Father of Stress" meets "Big Tobacco": Hans Selye and the tobacco industry. *American Journal of Public Health, 101*, 411–418.

Peuler, J. D., & Johnson, G. A. (1977). Simultaneous single isotope radioenzymatic assay of plasma norepinephrine, epinephrine and dopamine. *Life Sciences, 21*, 625–636.

Pfaffenseller, B., Kapczinski, F., Gallitano, A. L., & Klamt, F. (2018). EGR3 immediate early gene and the brain-derived neurotrophic factor in bipolar disorder. *Frontiers in Behavioral Neuroscience, 12*, 15.

Pfau, M. L., & Russo, S. J. (2015). Peripheral and central mechanisms of stress resilience. *Neurobiology of Stress, 1*, 66–79.

Phillips, M. L., & Kupfer, D. J. (2013). Bipolar disorder diagnosis: challenges and future directions. *Lancet, 381*, 1663–1671.

Pickles, A., & Angold, A. (2003). Natural categories or fundamental dimensions: on carving nature at the joints and the rearticulation of psychopathology. *Development and Psychopathology, 15*, 529–551.

Pieper, A. A., Xie, S., Capota, E., Estill, S. J., Zhong, J., Long, J. M., . . . McKnight, S. L. (2010). Discovery of a proneurogenic, neuroprotective chemical. *Cell, 142*, 39–51.

Pierce, K. L., Premont, R. T., & Lefkowitz, R. J. (2002). Seven-transmembrane receptors. *Nature Reviews Molecular and Cellular Biology, 3*, 639–650.

Pitman, R. K., Rasmusson, A. M., Koenen, K. C., Shin, L. M., Orr, S. P., Gilbertson, M. W., . . . Liberzon, I. (2012). Biological studies of post-traumatic stress disorder. *Nature Reviews Neuroscience, 13*, 769–787.

Pletnikov, M. V., Ayhan, Y., Nikolskaia, O., Xu, Y., Ovanesov, M. V., Huang, H., . . . Ross, C. A. (2008). Inducible expression of mutant human DISC1 in mice is associated with brain and behavioral abnormalities reminiscent of schizophrenia. *Molecular Psychiatry, 13*, 173–186.

Podhorna, J., & Didriksen, M. (2004). The heterozygous reeler mouse: behavioural phenotype. *Behavioural Brain Research, 153*, 43–54.

Polanczyk, G., Caspi, A., Williams, B., Price, T. S., Danese, A., Sugden, K., . . . Moffitt, T. E. (2009). Protective effect of CRHR1 gene variants on the development of adult depression following childhood maltreatment. *Archives of General Psychiatry, 66*, 978–985.

Polderman, T. J. C., Benyamin, B., de Leeuv, C. A., Sullivan, P. F., van Bochoven, A., Visscher, P. M., & Posthuma, D. (2015). Meta-analysis of the heritability of human traits based on fifty years of twin studies. *Nature Genetics, 47*, 702–709.

Pollak, D. D., Monje, F. J., Zuckerman, L., Denny, C. A., Drew, M. R., & Kandel, E. R. (2008). An animal model of a behavioral intervention for depression. *Neuron, 60*, 149–161.

Pollard, G. T., & Howard, J. L. (1979). The Geller-Seifter conflict paradigm with incremental shock. *Psychopharmacology, 62*, 117–121.

Popper, C. W., Chiueh, C. C., & Kopin, I. J. (1977). Plasma catecholamine concentrations in unanesthetized rats during sleep, wakefulness, immobilization and after decapitation. *Journal of Pharmacology and Experimental Therapeutics, 202*, 144–148.

Porsolt, R. D., Anton, G., Blavet, N., & Jalfre, M. (1978). Behavioural despair in rats: a new model sensitive to antidepressant treatments. *European Journal of Pharmacology, 47*, 379–391.

Porsolt, R. D., Le Pichon, M., & Jalfre, M. (1977). Depression: a new animal model sensitive to antidepressant treatments. *Nature, 266*, 730–732.

Post, R. M. (1992). Transduction of psychosocial stress into the neurobiology of recurrent affective disorder. *American Journal of Psychiatry, 149*, 999–1010.

Post, R. M. (2007). Role of BDNF in bipolar and unipolar disorder: clinical and theoretical implications. *Journal of Psychiatric Research, 41*, 979–990.

Post, R. M. (2016). Epigenetic basis of sensitization to stress, affective episodes, and stimulants: implications for illness progression and prevention. *Bipolar Disorders, 18*, 315–324.

Post, R. M., Leverich, G. S., Xing, G., & Weiss, S. R. B. (2001). Developmental vulnerabilities to the onset and course of bipolar disorder. *Development and Psychopathology, 13*, 581–598.

Potter, E., Behan, D. P., Linton, E. A., Lowry, P. J., Sawchenko, P. E., & Vale, W. W. (1992). The central distribution of a corticotropin-releasing factor (CRF)-binding protein predicts multiple sites and modes of interaction with CRF. *Proceedings of the National Academy of Sciences USA, 89*, 4192–4196.

Pouget, J. G., Gonçalves, V. F., Schizophrenia Working Group of the Psychiatric Genomics Consortium, Spain, S. L., Finucane, H. K., Raychaudhuri, S., . . . Knight, J. (2016). Genome-wide association studies suggest limited immune gene enrichment in schizophrenia compared to 5 autoimmune diseases. *Schizophrenia Bulletin, 42*, 1176–1184.

Powell, C. M., & Miyakawa, T. (2006). Schizophrenia-relevant behavioral testing in rodent models: a uniquely human disorder? *Biological Psychiatry, 59*, 1198–1207.

Powell, S. B., & Geyer, M. A. (2007). Overview of animal models of schizophrenia. *Current Protocols in Neuroscience, Unit 9.24*, 1–20.

Powell, S. B., Young, J. W., Ong, J. C., Caron, M. G., & Geyer, M. A. (2008). Atypical antipsychotics clozapine and quetiapine attenuate prepulse inhibition deficits in dopamine transporter knockout mice. *Behavioural Pharmacology, 19*, 562–565.

Power, R. A., Kyaga, S., Uher, R., MacCabe, J. H., Långström, N., Landen, M., . . . Svensson, A. C. (2013). Fecundity of patients with schizophrenia, autism, bipolar disorder, depression, anorexia nervosa, or substance abuse vs their unaffected siblings. *JAMA Psychiatry, 70*, 22–30.

Power, R. A., Steinberg, S., Bjornsdottir, G., Rietveld, C. A., Abdellaoui, A., Nivard, M. M., . . . Stefansson, K. (2015). Polygenic risk scores for schizophrenia and bipolar disorder predict creativity. *Nature Neuroscience, 18*, 953–955.

Praetorius, J., & Damkier, H. H. (2017). Transport across the choroid plexus epithelium. *American Journal of Physiology, 312*, C673–C686.

Prickaerts, J., Moechars, D., Cryns, K., Lenaerts, I., van Craenenbonck, H., Goris, I., . . . Steckler, T. (2006). Transgenic mice overexpressing glycogen synthase kinase 3β: a putative model of hyperactivity and mania. *Journal of Neuroscience, 26*, 9022–9029.

Priebe, K., Brake, W. G., Romeo, R. D., Sisti, H. M., Mueller, A., McEwen, B. S., & Francis, D. D. (2005). Maternal influences on adult stress and anxiety-like behavior in C57BL/6J and BALB/CJ mice: a cross-fostering study. *Developmental Psychobiology, 47*, 398–407.

Prince, C. R., & Anisman, H. (1984). Acute and chronic stress effects on performance in a forced-swim task. *Behavioral and Neural Biology, 42*, 99–119.

Proudfoot, J., Doran, J., Manicavasagar, V., & Parker, G. (2011). The precipitants of manic/hypomanic episodes in the context of bipolar disorder: a review. *Journal of Affective Disorders, 133*, 381–387.

Pruessner, M., Cullen, A. E., Aas, M., & Walker, E. F. (2017). The neural diathesis-stress model of schizophrenia revisited: an update on recent findings considering illness stage and neurobiological and methodological complexities. *Neuroscience and Biobehavioral Reviews, 73*, 191–218.

Prut, L., & Belzung, C. (2003). The open field as a paradigm to measure the effects of drugs on anxiety-like behaviors: a review. *European Journal of Pharmacology, 463*, 3–33.

Pryce, C. R., & Fuchs, E. (2017). Chronic psychosocial stressors in adulthood: studies in mice, rats and tree shrews. *Neurobiology of Stress, 6*, 94–103.

Psychiatric GWAS Consortium Bipolar Disorder Working Group (2011). Large-scale genome-wide association analysis of bipolar disorder identifies a new susceptibility locus near *ODZ4*. *Nature Genetics, 43*, 977–983.

Pucilowski, O., Overstreet, D. H., Rezvani, A. H., & Janowsky, D. S. (1993). Chronic mild stress-induced anhedonia: greater effect in a genetic rat model of depression. *Physiology and Behavior, 54*, 1215–1220.

Pullar, C. E., Rizzo, A., & Isseroff, R. R. (2006). Beta-adrenergic receptor antagonists accelerate skin wound healing: evidence for a catecholamine synthesis network in the epidermis. *Journal of Biological Chemistry, 281*, 21225–21235.

Quan, N., & Banks, W. A. (2007). Brain-immune communication pathways. *Brain, Behavior and Immunity, 21*, 727–735.

Rabkin, J. G. (1980). Stressful life events and schizophrenia: a review of the research literature. *Psychological Bulletin, 87*, 408–425.

Raczka, K. A., Gartmann, N., Mechias, M.-L., Reif, A., Büchel, C., Deckert, J., & Kalisch, R. (2010). A neuropeptide S receptor variant associated with overinterpretation of fear reactions: a potential neurogenetic basis for catastrophizing. *Molecular Psychiatry, 15*, 1067–1074.

Rader, K. A. (2004). *Making mice: standardizing animals for American biomedical research, 1900–1955*. Princeton, NJ: Princeton University Press.

Radley, J. J., Arias, C. M., & Sawchenko, P. E. (2006). Regional differentiation of the medial prefrontal cortex in regulating adaptive responses to acute emotional stress. *Journal of Neuroscience, 26*, 12967–12976.

Radley, J. J., Rocher, A. B., Rodriguez, A., Ehlenberger, D. B., Dammann, M., McEwen, B. S., . . . Hof, P. R. (2008). Repeated stress alters dendritic spine morphology in the rat medial prefrontal cortex. *Journal of Comparative Neurology, 507*, 1141–1150.

Radley, J. J., & Sawchenko, P. E. (2015). Evidence for involvement of a limbic paraventricular hypothalamic inhibitory network in hypothalamic-pituitary-adrenal axis adaptations to repeated stress. *Journal of Comparative Neurology, 523*, 2769–2787.

Rai, D., Golding, J., Magnusson, C., Steer, C., Lewis, G., & Dalman, C. (2012). Prenatal and early life exposure to stressful life events and risk of autism spectrum disorders: population-based studies in Sweden and England. *PLoS ONE, 7*, e38893.

Raichle, M. E., Macleod, A. M., Snyder, A. Z., Powers, W. J., Gusnard, D. A., & Shulman, G. L. (2001). A default mode of brain function. *Proceedings of the National Academy of Sciences USA, 98*, 676–682.

Raines, G. N. (1953). The new nomenclature. *American Journal of Psychiatry, 109*, 548–549.

Raison, C. L., Rutherford, R. E., Woolwine, B. J., Shuo, C., Shettler, P., Drake, D. F., . . . Miller, A. H. (2013). A randomized control trial of the tumor necrosis factor antagonist infliximab for treatment-resistant depression: the role of baseline inflammatory biomarkers. *JAMA Psychiatry, 70*, 31–41.

Rajagopal, S., Rajagopal, K., & Lefkowitz, R. J. (2010). Teaching old receptors new tricks: biasing seven-transmembrane receptors. *Nature Reviews Drug Discovery, 9,* 373–386.

Rakers, F., Rupprecht, S., Dreiling, M., Bergmeier, C., Witte, O. W., & Schwab, M. (2017). Transfer of maternal psychosocial stress to the fetus. *Neuroscience and Biobehavioral Reviews,* in press. http://dx.doi.org/10.1016/j.neurobiorev.2017.02.019.

Ralph-Williams, R. J., Paulus, M. P., Zhuang, X., Hen, R., & Geyer, M. A. (2003). Valproate attenuates hyperactive and perseverative behaviors in mutant mice with a dysregulated dopamine system. *Biological Psychiatry, 53,* 352–359.

Ramboz, S., Oosting, R., Amara, D. A., Kung, H. F., Blier, P., Mendelsohn, M., . . . Hen, R. (1998). Serotonin receptor 1A knockout: an animal model of anxiety-related disorder. *Proceedings of the National Academy of Sciences USA, 95,* 14476–14481.

Ramikie, T. S., & Ressler, K. J. (2018). Mechanisms of sex differences in fear and post-traumatic stress disorder. *Biological Psychiatry, 83,* 876–885.

Ranson, R. N., Motawei, K., Pyner, S., & Coote, J. H. (1998). The paraventricular nucleus of the hypothalamus sends efferents to the spinal cord of the rat that closely appose sympathetic preganglionic neurons projecting to the stellate ganglion. *Experimental Brain Research, 120,* 164–172.

Rao, A. R., Yourshaw, M., Christensen, B., Nelson, S. F., & Kerner, B. (2017). Rare deleterious mutations are associated with disease in bipolar disorder families. *Molecular Psychiatry, 22,* 1009–1014.

Rapoport, J. L., Giedd, J. N., & Gogtay, N. (2012). Neurodevelopmental model of schizophrenia: update 2012. *Molecular Psychiatry, 17,* 1228–1238.

Rathinam, V. A. K., Vanaja, S. K., & Fitzgerald, K. A. (2012). Regulation of inflammasome signaling. *Nature Immunology, 13,* 333–342.

Reading, A. J. (1966). Effect of maternal environment on the behavior of inbred mice. *Journal of Comparative and Physiological Psychology, 62,* 437–440.

Redrobe, J. P., Dumont, Y., Herzog, H., & Quirion, R. (2003). Neuropeptide Y (NPY) Y2 receptors mediate behavior in two animal models of anxiety: evidence from Y2 receptor knockout mice. *Behavioural Brain Research, 141,* 251–255.

Reichmann, F., & Holzer, P. (2016). Neuropeptide Y: a stressful review. *Neuropeptides, 55,* 99–109.

Reilly, J. N., McLaughlin, E. A., Stanger, S. J., Anderson, A. L., Hutcheon, K., Church, K., . . . Nixson, B. (2016). Characterisation of mouse epididymosomes reveals a complex profile of microRNAs and a potential mechanism for modification of the sperm epigenome. *Scientific Reports, 6,* 31794.

Reinscheid, R. K., Xu, Y.-L., Okamura, N., Zeng, J., Chung, S., Pai, R., . . . Civelli, O. (2005). Pharmacological characterization of human and murine neuropeptide S receptor variants. *Journal of Pharmacology and Experimental Therapeutics, 315,* 1338–1345.

Ren, Q., Ma, M., Ishima, T., Morisseau, C., Yang, J., Wagner, K. M., Zhang, J.-C., . . . Hashimoto, K. (2016). Gene deficiency and pharmacological inhibition of soluble epoxide hydrolase confers resilience to repeated social defeat stress. *Proceedings of the National Academy of Sciences USA, 113,* e1944–e1952.

Rentesi, G., Antoniou, K., Marselos, M., Syrrou, M., Papadopoulou-Daifoti, Z., & Konstandi, M. (2013). Early maternal deprivation-induced modifications in the neurobiological, neurochemical and behavioral profile of adult rats. *Behavioural Brain Research, 244,* 29–37.

Reppert, S. M., & Weaver, D. R. (2002). Coordination of circadian timing in mammals. *Nature, 418,* 935–941.

Rescorla, R. A. (1969). Conditioned inhibition of fear resulting from negative CS-US contingencies. *Journal of Comparative and Physiological Psychology, 67,* 504–509.

Ressler, K. J., Mercer, K. B., Bradley, B., Jovanovic, T., Mahan, A., Kerley, K., . . . May, V. (2011). Post-traumatic stress disorder is associated with PACAP and the PAC1 receptor. *Nature, 470,* 492–497.

Ressler, R. H. (1962). Parental handling in two strains of mice reared by foster parents. *Science, 137,* 129–130.

Ressler, R. H. (1963). Genotype-correlated parental influences in two strains of mice. *Journal of Comparative and Physiological Psychology, 56,* 882–886.

Reul, J. M., & de Kloet, E. R. (1985). Two receptor systems for corticosterone in rat brain: microdistribution and differential occupation. *Endocrinology, 117,* 2505–2511.

Reyes, T. M., Perrin, M. H., Kunitake, K. S., Vaughan, J., Arias, C. A., Hogenesch, J. B., . . . Sawchenko, P. E. (2001). Urocortin II: a member of the corticotropin-releasing factor (CRF) neuropeptide family that is selectively bound by type 2 CRF receptors. *Proceedings of the National Academy of Sciences USA, 98,* 2843–2848.

Rezin, G. T., Furlanetto, C. B., Scaini, G., Valvassori, S. S., Gonçalves, C. L., Ferreira, G. K., . . . Streck, E. L. (2014). Fenproporex increases locomotor activity and alters energy metabolism, and mood stabilizers reverse these changes: a proposal for a new animal model of mania. *Molecular Neurobiology, 49,* 877–892.

Richetto, J., Calabrese, F., Meyer, U., & Riva, M. A. (2013). Prenatal versus postnatal maternal factors in the development of infection-induced working memory impairments in mice. *Brain, Behavior, and Immunity, 33,* 190–200.

Richter, S. H., Zeuch, B., Riva, M. A., Gass, P., & Vollmayr, B. (2013). Environmental enrichment ameliorates depressive-like symptoms in young rats bred for learned helplessness. *Behavioural Brain Research, 252,* 287–292.

Rider, P., Voronov, E., Dinarello, C. A., Apte, R. N., & Cohen, I. (2017). Alarmins: feel the stress. *Journal of Immunology, 198,* 1395–1402.

Ritner, R. K. (2000). Innovations and adaptations in ancient Egyptian medicine. *Journal of Near Eastern Studies, 59,* 107–117.

Rivier, C., & Vale, W. (1983). Interaction of corticotropin-releasing factor and arginine vasopressin on adrenocorticotropin secretion in vivo. *Endocrinology, 113,* 939–942.

Robinson, E. B., St. Pourcain, B., Antilla, V., Kosmicki, J. A., Bulik-Sullivan, B., Grove, J., . . . Daly, M. J. (2016). Genetic risk for autism spectrum disorders and neuropsychiatric variation in the normal population. *Nature Genetics, 48,* 552–555.

Rodgers, A. B., Morgan, C. P., Bronson, S. L., Revello, S., & Bale, T. L. (2013). Paternal stress exposure alters sperm microRNA content and reprograms offspring HPA stress axis regulation. *Journal of Neuroscience, 33,* 9003–9012.

Rodgers, A. B., Morgan, C. P., Leu, N. A., & Bale, T. L. (2015). Transgenerational epigenetic programming via sperm microRNA recapitulates effects of paternal stress. *Proceedings of the National Academy of Sciences USA, 112,* 13699–13704.

Rodgers, R. J. (1997). Animal models of anxiety: where next? *Behavioural Pharmacology, 8,* 477–496.

Rodier, P. M., Ingram, J. L., Tisdale, B., Nelson, S., & Romano, J. (1996). Embryological origin for autism: developmental anomalies of the cranial nerve motor nuclei. *Journal of Comparative Neurology, 370,* 247–261.

Roeder, K., & State, M. W. (2015). Insights into autism spectrum disorder genetic architecture and biology from 71 risk loci. *Neuron, 87,* 1215–1233.

Rogers, J., Raveendran, M., Fawcett, G. L., Fox, A. S., Shelton, S. E., Oler, J. A., . . . Kalin, N. H. (2013). CRHR1 genotypes, neural circuits and the diathesis for anxiety and depression. *Molecular Psychiatry, 18,* 700–707.

Rogers, J. T., Zhao, L., Trotter, J. H., Rusiana, I., Peters, M. M., Li, Q., . . . Weeber, E. J. (2013). Reelin supplementation recovers sensorimotor gating, synaptic plasticity and associative learning deficits in the heterozygous reeler mouse. *Journal of Psychopharmacology, 27,* 386–394.

Roman, C. W., Sloat, S. R., & Palmiter, R. D. (2017). A tale of two circuits: CCKNTS neuron stimulation controls appetite and induces opposing motivational states by projections to distinct brain regions. *Neuroscience, 358,* 316–324.

Roozendaal, B. (2002). Stress and memory: opposing effects of glucocorticoids on memory consolidation and memory retrieval. *Neurobiology and Learning and Memory, 78,* 578–595.

Rosas-Vidal, L. E., Do-Monte, F. H., Sotres-Bayon, F., & Quirk, G. J. (2014). Hippocampal-prefrontal BDNF and memory for fear extinction. *Neuropsychopharmacology, 39,* 2161–2169.

Rose, D. R., Careaga, M., Van de Water, J., McAllister, K., Bauman, M. D., & Ashwood, P. (2017). Long-term altered immune responses following fetal priming in a non-human primate model of maternal immune activation. *Brain, Behavior, and Immunity, 63,* 60–70.

Roseboom, P. H., Nanda, S. A., Fox, A. S., Oler, J. A., Shackman, A. J., Shelton, S. E., . . . Kalin, N. H. (2014). Neuropeptide Y receptor gene expression in the primate amygdala predicts anxious temperament and brain metabolism. *Biological Psychiatry, 76,* 850–857.

Rosen, A. M., Spellman, T., & Gordon, J. A. (2015). Electrophysiological endophenotypes in rodent models of schizophrenia and psychosis. *Biological Psychiatry, 77,* 1041–1049.

Rosenblueth, A., & Cannon, W. B. (1932). Studies on conditions of activity in endocrine organs. XXVIII. Some effects of sympathin on the nictitating membrane. *American Journal of Physiology, 99,* 398–407.

Rosenhan, D. L. (1973). On being sane in insane places. *Science, 179,* 250–259.

Rosenthal, D. (1963). *The Genain quadruplets: a case study and theoretical analysis of heredity and environment in schizophrenia.* New York, NY: Basic Books.

Rosenthal, N., & Brown, S. (2007). The mouse ascending: perspectives for human-disease models. *Nature Cell Biology, 9,* 993–999.

Rosenthal, S. J., & McCarty, R. (2019). Switching winter and summer photoperiods in an animal model of bipolar disorder. *Neuropsychopharmacology, 44,* 1677–1678.

Ross, R. G., Hunter, S. K., McCarthy, L., Beuler, J., Hutchison, A. K., Wagner, B. D., . . . Freedman, R. (2013). Perinatal choline effects on neonatal pathophysiology related to later schizophrenia risk. *American Journal of Psychiatry, 170,* 290–298.

Roth, B. L. (2016). DREADDs for neuroscientists. *Neuron, 89,* 683–694.

Roth, T. L., & Sweatt, J. D. (2010). Annual research review: epigenetic mechanisms and environmental shaping of the brain during sensitive periods of development. *Journal of Child Psychology and Psychiatry, 52,* 398–408.

Roullet, F. I., Lai, J. K. Y., & Foster, J. A. (2013). In utero exposure to valproic acid and autism: a current review of clinical and animal studies. *Neurotoxicology and Teratology, 36,* 47–56.

Roy, B., Dunbar, M., Shelton, R. C., & Dwivedi, Y. (2017). Indentification of microRNA-124-3p as a putative epigenetic signature of major depression. *Neuropsychopharmacology, 42*, 864–875.

Roybal, K., Theobold, D., Graham, A., Dinieri, J. A., Russo, S. J., Krishnan, V., . . . McClung, C. A. (2007). Mania-like behavior induced by disruption of *CLOCK. Proceedings of the National Academy of Sciences USA, 104*, 6406–6411.

Ruby, E., Polito, S., McMahon, K., Gorovita, M., Corcoran, C., & Malaspina, D. (2014). Pathways associating childhood trauma to the neurobiology of schizophrenia. *Frontiers in Psychological and Behavioral Science, 3*, 1–17.

Rudisch, B., & Nemeroff, C. B. (2003). Epidemiology of comorbid coronary artery disease and depression. *Biological Psychiatry, 54*, 227–240.

Russo, S. J., Murrough, J. W., Han, M.-H., Charney, D. S., & Nestler, E. J. (2012). Neurobiology of resilience. *Nature Neuroscience, 15*, 1475–1484.

Rutkowski, T. P., Purcell, R. H., Pollak, R. M., Grewenow, S. M., Gafford, G. M., Malone, T., Mulle, J. G. (2019). Behavioral changes and growth deficits in a CRISPR engineered mouse model of the schizophrenia-associated 3q29 deletion. *Molecular Psychiatry*, in press. doi:10.1038/s41380-019-0413-5

Rutter, M. (1979). Protective factors in children's responses to stress and disadvantage. In M. W. Kent & J. E. Rolf (Eds.), *Primary prevention of psychopathology*: Vol. 3. *Social competence in children* (pp. 49–74). Hanover, NH: University Press of New England.

Rutter, M. (1981). Stress, coping and development: some issues and some questions. *Journal of Child Psychology and Psychiatry, 22*, 323–356.

Rutter, M. (2012). Resilience as a dynamic concept. *Development and Psychopathology, 24*, 335–344.

Ruzza, C., Pulga, A., Rizzi, A., Marzola, G., Guerrini, R., & Calo, G. (2012). Behavioural phenotypic characterization of CD-1 mice lacking the neuropeptide S receptor. *Neuropharmacology, 62*, 1999–2009.

Saavedra-Rodríguez, L., & Feig, L. A. (2013). Chronic social instability induces anxiety and defective social interactions across generations. *Biological Psychiatry, 73*, 44–53.

Sabban, E. L., Alaluf, L. G., & Serova, L. I. (2016). Potential of neuropeptide Y for preventing or treating post-traumatic stress disorder. *Neuropeptides, 56*, 19–24.

Sachs, B. D., Ni, J. R., & Caron, M. G. (2014). Sex differences in response to chronic mild stress and congenital serotonin deficiency. *Psychoneuroendocrinology, 40*, 123–129.

Sachs, B. D., Ni, J. R., & Caron, M. G. (2015). Brain 5-HT deficiency increases stress vulnerability and impairs antidepressant responses following psychosocial stress. *Proceedings of the National Academy of Sciences USA, 112*, 2557–2562.

Sachs, N. A., Sawa, A., Holmes, S. E., Ross, C. A., DeLisi, L. E., & Margolis, R. L. (2005). A frameshift mutation in Disrupted in Schizophrenia 1 in an American family with schizophrenia and schizoaffective disorder. *Molecular Psychiatry, 10*, 758–764.

Saha, S. (2005). Role of the central nucleus of the amygdala in the control of blood pressure: descending pathways to medullary cardiovascular nuclei. *Clinical and Experimental Pharmacology and Physiology, 32*, 450–456.

Sala, C., Vicidomini, C., Bigi, I., Mossa, A., & Verpelli, C. (2015). Shank synaptic scaffold proteins: keys to understanding the pathogenesis of autism and other synaptic disorders. *Journal of Neurochemistry, 135*, 849–858.

Sala, M., Braida, D., Lentini, D., Busnelli, M., Bulgheroni, E., Capurro, V., . . . Chini, B. (2011). Pharmacological rescue of impaired cognitive flexibility, social deficits, increased aggression, and seizure susceptibility in oxytocin receptor null mice: a neurobehavioral model of autism. *Biological Psychiatry, 69,* 875–882.

Salatino-Oliveira, A., Rohde, L. A., & Hutz, M. H. (2018). The dopamine transporter role in psychiatric phenotypes. *American Journal of Medical Genetics B, 177B,* 211–231.

Salery, M., Dos Santos, M., Saint-Jour, E., Moumné, L., Pagès, C., Kappès, V., . . . Vanhoutte, P. (2017). Activity-regulated cytoskeleton-associated protein accumulates in the nucleus in response to cocaine and acts as a brake on chromatin remodeling and long-term behavioral alterations. *Biological Psychiatry, 81,* 573–584.

Sales, A. J., & Joca, S. R. L. (2018). Antidepressant administration modulates stress-induced DNA methylation and DNA methyltransferase expression in rat prefrontal cortex and hippocampus. *Behavioural Brain Research, 343,* 8–15.

Salmaso, N., Stevens, H. E., Mcneill, J., El Sayed, M., Ren, Q., Maragnoli, M. E., . . . Vaccarino, F. M. (2016). Fibroblast growth factor 2 modulates hypothalamic pituitary axis activity and anxiety behavior through glucocorticoid receptors. *Biological Psychiatry, 80,* 479–489.

Salmon, T. W., Copp, O., May, J. V., Abbot, E. S., & Cotton, H. A. (1917). Report of the Committee on Statistics of the American Medico-Psychological Association. *American Journal of Insanity, 74,* 255–260.

Salomé, N., Salchner, P., Viltart, O., Sequeira, H., Wigger, A., Landgraf, R., & Singewald, N. (2004). Neurobiological correlates of high (HAB) versus low anxiety-related behavior (LAB): differential Fos expression in HAB and LAB rats. *Biological Psychiatry, 55,* 715–723.

Salomé, N., Tasiemski, A., Dutriez, I., Wigger, A., Landgraf, R., & Viltart, O. (2008). Immune challenge induces differential corticosterone and interleukin-6 responsiveness in rats bred for extremes in anxiety-related behavior. *Neuroscience, 151,* 1112–1118.

Salomé, N., Viltart, O., Darnaudéry, M., Salchner, P., Singewald, N., Landgraf, R., . . . Wigger, A. (2002). Reliability of high and low anxiety-related behavior: influence of laboratory environment and multifactorial analysis. *Behavioural Brain Research, 136,* 227–237.

Salvadore, G., Quiroz, J. A., Machado-Vieira, R., Henter, I. D., Manji, H. K., & Zarate, C. A., Jr. (2010). The neurobiology of the switch process in bipolar disorder: a review. *Journal of Clinical Psychiatry, 71,* 1488–1501.

Sánchez-Blázquez, P., Cortés-Montero, E., Rodríguez-Muñoz, M., & Garzón, J. (2018). Sigma 1 receptor antagonists inhibit manic-like behaviors in two congenital strains of mice. *International Journal of Neuropsychopharmacology, 21,* 938–948.

Sanders, S. J., He, X., Willsey, A. J., Ercan-Sencicek, A. G., Samocha, K. E., Cicek, A. E., . . . State, M. W. (2015). Insights into autism spectrum disorder genomic architecture and biology from 71 risk loci. *Neuron, 87,* 1215–1233.

Sanders, S. J., He, X., Willsey, A. J., Ercan-Sencicek, A. G., Samocha, K. E., Cicek, A. E., . . . Schmidt, M. V. (2014). Evidence supporting the match/mismatch hypothesis of psychiatric disorders. *European Neuropsychopharmacology, 24,* 907–918.

Santarelli, S., Wagner, K. V., Labermaier, C., Uribe, A., Dournes, C., Balsevich, G., . . . Schmidt, M. V. (2016). SLC6A15, a novel stress vulnerability candidate, modulates anxiety and depression-like behavior: involvement of the glutamatergic system. *Stress, 19,* 83–90.

Santarelli, S., Zimmermann, C., Kalideris, G., Lesuis, S. L., Arloth, J., Uribe, A., . . . Schmidt, M. V. (2017). An adverse early life environment can enhance stress resilience in adulthood. *Psychoneuroendocrinology, 78,* 213–221.

Saper, C. B. (2002). The central autonomic nervous system: conscious visceral perception and autonomic pattern generation. *Annual Review of Neuroscience, 25*, 433–469.

Saper, C. B., Loewy, A. D., Swanson, L. W., & Cowan, W. M. (1976). Direct hypothalamo-autonomic connections. *Brain Research, 117*, 305–312.

Saper, C. B., & Stornetta, R. L. (2015). Central autonomic system. In G. Paxinos (Ed.), *The rat nervous system* (4th ed.) (pp. 629–673). Amsterdam, The Netherlands: Elsevier.

Sapienza, J. K., & Masten, A. S. (2011). Understanding and promoting resilience in children and youth. *Current Opinion in Psychiatry, 24*, 267–273.

Sapolsky, R. M. (1992). *Stress, the aging brain, and the mechanisms of neuron death.* Cambridge, MA: MIT Press.

Sapolsky, R. M., & Meaney, M. J. (1986). Maturation of the adrenocortical stress response: neuroendocrine control mechanisms and the stress hyporesponsive period. *Brain Research Reviews, 11*, 65–76.

Sartor, C. E., McCutcheon, V. V., Pommer, N. E., Nelson, E. C., Grant, J. D., Duncan, A. E., . . . Heath, A. C. (2011). Common genetic and environmental contributions to posttraumatic stress disorder and alcohol dependence in young women. *Psychological Medicine, 41*, 1497–1505.

Sartorius, A., Kiening, K. L., Kirsch, P., von Gall, C. C., Haberkorn, U., Unterberg, A. W., . . . Meyer-Lindenberg, A. (2010). Remission of major depression under deep brain stimulation of the lateral habenula in a therapy-refractory patient. *Biological Psychiatry, 67*, e9–e11.

Saul, M. C., Gessay, G. M., & Gammie, S. C. (2012). A new mouse model for mania shares genetic correlates with human bipolar disorder. *PLoS ONE, 7*, e38128.

Saul, M. C., Stevenson, S. A., & Gammie, S. C. (2013). Sexually dimorphic, developmental, and chronobiological behavioral profiles of a mouse mania model. *PLoS ONE, 8*, e72125.

Saul, M. C., Stevenson, S. A., Zhao, C., Driessen, T. M., Eisinger, B. E., & Gammie, S. C. (2018). Genomic variants in an inbred mouse model predict mania-like behaviors. *PLoS ONE, 13*, e0197624.

Saunderson, E. A., Spiers, H., Mifsud, K. R., Gutierrez-Micinas, M., Trollope, A. F., Shaikh, A., . . . Reul, J. M. H. M. (2016). Stress-induced gene expression and behavior are controlled by DNA methylation and methyl donor availability in the dentate gyrus. *Proceedings of the National Academy of Sciences USA, 113*, 4830–4835.

Sawamura, N., Ando, T., Maruyama, Y., Fujimuro, M., Mochizuki, H., Hono, K., . . . Sawa, A. (2008). Nuclear DISC1 regulates CRE-mediated gene transcription and sleep homeostasis in the fruit fly. *Molecular Psychiatry, 13*, 1138–1148.

Scattoni, M. L., Gandhy, S. U., Ricceri, L., & Crawley, J. N. (2008). Unusual repertoire of vocalizations in the BTBR T+tf/J mouse model of autism. *PLoS ONE, 3*, e3067.

Scattoni, M. L., Martire, A., Cartocci, G., Ferrante, A., & Ricceri, L. (2013). Reduced social interaction, behavioural flexibility and BDNF signaling in the BTBR T+tf/J strain, a mouse model of autism. *Behavioural Brain Research, 251*, 35–40.

Scattoni, M. L., Ricceri, L., & Crawley, J. N. (2011). Unusual repertoire of vocalizations in adult BTBR T+tf/J mice during three types of social encounters. *Genes, Brain and Behavior, 10*, 44–56.

Schaafsma, S. M., & Pfaff, D. W. (2014). Etiologies underlying sex differences in Autism Spectrum Disorders. *Frontiers in Neuroendocrinology, 35*, 255–271.

Schafe, G. E., Nader, K., Blair, H. T., & LeDoux, J. E. (2001). Memory consolidation of Pavlovian fear conditioning: a cellular and molecular perspective. *Trends in Neurosciences, 24*, 540–546.

Schaller, G. B. (2010). *The year of the gorilla*. Chicago, IL: University of Chicago Press.

Scharf, S. H., & Schmidt, M. V. (2012). Animal models of stress vulnerability and resilience in translational research. *Current Psychiatry Reports, 14*, 159–165.

Schildkraut, J. J. (1965). The catecholamine hypothesis of affective disorders: a review of supporting evidence. *American Journal of Psychiatry, 122*, 509–522.

Schiller, J. (1967). Claude Bernard and vivisection. *Journal of the History of Medicine and Allied Sciences, 22*, 246–260.

Schinner, S., & Bornstein, S. R. (2005). Cortical-chromaffin cell interactions in the adrenal gland. *Endocrine Pathology, 16*, 91–98.

Schizophrenia Working Group of the Psychiatric Genomics Consortium (2014). Biological insights from 108 schizophrenia-associated genetic loci. *Nature, 511*, 421–427.

Schmidt, M. V. (2011). Animal models for depression and the mismatch hypothesis of disease. *Psychoneuroendocrinology, 36*, 330–338.

Schmidt, M. V., Sterlemann, V., Ganea, K., Liebl, C., Alam, S., Harbich, D., . . . Müller, M. B. (2007). Persistent neuroendocrine and behavioral effects of a novel, etiologically relevant mouse paradigm for chronic social stress during adolescence. *Psychoneuroendocrinology, 32*, 417–429.

Schmitz, C., Rhodes, M. E., Bludau, M., Kaplan, S., Ong, P., Ueffing, I., . . . Frye, C. A. (2002). Depression: reduced number of granule cells in the hippocampus of female, but not male, rats due to prenatal restraint stress. *Molecular Psychiatry, 7*, 810–813.

Schneider, T., Turczak, J., & Przewlocki, R. (2006). Environmental enrichment reverses behavioral alterations in rats prenatally exposed to valproic acid: issues for a therapeutic approach to autism. *Neuropsychopharmacology, 31*, 36–46.

Schoenfeld, T. J., & Cameron, H. A. (2015). Adult neurogenesis and mental illness. *Neuropsychopharmacology Reviews, 40*, 113–128.

Schöner, J., Heinz, A., Endres, M., Gertz, K., & Kronenberg, G. (2017). Post-traumatic stress disorder and beyond: an overview of rodent stress models. *Journal of Cellular and Molecular Medicine, 21*, 2248–2256.

Schork, A. J., Won, H., Appadurai, V., Nudel, R., Gandal, M., Delaneau, O., . . . Werge, T. (2019). A genome-wide association study of shared risk across psychiatric disorders implicates gene regulation during fetal neurodevelopment. *Nature Neuroscience, 22*, 353–361.

Schroeder, A., Buret, L., Hill, R. A., & van den Buuse, M. (2015). Gene-environment interaction of reelin and stress in cognitive behaviours in mice: implications for schizophrenia. *Behavioural Brain Research, 287*, 304–314.

Schuebel, K., Gitik, M., Domschke, K., & Goldman, D. (2016). Making sense of epigenetics. *International Journal of Neuropsychopharmacology, 19*, 1–10.

Schumann, G., Binder, E. B., Holte, A., de Kloet, E. R., Oedegaard, K. J., Robbins, T. W., . . . Wittchen, H. U. (2014). Stratified medicine for mental disorders. *European Neuropsychopharmacology, 24*, 5–50.

Schwartz, M., & Baruch, K. (2014). The resolution of neuroinflammation in neurodegeneration: leucocyte recruitment via the chroid plexus. *EMBO Journal, 33*, 7–22.

Schwartzer, J. J., Careaga, M., Onore, C. E., Rushakoff, J. A., Berman, R. F., & Ashwood, P. (2013). Maternal immune activation and strain specific interactions in the development of autism-like behaviors in mice. *Translational Psychiatry, 3*, e240.

Scott, J., Leboyer, M., Hickie, I., Berk, M., Kapczinski, F., Frank, E., . . . McGorry, P. (2013). Clinical staging in psychiatry: a cross-cutting model of diagnosis with heuristic and practical value. *British Journal of Psychiatry, 202,* 243–245.

Scotti, M.-A. L., Lee, G., Stevenson, S. A., Ostromecki, A. M., Wied, T. J., Kula, D. J., . . . Gammie, S. C. (2011). Behavioral and pharmacological assessment of a potential new mouse model for mania. *Physiology and Behavior, 103,* 376–383.

Scourzic, L., Mouly, E., & Bernard, O. A. (2015). TET proteins and the control of cytosine demethylation in cancer. *Genome Medicine, 7,* 9.

Seckl, J. R., & Holmes, M. C. (2007). Mechanisms of disease: glucocorticoids, their placental metabolism and 'fetal' programming of adult pathophysiology. *Nature Clinical Practice Endocrinology and Metabolism, 3,* 479–488.

Seese, R. R., Chen, L. Y., Cox, C. D., Schulz, D., Babayan, A. H., Bunney, W. E., . . . Lynch, G. (2013). Synaptic abnormalities in the infralimbic cortex of a model of congenital depression. *Journal of Neuroscience, 33,* 13441–13448.

Sekar, A., Bialas, A. R., de Rivera, H., Davis, A., Hammond, T. R., Kamitaki, N., . . . McCarroll, S. A. (2016). Schizophrenia risk from complex variation of complement component 4. *Nature, 530,* 177–183.

Selemon, L. D., & Zecevic, N. (2015). Schizophrenia: a tale of two critical periods for prefrontal cortical development. *Translational Psychiatry, 5,* e623.

Seligman, M. E. P., & Maier, S. F. (1967). Failure to escape traumatic shock. *Journal of Experimental Psychology, 74,* 1–9.

Selimbeyoglu, A., Kim, C. K., Inoue, M., Lee, S. Y., Hong, A. S. O., Kauvar, I., . . . Deisseroth, K. (2017). Modulation of prefrontal cortex excitation/inhibition balance rescues social behavior in *CNTNAP2*-deficient mice. *Science Translational Medicine, 9,* eaah6733.

Sellgren, C. M., Gracias, J., Watmuff, B., Biag, J. D., Thanos, J. M., Whittredge, P. B., . . . Perlis, R. H. (2019). Increased synapse elimination by microglia in schizophrenic patient-derived models of synaptic pruning. *Nature Neuroscience, 22,* 374–385.

Selten, J.-P., Booij, J., Buwalda, B., & Meyer-Lindenberg, A. (2017). Biological mechanisms whereby social exclusion may contribute to the etiology of psychosis: a narrative review. *Schizophrenia Bulletin, 43,* 287–292.

Selten, J.-P., van der Ven, E., Rutten, B. P. F., & Cantor-Graae, E. (2013). The social defeat hypothesis of schizophrenia: an update. *Schizophrenia Bulletin, 39,* 1180–1186.

Selye, H. (1936a). Thymus and adrenals in the response of the organism to injuries and intoxications. *British Journal of Experimental Pathology, 17,* 234–248.

Selye, H. (1936b). A syndrome produced by diverse nocuous agents. *Nature, 138,* 32.

Selye, H. (1941). Anesthetic effect of steroid hormones. *Experimental Biology and Medicine, 46,* 116–121.

Selye, H. (1946). The General Adaptation Syndrome and the diseases of adaptation. *Journal of Clinical Endocrinology, 6,* 117–230.

Selye, H. (1950). *The physiology and pathology of exposure to stress: a treatise based on the concepts of the general-adaptation-syndrome and the diseases of adaptation.* Montreal, Quebec, Canada: Acta.

Selye, H. (1951). The general-adaptation-syndrome. *Annual Review of Medicine, 2,* 327–342.

Selye, H. (1955). Stress and disease. *Science, 122,* 625–631.

Selye, H. (1956). What is stress? *Metabolism, 5,* 525–530.

Selye, H. (1973). The evolution of the stress concept. *American Scientist, 61,* 692–699.

Selye, H. (1975). Confusion and controversy in the stress field. *Journal of Human Stress, 1*, 37–44.

Selye, H. (1977). *The stress of my life: a scientist's memoirs.* Toronto, Ontario, Canada: McClelland and Stewart.

Selye, H. (1978). *The stress of life* (rev. ed.). New York, NY: McGraw-Hill.

Serova, L., Mulhall, H., & Sabban, E. (2017). NPY1 receptor agonist modulates development of depressive-like behavior and gene expression in hypothalamus in SPS rodent PTSD model. *Frontiers in Neuroscience, 11*, 203.

Serova, L .I., Nwokafor, C., Van Bockstaele, E. J., Reyes, B. A. S., Lin, X., & Sabban, E. L. (2019). Single prolonged stress PTSD model triggers progressive severity of anxiety, altered gene expression in locus coeruleus and hypothalamus and effected sensitivity to NPY. *European Neuropsychopharmacology, 29*, 482–492.

Serova, L. I., Tillinger, A., Alaluf, L. G., Laukova, M., Keegan, K., & Sabban, E. L. (2013). Single intranasal neuropeptide Y infusion attenuates development of PTSD-like symptoms to traumatic stress in rats. *Neuroscience, 236*, 298–312.

Shackman, A. J., Fox, A. S., Oler, J. A., Shelton, S. E., Davidson, R. J., & Kalin, N. H. (2013). Neural mechanisms underlying heterogeneity in the presentation of anxious temperament. *Proceedings of the National Academy of Sciences USA, 110*, 6145–6150.

Shackman, A. J., Fox, A. S., Oler, J. A., Shelton, S. E., Oakes, T. R., Davidson, R. J., & Kalin, N. H. (2017). Heightened extended amygdala metabolism following threat characterizes the early phenotypic risk to develop anxiety-related psychopathology. *Molecular Psychiatry, 22*, 724–732.

Shallcross, R., Bromley, R. L., Irwin, B., Bonnett, L. J., Morrow, J., & Baker, G. A. (2011). Child development following in utero exposure: levetiracetam vs sodium valproate. *Neurology, 76*, 383–389.

Shaltiel, G., Chen, G., & Manji, H. K. (2007). Neurotrophic signaling cascades in the pathophysiology and treatment of bipolar disorder. *Current Opinion in Pharmacology, 7*, 22–26.

Shang, K., Talmage, D. A., & Karl, T. (2017). Parent-of-origin effects on schizophrenia-relevant behaviours of type III neuregulin 1 mutant mice. *Behavioural Brain Research, 332*, 250–258.

Shansky, R. M. (2019). Are hormones a "female problem" for animal research? *Science, 364*, 825–826.

Shansky, R. M., Hamo, C., Hof, P. R., Lou, W., McEwen, B. S., & Morrison, J. H. (2010). Estrogen promotes stress sensitivity in a prefrontal cortex-amygdala pathway. *Cerebral Cortex, 20*, 2560–2567.

Shansky, R. M., Hamo, C., Hof, P. R., McEwen, B. S., & Morrison, J. H. (2009). Stress-induced dendritic remodeling in the prefrontal cortex is circuit specific. *Cerebral Cortex, 19*, 2479–2484.

Shapero, B. G., Weiss, R. B., Burke, T. A., Boland, E. M., Abramson, L. Y., & Alloy, L. B. (2017). Kindling of life stress in bipolar disorder: effects of early adversity. *Behavior Therapy, 48*, 322–334.

Shapiro, S. J. (2010). Animal models for human behavior. In J. Hann & S. J. Shapiro (Eds.), *Handbook of laboratory animal science*: Vol. 2. *Animal models* (3rd ed.) (pp. 11–27). New York, NY: CRC Press.

Sharma, A. N., Fries, G. R., Galvez, J. F., Valvassori, S., Soares, J. C., Carvalho, A. F., & Quevedo, J. (2016). Modeling mania in preclinical settings: a comprehensive review. *Progress in Neuro-Psychopharmacology and Biological Psychiatry, 66*, 22–34.

Sharon, G., Sampson, T. R., Geschwind, D. H., & Mazmanian, S. K. (2016). The central nervous system and the gut microbiome. *Cell, 167*, 915–932.

Shay, J. (1994). *Achilles in Vietnam: combat trauma and the undoing of character.* New York, NY: Scribner.

Shekhar, A., McCann, U. D., Meaney, M. J., Blanchard, D. C., Davis, M., Frey, K. A., . . . Winsky, L. (2001). Summary of a National Institute of Mental Health workshop: developing animal models of anxiety disorders. *Psychopharmacology, 157*, 327–339.

Shephard, R. A., & Broadhurst, P. L. (1982). Hyponeophagia and arousal in rats: effects of diazepam, 5-methoxy-N,N-dimethyltryptamine, d-amphetamine and food deprivation. *Psychopharmacology, 78*, 368–372.

Sherman, J. A. (2012). Evolutionary origin of bipolar disorder-revised (EOBD-R). *Medical Hypotheses, 78*, 113–122.

Shi, L., Fatemi, S. H., Sidwell, R. W., & Patterson, P. H. (2003). Maternal influenza infection causes marked behavioral and pharmacological changes in the offspring. *Journal of Neuroscience, 23*, 297–302.

Shively, C. A., Laber-Laird, K., & Anton, R. F. (1997). Behavior and physiology of social stress and depression in female cynomolgous monkeys. *Biological Psychiatry, 41*, 871–882.

Shively, C. A., Silverstein-Metzler, M., Justice, J., & Willard, S. L. (2017). The impact of treatment with selective serotonin reuptake inhibitors on primate cardiovascular disease, behavior, and neuroanatomy. *Neuroscience and Biobehavioral Reviews, 74*, 433–443.

Shoener, J. A., Baig, R., & Page, K. C. (2006). Prenatal exposure to dexamethasone alters hippocampal drive on hypothalamic-pituitary-adrenal axis activity in adult male rats. *American Journal of Physiology, 290*, R1366–R1373.

Short, A. K., Fennell, K. A., Perreau, V. M., Fox, A., O'Bryan, M. K., Kim, J. H., . . . Hannan, A. J. (2018). Elevated paternal glucocorticoid exposure alters the small noncoding RNA profile in sperm and modifies anxiety and depressive phenotypes in the offspring. *Translational Psychiatry, 6*, e837.

Si, Y., Song, Z., Sun, X., & Wang, J.-H. (2018). MicroRNA and mRNA profiles in nucleus accumbens underlying depression versus resilience in response to chronic stress. *American Journal of Medical Genetics B, 177B*, 563–579.

Sidor, M. M., Spencer, S. M., Dzirasa, K., Parekh, P. K., Tye, K. M., Warden, M. R., . . . McClung, C. A. (2015). Daytime spikes in dopaminergic activity drive rapid mood-cycling in mice. *Molecular Psychiatry, 20*, 1406–1419.

Silberg, J., Pickles, A., Rutter, M., Hewitt, J., Simonoff, E., Maes, H., . . . Eaves, L. (1999). The influence of genetic factors and life stress on depression among adolescent girls. *Archives of General Psychiatry, 56*, 225–232.

Silbersweig, D., & Loscalzo, J. (2017). Precision psychiatry meets network medicine. Network Psychiatry. *JAMA Psychiatry, 74*, 665–666.

Sillivan, S. E., Joseph, N. F., Jamieson, S., King, M. L., Chévere-Torres, I., Fuentes, I., . . . Miller, C. A. (2017). Susceptibility and resilience to posttraumatic stress disorder-like behaviors in inbred mice. *Biological Psychiatry, 82*, 924–933.

Silva, A. P., Cavadas, C., & Grouzmann, E. (2002). Neuropeptide Y and its receptors as potential therapeutic drug targets. *Clinica Chimica Acta, 326*, 3–25.

Silverman, J. L., Yang, M., Lord, C., & Crawley, J. N. (2010). Behavioural phenotyping assays for mouse models of autism. *Nature Reviews Neuroscience, 11*, 490–502.

Silverman, J. L., Yang, M., Turner, S. M., Katz, A. M., Bell, D. B., Koenig, J. I., & Crawley, J. N. (2010). Low stress reactivity and neuroendocrine factors in the BTBR T+tf/J mouse model of autism. *Neuroscience, 171,* 1197–1208.

Simon, G. E. (2019). Big data from health records in mental health care: hardly clairvoyant but already useful. *JAMA Psychiatry, 76,* 349–350.

Singer, H. S., Morris, C., Gause, C., Pollard, M., Zimmerman, A. W., & Pletnikov, M. (2009). Prenatal exposure to antibodies from mothers of children with autism produces neurobehavioral alterations: a pregnant dam mouse model. *Journal of Neuroimmunology, 211,* 39–48.

Singewald, G. M., Rjabokon, A., Singewald, N., & Ebner, K. (2011). The modulatory role of the lateral septum on neuroendocrine and behavioral stress responses. *Neuropsychopharmacology, 36,* 793–804.

Singh, M. M. (1970). A unifying hypothesis on the biochemical basis of affective disorder. *Psychiatric Quarterly, 44,* 706–724.

Skolnick, N. J., Ackerman, S. H., Hofer, M. A., & Weiner, H. (1980). Vertical transmission of acquired ulcer susceptibility in the rat. *Science, 208,* 1161–1163.

Slattery, D. A., & Cryan, J. R. (2017). Modelling depression in animals: at the interface of reward and stress pathways. *Psychopharmacology, 234,* 1451–1465.

Slattery, D. A., Naik, R. R., Grund, T., Yen, Y.-C., Sartori, S. B., Füchsl, A., . . . Neumann, I. D. (2015). Selective breeding for high anxiety introduces a synonymous SNP that increases neuropeptide S receptor activity. *Journal of Neuroscience, 35,* 4599–4613.

Slavich, G. M., & Irwin, M. R. (2014). From stress to inflammation and major depressive disorder: a social signal transduction theory of depression. *Psychological Bulletin, 140,* 774–815.

Slavich, G. M., Taylor, S., & Picard, R. W. (2019). Stress measurement using speech: recent advances, validation issues, and ethical and privacy concerns. *Stress, 22,* 408–413.

Slotnikov, S. V., Markt, P. O., Malik, V., Chekmareva, N. Y., Naik, R. R., Sah, A., . . . Landgraf, R. (2014a). Bidirectional rescue of extreme genetic predispositions to anxiety: impact of CRH receptor 1 as epigenetic plasticity gene in the amygdala. *Translational Psychiatry, 4,* e359.

Slotnikov, S., Wittmann, A., Bunck, M., Bauer, S., Deussing, J., Schmidt, M., Touma, C., Landgraf, R., & Czibere, L. (2014b). Blunted HPA axis reactivity reveals glucocorticoid system dysbalance in a mouse model of high anxiety-related behavior. *Psychoneuroendocrinology, 48,* 41–51.

Smemo, S., Tena, J. J., Kim, K.-H., Gamazon, E. R., Sakabe, N., Gómez-Marin, C., . . . Nóbrega, M. A. (2014). Obesity-associated variants within FTO form long-range functional connections with IRX3. *Nature, 507,* 371–375.

Smith, C. B., & Eiden, L. E. (2012). Is PACAP the major neurotransmitter for stress transduction at the adrenomedullary synapse? *Journal of Molecular Neuroscience, 48,* 403–412.

Smith, K. L., Patterson, M., Dhillo, W. S., Patel, S. R., Semjonous, N. M., Gardiner, J. V., . . . Bloom, S. R. (2006). Neuropeptide S stimulates the hypothalamo-pituitary-adrenal axis and inhibits food intake. *Endocrinology, 147,* 3510–3518.

Smith, M. A., Makino, S., Kvetnansky, R., & Post, R. M. (1995). Stress and glucocorticoids affect the expression of brain-derived neurotrophic factor and neurotrophin-3 mRNAs in the hippocampus. *Journal of Neuroscience, 15,* 1768–1777.

Smits, S. M., Ponnio, T., Conneely, O. M., Burbach, J. P. H., & Smidt, M. P. (2003). Involvement of Nurr1 in specifying the neurotransmitter identity of ventral midbrain dopaminergic neurons. *European Journal of Neuroscience, 18,* 1731–1738.

Smoller, J. W. (2013). Disorders and borders: psychiatric genetics and nosology. *American Journal of Medical Genetics B, 162B,* 559–578.

Smoller, J. W. (2016). The genetics of stress-related disorders: PTSD, depression, and anxiety disorders. *Neuropsychopharmacology Reviews, 41,* 297–319.

Smoller, J. W., Andreassen, O. A., Edenberg, H. J., Faraone, S. V., Glatt, S. J., & Kendler, K. S. (2019). Psychiatric genetics and the structure of psychopathology. *Molecular Psychiatry, 24,* 409–420.

Smoller, J., Cerrato, F., & Weatherall, S. (2015). The genetics of anxiety disorders. In D. Pine, B. Rothbaum, K. Ressler, & A. Muskin (Eds.), *Anxiety disorders: translational perspectives on diagnosis and treatment* (pp. 47–61). Oxford, UK: Oxford University Press.

Solberg Woods, L. C. (2014). QTL mapping in outbred populations: successes and challenges. *Physiological Genomics, 46,* 81–90.

Solomon, E., Avni, R., Hadas, R., Raz, T., Garbow, J. R., Bendel, P., . . . Neeman, M. (2014). Major mouse placenta compartments revealed by diffusion-weighted, contrast-enhanced MRI, and fluorescence imaging. *Proceedings of the National Academy of Sciences USA, 111,* 10353–10358.

Son, G. H., Cha, H. K., Chung, S., & Kim, K. (2018). Multimodal regulation of circadian glucocorticoid rhythm by central and adrenal clocks. *Journal of the Endocrine Society, 2,* 444–459.

Southwick, S. M., & Charney, D. S. (2012). The science of resilience: implications for the prevention and treatment of depression. *Science, 338,* 79–82.

Souza, R. R., Noble, L. J., & McIntyre, C. K. (2017). Using the single prolonged stress model to examine the pathophysiology of PTSD. *Frontiers in Pharmacology, 8,* 615.

Sparrow, R. A., & Coupland, R. E. (1987). Blood flow to the adrenal gland of the rat: its distribution between the cortex and the medulla before and after haemorrhage. *Journal of Anatomy, 155,* 51–61.

Spencer, R. L., & Deak, T. (2017). A user's guide to HPA axis research. *Physiology and Behavior, 178,* 43–65.

Spitz, R. A. (1945). Hospitalism; an inquiry into the genesis of psychiatric conditions in early childhood. *Psychoanalytic Study of the Child, 1,* 53–74.

Spitzer, R. L. (1975). On pseudoscience in science, logic in remission, and psychiatric diagnosis: a critique of Rosenhan's "On being sane in insane places." *Journal of Abnormal Psychology, 84,* 442–452.

Spitzer, R. L., & Wilson, P. T. (1968). A guide to the American Psychiatric Association's new diagnostic nomenclature. *American Journal of Psychiatry, 124,* 1619–1629.

Spratt, E. G., Nicholas, J. S., Brady, K. T., Carpenter, L. A., Hatcher, C. R., Meekins, K. A., . . . Charles, J. M. (2012). Enhanced cortisol responses to stress in children in autism. *Journal of Autism and Developmental Disorders, 42,* 75–81.

Srinivasan, S., Bettella, F., Mattingsdal, M., Wang, Y., Witoelar, A., Schork, A. J., . . . Andreassen, O. A. (2016). Genetic markers of human evolution are enriched in schizophrenia. *Biological Psychiatry, 80,* 284–292.

Stafford, N. P., Jones, A. M., & Drugan, R. C. (2015). Ultrasonic vocalizations during intermittent swim stress forecasts resilience in a subsequent juvenile exploration test of anxiety. *Behavioural Brain Research, 287,* 196–199.

St. Clair, D., Blackwood, D., Muir, W., Carothers, A., Walker, M., Spowart, G., . . . Evans, H. J. (1990). Association within a family of a balanced autosomal translocation with major mental illness. *Lancet, 336,* 13–16.

Stead, J. D. H., Clinton, S., Neal, C., Schneider, J., Jama, A., Miller, S., . . . Akil. H. (2006). Selective breeding for divergence in novelty-seeking traits: heritability and enrichment in spontaneous anxiety-related behaviors. *Behavior Genetics, 36*, 697–712.

Stedenfeld, K. A., Clinton, S. M., Kerman, I. A., Akil, H., Watson, S. J., & Sved, A. F. (2011). Novelty-seeking behavior predicts vulnerability in a rodent model of depression. *Physiology and Behavior, 103*, 210–216.

Stefansson, H., Sigurdsson, E., Steinthorsdottir, V., Bjornsdottir, S., Sigmundsson, T., Ghosh, S., . . . Stefansson, K. (2002). *Neuregulin 1* and susceptibility to schizophrenia. *American Journal of Human Genetics, 71*, 877–892.

Steffens, A. B. (1969). A method for frequent sampling blood and continuous infusion of fluids in the rat without disturbing the animal. *Physiology and Behavior, 4*, 833–836.

Steimer, T. (2011). Animal models of anxiety disorders in rats and mice: some conceptual issues. *Dialogues in Clinical Neuroscience, 13*, 495–506.

Stein, D. J., Craske, M. A., Friedman, M. J., & Phillips, K. A. (2014). Anxiety disorders, obsessive-compulsive and related disorders, trauma- and stressor-related disorders, and dissociative disorders in DSM-5. *American Journal of Psychiatry, 171*, 611–613.

Stein, D. J., Lund, C., & Nesse, R. M. (2013). Classification systems in psychiatry: diagnosis and global mental health in the era of DSM-5 and ICD-11. *Current Opinion in Psychiatry, 26*, 493–497.

Stein, D. J., Phillips, K. A., Bolton, D., Fulford, K. W. M., Sadler, J. Z., & Kendler, K. S. (2010). What is a mental/psychiatric disorder? From DSM-IV to DSM-V. *Psychological Medicine, 40*, 1759–1765.

Stein, M. B., Jang, K. L., Taylor, S., Vernon, P. A., & Livesley, W. J. (2002). Genetic and environmental influences on trauma exposure and posttraumatic stress disorder symptoms: a twin study. *American Journal of Psychiatry, 159*, 1675–1681.

Stephan, A. H., Barres, B. A., & Stevens, B. (2012). The complement system: an unexpected role in synaptic pruning during development and disease. *Annual Review of Neuroscience, 35*, 369–389.

Stephan, K. E., Bach, D. R., Fletcher, P. C., Flint, J., Frank, M. J., Friston, K. J., . . . Breakspear, M. (2016). Charting the landscape of priority problems in psychiatry, part 1: classification and diagnosis. *Lancet Psychiatry, 3*, 77–83.

Sterling, P., & Eyer, J. (1981). Biological basis of stress-related mortality. *Social Science and Medicine, Part E. Medical Psychology, 15*, 3–42.

Sterling, P., & Eyer, J. (1988). Allostasis: a new paradigm to explain arousal pathology. In S. Fisher & J. Reason (Eds.), *Handbook of life stress, cognition and health* (pp. 629–649). New York, NY: Wiley.

Stern, S., Santos, R., Marchetto, M. C., Mendes, A. P. D., Rouleau, G. A., Biesmans, S., . . . Gage, F. H. (2018). Neurons derived from patients with bipolar disorder divide into intrinsically different sub-populations of neurons, predicting the patients' responsiveness to lithium. *Molecular Psychiatry, 23*, 1453–1565.

Sternson, S. M., & Roth, B. L. (2014). Chemogenetic tools to interrogate brain functions. *Annual Review of Neuroscience, 37*, 387–407.

Steullet, P., Cabungcal, J.-H., Coyle, J., Didriksen, M., Gill, K., Grace, A. A., . . . Do, K. Q. (2017). Oxidative stress-driven parvalbumin interneuron impairment as a common mechanism in models of schizophrenia. *Molecular Psychiatry, 22*, 936–943.

Stewart, A. M., Braubach, O., Spitsbergen, J., Gerlai, R., & Kalueef, A. V. (2014). Zebrafish models for translational neuroscience research: from tank to bedside. *Trends in Neurosciences, 37*, 264–278.

Stewart, A. M., & Kalueff, A. V. (2015). Developing better and more valid animal models of brain disorders. *Behavioural Brain Research, 276,* 28–31.

Stewart, A. M., Nguyen, M., Wong, K., Poudel, M. K., & Kalueff, A. V. (2014). Developing zebrafish models of autism spectrum disorder (ASD). *Progress in Neuro-Psychopharmaqology and Biological Psychiatry, 50,* 27–36.

Stewart, A. M., Ullmann, J. F. P., Norton, W. H. J., Parker, M. O., Brennan, C. H., Gerlai, R., & Kalueff, A. V. (2015). Molecular psychiatry of zebrafish. *Molecular Psychiatry, 20,* 2–17.

Stiller, A. L., Drugan, R. C., Hazi, A., & Kent, S. P. (2011). Stress resilience and vulnerability: the association with rearing conditions, endocrine function, immunology, and anxious behavior. *Psychoneuroendocrinology, 36,* 1383–1395.

Stoodley, C. J., D'Mello, A. M., Ellegood, J., Jakkamsetti, V., Piu, P., Bebel, M. B., . . . Tsai, P. T. (2017). Altered cerebellar connectivity in autism and cerebellar-mediated rescue of autism-related behaviors in mice. *Nature Neuroscience, 20,* 1744–1751.

Stornetta, R. L., & Guyenet, P. G. (2018). C1 neurons: a nodal point for stress? *Experimental Physiology, 103,* 332–336.

Strahl, B. D., & Allis, C. D. (2000). The language of covalent histone modifications. *Nature, 403,* 41–45.

Strittmatter, W. J., Davis, J. N., & Lefkowitz, R. J. (1977). Alpha-adrenergic receptors in rat parotid cells II. Desensitization of receptor binding sites and potassium release. *Journal of Biological Chemistry, 252,* 5478–5482.

Su, W.-J., Zhang, Y., Chen, Y., Gong, H., Lian, Y-J., Peng, W., . . . Jiang, C.-L. (2017). NLRP3 gene knockout blocks NF-κB and MAPK signaling pathway in CUMS-induced depression mouse model. *Behavioural Brain Research, 322,* 1–8.

Subbarayappa, B. V. (2001). The roots of ancient medicine: an historical outline. *Journal of Biosciences, 26,* 135–144.

Suderman, M., McGowan, P. O., Sasaki, A., Huang, T. C. T., Hallett, M. T., Meaney, M. J., . . . Szyf, M. (2012). Conserved epigenetic sensitivity to early life experience in the rat and human hippocampus. *Proceedings of the National Academy of Sciences USA, 109,* 17266–17272.

Sullivan, P. F. (2013). Questions about *DISC-1* as a genetic risk factor for schizophrenia. *Molecular Psychiatry, 18,* 1050–1052.

Sullivan, P. F., Kendler, K. S., & Neale, M. C. (2003). Schizophrenia as a complex trait: evidence from a meta-analysis of twin studies. *Archives of General Psychiatry, 60,* 1187–1192.

Sullivan, P. F., & Psychiatric Genomics Consortium (2012). Don't give up on GWAS. *Molecular Psychiatry, 17,* 2–3.

Sullivan, R. (2015). Epididymosomes: a heterogeneous population of microvesicles with multiple functions in sperm maturation and storage. *Asian Journal of Andrology, 17,* 726–729.

Sullivan, R., & Saez, F. (2013). Epididymosomes, prostasomes, and liposomes: their roles in mammalian male reproductive physiology. *Reproduction, 146,* R21–R35.

Sun, H., Kennedy, P. J., & Nestler, E. J. (2013). Epigenetics and the depressed brain: role of histone acetylation and methylation. *Neuropsychopharmacology Reviews, 38,* 124–137.

Suo, L., Zhao, L., Si, J., Liu, J., Zhu, W., Chai, B., . . . Lu, L. (2013). Predictable chronic mild stress in adolescence increases resilience in adulthood. *Neuropsychopharmacology, 38,* 1387–1400.

Suomi, S. J., & Leroy, H. A. (1982). In memorium: Harry F. Harlow (1905–1981). *American Journal of Primatology, 2,* 319–342.

Susser, E., Neugebauer, R., Hoek, H. W., Brown, A. S., Lin, S., Labovitz, D., & Gorman, J. M. (1996). Schizophrenia after famine: further evidence. *Archives of General Psychiatry*, *53*, 25–31.

Susser, E. S., Schaefer, C. A., Brown, A. S., Begg, M. D., & Wyatt, R. J. (2000). The design of the Prenatal Determinants of Schizophrenia Study. *Schizophrenia Bulletin*, *26*, 257–273.

Suvisaari, J., Haukka, J., Tanskanen, A., Hovi, T., & Lönnqvist, J. (1999). Association between prenatal exposure to poliovirus infection and adult schizophrenia. *American Journal of Psychiatry*, *156*, 1100–1102.

Swartz, J. R., Knodt, A. R., Radtke, S. R., & Hariri, A. R. (2015). A neural biomarker of psychological vulnerability to future life stress. *Neuron*, *85*, 505–511.

Sweatt, J. D., & Taminga, C. A. (2016). An epigenomics approach to individual differences and its translation to neuropsychiatric conditions. *Dialogues in Clinical Neuroscience*, *18*, 289–298.

Swerdlow, N. R., Braff, D. L., & Geyer, M. A. (2016). Sensorimotor gating of the startle reflex: what we said 25 years ago, what has happened since then, and what comes next. *Journal of Psychopharmacology*, *30*, 1072–1081.

Syed, S. A., & Nemeroff, C. B. (2017). Early life stress, mood, and anxiety disorders. *Chronic Stress*, *1*, 1–16.

Szablowski, J. O., Lee-Gosselin, A., Lue, B., Malounda, D., & Shapiro, M. G. (2018). Acoustically targeted chemogenetics for the non-invasive control of neural circuits. *Nature Biomedical Engineering*, *2*, 475–484.

Szabo, S., Taché, Y., & Somogyi, A. (2012). The legacy of Hans Selye and the origins of stress research: a retrospective 75 years after his landmark brief "Letter" to the Editor of *Nature*. *Stress*, *15*, 472–478.

Szasz, T. (1961). *The myth of mental illness: foundations of a theory of personal conduct*. New York, NY: Harper & Row.

Taché, J., & Selye, H. (1985). On stress and coping mechanisms. *Issues in Mental Health Nursing*, *7*, 3–24.

Tagliavini, A., Tabak, J., Bertram, R., & Peterson, M. G. (2016). Is bursting more effective than spiking in evoking pituitary hormone secretion? A spatiotemporal simulation study of calcium and granule dynamics. *American Journal of Physiology*, *310*, E515–E525.

Takahashi, A., Chung, J.-R., Zhang, S., Zhang, H., Grossman, Y., Aleyasin, H., . . . Russo, S. J. (2017). Establishment of a repeated social defeat stress model in female mice. *Scientific Reports*, *7*, 12838.

Takei, S., Morinobu, S., Yamamoto, S., Fuchikami, M., Matsumoto, T., & Yamawaki, S. (2011). Enhanced hippocampal BDNF/TrkB signaling in response to fear conditioning in an animal model of posttraumatic stress disorder. *Journal of Psychiatric Research*, *45*, 460–468.

Taliaz, D., Loya, A., Gersner, R., Haramati, S., Chen, A., & Zangen, A. (2011). Resilience to chronic stress is mediated by hippocampal brain-derived neurotrophic factor. *Journal of Neuroscience*, *31*, 4475–4483.

Tandon, R., Gaebel, W., Barch, D. M., Bustillo, J., Gur, R. E., Heckers, S., . . . Carpenter, W. (2013). Definition and description of schizophrenia in the DSM-5. *Schizophrenia Research*, *150*, 3–10.

Taneja, M., Salim, S., Saha, K., Happe, H. K., Qutna, N., Petty, F., . . . Eikenburg, D. C. (2011). Differential effects of inescapable stress on locus coeruleus GRK3, alpha2-adrenoceptor and CRF1 receptor levels in learned helpless and non-helpless rats: a potential link to stress resilience. *Behavioural Brain Research, 221,* 25–33.

Tang, X., Wang, Y., Luo, J., & Liu, M. (2012). Orphan G protein-coupled receptors: GPCRs): biological functions and potential drug targets. *Acta Pharmacologica Sinica, 33,* 363–371.

Tarantino, L., & Bucan, M. (2000). Dissection of behavior and psychiatric disorders using the mouse as a model. *Human Molecular Genetics, 9,* 953–965.

Tasan, R. O., Nguyen, N. K., Weger, S., Sartori, S. B., Singewald, N., Heilbronn, R., . . . Sperk, G. (2010). The central and basolateral amygdala are critical sites of neuropeptide Y/Y2 receptor-mediated regulation of anxiety and depression. *Journal of Neuroscience, 30,* 6282–6290.

Tasker, J. G., & Herman, J. P. (2011). Mechanisms of rapid glucocorticoid feedback inhibition of the hypothalamic-pituitary-adrenal axis. *Stress, 14,* 398–406.

Tatemoto, K., Carlquist, M., & Mutt, V. (1982). Neuropeptide Y: a novel brain peptide with structural similarities to peptide YY and pancreatic polypeptide. *Nature, 296,* 659–660.

Teixeira, C. M., Martin, E. D., Sahún, I., Masachs, N., Pujadas, L., Corvelo, A., . . . Soriano, E. (2011). Overexpression of reelin prevents the manifestation of behavioral phenotypes related to schizophrenia and bipolar disorder. *Neuropsychopharmacology, 36,* 2395–2405.

Tejani-Butt, S. M., Pare, W. P., & Yang, J. (1994). Effect of repeated novel stressors on depressive behavior and brain norepinephrine receptor system in Sprague-Dawley and Wistar Kyoto (WKY) rats. *Brain Research, 649,* 27–35.

Temkin, O. (1953). Greek medicine as science and craft. *Isis, 44,* 213–225.

Teng, B. L., Nonneman, R. J., Agster, K. L., Kiolova, V. D., Davis, T. T., Riddick, N. V., . . . Moy, S. S. (2013). Prosocial effects of oxytocin in two mouse models of autism spectrum disorders. *Neuropharmacology, 72,* 187–196.

The Autism Spectrum Disorders Working Group of the Psychiatric Genomics Consortium (2017). Meta-analysis of GWAS of over 16,000 individuals with autism spectrum disorder highlights a novel locus at 10q24.32 and a significant overlap with schizophrenia. *Molecular Autism, 8,* 21.

The Brainstorm Consortium (2018). Analysis of shared heritability in common disorders of the brain. *Science, 360,* eaap8757.

The C. elegans Sequencing Consortium (1999). Genome sequence of the nematode C. elegans: a platform for investigating biology. *Science, 282,* 2012–2018.

Tkach, M., & Théry, C. (2016). Communication by extracellular vesicles: where we are and where we need to go. *Cell, 164,* 1226–1232.

Tobe, B. T. D., Crain, A. M., Winquist, A. M., Calabrese, B., Makihara, H., Zhao, W., . . . Snyder, E. Y. (2017). Probing the lithium-response pathway in hiPSCs implicates the phosphoregulatory set-point for a cytoskeletal modulatory in bipolar pathogenesis. *Proceedings of the National Academy of Sciences USA, 114,* E4462–E4471.

Tobler, P. N., Fiorillo, C. D., & Schultz, W. (2005). Adaptive coding of reward value by dopamine neurons. *Science, 307,* 1642–1645.

Toledano, D., & Gisquet-Verrier, P. (2014). Only susceptible rats exposed to a model of PTSD exhibit reactivity to trauma-related cues and other symptoms: an effect abolished by a single amphetamine injection. *Behavioural Brain Research, 272,* 165–174.

Tordjman, S., Somogyi, E., Coulon, N., Kermarrec, S., Cohen, D., Bronsard, G., . . . Xavier, J. (2014). Gene x environment interactions in autism spectrum disorders: role of epigenetic mechanisms. *Frontiers in Psychiatry, 5,* 53.

Torrey, E. F., Bartko, J. J., & Yolken, R. H. (2012). Toxoplasma gondii and other risk factors for schizophrenia: an update. *Schizophrenia Bulletin, 38*, 642–647.

Treccani, G., Musazzi, L., Peregro, L., Milanese, M., Nava, N., Bonifacino, T., . . . Popoli, M. (2014). Stress and corticosterone increase the readily releasable pool of glutamate vesicles in synaptic nerve terminals of prefrontal and frontal cortex. *Molecular Psychiatry, 19*, 433–443.

Treit, D., Engin, E., & McEown, K. (2010). Animal models of anxiety and anxiolytic drug action. In M. B. Stein & T. Steckler (Eds.), *Behavioral neurobiology of anxiety and its treatment. Current topics in behavioral neurosciences*, vol. 2 (pp. 121–160). Berlin, Germany: Springer-Verlag.

Treit, D., Pinel, J. P. J., & Fibiger, H. C. (1981). Conditioned defensive burying: a new paradigm for the study of anxiolytic agents. *Pharmacology, Biochemistry and Behavior, 15*, 619–626.

Trivedi, M. H. (2016). Right patient, right treatment, right time: biosignatures and precision medicine in psychiatry. *World Psychiatry, 15*, 237–238.

Trotman, H. D., Holtzman, C. W., Walker, E. F., Addington, J. M., Bearden, C. E., Cadenhead, K. S., . . . McGlashan, T. H. (2014). Stress exposure and sensitivity in the clinical high-risk syndrome: initial findings from the North American Prodrome Longitudinal Study (NAPLS). *Schizophrenia Research, 160*, 104–109.

Trusheim, M. R., Berndt, E. R., & Douglas, F. L. (2007). Stratified medicine: strategic and economic implications of combining drugs and clinical biomarkers. *Nature Reviews Drug Discovery, 6*, 287–293.

Tsai, P. T., Hull, C., Chu, Tsai, P. T., Hull, C., Chu, Y., . . . Sahin, M. (2012). Autistic-like behavior and cerebellar dysfunction in Purkinje cell Tsc1 mutant mice. *Nature, 488*, 647–651.

Tsankova, N., Renthal, W., Kumar, A., & Nestler, E. J. (2007). Epigenetic regulation in psychiatric disorders. *Nature Reviews Neuroscience, 8*, 355–367.

Tseng, K. Y., Chambers, R. A., & Lipska, B. K. (2009). The neonatal ventral hippocampal lesion as a heuristic neurodevelopmental model of schizophrenia. *Behavioural Brain Research, 204*, 295–305.

Tsui, C. C., Copeland, N. G., Gilbert, D. J., Jenkins, N. A., Barnes, C., & Worley, P. F. (1996). Narp, a novel member of the pentraxin family, promotes neurite outgrowth and is dynamically regulated by neuronal activity. *Journal of Neuroscience, 16*, 2463–2478.

Tu, Z., Zhao, H., Li, B., Yan, S., Wang, L., Tang, Y., . . . Li, X.-J. (2019). CRISPR/Cas9-mediated disruption of SHANK3 in monkey leads to drug-treatable autism-like symptoms. *Human Molecular Genetics, 28*, 561–571.

Tucker, D. C., & Saper, C. B. (1985). Specificity of spinal projections from hypothalamic and brainstem areas which innervate sympathetic preganglionic neurons. *Brain Research, 360*, 159–164.

Tulogdi, A., Biro, L., Barsvari, B., Stankovic, & Tot, M. (2015). Neural mechanisms of predatory aggression in rats: implications for abnormal intraspecific aggression. *Behavioural Brain Research, 283*, 108–115.

Turnbull, A. V., & Rivier, C. L. (1999). Regulation of the hypothalamic-pituitary-adrenal axis by cytokines: actions and mechanisms of action. *Physiological Reviews, 79*, 1–71.

Turner, C. A., Clinton, S. M., Thompson, R. C., Watson, S. J., & Akil, H. (2011). Fibroblast growth factor-2 (FGF2) augmentation early in life alters hippocampal development and rescues the anxiety phenotype in vulnerable animals. *Proceedings of the National Academy of Sciences USA, 108*, 8021–8025.

Turner, C. A., Watson, S. J., & Akil, H. (2012). Fibroblast growth factor-2: an endogenous antidepressant and anxiolytic molecule? *Biological Psychiatry, 72*, 254–255.

Turner, C. A., Watson, S. J., & Akil, H. (2016). Fibroblast growth factor 2 sits at the interface of stress and anxiety. *Biological Psychiatry, 80*, 419–421.

Tye, K. M., Mirzabekov, J. J., Warden, M. R., Ferenczi, E. A., Tsai, H.-C., Finkelstein, J., . . . Deisseroth, K. (2013). Dopamine neurons modulate neural encoding and expression of depression-related behaviour. *Nature, 493*, 537–541.

Tyzio, R., Nardou, R., Ferrari, D. C., Tsintsadze, T., Shahrokhi, A., Eftekhari, I., . . . Ben-Ari, Y. (2014). Oxytocin-mediated GABA inhibition during delivery attenuates autism pathogenesis in rodent offspring. *Science, 343*, 675–679.

Ulrich-Lai, Y. M., & Herman, J. P. (2009). Neural regulation of endocrine and autonomic stress responses. *Nature Reviews Neuroscience, 10*, 397–409.

Umemura, S., Imai, S., Mimura, A., Fijiwara, M., & Ebihara, S. (2015). Impaired maternal behavior in Usp46 mutant mice: a model for trans-generational transmission of maternal care. *PLoS One, 10*, e1036016.

Uno, H., Tarara, R., Else, J. G., Suleman, M. A., & Sapolsky, R. M. (1989). Hippocampal damage associated with prolonged and fatal stress in primates. *Journal of Neuroscience, 9*, 1705–1711.

Urban, D. J., & Roth, B. L. (2015). DREADDs (Designer Receptors Exclusively Activated by Designer Drugs): chemogenetic tools with therapeutic utility. *Annual Review of Pharmacology and Toxicology, 55*, 399–417.

Urs, N. M., Peterson, S. M., & Caron, M. G. (2017). New concepts in dopamine D2 receptor biased signaling and implications for schizophrenia therapy. *Biological Psychiatry, 81*, 78–85.

Ursini, G., Punzi, G., Chen, Q., Marenco, S., Robinson, J. F., Porcelli, A., . . . Weinberger, D. R. (2018). Convergence of placenta biology and genetic risk for schizophrenia. *Nature Medicine, 24*, 792–801.

Vale, W., Spiess, J., Rivier, C., & Rivier, J. (1981). Characterization of a 41-residue ovine hypothalamic peptide that stimulates secretion of corticotropin and β-endorphin. *Science, 213*, 1394–1397.

Valjent, E., Pascoli, V., Svenningsson, P., Paul, S., Enslen, H., Corvol, J.-C., . . . Girault, J.-A. (2005). Regulation of a protein phosphatase cascade allows convergent dopamine and glutamate signals to activate ERK in the striatum. *Proceedings of the National Academy of Sciences USA, 102*, 491–496.

Valvassori, S. S., Dal-Pont, G. C., Resende, W. R., Jornada, L. K., Peterle, B. R., Machado, A. G., . . . Quevedo, J. (2017). Lithium and valproate act on the GSK-3β signaling pathway to reverse manic-like behavior in an animal model of mania induced by ouabain. *Neuropharmacology, 117*, 447–459.

Valvassori, S. S., Resende, W. R., Lopes-Borges, J., Mariot, E., Dal-Pont, G. C., Vitto, M. F., . . . Quevedo, J. (2015). Effects of mood stabilizers on oxidative stress-induced cell death signaling pathways in the brains of rats subjected to the ouabain-induced animal model of mania: mood stabilizers exert protective effects against ouabain-induced activation of the cell death pathway. *Journal of Psychiatric Research, 65*, 63–70.

van Alphen, B., & van Swinderen, B. (2013). Drosophila strategies to study psychiatric disorders. *Brain Research Bulletin, 92*, 1–11.

van Bogaert, M., Oosting, R., Toth, M., Groenink, L., van Oorschot, R., & Olivier, B. (2006). Effects of genetic background and null mutation of 5-HT1A receptors on basal and stress-induced body temperature: modulation by serotonergic and GABAA-ergic drugs. *European Journal of Pharmacology, 550*, 84–90.

van den Buuse, M., Lee, J. J. W., & Jaehne, E. (2018). Interaction of brain-derived neurotrophic factor Val66Met genotype and history of stress in regulation of prepulse inhibition in mice. *Schizophrenia Research, 198*, 60–67.

van den Pol, A. N., Wuarin, J.-P., & Dudek, F. E. (1990). Glutamate, the dominant excitatory transmitter in neuroendocrine regulation. *Science, 250*, 1276–1278.

Van Der Heydena, J. A. M., Zethofa, T. J. J., Olivier, B. (1997). Stress-induced hyperthermia in singly housed mice. *Physiology and Behavior, 62*, 463–470.

Van der Kolk, B. A. (1998). Trauma and memory. *Psychiatry and Clinical Neurosciences, 52*, S52–S64.

Van der Kolk, B., Greenberg, M., Boyd, H., & Krystal, J. (1985). Inescapable shock, neurotransmitters, and addiction to trauma: toward a psychobiology of post traumatic stress. *Biological Psychiatry, 20*, 314–325.

van der Staay, F. J. (2006). Animal models of behavioral dysfunctions: basic concepts and classifications, and an evaluation strategy. *Brain Research Reviews, 52*, 131–159.

van der Staay, F. J., Arndt, S. S., & Nordquist, R. E. (2009). Evaluation of animal models of neurobehavioral disorders. *Behavioral and Brain Functions, 5*, 11.

van Dongen, J., & Boomsma, D. I. (2013). The evolutionary paradox and the missing heritability of schizophrenia. *American Journal of Medical Genetics B, 162B*, 122–136.

Van Enkhuizen, J., Henry, B. L., Minassian, A., Perry, W., Milienne-Petiot, M., Higa, K. K., Geyer, M. A., & Young, J. W. (2014). Reduced dopamine transporter functioning induces high-reward risk-preference consistent with bipolar disorder. *Neuropsychopharmacology, 39*, 3112–3122.

Van Enkhuizen, J., Janowsky, D. S., Olivier, B., Minassian, A., Perry, W., Young, J. W., & Geyer, M. A. (2015). The catecholaminergic-cholinergic balance hypothesis of bipolar disorder revisited. *European Journal of Pharmacology, 753*, 114–126.

Van Enkhuizen, J., Minassian, A., & Young, J. W. (2013). Further evidence for ClockΔ19 mice as a model for bipolar disorder mania using cross-species tests for exploration and sensorimotor gating. *Behavioural Brain Research, 249*, 44–54.

Van Hasselt, F. N., Boudewijns, Z. S. R. M., van der Knapp, N. J. F., & Joëls, M. (2011). Maternal care received by individual pups correlates with adult CA1 dendritic morphology and synaptic plasticity in a sex-dependent manner. *Journal of Neuroendocrinology, 24*, 331–340.

Van Hasselt, F. N., Cornelisse, S., Zhang, T. Y., Meaney, M. J., Velzing, E. H., Krugers, H. J., & Joëls, M. (2012b). Adult hippocampal glucocorticoid receptor expression and dentate synaptic plasticity correlate with maternal care received by individuals early in life. *Hippocampus, 22*, 255–266.

Van Hasselt, F. N., de Visser, L., Tieskens, J. M., Cornelisse, S., Baars, A. M., Lavrijsen, M., . . . Joëls, M. (2012c). Individual variations in maternal care early in life correlate with later life decision-making and c-Fos expression in prefrontal regions of rats. *PLoS One, 7*, e37820.

Van Hasselt, F. N., Tieskens, J. M., Trezza, V., Krugers, H. J., Vanderschuren, L. J. M. J., & Joëls, M. (2012a). Within-litter variation in maternal care received by individual pups correlates with adolescent play behavior in male rats. *Physiology and Behavior, 106*, 701–706.

van Os, J., & Selten, J.-P. (1998). Prenatal exposure to maternal stress and subsequent schizophrenia: the May 1940 invasion of The Netherlands. *British Journal of Psychiatry, 172*, 324–326.

Van Steenwyk, G., Roszkowski, M., Manuella, F., Franklin, T. B., & Mansuy, I. M. (2018). Transgenerational inheritance of behavioral and metabolic effects of paternal exposure to traumatic stress in early postnatal life: evidence in the 4th generation. *Environmental Epigenetics, 4,* dvy023.

van Vugt, R. W., Meyer, F., van Hulten, J. A., Vernooij, J., Cools, A. R., Verheij, M. M., & Martens, G. J. (2014). Maternal care affects the phenotype of a rat model for schizophrenia. *Frontiers in Behavioral Neuroscience, 8,* 268.

van Winkel, R., Stefanis, N. C., & Myin-Germeys, I. (2008). Psychosocial stress and psychosis: a review of the neurobiological mechanisms and the evidence for gene-stress interaction. *Schizophrenia Bulletin, 34,* 1095–1105.

Varatharaj, A., & Galea, I. (2017). The blood-brain barrier in systemic inflammation. *Brain, Behavior, and Immunity, 60,* 1–12.

Vardy, E., Robinson, J. E., Li, C., Olsen, R. H. J., DiBerto, J. F., Giguere, P. M., . . . Roth, B. L. (2015). A new DREADD facilitates the multiplexed chemogenetic interrogation of behavior. *Neuron, 86,* 936–946.

Varese, F., Smeets, F., Drukker, M., Lieverse, R., Lataster, T., Viechtbauer, W., . . . Bentall, R. P. (2012). Childhood adversities increase the risk of psychosis: a meta-analysis of patient-control, prospective- and cross-sectional cohort studies. *Schizophrenia Bulletin, 38,* 661–671.

Varmus, H., Klausner, R., Zerhouni, E., Acharya, T., Daar, A. S., & Singer, P. A. (2003). Grand challenges in global health. *Science, 302,* 398–399.

Vaughn, J., Donaldson, C., Bittencourt, J., Perrin, M. H., Lewis, K., Sutton, S., . . . Vale, W. (1995). Urocortin, a mammalian neuropeptide related to fish urotensin I and to corticotropin-releasing factor. *Nature, 378,* 287–292.

Veening, J. G., Swanson, L. W., & Sawchenko, P. E. (1984). The organization of projections from the central nucleus of the amygdala to brainstem sites involved in central autonomic regulation: a combined retrograde transport-immunohistochemical study. *Brain Research, 303,* 337–357.

Veenstra-Vanderweele, J, Muller, C. L., Iwamoto, H., Sauer, J. E., Owens, W. A., Shah, C. R., . . . Blakely, R. D. (2016). Autism gene variant causes hyperserotonemia, serotonin receptor hypersensitivity, social impairment and repetitive behavior. *Proceedings of the National Academy of Sciences USA, 109,* 5469–5474.

Venter, J. C., Adams, M. D., Myers, E. W., Li, P. W., Mural, R. J., Sutton, G.G., . . . Zhu, X. (2001). The sequence of the human genome. *Science, 291,* 1304–1351.

Ventura, J., Nuechterlein, K. H., Lukoff, D., & Hardesty, J. P. (1989). A prospective study of stressful life events and schizophrenic relapse. *Journal of Abnormal Psychology, 98,* 407–411.

Vetere, G., Kenney, J. W., Tran, L. M., Xia, F., Steadman, P. E., Parkinson, J., . . . Frankland, P. W. (2017). Chemogenetic interrogation of a brain-wide fear memory network in mice. *Neuron, 94,* 363–374.

Vialou, V., Maze, I., Renthal, W., LaPlant, Q. C., Watts, E. L., Mouzon, E., . . . Nestler, E. J. (2010a). Serum response factor promotes resilience to chronic social stress through the induction of ΔFosB. *Journal of Neuroscience, 30,* 14585–14592.

Vialou, V., Robison, A. J., LaPlant, Q. C., Covington, H. E., III, Dietz, D. M., Ohnishi, Y. N., . . . Nestler, E. J. (2010b). ΔFosB in brain reward circuits mediates resilience to stress and antidepressant responses. *Nature Neuroscience, 13,* 745–752.

Vieta, E., Berk, M., Schulze, T. G., Carvalho, A. F., Suppes, T., Calabrese, J. R., . . . Grande, I. (2018). Bipolar disorders. *Nature Reviews Disease Primers, 4,* 18008.

Viner, R. (1999). Putting stress in life: Hans Selye and the making of stress theory. *Social Studies of Science, 29,* 391–410.

Vitaterna, M. H., King, D. P., Chang, A.-M., Kornhauser, J. M., Lowrey, P. L., McDonald, J. D., . . . Takahashi, J. S. (1994). Mutagenesis and mapping of a mouse gene, *Clock,* essential for circadian behavior. *Science, 264,* 719–725.

Vitkovic, L., Konsman, J. P., Bockaert, J., Dantzer, R., Homburger, V., & Jacque, C. (2000). Cytokine signals propagate through the brain. *Molecular Psychiatry, 5,* 604–615.

Vogel, J. R., Beer, B., & Clody, D. E. (1971). A simple and reliable conflict procedure for testing anti-anxiety agents. *Psychopharmacologia, 21,* 1–7.

Voineagu, I., Wang, X., Johnston, P., Lowe, J. K., Tian, Y., Horvath, S., . . . Geschwind, D. H. (2011). Transcriptomic analysis of autistic brain reveals convergent molecular pathology. *Nature, 474,* 380–384.

Vollmayr, B., & Gass, P. (2013). Learned helplessness: unique features and translational value of a cognitive depression model. *Cell and Tissue Research, 354,* 171–178.

Vollmayr, B., Mahlstedt, M. M., & Henn, F. A. (2007). Neurogenesis and depression: what animal models tell us about the link. *European Archives of Psychiatry and Clinical Neuroscience, 257,* 300–303.

von Euler, U. S. (1948). Identification of the sympathomimetic ergone in adrenergic nerves of cattle (Sympathin N) with laevo-noradrenaline. *Acta Physiologica Scandinavica, 16,* 63–74.

Von Hohenberg, C. C., Weber-Fahr, W., Lebhardt, P., Ravi, N., Braun, U., Gass, N., . . . Sartorius, A. (2018). Lateral habenula perturbation reduces default-mode network connectivity in a rat model of depression. *Translational Psychiatry, 8,* 68.

Vrshek-Schallhorn, S., Mineka, S., Zinbarg, R. E., Craske, M. G., Griffith, J. W., Sutton, J., . . . Adam, E. K. (2014). Refining the candidate environment: interpersonal stress, the serotonin transporter polymorphism, and gene-environment interactions in major depression. *Clinical Psychological Science, 2,* 235–248.

Vuillermot, S., Joodmardi, E., Perlmann, T., Ögren, S. O., Feldon, J., & Meyer, U. (2012). Prenatal immune activation interacts with genetic *Nurr1* deficiency in the development of attentional impairments. *Journal of Neuroscience, 32,* 436–451.

Vyas, A., Mitra, R., Shankaranarayana Rao, B. S., & Chattarji, S. (2002). Chronic stress induces contrasting patterns of dendritic remodeling in hippocampal and amygdaloid neurons. *Journal of Neuroscience, 22,* 6810–6818.

Wachter, S. B., & Gilbert, E. M. (2012). Beta-adrenergic receptors, from their discovery and characterization through their manipulation to beneficial clinical application. *Cardiology, 122,* 104–112.

Waddington, C. H. (1942). The epigenotype. *Endeavour, 1,* 18–20.

Wahlsten, D., Backmanov, A., Finn, D. A., & Crabbe, J. C. (2006). Stability of mouse strain differences in behavior and brain size between laboratories and across decades. *Proceedings of the National Academy of Sciences USA, 103,* 16364–16369.

Wahlsten, D., Metten, P., & Crabbe, J. C. (2003). Survey of 21 inbred mouse strains in two laboratories reveals that BTBR T/+tf/tf has severely reduced hippocampal commissure and absent corpus callosum. *Brain Research, 971,* 47–54.

Walker, A. K., Hawkins, G., Sominsky, L., & Hodgson, D. M. (2012). Transgenerational transmission of anxiety induced by neonatal exposure to lipopolysaccharide: implications for male and female germ lines. *Psychoneuroendocrinology, 37,* 1320–1335.

Walker, A. K., Rivera, P. D., Wang, Q., Chuang, J.-C., Tran, S., Osborne-Lawrence, S., . . . Zigman, J. M. (2015). The P7C3 class of neuroprotective compounds exerts antidepressant efficacy in mice by increasing hippocampal neurogenesis. *Molecular Psychiatry, 20,* 500–508.

Walker, E., Mittal, V., & Tessner, K. (2008). Stress and the hypothalamic pituitary adrenal axis in the developmental course of schizophrenia. *Annual Review of Clinical Psychology, 4,* 189–216.

Walker, E. F., & Diforio, D. (1997). Schizophrenia: a neural diathesis-stress model. *Psychological Review, 104,* 667–685.

Walker, E. F., Trotman, H. D., Pearce, B. D., Addington, J., Cadenhead, K. S., Cornblatt, B. A., . . . Woods, S. W. (2013). Cortisol levels and risk for psychosis: initial findings from the North American prodrome longitudinal study. *Biological Psychiatry, 74,* 410–417.

Walker, J. J., Spiga, F., Gupta, R., Zhao, Z., Lightman, S. L., & Terry, J. R. (2015). Rapid intra-adrenal feedback regulation of glucocorticoid synthesis. *Journal of the Royal Society Interface, 12,* 20140875.

Walker, E. R., McGee, R. E., & Druss, B. G. (2015). Mortality in mental disorders and global disease burden implications. A systematic review and meta-analysis. *JAMA Psychiatry, 72,* 334–341.

Wall, P. M., & Messier, C. (2001). Methodological and conceptual issues in the use of the elevated plus-maze as a psychological measurement instrument of animal anxiety-like behavior. *Neuroscience and Biobehavioral Reviews, 25,* 275–286.

Walsh, J. J., Christoffel, D. J., Heifets, B. D., Ben-Dor, G. A., Selimbeyoglu, A., Hung, L. W., . . . Malenka, R. C. (2018). 5-HT release in nucleus accumbens rescues social deficits in mouse autism model. *Nature, 560,* 589–593.

Walsh, R. M., Shen, E. Y., Bagot, R. C., Anselmo, A., Jiang, Y., Javidfar, B., . . . Hochedlinger, K. (2017). *Phf8* loss confers resistance to depression-like and anxiety-like behaviors in mice. *Nature Communications, 8,* 15142.

Walsh, R. N., & Cummins, R. A. (1976). The open-field test: a critical review. *Psychological Bulletin, 83,* 482–504.

Wang, B., & Chen, D. (2013). Evidence for seasonal mania: a review. *Journal of Psychiatric Practice, 19,* 301–308.

Wang, L., McLeod, H. L., & Weinshilboum, R. M. (2011). Genomics and drug response. *New England Journal of Medicine, 364,* 1144–1153.

Wang, M., Perova, Z., Arenkiel, B. R., & Li, B. (2014). Synaptic modifications in the medial prefrontal cortex in susceptibility and resilience to stress. *Journal of Neuroscience, 34,* 7485–7492.

Warren, B. L., Vialou, V. F., Iñiguez, S. D., Alcantara, L. F., Wright, K. N., Feng, J., . . . Bolaños-Guzmán, C. A. (2013). Neurobiological sequelae of witnessing stressful events in adult mice. *Biological Psychiatry, 73,* 7–14.

Warthan, M. D., Freeman, J. G., Loesser, K. E., Lewis, C. W., Hong, M., Conway, C. M., & Stewart, J. K. (2002). Phenylethanolamine N-methyl transferase expression in mouse thymus and spleen. *Brain, Behavior and Immunity, 16,* 493–499.

Washburn, S. L., & DeVore, I. (1961). The social life of baboons. *Scientific American, 204,* 62–71.

Wasserstein, A. G. (1996). Death and the internal milieu: Claude Bernard and the origins of experimental medicine. *Perspectives in Biology and Medicine, 39,* 313–326.

Watanabe, Y., Gould, E., Cameron, H. A., Daniels, D. C., & McEwen, B. S. (1992a). Phenytoin prevents stress- and corticosterone-induced atrophy of CA3 pyramidal neurons. *Hippocampus, 2,* 431–436.

Watanabe, Y., Gould, E., Daniels, D. C., Cameron, H., & McEwen, B. S. (1992c). Tianeptine attenuates stress-induced morphological changes in the hippocampus. *European Journal of Pharmacology, 222*, 157–162.

Watanabe, Y., Gould, E., & McEwen, B. S. (1992b). Stress induces atrophy of apical dendrites of hippocampal CA3 pyramidal neurons. *Brain Research, 588*, 341–345.

Watson, J. D., & Crick, F. H. C. (1953). A structure for deoxyribose nucleic acid. *Nature, 171*, 737–738.

Watson, P. J., & Andrews, P. W. (2002). Toward a revised evolutionary adaptationist analysis of depression: the social navigation hypothesis. *Journal of Affective Disorders, 72*, 1–14.

Weaver, I. C. G., Cervoni, N., Champagne, F. A., D'Alessio, A. C., Sharma, S., Seckl, J. R., . . . Meaney, M. J. (2004). Epigenetic programming by maternal behavior. *Nature Neuroscience, 7*, 847–854.

Weaver, I. C. G., D'Alessio, A. C., Brown, S. E., Hellstrom, I. C., Dymov, S., Sharma, S., . . . Meaney, M. J. (2007). The transcription factor nerve growth factor-inducible protein A mediates epigenetic programming: altering epigenetic marks by immediate-early genes. *Journal of Neuroscience, 27*, 1756–1768.

Weaver, I. C. G., Korgan, A. C., Lee, K., Wheeler, R. V., Hundert, A. S., & Goguen, D. (2017). Stress and the emerging roles of chromatin remodeling in signal integration and stable transmission of reversible phenotypes. *Frontiers in Behavioral Neuroscience, 11*, 41.

Weaver, I. C. G., Meaney, M. J., & Szyf, M. (2006). Maternal care effects on the hippocampal transcriptome and anxiety-mediated behaviors in the offspring that are reversible in adulthood. *Proceedings of the National Academy of Sciences USA, 103*, 3480–3485.

Weber, M. D., Frank, M. G., Sobesky, J. L., Watkins, L. R., & Maier, S. F. (2013). Blocking toll-like receptor 2 and 4 signaling during a stressor prevents stress-induced priming of neuroinflammatory responses to a subsequent immune challenge. *Brain, Behavior and Immunity, 32*, 112–121.

Weber, M. D., Frank, M. G., Tracey, K. J., Watkins, L. R., & Maier, S. F. (2015). Stress induces the danger-associated molecular pattern HMGB-1 in the hippocampus of male Sprague-Dawley rats: a priming stimulus of microglia and the NLRP3 inflammasome. *Journal of Neuroscience, 35*, 316–324.

Weber, M. D., McKim, D. B., Niraula, A., Witcher, K. G., Yin, W., Sobol, C. G., . . . Godbout, J. P. (2019). The influence of microglial elimination and repopulation on stress sensitization induced by repeated social defeat. *Biological Psychiatry, 85*, 667–678.

Weber-Stadlbauer, U., Richetto, J., Labouesse, M. A., Bohacek, J., Mansuy, I. M., & Meyer, U. (2017). Transgenerational transmission and modification of pathological traits induced by prenatal immune activation. *Molecular Psychiatry, 22*, 102–112.

Weeke, P., & Roden, D. M. (2014). Applied pharmacogenomics in cardiovascular medicine. *Annual Review of Medicine, 65*, 81–94.

Wegener, G., Harvey, B. H., Bonefeld, B., Müller, H. K., Volke, V., Overstreet, D. H., & Elfving, B. (2010). Increased stress-evoked nitric oxide signaling in the Flinders sensitive line (FSL) rat: a genetic animal model of depression. *International Journal of Neuropsychopharmacology, 13*, 461–473.

Wei, J., Yuen, E. Y., Liu, W., Li, X., Zhong, P., Karatsoreos, I. N., . . . Yan, Z. (2014). Estrogen protects against the detrimental effects of repeated stress on glutamatergic transmission and cognition. *Molecular Psychiatry, 19*, 588–598.

Weickert, C. S., Hyde, T. M., Lipska, B. K., Herman, M. M., Weinberger, D. R., & Kleinman, J. E. (2003). Reduced brain-derived neurotrophic factor in prefrontal cortex of patients with schizophrenia. *Molecular Psychiatry*, 8, 592–610.

Weiling, F. (1991). Historical study: Johann Gregor Mendel 1822–1884. *American Journal of Medical Genetics*, 40, 1–25.

Weinberger, D. R. (1987). Implications of normal brain development for the pathogenesis of schizophrenia. *Archives of General Psychiatry*, 44, 660–669.

Weinberger, D. R., Glick, I. D., & Klein, D. F. (2015). Whither Research Domain Criteria (RDoc)? The good, the bad, and the ugly. *JAMA Psychiatry*, 72, 1161–1162.

Weinstock, M. (2008). The long-term behavioural consequences of prenatal stress. *Neuroscience and Biobehavioral Reviews*, 32, 1073–1086.

Weinstock, M. (2017). Prenatal stressors in rodents: effects on behavior. *Neurobiology of Stress*, 6, 3–13.

Weir, R. K., Forghany, R., Smith, S. E. P., Patterson, P. H., McAllister, A. K., Schumann, C. M., & Bauman, M. D. (2015). Preliminary evidence of neuropathology in nonhuman primates prenatally exposed to maternal immune activation. *Brain, Behavior, and Immunity*, 48, 139–146.

Weiss, I. C., & Feldon, J. (2001). Environmental animal models for sensorimotor gating deficiencies in schizophrenia: a review. *Psychopharmacology*, 156, 305–326.

Weiss, R. B., Stange, J. P., Boland, E. M., Black, S. K., LaBelle, D. R., Abramson, L. Y., & Alloy, L. B. (2015). Kindling of life stress in bipolar disorder: comparison of sensitization and autonomy models. *Journal of Abnormal Psychology*, 124, 4–16.

Welberg, L. A. M., & Seckl, J. R. (2001). Prenatal stress, glucocorticoids and the programming of the brain. *Journal of Neuroendocrinology*, 13, 113–128.

Welberg, L. A. M., Seckl, J. R., & Holmes, M. C. (2000). Inhibition of 11β-hydroxysteroid dehydrogenase, the foeto-placental barrier to maternal glucocorticoids, permanently programs amygdala GR mRNA expression and anxiety-like behaviour in the offspring. *European Journal of Neuroscience*, 12, 1047–1054.

Wendeln, A.-C., Degenhardt, K., Kaurani, L., Gertig, M., Ulas, T., Jain, G., ... Neher, J. J. (2018). Innate immune memory in the brain shapes neurological disease hallmarks. *Nature*, 556, 332–338.

Weninger, S. C., Peter, L. L., & Majzoub, J. A. (2000). Urocortin expression in the Edinger-Westphal nucleus is up-regulated by stress and corticotropin-releasing hormone deficiency. *Endocrinology*, 141, 256–263.

Wertz, J., & Pariante, C. M. (2014). Invited commentary on ... psychiatric resilience: longitudinal twin study. *British Journal of Psychiatry*, 205, 281–282.

Whiteford, H. A., Degenhardt, L., Rehm, J., Baxter, A. J., Ferrari, A. J., Erskine, H. E., ... Vos, T. (2013). Global burden of disease attributable to mental and substance use disorders: findings from the Global Burden of Disease Study 2010. *Lancet*, 382, 1575–1586.

Widom, C. S., Weiler, B. L., & Cottler, L. B. (1999). Childhood victimization and drug abuse: a comparison of prospective and retrospective findings. *Journal of Consulting and Clinical Psychology*, 67, 867–880.

Wigger, A., Loerscher, P., Weissenbacher, P., Holsboer, F., & Landgraf, R. (2001). Cross-fostering and cross-breeding of HAB and LAB rats: a genetic rat model of anxiety. *Behavior Genetics*, 31, 371–382.

Wigger, A., Sánchez, M. M., Mathys, K. C., Ebner, K., Frank, E., Liu, D., ... Landgraf, R. (2004). Alterations in central neuropeptide expression, release, and receptor binding in rats bred for high anxiety: critical role of vasopressin. *Neuropsychopharmacology*, *29*, 1–14.

Wightman, B., Ha, I., & Ruvkun, G. (1993). Posttranscriptional regulation of the heterochronic gene *lin-14* by *lin-4* mediates temporal pattern formation in C. elegans. *Cell*, *75*, 855–862.

Wilkinson, M. B., Xiao, G., Kumar, A., LaPlant, Q., Renthal, W., Sikder, D., . . . Nestler, E. J. (2009). Imipramine treatment and resiliency exhibit similar chromatin regulation in the mouse nucleus accumbens in depression models. *Journal of Neuroscience*, *29*, 7820–7832.

Will, C. C., Aird, F., & Redei, E. E. (2003). Selectively bred Wistar-Kyoto rats: an animal model of depression and hyper-responsiveness to antidepressants. *Molecular Psychiatry*, *8*, 925–932.

Willard, S. L., & Shively, C. A. (2012). Modeling depression in adult female cynomolgus monkeys (*Macaca fascicularis*). *American Journal of Primatology*, *74*, 528–542.

Willi, R., Harmeier, A., Giovanoli, S., & Meyer, U. (2013). Altered GSK3β signaling in an infection-based mouse model of developmental neuropsychiatric disease. *Neuropharmacology*, *73*, 56–65.

Willner, P. (1986). Validation criteria for animal models of human mental disorders: learned helplessness as a paradigm case. *Progress in Neuro-Psychopharmacology and Biological Psychiatry*, *10*, 677–690.

Willner, P. (2017). The chronic mild stress (CMS) model of depression: history, evaluation and usage. *Neurobiology of Stress*, *6*, 78–93.

Willner, P., & Belzung, C. (2015). Treatment-resistant depression: are animal models of depression fit for purpose? *Psychopharmacology*, *232*, 3473–3495.

Willner, P., Towell, A., Sampson, D., Muscat, R., & Sophokleous, S. (1987). Reduction of sucrose preference by chronic mild stress and its restoration by a tricyclic antidepressant. *Psychopharmacology*, *93*, 358–364.

Willnow, T. E., & Nykjaer, A. (2010). Cellular uptake of steroid carrier proteins: mechanisms and implications. *Cellular and Molecular Endocrinology*, *316*, 93–102.

Wilson, E. O. (1975). *Sociobiology: the new synthesis*. Cambridge, MA: Belknap Press.

Wilson, E. O. (1981). *On human nature*. Cambridge, MA: Harvard University Press.

Wilson, M. (1993). DSM-III and the transformation of American psychiatry: a history. *American Journal of Psychiatry*, *150*, 399–410.

Windle, R. J., Wood, S. A., Shanks, N., Lightman, S. L., & Ingram, C. D. (1998). Ultradian rhythm of basal corticosterone release in the female rat: dynamic interaction with the response to acute stress. *Endocrinology*, *139*, 443–450.

Winslow, J. T., & Insel, T. R. (2002). The social deficits of the oxytocin knockout mouse. *Neuropeptides*, *36*, 221–229.

Winter, C., Vollmayr, B., Djodari-Irani, A., Klein, J., & Sartorius, A. (2011). Pharmacological inhibition of the lateral habenula improves depressive-like behavior in an animal model of treatment resistant depression. *Behavioural Brain Research*, *216*, 463–465.

Wischhof, L., Irrsack, E., Osorio, C., & Koch, M. (2015). Prenatal LPS-exposure—a neurodevelopmental rat model of schizophrenia—differentially affects cognitive functions, myelination and parvalbumin expression in male and female offspring. *Progress in Neuro-Psychopharmacology & Biological Psychiatry*, *57*, 17–30.

Wohleb, E. S. (2016). Neuron-microglia interactions in mental health disorders: "for better, and for worse." *Frontiers in Immunology*, *7*, 544.

Wohleb, E. S., Franklin, T., Iwata, M., & Duman, R. S. (2016). Integrating neuroimmune systems in the neurobiology of depression. *Nature Reviews Neuroscience, 17*, 497–511.

Wohleb, E. S., McKim, D. B., Sheridan, J. F., & Godbout, J. P. (2015). Monocyte trafficking to the brain with stress and inflammation: a novel axis of immune-to-brain communication that influences mood and behavior. *Frontiers in Neuroscience, 8*, 447.

Wöhr, M., Roullet, F. I., & Crawley, J. N. (2011). Reduced scent marking and ultrasonic vocalizations in the BTBR T+tf/J mouse model of autism. *Genes, Brain and Behavior, 10*, 35–43.

Wöhr, M., Silverman, J. L., Scattoni, M. L., Turner, S. M., Harris, M. J., Saxena, R., & Crawley, J. N. (2013). Developmental delays and reduced pup ultrasonic vocalizations but normal sociability in mice lacking the postsynaptic cell adhesion protein neuroligin2. *Behavioural Brain Research, 251*, 50–64.

Wolf, S. A., Boddeke, H. W. G. M., & Kettenmann, H. (2017). Microglia in physiology and disease. *Annual Review of Physiology, 79*, 619–643.

Wolosker, H., Sheth, K. N., Takahashi, M., Mothet, J.-P., Brady, R. O., Jr., Ferris, C. D., & Snyder, S. H. (1999). Purification of serine racemase: biosynthesis of the neuromodulator D-serine. *Proceedings of the National Academy of Sciences USA, 96*, 721–725.

Woloszynowska-Fraser, M. U., Wulff, P., & Riedel, G. (2017). Parvalbumin-containing GABA cells and schizophrenia: experimental model based on targeted gene delivery through adreno-associated viruses. *Behavioural Pharmacology, 28*, 630–641.

Wong, A. H. C., & Josselyn, S. A. (2016). Caution when diagnosing your mouse with schizophrenia: the use and misuse of model animals for understanding psychiatric disorders. *Biological Psychiatry, 79*, 32–38.

Wong, M.-L., Arcos-Burgos, M., Liu, S., Vélez, J. L., Baune, B. T., Jawahar, M. C., . . . Licinio, J. (2017). The PHF21B gene is associated with major depression and modulates the stress response. *Molecular Psychiatry, 22*, 1015–1025.

Wong, M.-L., & Licinio, J. (2001). Research and treatment approaches to depression. *Nature Reviews Neuroscience, 2*, 343–351.

Wood, M., Adil, O., Wallace, T., Fourman, S., Wilson, S. P., Herman, J. P., & Myers, B. (2019). Infralimbic prefrontal cortex structural and functional connectivity with the limbic forebrain: a combined viral genetic and optogenetic analysis. *Brain Structure and Function, 224*, 73–97.

Wood, S. K., Walker, H. E., Valentino, R. J., & Bhatnagar, S. (2010). Individual differences in reactivity to social stress predict susceptibility and resilience to a depressive phenotype: role of corticotropin-releasing factor. *Endocrinology, 151*, 1795–1805.

Wood, S. K., Wood, C. S., Lombard, C. M., Lee, C. S., Zhang, X.-Y., Finnell, J. E., & Valentino, R. J. (2015). Inflammatory factors mediate vulnerability to a social stress-induced depressive-like phenotype in passive coping rats. *Biological Psychiatry, 78*, 38–48.

Woolf, S. H. (2008). The meaning of translational research and why it matters. *Journal of the American Medical Association, 299*, 211–213.

Woolley, C. S., Gould, E., Frankfurt, M., & McEwen, B. S. (1990). Naturally occurring fluctuations in dendritic spine density on adult hippocampal pyramidal neurons. *Journal of Neuroscience, 10*, 4035–4039.

Woolley, C. S., Gould, E., & McEwen, B. S. (1990). Exposure to excess glucocorticoids alters dendritic morphology of adult hippocampal pyramidal neurons. *Brain Research, 531*, 225–231.

Wray, N. R., Ripke, S., Mattheisen, M., Trzaskowski, M., Byrne, E. M., Abdellaoui, A., . . . the Major Depressive Disorder Working Group of the Psychiatric Genomics Consortium (2018). Genome-wide association analyses identify 44 risk variants and refine the genetic architecture of major depression. *Nature Genetics, 50*, 668–681.

World Health Organization (2019). *ICD-11. International Classification of Diseases, 11th Revision*. Retrieved March 21, 2019, from, https://icd.who.int/

Wright, C., Rose, D. A., & Weinberger, D. R. (2018). Small RNAs may answer big questions in mental illness. *Biological Psychiatry, 83*, e1–e3.

Wu, Y. C., Hill, R. A., Gogos, A., & van den Buuse, M. (2013). Sex differences and the role of estrogen in animal models of schizophrenia: interaction with BDNF. *Neuroscience, 239*, 67–83.

Wurtman, R. J. (2002). Stress and adrenocortical control of epinephrine synthesis. *Metabolism, 51* (Suppl. 1), 11–14.

Wurtman, R. J., & Axelrod, J. (1965). Adrenaline synthesis: control by the pituitary gland and adrenal glucocorticoids. *Science, 150*, 1464–1465.

Xu, F., Wu, Q., Xie, L., Gong, W., Zhang, J., Zheng, P., . . . Xie, P. (2015). Macaques exhibit a naturally-occurring depression similar to humans. *Scientific Reports, 5*, 9220.

Xu, Y.-L., Gall, C. M., Jackson, V. R., Civelli, O., & Reinscheid, R. K. (2007). Distribution of neuropeptide S receptor mRNA and neurochemical characteristics of neuropeptide S-expressing neurons in the rat brain. *Journal of Comparative Neurology, 500*, 84–102.

Xu, Y.-L., Reinscheid, R. K., Huitron-Resendiz, S., Clark, S. D., Wang, Z., Lin, S. H., . . . Civelli, O. (2004). Neuropeptide S: a neuropeptide promoting arousal and anxiolytic-like effects. *Neuron, 43*, 487–497.

Yamaguchi, I., & Kopin, I. J. (1979). Plasma catecholamine and blood pressure responses to sympathetic stimulation in pithed rats. *American Journal of Physiology, 237*, H305–H310.

Yamamoto, S., Morinobu, S., Iwamoto, Y., Ueda, Y., Takei, S., Fujita, Y., & Yamawaki, S. (2010). Alterations in the hippocampal glycinergic system in an animal model of post-traumatic stress disorder. *Journal of Psychiatric Research, 44*, 1069–1074.

Yamamoto, S., Morinobu, S., Takei, S., Fuchikami, M., Matsuki, A., Yamawaki, S., & Liberzon, I. (2009). Single prolonged stress: toward an animal model of posttraumatic stress disorder. *Depression and Anxiety, 26*, 1110–1117.

Yang, C., Shirayama, Y., Zhang, J., Ren, Q., & Hashimoto, K. (2015). Regional differences in brain-derived neurotrophic factor levels and dendritic spine density confer resilience to inescapable stress. *International Journal of Neuropsychopharmacology, 18*, pyu121.

Yang, M., Zhodzishsky, V., & Crawley, J. N. (2007). Social deficits in BTBR T + tf/J mice are unchanged by cross-fostering with C57BL/6J mothers. *International Journal of Developmental Neuroscience, 25*, 515–521.

Yang, Z., Han, D., & Coote, J. H. (2009). Cardiac sympatho-excitatory action of PVN-spinal oxytocin neurons. *Autonomic Neuroscience, 147*, 80–85.

Yee, C. M., Javitt, D. C., & Miller, G. A. (2015). Replacing *DSM* categorical analyses with dimensional analyses in psychiatry research. The Research Domain Criteria Initiative. *JAMA Psychiatry, 72*, 1159–1160.

Yehuda, R. (2002). Post-traumatic stress disorder. *New England Journal of Medicine, 346*, 108–114.

Yehuda, R., & Antelman, S. M. (1993). Criteria for rationally evaluating animal models of posttraumatic stress disorder. *Biological Psychiatry, 33*, 479–486.

Yehuda, R., Daskalakis, N. P., Lehrner, A., Desarnaud, F., Bader, H. N., Makotkine, I., . . . Meaney, M. J. (2014). Influences of maternal and paternal PTSD on epigenetic regulation of the glucocorticoid receptor gene in Holocaust survivor offspring. *American Journal of Psychiatry, 171*, 872–880.

Yehuda, R., Hoge, C. W., McFarlane, A. C., Vermetten, E., Lanius, R. A., Nievergelt, C. M., . . . Hyman, S. E. (2015). Post-traumatic stress disorder. *Nature Reviews Disease Primers, 1*, 15057.

Yehuda, R., & LeDoux, J. (2007). Response variation following trauma: a translational neuroscience approach to understanding PTSD. *Neuron, 56*, 19–32.

Yilmazer-Hanke, D. M., Wigger, A., Linke, R., Landgraf, R., & Schwegler, H. (2004). Two Wistar rat lines selectively bred for anxiety-related behavior show opposite reactions in elevated plus maze and fear-sensitized acoustic startle tests. *Behavior Genetics, 34*, 309–318.

Yim, Y. S., Park, A., Berrios, J., Lafourcade, M., Pascual, L. M., Soares, N., . . . Choi, G. B. (2017). Reversing behavioural abnormalities in mice exposed to maternal inflammation. *Nature, 549*, 482–487.

Yin, Y., Li, Y., & Zhang, W. (2014). The growth hormone secretagogue receptor: its intracellular signaling and regulation. *International Journal of Molecular Science, 15*, 4837–4855.

Yin, X., Guven, N., & Dietis, N. (2016). Stress-based animal models of depression: do we actually know what we are doing? *Brain Research, 1652*, 30–42.

Young, J. W., Cope, Z. A., Romoli, B., Schrurs, E., Joosen, A., van Enkhuizen, J., . . . Dulcis, D. (2018). Mice with reduced DAT levels recreate seasonal-induced switching between states in bipolar disorder. *Neuropsychopharmacology, 43*, 1721–1731.

Young, J. W., & Dulcis, D. (2015). Investigating the mechanism(s) underlying switching between states in bipolar disorder. *European Journal of Pharmacology, 759*, 151–162.

Young, J. W., Minassian, A., Paulus, M. P., Geyer, M. A., & Perry, W. (2007). A reverse-translational approach to bipolar disorder: rodent and human studies in the behavioral pattern monitor. *Neuroscience and Biobehavioral Reviews, 31*, 882–896.

Young, J. W., van Enkhuizen, J., Winstanley, C. A., & Geyer, M. A. (2011). Increased risk-taking behavior in dopamine transporter knockdown mice: further support for a mouse model of mania. *Journal of Psychopharmacology, 25*, 934–943.

Yousufzai, M. I., Harmatz, E. S., Shah, M., Malik, M. O., & Goosens, K. A. (2018). Ghrelin is a persistent biomarker for chronic stress exposure in adolescent rats and humans. *Translational Psychiatry, 8*, 74.

Yu, H.-S., Kim, S. H., Park, H. G., Kim, Y. S., & Ahn, Y. M. (2010). Activation of Akt signaling in rat brain by intracerebroventricular injection of ouabain: a rat model for mania. *Progress in Neuro-Psychopharmacology and Biological Psychiatry, 34*, 888–894.

Yuen, R. K. C., Thiruvahindrapuram, B., Merico, D., Walker, S., Tammimies, K., Hoang, N., . . . Scherer, S. W. (2015). Whole-genome sequencing of quartet families with autism spectrum disorder. *Nature Medicine, 21*, 185–191.

Zablotsky, B., Black, L. I., Maenner, M. J., Schieve, L. A., & Blumberg, S. J. (2015). Estimated prevalence of autism and other developmental disabilities following questionnaire changes in the 2014 National Health Interview Survey. *National Health Statistics Reports, 87*, pp. 1–20.

Zaccaria, K. J., Lagace, D. C., Eisch, A. J., & McCasland, J. S. (2010). Resistance to change and vulnerability to stress: autistic-like features of *GAP43*-deficient mice. *Genes, Brain and Behavior, 9*, 985–996.

Zamponi, G. W., Striessnig, J., Koschak, A., & Dolphin, A. C. (2015). The physiology, pathology, and pharmacology of voltage-gated calcium channels and their future therapeutic potential. *Pharmacological Reviews, 67*, 821–890.

Zannas, A. S., & West, A. E. (2014). Epigenetics and the regulation of stress vulnerability and resilience. *Neuroscience, 264*, 157–170.

Zeggini, E., Gloyn, A.L., Barton, A.C., & Wain, L.V. (2019). Translational genomics and precision medicine: moving from the lab to the clinic. *Science, 365*, 1409-1413.

Zeier, Z., Carpenter, L. L., Kalin, N. H., Rodriguez, C. I., McDonald, W. M., Widge, A. S., & Nemeroff, C. B. (2018). Clinical implementation of pharmacogenetic decision support tools for antidepressant drug prescribing. *American Journal of Psychiatry, 175*, 873–886.

Zhang, F., Gardinaru, V., Adamantidis, A. R., Durand, R., Airan, R. D., de Lecea, L., & Deisseroth, K. (2010). Optogenetic interrogation of neural circuits: technology for probing mammalian brain structures. *Nature Protocols, 5*, 439–456.

Zhang, H., Chaudhury, D., Nectow, A. R., Friedman, A. K., Zhang, S., Juarez, B., . . . Han, M.-H. (2019). α1- and β3-adrenergic receptor-mediated mesolimbic homeostatic plasticity confers resilience to social stress in susceptible mice. *Biological Psychiatry, 85*, 226–236.

Zhang, R., Asai, M., Mahoney, C. E., Joachim, M., Shen, Y., Gunnar, G., & Majzoub, J. A. (2017). Loss of hypothalamic corticotropin-releasing hormone markedly reduces anxiety behaviors in mice. *Molecular Psychiatry, 22*, 733–744.

Zhang, T.-Y., Hellstrom, I. C., Bagot, R. C., Wen, X., Diorio, J., & Meaney, M. J. (2010). Maternal care and DNA methylation of a glutamic acid decarboxylase 1 promoter in rat hippocampus. *Journal of Neuroscience, 30*, 13130–13137.

Zhang, Y., Ghandi, P. R., & Standifer, K. M. (2012). Increased nociceptive sensitivity and nociceptin/orphanin FQ levels in a rat model of PTSD. *Molecular Pain, 8*, 76.

Zhang, Y., Liu, L., Liu, Y.-Z., Shen, X.-L., Wu, T.-Y., Zhang, T., . . . Jiang, C.-L. (2015). NLRP3 inflammasome mediates chronic mild stress-induced depression in mice via neuroinflammation. *International Journal of Neuropsychopharmacology, 18*, pyv006.

Zhu, H., & Roth, B. L. (2015). DREADD: a chemogenetic GPCR signaling platform. *International Journal of Neuropsychopharmacology, 18*, pyu007.

Zhu, S., Cordner, Z. A., Xiong, J., Chiu, C.-T., Artola, A., Zuo, Y., . . . Ross, C. A. (2017). Genetic disruption of ankyrin-G in adult mouse forebrain causes cortical synapse alteration and behavior reminiscent of bipolar disorder. *Proceedings of the National Academy of Sciences USA, 114*, 10479–10484.

Zhuang, X., Oosting, R. S., Jones, S. R., Gainetdinov, R. R., Miller, G. W., Caron, M. G., & Hen, R. (2001). Hyperactivity and impaired response habituation in hyperdopaminergic mice. *Proceedings of the National Academy of Sciences USA, 98*, 1982–1987.

Zimbler-Delorenzo, H. S., & Stone, A. I. (2011). Integration of field and captive studies for understanding the behavioral ecology of the squirrel monkey (*Saimiri* Sp.). *American Journal of Primatology, 73*, 607–622.

Zimmerman, A. W., & Connors, S. L. (2014). Could autism be treated prenatally? *Science, 343*, 620–621.

Zimmerman, A. W., Connors, S. L., Matteson, K. J., Lee, L.-C., Singer, H. S., Castaneda, J. A., & Pearce, D. A. (2007). Maternal antibrain antibodies in autism. *Brain, Behavior, and Immunity, 21*, 351–357.

Zimmerman, E. C., Bellaire, M., Ewing, S. G., & Grace, A. A. (2013). Abnormal stress responsivity in a rodent developmental disruption model of schizophrenia. *Neuropsychopharmacology, 38,* 2131–2139.

Zink, M., Vollmayr, B., Gebicke-Haerter, P. J., & Henn, F. A. (2010). Reduced expression of glutamate transporters vGluT1, EAAT2, and EAAT4 in learned helpless rats, an animal model of depression. *Neuropharmacology, 58,* 465–473.

Ziv, Y., Ron, N., Butovsky, O., Landa, G., Sudai, E., Greenberg, N., . . . Schwartz, M. (2006). Immune cells contribute to the maintenance of neurogenesis and spatial learning abilities in adulthood. *Nature Neuroscience, 9,* 268–275.

Zohar, J., Yahalom, H., Kozlovsky, N., Cwikel-Hamzany, S., Matar-M. A., Kaplan, Z., . . . Cohen, H. (2011). High dose hydrocortisone immediately after trauma may alter the trajectory of PTSD: interplay between clinical and animal studies. *European Neuropsychopharmacology, 21,* 796–809.

Zorumski, C. F., Paul, S. M., Izumi, Y., Covey, D. F., & Mennerick, S. (2013). Neurosteroids, stress and depression: potential therapeutic opportunities. *Neuroscience and Biobehavioral Reviews, 37,* 109–122.

Zovkic, I. B., & Sweatt, J. D. (2013). Epigenetic mechanisms in learned fear: implications for PTSD. *Neuropsychopharmacology, 38,* 77–93.

Zubin, J., & Spring, B. (1977). Vulnerability: a new view of schizophrenia. *Journal of Abnormal Psychology, 86,* 103–126.

Zuckerman, L., Rehavi, M., Nachman, R., & Weiner, I. (2003). Immune activation during pregnancy in rats leads to a postpubertal emergence of disrupted latent inhibition, dopaminergic hyperfunction, and altered limbic morphology in the offspring: a novel neurodevelopmental model of schizophrenia. *Neuropsychopharmacology, 28,* 1778–1789.

Zukowska-Grojec, Z. (1995). Neuropeptide Y: a novel sympathetic stress hormone and more. *Annals of the New York Academy of Sciences, 771,* 219–233.

Zukowska-Grojec, Z., Konarska, M., & McCarty, R. (1988). Differential plasma catecholamine and neuropeptide Y responses to acute stress in rats. *Life Sciences, 42,* 1615–1624.

Żurawek, D., Faron-Górecka, A., Kuśmider, M., Kolasa, M., Gruca, P., Papp, M., & Dziedzicka-Wasylewska, M. (2013). Mesolimbic dopamine D2 receptor plasticity contributes to stress resilience in rats subjected to chronic mild stress. *Psychopharmacology, 227,* 583–593.

Index

Tables and figures are indicated by *t* and *f* following the page number

For the benefit of digital users, indexed terms that span two pages (e.g., 52–53) may, on occasion, appear on only one of those pages.